Chain of Friendship

Selected Letters of Dr. John Fothergill
1735–1780

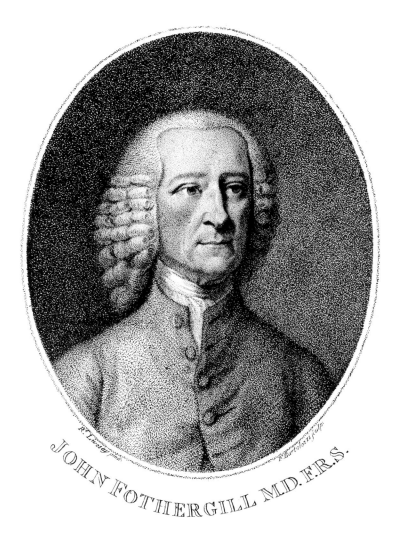

JOHN FOTHERGILL M.D. F.R.S.

Cui suas artes, sua dona lactus
Et herbam et Venae salientis ictum
Scire concessit, celerem et medendi
　　　　　Delius usum.

Chain of Friendship

*Selected Letters of Dr. John Fothergill
of London, 1735-1780*

*With Introduction and Notes by
Betsy C. Corner
& Christopher C. Booth*

*The Belknap Press of
Harvard University Press
Cambridge, Massachusetts, 1971*

Published in Great Britain by
Oxford University Press
London

Library of Congress Catalog Card Number 75-127877
SBN 674-10660-1

Printed in the United States of America

Preface

The letters written by Dr. John Fothergill, eminent London physi·
cian, friend of the American Colonies, Quaker internationalist, are a
collection without parallel from the pen of any other eighteenth century
doctor. The body of his correspondence is small but significant. Less
than four hundred letters have been found, widely scattered in England,
Scotland, and the United States. The editors have chosen for publication
some two hundred of these letters in which Dr. Fothergill's account of
his activities, interests, opinions, and friendships constitutes an informal
autobiography covering more than forty years of his professional life.
His letters cover a wide field of interest. Some of them were written to
relatives and friends of his youth, most of whom lived in Yorkshire or
Lancashire; some to colleagues and acquaintances he seldom met in
person because they lived far from London; others were directed to men
prominent in public affairs, such as Lord Dartmouth and Benjamin
Franklin. A long important series went to American colonists on political, cultural, and botanical subjects.

Dr. Fothergill's character shines through his letters. He recognizes the
individuality of each correspondent. To him a letter was a bridge of
communication with a distant friend eagerly awaiting a message. He
usually wrote at night in the quiet of his study after fatiguing days of
visits to sickrooms. He never tried for literary effect, though sometimes
he achieved it when pleading a cause to which he was devoted with mind
and heart. His sincerity and idealism are particularly evident when first
he seeks a peaceful settlement of the increasing difficulties between Great
Britain and the American Colonies — and perhaps in the end a cure for
the ills of the world by outlawing war.

Recognized in his maturity as one of London's foremost physicians, sought by patients of every occupation and social class because of the warmth of his humanity, he was highly respected by professional colleagues, active in scientific circles, and honored by learned societies on both sides of the sea. Always loyal to the Society of Friends in its concern for human welfare, he enjoyed the pursuits of a singularly varied life to which he contributed the qualities which won him phenomenal success.

What he achieved is vividly emphasized by comparison of the first and the last letters in this volume. The first letter was written in 1735 by John Fothergill, Jr., aged twenty-three, at the end of his first year as a medical student in the University of Edinburgh. He was down in pocket to his last guinea, and wrote to his father tactfully for "what thou pleases further" to enable him to spend the summer in London at work in a hospital or in an apothecary's shop.

The last letter in this volume was written in 1780 by Dr. Fothergill, aged sixty-eight, to his longtime friend and patient, Benjamin Franklin, Minister Plenipotentiary from the United States to the Court of Louis XVI of France. Dr. Fothergill answered a query Franklin had made about his health. Advice for alleviation of Franklin's difficulty was followed by a proposal conceived with Fothergillian idealism, nothing less than a concerted effort for the abolition of wars by the institution of a College of Justice where the claims of disputing nations might be weighed and adjusted without recourse to barbaric slaughter. "No man," he wrote, "has it so much in his power as my honoured Friend to infuse this thought into the breasts of Princes or those who rule them and their affairs."

To assemble and edit a collection of letters as widely diverse in subject matter and interest as those written by Dr. Fothergill might challenge a team of several experts versed in the disciplines of medicine, history, religion, and science. By virtue of their discovery, however, and the recognition of their value, the privilege of introducing them to the public has been claimed by the present editors, Dr. Booth of London and Mrs. Corner of Philadelphia, thus making possible an Anglo-American collaboration in the two cities where most of Dr. Fothergill's letters are now found. Dr. Booth, like Dr. Fothergill, was educated at Sedbergh School and received a medical degree from a Scottish medical school. He is a Fellow of the Royal College of Physicians of London and is now Professor of Medicine in the Royal Postgraduate School of Medicine, London. The senior editor was born in Massachusetts and grew up in the region where the first battles of the War for Independence took place. She is familiar with English life and institutions, having resided in both London and Oxford, where she has pursued historical research.

She now lives in Philadelphia, where many of Dr. Fothergill's correspondents had their homes in the eighteenth century.

Dr. Fothergill died while the two countries he loved were still engaged in a bitter war which he had tried to avert. He would have rejoiced could he have known that two centuries after he lived and worked and penned his letters, scholars on both sides of the Atlantic, seeing in his correspondence much of interest and benefit for our own time, have joined forces to make these letters available to modern readers.

Betsy C. Corner, Philadelphia
Christopher C. Booth, London
1970

Contents

I. Dr Fothergill's ancestry and education — II. The Fothergill brothers — III. The Doctor, his profession, and his patients — IV. Botanical friendships and a garden — V. Dr. Fothergill's library — VI. War and peace — VII. The Society of Friends; Quaker meetings — VIII. Ackworth School — IX. Last days.

Medical student in Edinburgh — "Walking the wards" in London — First botanical correspondence — Young Friends from America — Tour to the Low Countries and Bremen.

Setting up practice in London — Friendship with eminent botanists — Appointed correspondent for London Meeting with Pennsylvania Quakers — Political problems of Pennsylvania — Threat of war with France over the Austrian Succession — A doctor's life in London — Scientific queries for John Bartram — Dr. Fothergill thought too liberal about out-of-meeting marriages — Made Licentiate of the Royal College of Physicians — Death of John Fothergill, Senior.

Pennsylvania treaties with the Indians — The Rebellion of '45 — Quaker

Contents

reconciliation with the Colonies — Letter to Franklin in France — Dr. Fothergill painfully ill — Alexander's financial difficulties — Founding of Ackworth School — Proposal to Franklin of an international court to avert wars — Franklin's affectionate memory of Dr. Fothergill.

Illustrations

Illustrations

xiv

Acknowledgments

To name all those who have given valuable help during the progress of assembling and preparing material for this book would be impossible. The interest and assistance of many on both sides of the sea has been an inspiration. Both editors have been particularly fortunate in the friendship of Mrs. Amy E. Wallis of Darlington, County Durham, who has in her keeping a varied collection of Fothergill family papers. She has a long line of Quaker ancestry, and has become an authority on Quaker genealogy. Since the editors are neither of them Quakers, acquaintance with Mrs. Wallis, for at least forty years a devoted member of the Meeting for Sufferings of London Yearly Meeting of the Society of Friends, has been especially instructive and rewarding. Special thanks are due to Mrs. Wallis for her generosity in providing the editors with photographic copies of the letters of Dr. Fothergill in her care.

In Philadelphia, Mrs. Corner has had the benefit of correspondence and consultation with Professor Frederick B. Tolles, Director of the Friends Historical Library of Swarthmore College and author of books of eighteenth-century importance, and Dr. Henry J. Cadbury, Hollis Professor Emeritus of Divinity at Harvard University, Quaker historian. Their comment after reading certain sections of the Introduction was a favor especially appreciated. At the Library of the Society of Friends, London, which contains the Society's historical archives, the Librarian, Edward H. Milligan, with his staff has been most responsive to every request and every question of both editors during the long period of research. In the early stages of preparation, Miss Muriel Hicks provided capable assistance, particularly to Dr. Booth by arranging for photography of the collection of Fothergill letters in the library at Friends House.

Generous assistance has been rendered by the staff of the Library of the American Philosophical Society, to whom Mrs. Corner is greatly indebted, particularly to Mrs. Gertrude D. Hess, Mrs. Ruth Duncan, and

Acknowledgments

Mr. Murphy D. Smith for supplying books, making available important eighteenth-century manuscripts, and securing exact titles of books now long out of print. Thanks are also due to a succession of A.P.S. typists, especially to Mrs. Julianne W. Pearson and Mrs. Lillian Leidy Silberman.

At the Historical Society of Pennsylvania Mr. J. Harcourt Givens, his successor Mr. Conrad Wilson, and their assistants have been tireless in searching among their large collection for Fothergill letters. Their help is heartily appreciated.

Publication of a letter written by Dr. Fothergill in 1751 to his friend of Edinburgh days, Dr. William Cuming, owes its appearance in this volume to the thoughtfulness and generosity of its discoverer, Dr. Whitfield J. Bell, Librarian of the American Philosophical Society, who found it in Richmond, Virginia.

Gratitude is expressed to the President of the Pennsylvania Hospital, Mr. T. Truxton Hare, for permission to consult the early Minute Books of the Board of Managers of the Hospital. This gave Mrs. Corner opportunity to procure data concerning investments made in London chiefly through the exertions of Dr. Fothergill, Benjamin Franklin, and David Barclay to enable the first hospital established in the American Colonies to maintain its services during its early days of difficulty.

Search for letters during 1952–1953, while Dr. and Mrs. Corner were residing in Oxford, led by special arrangement to the privilege of examining the Dartmouth Papers then in possession of the seventh Earl of Dartmouth at Patshull House near Wolverhampton. Two days of intensive research, combined with gracious hospitality, gave opportunity to review the huge mass of correspondence which the second Earl of Dartmouth (Dr. Fothergill's patient and friend) had received while Secretary of State for the Northern Department (American Colonies) during the fateful years of 1772–1775. Seven letters of exceptional interest were found at this time, and permission to publish given *viva voce* by the seventh Lord Dartmouth. Written permission has since been received through the courtesy of the ninth Earl of Dartmouth. His Lordship has kindly contributed a photograph of a portrait of his illustrious ancestor, who as a young man sat for a likeness by Thomas Gainsborough.

Dr. Booth had the pleasure of acquaintance with the late Quintin Gurney, Esq., of Bawdeswell Hall, not far from Norwich, England, thereby gaining the privilege of examining the David Barclay Papers which Mr. Gurney inherited.

During one of several visits to Mrs. Wallis of Darlington, County Durham, an opportunity occurred to meet the late Dr. W. Crichton Fothergill, a well-known radiologist of that city, who was a lineal descendant of Dr. Fothergill's brother Alexander. A pleasant evening was spent listening to family lore past and present, and viewing family treasures in his possession. Two of Dr. Fothergill's letters had been previously sent by Dr. W. Crichton Fothergill to Dr. Booth, one of which is found on p. 129 of this volume. Friends in Wensleydale were particularly helpful. Mr. Frank Outhwaite and his late wife, until recently residing at Carr End, Dr. Fothergill's birthplace, kindly showed the house and farm. Miss Joan Ingilby and Miss Marie Hartley of Askrigg, whose literary-artistic partnership has resulted in a series of books about the surrounding country and its people, generously contributed local information.

In London the Registrar of the Royal College of Physicians, Sir Kenneth Robson, and the Librarian, Mr. L. M. Payne, have very kindly provided extracts from the records of the College. At the Linnean Society, the Librarian helpfully drew the Editors' attention to Dr. Fothergill's correspondence with John Ellis.

In Scotland through the assistance of Dr. Douglas Guthrie, Edinburgh's medical historian, sixteen letters written by young Dr. Fothergill to his revered teacher, Dr. Charles Alston, were found in the library of the University of Edinburgh. Another letter, describing a visit to Scarborough's Spa, was discovered in the National Library of Scotland.

At Edinburgh also the late Miss Mabyn Fothergill, another descendant of Alexander, lent to the editors from her collection of family papers the original drafts of a number of Dr. John Fothergill's letters. Miss Fothergill's brother, Edward Rimington Fothergill of Edinburgh, survives her and has furnished Dr. Booth with other letters.

Two small grants from the Penrose Fund of the American Philosophical Society, gratefully received when the letters were first being assembled, made possible photocopying of original manuscripts in many collections.

The senior editor's husband, Dr. George W. Corner, Sr., by his knowledge of medical history and his editorial experience has given invaluable assistance.

Special gratitude is owed to Mrs. L. J. Kewer, Chief Editor for Special Projects of Harvard University Press, for the literary skill and historical learning which she has devoted to the preparation of the manuscript for press. Her contribution, far exceeding the ordinary demands of such a task, has added to the precision and cogency of the annotation.

Editorial Procedures

The editors, in transcribing Dr. Fothergill's letters, have followed the originals closely. His spelling, excellent for the period, is in the main retained. Capitalization has been somewhat modernized, but capitals are retained in titles of rank or respect and abstract terms of special significance. Punctuation, variable in letters of the period, has been simplified and a number of exceptionally long complex sentences have been divided into shorter complete sentences, with gain in clarity.

Some overlong letters have been shortened by the omission of irrelevant introductory passages, pious exhortations not related to the subject in hand, and passages dealing with topics amply discussed in other letters. Such deletions are indicated by the words *passage omitted* within square brackets. Brief deletions, of a few redundant or irrelevant words, are indicated by suspension points (. . .). When a word or phrase cannot be deciphered, either a conjectural replacement or the word *illegible* is inserted within square brackets.

A few letters which are known only from printed versions are reprinted literally, with corrections only of obvious misprints. Omissions not indicated by the original editors of these printed letters are mentioned after the provenance of each letter requiring such explanation.

The dating of Dr. Fothergill's letters calls for a special statement. Puritans and Quakers of the eighteenth century did not use the "pagan" names of the months, but instead numbered them from 1 to 12. In the Julian calendar, which in Great Britain and her colonies was not replaced by the Gregorian calendar until 1752, March was the first month, making February the twelfth month of the year. For example,

29.1.1744 or 1 mo. 29, 1744 was written for 29 March 1744
13.4.1746 or 4 mo. 13, 1746 was written for 13 June 1746

In England, from the twelfth century until 1752, New Year's Day was celebrated on 25 March. All dates in January (11th month), February (12th month), and up to 24 March were usually assigned to the old year. It was therefore customary to indicate, in letters written during these months, both the old year and the approaching new year. Thus

4 January 1730 (Old Style) would be written 4.11.1730/1; 15 February 1732 (O.S.) would be written 15.12.1732/3; 7 March 1745 (O.S.) would be written 7.1.1745/6; but 26 March 1748 (O.S.) would be written 26.1.1748.

Great Britain and her American colonies adopted the Gregorian calendar on 3 September 1752, Old Style. To compensate for astronomical inaccuracy in the Julian calendar, that day became 14 September New Style. From 1752, January instead of March was recognized as the first month of the year; and instead of February, December became the last month. A clear statement of this subject is found in the *Harvard Guide to American History* (Cambridge, Mass., Harvard University Press, 1955), 92.

Dr. Fothergill, when writing to Friends, regularly used the Quaker style, indicating the months by number, but in his letters to non-Quakers he frequently used the traditional names of the months. His letters published in this book are dated as he wrote them, Old Style or New Style according to the time when they were written.

Abbreviations Used in the Notes

APS	American Philosophical Society
Coll. Phys.	College of Physicians, Philadelphia
DAB	*Dictionary of American Biography*
DNB	*Dictionary of National Biography*
HSP	Historical Society of Pennsylvania
LSFL	Library of the Society of Friends, London
NCMH	New Cambridge Modern History
Phil. Trans. R.S.	*Philosophical Transactions* of the Royal Society of London
Port.	Portfolio
UEL	University of Edinburgh Library

Brief Chronology

1774–1775	Conciliation efforts, with Benjamin Franklin and David Barclay
1776	Foreign Associate, Société Royale de Médicine, Paris; member, Committee to visit Friends' meetings in the Northern Counties
1778	Serious illness
1779	Clerk, London Yearly Meeting
1779	Founds Ackworth School, near Pontefract, Yorkshire
26 December 1780	Death from prostatic obstruction, London

Dr. Fothergill's London

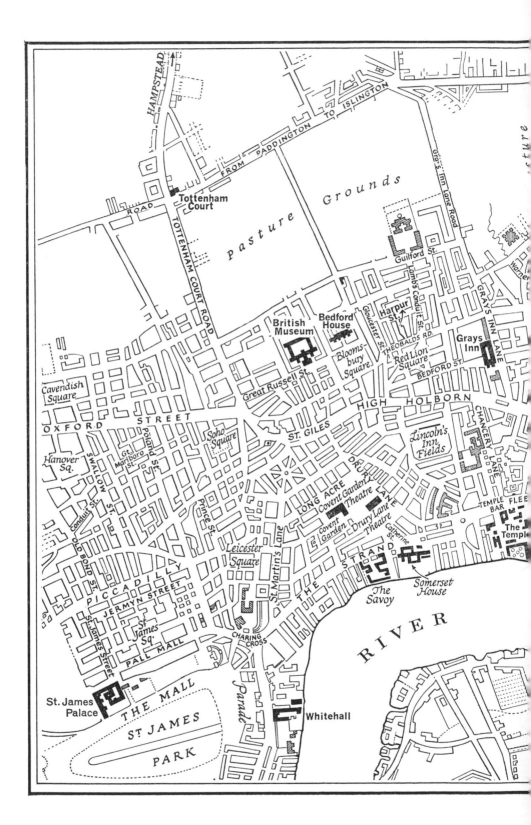

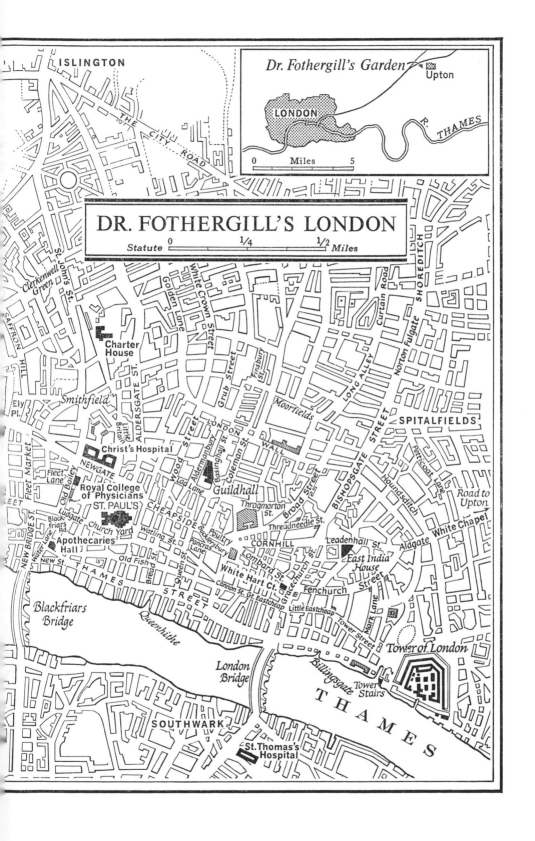

DR. FOTHERGILL'S LONDON

Statute 0 ¼ ½ Miles

Dr. Fothergill's Garden Upton

LONDON

R. THAMES

0 Miles 5

ISLINGTON

THE CITY ROAD

Clerkenwell Green

St. John's St.

SAFFRON HILL

Ely Pl.

Smithfield

Charter House

ALDERSGATE ST.

Golden Lane

White Crown Street

Grub Street

Finsbury St.

Moorfields

LONG ALLEY

Curtain Road

Norton Fulgate

SHOREDITCH

SPITALFIELDS

Christ's Hospital

NEWGATE

Fleet Lane

Old Bailey

Fleet Market

Royal College of Physicians

ST. PAUL'S

Church Yard

Blackfriars Rd.

Ludgate

Apothecaries' Hall

New St.

NEW BRIDGE ST.

Water Lane

THAMES STREET

CHEAPSIDE

Watling St.

Old Fish St.

Bread St.

Queen St.

Wood Street

Lad Lane

Aldermanbury

Basinghall St.

Coleman St.

LONDON WALL

Guildhall

Throgmorton St.

Broad Street

Threadneedle St.

Poultry

Buckersbury

Pancras Lane

Lombard St.

CORNHILL

White Hart Ct.

Cannon St. Gt. Eastcheap

Grace Church St.

Fenchurch

Little Eastcheap

BISHOPSGATE STREET

Houndsditch

Petticoat Lane

Leadenhall St.

East India House

Street

Aldgate

White Chapel

Road to Upton

Tower Street

Tower Hill

Tower Mark Lane

Blackfriars Bridge

Queenhithe

London Bridge

Billingsgate

Tower Stairs

Tower of London

THAMES

SOUTHWARK

St. Thomas's Hospital

THAMES

Chain of Friendship

Selected Letters of Dr. John Fothergill
1735–1780

"Don't let us suffer the fire to go
wholly out, nor the chain to grow
rusty but as little as we can."

To Israel Pemberton, 25 April 1748

Introduction

I. Dr. Fothergill's Ancestry and Education

Three generations of Fothergills had lived on the Yorkshire farm in Wensleydale where John Fothergill, Jr., the future doctor, was born March 8, 1712, to John Fothergill, a Quaker minister, and his wife Margaret Hough. The Fothergills possessed some two hundred acres of desirable land and a substantial stone farmhouse, erected in 1667 by John Jr.'s great-grandfather, the first Quaker of their line. By acquiring this property, known as Carr End, great-grandfather John had taken the first step toward advancing the Fothergills to the ranks of the middle class as landowners.

John Fothergill, Jr., was unable to trace his ancestry beyond the accomplishment and worth of his great-grandfather, from whom he could claim inheritance of name, birthplace, religion, and the characteristics of ambition and determination which served throughout a lifetime to bring him distinction in the profession of his choice.

In the middle of the seventeenth century, while George Fox was arousing dwellers in the North of England by his fervent evangelistic preaching, great-grandfather John had become a convinced Quaker. He suffered persecution for his religious dissent, a fate shared in the next generation by his son Alexander, who in the course of time inherited Carr End. Each of them in his day had steadfastly refused to support what they termed the "hireling ministry" of the established church: for this refusal to pay their tithes they each paid the penalty of imprisonment. Prolonged confinement in an unheated, vermin-infested cell, with a diet insufficient to maintain health, failed to make either of them repentant but shortened the lives of each in succession.

In 1695, Alexander's son John succeeded his father, becoming the third

3

owner of Carr End when he was barely twenty. His mother's death having preceded his father's, the burden of running the farm with supervision of two younger children became suddenly his responsibility. Shiftless servants in the house and on the farm took advantage of his inexperience. Led astray in his lonely youth of hardship, and being deeply troubled, he at last found anchorage in the faith of his fathers. He had a mystical experience in a Quaker meeting, becoming suddenly convinced that the gift of the ministry had been bestowed upon him. His obvious sincerity, his fluency of speech, his air of youthful dedication, made him an exceptional preacher and he was soon called upon to visit many parts of England to rouse his hearers to a better life.

It was in silent expectant corporate worship that Quakers became accustomed to receive intimations of divine leadings: these intimations they habitually tested by reference to their fellow-members in meetings for church affairs, local, county, or national. In 1705, John Fothergill experienced in this way a strong call to visit the American Colonies. At this time, British Quakers felt it necessary to strengthen religious ties between London, the center of British Quakerism, and Philadelphia, still regarded as William Penn's City of Brotherly Love. A fund maintained for charitable needs and frequently drawn upon for religious visits provided financial support for John Fothergill's journey and for a companion, William Armistead.

Their tedious ten-weeks' voyage on a tumultuous sea was followed by arduous travel on horseback to isolated settlements in southern colonies — mile after mile through unsettled country where roads were merely rough forest tracks. Courage and determination, however, accomplished what the Society of Friends deemed necessary — a survey of the extent, conditions, and needs of colonial American Quakerism. When this phase of the religious visit came to an end, Philadelphia's warm welcome was a blessing. It was an encouraging experience to visit important Quaker centers long established in Pennsylvania, Maryland, New Jersey, New York, and Long Island.

After two years of effort, John Fothergill returned to England, made his reports, and found himself quite ready for a more settled existence. In 1709, he married Margaret Hough, a Quakeress two years his junior, daughter of a prosperous family of Cheshire Quakers of high standing, and took her to live at Carr End.

By 1718, their family of children numbered seven: Alexander, Thomas, John, Jr., the future doctor, Joseph, William, Samuel, and Ann. The mother was again pregnant, but in 1719 she and her child both died in her eighth childbirth.

In 1721, American Quakers expressed hope for another visit from the trusted leader who had visited them more than a decade earlier. The gains John Fothergill had secured in the Colonies needed revival and consolidation, particularly in small, remote communities. He felt it was his duty to undertake the task. Little Ann was put under the care of Ruth Gorton, a woman devoted to the Fothergills and called a cousin. Some of the boys may have stayed at Carr End, which was leased to a tenant farmer. Margaret's brother, Thomas Hough, took his nephews John, nearing ten, and Samuel, three years younger, to live in Marsh Gate, his Cheshire home, and attend school nearby in Frodsham.

When the father returned to his home in 1724, he found that Uncle Hough had made arrangements for young John to enter Sedbergh Grammar School, some twenty miles from Carr End. Samuel was still to be John's companion, receiving more elementary instruction. Both boys would live with a Quaker family at Brigflatts, within walking distance of the school. Thus, surrounded by Quaker influences, they would benefit from the best secular education available in the North of England.

Sedbergh School was fortunate in having a remarkably able headmaster, the Reverend Samuel Saunders, late Fellow of St. John's, Cambridge, who had come to the school in 1709. A classicist, he had an enviable reputation with the dons of Oxford and Cambridge for sending them pupils with superior preparation for university studies. Although John and Samuel Fothergill, as dissenters, would never be admitted to those Anglican centers of learning, John, an eager student, profited from all that Sedbergh offered for his individual development.

In 1728 school days came to an end for the two brothers. Their father, who had made a second marriage to a worthy spinster, Elizabeth Buck, now arranged for each of these two sons the usual seven years of apprenticeship. Young John would remain in Yorkshire, going to Bradford to acquire the skills of an apothecary from Benjamin Bartlett, his father's friend. Samuel, less bookish than John, was apprenticed to a shopkeeper of Stockport in Cheshire, to learn merchandising.

The years John Fothergill, Jr., spent in Bradford with Benjamin Bartlett brought happiness and absorbing occupations. John apparently lived in the hospitable Bartlett home, where a daughter, Betty, and her younger brother were growing up and many visitors were entertained. Benjamin Bartlett, in addition to an apothecary's shop, kept a bookstore and received regular shipments of volumes from London, especially books on scientific subjects and occasional rarities of special interest, to all of which John had access. In his daily work the young apprentice

5

studied the properties of drugs commonly in use and learned how to compound medicines with the exactitude Bartlett required. Since apothecaries of the eighteenth century customarily gave medical advice to those who bought their remedies, and even visited those afflicted by illness, John had an opportunity to see on a small scale what the problems of medical practice were like.

Perhaps it was Bartlett, impressed by his pupil's industry, versatility, and ambition, who first brought to John Fothergill's attention that he was acquiring sufficient preparation to gain admission to Edinburgh's medical school, where possibly within a year he could acquire the precise knowledge and skills of a master apothecary. Since the established Church of Scotland was Presbyterian, there were no barriers against the admission of dissenters to the University of Edinburgh. Latin was the language of Scotland's halls of higher learning as in the Anglican colleges of Oxford and Cambridge. Thanks to the Rev. Dr. Saunders, Latin was already a living language to John Fothergill, to speak as well as to read and write. Benjamin Bartlett, eager for the young man's success, generously offered to release his pupil before the end of his indentured apprenticeship and gladly supplied necessary recommendations for his admission to Edinburgh's school of medicine.

As soon as the young man received news of his acceptance, he made ready to go to Carr End for a visit of respect to his father. Upon receiving the parental blessing, John started his long ride on horseback to Scotland's capital. What he would need on the road he packed into saddlebags; heavy luggage would be shipped to his lodgings. Grandfather Hough's legacy of £120 to further his grandson's education was tapped for £20; the rest would be divided into installments to last, if possible, through the two years of his course, though his father would help with necessary expenses. A little account book John kept shows that he laid out only seventeen shillings and sixpence during a three-days' journey to Edinburgh, secured student lodgings for half a crown a week, and sold his horse for four guineas.

Educationally, fortune favored this young man. He entered Edinburgh's medical school in 1734 while the curriculum was undergoing radical reform led by a faculty trained in Leyden. There Hermann Boerhaave, the greatest medical teacher of the age, competent in many disciplines of learning, had stressed new ways of study and thinking. Scotland's foremost medical leaders, profiting from this example, released their students from complete bondage to the ancient authority of textbooks. John Fothergill and his fellow students, with an armamentarium of facts well in mind, were encouraged to seek for themselves the answers to problems which the study of disease never ceases to present.

John Fothergill began his medical studies with Alexander Monro, Primus, Professor of Anatomy, the first of three Alexanders of a family who in three successive generations held this chair for 126 years. He had studied medicine under some of the most noted teachers of the age, in London, Paris, and Leyden. In later years Dr. Fothergill remembered Monro's almost fatherly concern for the young men then coming from England, Ireland, and the West Indies — and increasingly from the American Colonies — to secure in Edinburgh the best medical education obtainable short of the Continent. John Fothergill testifies that Professor Monro was the first person who advised him to continue his studies, take a medical diploma, and practice medicine.

By the attraction of kindred interests, Dr. Charles Alston, Professor of Materia Medica and the Regius Professor of Botany, a Leyden graduate in his fifties, won admiration for his attainments from the Yorkshire student less than half his age. Alston's instruction and stimulating friendship had a strong formative influence upon John Fothergill's development, and the friendship was continued for some time by correspondence after Fothergill went to London.

Two years of steady application to the theoretical background of medicine as understood in the eighteenth century, plus public delivery of a Latin dissertation before a full assembly of the faculty of Edinburgh's medical school, brought John Fothergill the coveted medical degree. In the summer of 1736 he went directly to London to gain clinical experience by "walking the wards" of St. Thomas's Hospital, under the tutelage of Dr. Edward Wilmot (later Sir Edward), who was influential in the counsels of the Royal College of Physicians and a Fellow of the Royal Society of London. After demonstrating ability in this phase of medical work, Dr. John began seeing a few patients of his own, and in 1740 he moved to 2 White Hart Court, off Gracechurch Street, to begin independent practice.

II. The Fothergill Brothers

The letters between Dr. John Fothergill in London and his brothers Joseph, Samuel, and Alexander, and other family letters and records left by the Fothergills of Carr End, provide material for a sociological study of considerable detail, depicting eighteenth century life, occupations, and moral principles in the rise of a Quaker family of exceptional ability

7

from an ancestral background of yeoman farmers to middle-class status —
John to professional rank, Samuel and Alexander to semi-professional
activities.

Both Joseph and Samuel settled in Lancashire. Alexander remained
in Wensleydale; Dr. John came to have a busy practice in London.
Exchange of letters was the only way to keep the sense of family unity
alive.

Dr. John's early letters show a lightness of mood which vanished later
as responsibilities of maturity burdened him. While young, he often
depended upon Samuel and Alexander for practical assistance. As they
all grew older, Samuel and Alexander came to rely upon Dr. John's
wisdom and experience.

Dr. John never married. Late in 1749 he invited his sister Ann to visit
him in London. Ann was a dutiful spinster who had suffered from poor
health and depression after caring for her father during his last illness.
She came to make John a visit and remained a resident of London the
rest of her life, devoting herself to her brother's comfort for more than
thirty years. In 1765 Dr. Fothergill leased a summer home, Lea Hall,
in Cheshire, and in 1767, he and his sister moved from White Hart Court
out of the City to a pleasant new house in Harpur Street, Bloomsbury,
near Red Lion Square, where they could look across green fields to the
hills with the twin villages of Highgate and Hampstead. Dr. John,
whose tastes and temperament were those of a scholar, enjoyed many
quiet evenings at home in his study, engaged in literary pursuits,
in arranging new acquisitions for his library, cataloguing his collections
of prints, shells, and corals, or writing to far-distant friends. Dr. Benjamin Rush, a visitor from Philadelphia in 1768, described Ann Fothergill as a woman of good sense and great worth, who added greatly to the
pleasure of guests at her brother's table by her sensible conversation.

Joseph, the brother next younger than John, became the successful
head of an iron industry large enough in scale "to find work and wages
for 140 families," he wrote in a letter of 1748. He lived in Warrington,
Lancashire, a pleasant non-corporate town favored by early Quakers
because of its freedom from religious prejudice. In such non-corporate
towns, dissenters were allowed to set up business for themselves, while
many larger corporate towns restricted trade to members of the corporation. Joseph married Hannah Kelsall, whose surname suggests connection with a family important in the iron industry of Wales. Nine
children were born to them, but a son and a daughter died in early
childhood. By 1761, both Joseph and his wife had died. Henry, the surviving son, succeeded his father as head of the business. By the time of

his death in 1769, three of his sisters — Margaret, Sarah, and Hannah — were married. The three younger sisters — Ann, Mary, and Elizabeth — were placed under the guardianship of their uncle Samuel. Betty, aged seventeen, was invited to visit her aunt and uncle in London, and her diary, kept during a stay of several months, is the only known record of everyday happenings in the famous Quaker doctor's household.

Samuel, youngest of the four brothers, entered upon an apprenticeship of labor without educational advantages when he went to Stockport to learn merchandising in a small shop. His easy sociability led him astray, and in 1736 his father threatened to disown him. But while John Fothergill Senior was absent on his third and last visit to the American colonies, Samuel surprisingly reformed, largely because of the influence of a Quaker woman preacher, Susanna Croudson. Although she was fifteen years his senior, Samuel married her in 1738 and they went to live in Warrington, where they set up a shop supplying a variety of goods. Susanna soon gave up itinerant preaching entirely in order to take over management of their business, leaving her husband free to exercise more widely his newly discovered gifts as a preacher. With the encouragement of his fellow Quakers, Samuel traveled to many parts of England and to Ireland. In 1754, he voyaged to America and traveled thousands of miles on horseback, like his father before him, to visit most of the thirteen colonies. In Boston, where Quakers had been persecuted and had suffered martyrdom in the seventeenth century, he received an overwhelming welcome; two thousand people crowded Faneuil Hall to hear him. In Newport, Rhode Island, where he also drew crowds, he probably saw his British cousin, Hannah Proud, now married to Timothy Waterhouse, and no doubt admired their small son Benjamin, who was to become a famous New England physician.

Returning to England in July 1756, Samuel found himself highly acclaimed among the Quakers. He had a following similar to that of John Wesley among Methodists, though not as numerous. His most popular sermons were soon published, and as late as the first quarter of the nineteenth century, his religious discourses were still being issued from the press in Philadelphia; in Wilmington, Delaware; in Salem, Massachusetts, and in Newport, Rhode Island, and were in demand in every Quaker settlement.

Samuel's public career was increasingly interrupted after 1769 by illness — a so-called dropsical condition involving both heart and kidneys — and in June 1772 he died.

Alexander Fothergill, unlike his brothers, never left home for a term of apprenticeship. Since he was the oldest son, the family estate was his inheritance and it became his burden. He married at twenty-four, and in two years' time was a widower with an infant daughter. A second marriage a year later, to Margaret Thistlethwaite of Harbour Gill, Dent, Yorkshire, brought him a capable, healthy wife, who became the mother of four sons and two daughters. The great sorrow they shared was the loss at the age of twelve of their firstborn child, a promising boy who died after a short illness from smallpox, the scourge of eighteenth-century England.

Alexander early won a reputation as a man who could carry responsibilities effectively. Chosen as clerk and assistant by Thomas Metcalfe, a highly respected Justice of the Peace, he was apparently given the run of the Justice's library of law books. He learned to prepare writs, deeds, and wills, and became familiar with the details of property transfers, boundary questions, and marriage settlements. Dr. John opposed this employment, which would inevitably lead, he feared, to Alexander's neglect of Carr End and his family.

Quakers, moreover, disapproved of litigation and judicial oaths, with which Alexander as a law clerk would be much engaged. Alexander, however, paid slight attention to Dr. John's objections. Association with Justice Metcalfe had given him the privilege of friendship with a cultivated man of the world. The whole experience had broadened his outlook as he took part in neighborhood business. When, in 1751, Parliament passed a Turnpike Act for construction of a road between Richmond and Lancaster which would greatly facilitate Wensleydale's access to the outside world, the Trustees unanimously elected Alexander Fothergill surveyor-in-chief of the turnpike project.

Building this road was a tremendous undertaking, with its course laid over moors and fenland, across hills and vales, through sixty or seventy miles of the roughest part of Yorkshire, to reach its terminus in Lancashire. Parliament had specified twenty-one years for completion. Alexander was forty-two when the work started and sixty-five before he could ride the full length of the road. When the turnpike was almost finished, in midsummer of 1774, a storm of criticism took him completely by surprise. He was accused of making arbitrary decisions without referring to the Trustees for advice, and was charged with flagrant dishonesty for failure to pay construction bills with sums provided for the purpose. A demand was made that he should place a sizeable sum of money on the table, and he could not at once comply. Unable to endure further opposition, he resigned.

Meanwhile other pressures were troubling him. His personal finances were in a tangle; Carr End was heavily mortgaged. One First Day, as he was leaving Friends Meeting, two prominent local members of the Society approached him to deliver a charge of gross misconduct and the paternity of at least two bastard children. Alexander declared that these charges were groundless malicious gossip, but in the weeks that followed, he was "read out of Meeting." Scandal had never before touched the Fothergill name. Alexander's legal experience made him wary; he refused to discuss definite accusations placed against him unless persons, places, and dates of misconduct were specifically stated. No such evidence could be procured.

In September 1774, Dr. John sent word that he and Ann, on their way back to London from their summer home in Cheshire, were coming to see their brother, but not to Carr End. They preferred to meet him at Knaresborough, safe from curious eyes, where they could be together for private conversation. When this reunion took place, confidence and affection marked the meeting. Not one word of remonstrance was uttered. Alexander's diary records, "Brother and Sister manifested the highest regard . . . in advising for my good . . . and this in the most tender and affecting manner, not 'obraidingly.' " The next morning the three went together to nearby Scotton, stood beside their beloved father's grave in silent contemplation, then spoke their brief farewells and were soon on their separate ways homeward.

Suspense and anxiety, however, still clouded Alexander's days. Perplexed and grief-stricken because sensational gossip seemingly outweighed his record of valuable public service, he sought reinstatement in the Society of Friends. He had to prepare for the Society's careful study a confession of his wrongdoing, together with an expression of his earnest resolve to amend his way of life. In this remarkable document, he confessed only that for a long time he had become completely absorbed in worldly concerns to the consequent neglect of religious duties and greatly to his own detriment. He begged contritely for forgiveness and for assistance which only the Society of Friends could render in his penitent determination to live honorably by his own wish, following Quaker standards. Submitted to Wensleydale Preparative Meeting, the document was passed on to Richmond Monthly Meeting, and after a prolonged period of probation, Alexander was at last restored as he wished to the Quaker fold. The scandal died down, never proven.

With public duties no longer claiming his powers, Alexander suddenly felt old, but he lived longer than Dr. John. William, a son with a taste for farming, took over the management of Carr End. The family property was always saddled with debt, but Alexander had a few years of comparative comfort before his death in 1788 at the age of seventy-nine.

11

Margaret, his wife, seems never to have lost faith in him. She survived her husband by a decade, and had the joy of seeing a sixth generation of Fothergills of Carr End at play on the pleasant acreage of the Wensleydale homestead. Carr End was owned by the family until 1841.

III. The Doctor, His Profession and His Patients

Dr. Fothergill's contributions to medical literature were gathered together soon after his death by his protegé, Dr. John Coakley Lettsom, in a three-volume edition. Among the articles included were a series of early letters on "Weather" and "Disease" from the *Gentleman's Magazane*, and five papers read at sessions of the Royal Society. One of these, originally written in Latin, presents what is apparently the earliest description of a diaphragmatic hernia. Dr. Fothergill describes, not without feeling (the patient was a child), the onset, progress, and fatal outcome of a condition then impossible to correct.

His medical reputation was established when at the age of thirty-five he prepared a careful *Account of the Sore-Throat attended with Ulcers*, published a year later, in 1748. The first part of this work is a history of a disease that had spread like a plague through southern Europe almost a century before. The second part expounds a new method of treatment he had found generally successful during the outbreak of a similar disease which reached the proportions of an epidemic with high mortality in London and adjacent localities during the autumn and early winter of 1747. His book won immediate attention and continued in demand during the next three decades while there were periodic outbreaks of this alarming malady. Seven editions of the *Account* had been issued by 1777.

From Dr. Fothergill's clear and full description, it seems probable that he was describing an ulcerative sore throat of streptococcal origin. He certainly saw also cases of scarlet fever and what is now known to be diphtheria, in his time not easily distinguishable from streptococcal sore throat. His treatment of this serious disease was radically new in an age of excessively vigorous therapy. Patients were customarily dosed heavily with "the bark" (quinine) and with opium. They were given powerful emetics, copiously bled or cupped, frequently purged, often blistered and clystered. Dr. Fothergill rejected this depleting system of treatment. He prescribed a mild sustaining diet. He considered bleeding an excessive and unnecessary strain upon a patient's "natural strength of constitution," and thought purging was actually injurious. He opposed scarification of the tonsils. He stressed what seems more commonplace today, such as "free, but not cold air," constant attention to cleanliness and change of linen, and frequent washing of the mouth and throat with homemade gargles. He used warm, aromatic, gently stimulating medicines. Toward the end of the eighteenth century, these less drastic methods of treatment, advocated as early as 1748 by Dr. Fothergill, had been generally accepted by progressive British physicians. In 1793, William Withering, himself a renowned innovator by his introduction of digitalis in the treatment of heart failure, paid a grateful tribute to Dr. Fothergill when calling to mind "how many lives were lost until Dr. Fothergill and Dr. Wall taught us to withhold the lancet and the purge."

The second volume of Dr. Fothergill's *Works* contains more than twenty of his papers, of which three, especially, show the scope and variety of his professional interest during the busiest years of his practice. In 1773 his account of *A Painful Affection of the Face*, later named *tic douloureux* and more recently trigeminal neuralgia, laid the foundation for further investigation by his great-nephew, Dr. Samuel Fothergill, who in 1804 correctly located the seat of the disease in the fifth cranial nerve. Today this extremely painful condition is frequently designated "Fothergill's disease" in Great Britain.

In two other papers, brief but of outstanding importance published in 1776, Dr. Fothergill displayed a high degree of diagnostic insight. Each of these describes a fatal attack of angina pectoris with a complete case history of the patient and a report of pathological conditions found at autopsy. Dr. Fothergill had already observed that patients suffering from this disease usually had "an irregular and intermittent pulse." For this reason he urged the physician who performed the postmortem in the first case "to attend to the condition of the heart with all possible accuracy." The only abnormal finding, a cicatrice or scar-like appearance on the wall of the heart, was no doubt the first cardiac infarction ever seen in a case of death from angina pectoris. Dr. Fothergill's conclusion that "time and further opportunity must inform us of the rest" was prophetic. Only a year later, another patient, "a gentleman inclined to corpulency, but active and of a very irritable habit," died quite suddenly from angina pectoris "in a fit of anger." At Dr. Fothergill's request, John Hunter, "that skillful and accurate anatomist," agreed to perform the postmortem. Hunter's examination brilliantly confirmed Dr. Fothergill's conjecture that angina pectoris is related to disease of the heart, and pointed to an occluded coronary artery as the precise seat of the disease.

No list of Dr. Fothergill's patients has ever been located, nor any record of his professional accounts. Possibly his sister Ann, his careful housekeeper for many years, destroyed whatever she found in his desk

13

which seemed no longer needed. It is certain, however, that he had an extensive and lucrative practice, estimated at its height to provide an income of between £7000 and £10,000 annually, a sum of much greater economic value than now. He never had, however, what is called "a fashionable practice." Many people of wealth and title sought his services, but the solid majority of his patients were Quakers and other dissenters, some well placed and prosperous, others struggling for maintenance, some wretchedly poor. Leading Quaker merchants of London, captains of industry such as the Hanburys of the Virginia tobacco company, the apothecaries Sylvanus and Timothy Bevan, the bankers David Barclay, Henton Brown, and Brown's son-in-law Thomas Collinson, regularly sought Dr. Fothergill's services. Many county families, like the Gurneys of Norfolk, came to London periodically to consult him, as did Quaker merchants from Philadelphia when in London on business. He was a familiar figure to members of Parliament. Lord Dartmouth employed him as family physician. The Marquis of Rockingham was attracted to him because he was a Yorkshireman. The Honourable Thomas Penn called Dr. Fothergill to his country home in Braywick when Lady Juliana fell ill, and kept him there overnight. Horace Walpole reports that Lord Clive in his days of departed glory was last visited by the compassionate Quaker doctor. In 1757, Benjamin Franklin, in London on a political mission, became Doctor Fothergill's patient.

Dr. Fothergill was always hospitable to young physicians and students of medicine, and to travellers from America. Through his eagerness to help some visitors who possessed both these claims upon his interest he rendered what was perhaps his greatest service to his profession, that of encouraging the organization of the Pennsylvania Hospital and the Medical School of the University of Pennsylvania. In 1738, when he had been in practice for only two years, he entertained at his home Thomas Bond, who later was the first to propose the creation of a hospital in Philadelphia (chartered in 1751) and became one of its staff physicians. Two decades later three other young Philadelphians who came to study medicine in London and Edinburgh were his guests at breakfast, the only time of day his busy practice allowed him for such visits. The first of these was William Shippen junior, who in 1759 told the Doctor of his ambition to teach anatomy and midwifery in Philadelphia. In May 1760, John Morgan was in London on his way to Edinburgh. Dr. Fothergill and the two young men talked together about plans for a school of medicine in which Morgan would have the chair of physic. Two years later Benjamin Rush, in London for medical study, was welcomed at Dr. Fothergill's breakfast table once a week for several months. He returned to Philadelphia to take the medical professorship of chemistry. Thomas Bond, already well established in practice, became lecturer in medicine, and thus all four of the first faculty of the University of Pennsylvania School of Medicine had been encouraged and advised by Dr. Fothergill. To aid Shippen's teaching, Dr. Fothergill presented to the Pennsylvania Hospital a handsome set of anatomical drawings by Jan van Rymsdyk, plus cash to a total value of £350, equivalent to some thousands of dollars today. The drawings, still preserved by the Hospital, are a permanent memorial of Dr. Fothergill's help in founding the first general hospital and the first medical school in the American Colonies.

After moving to Harpur Street in 1767, Dr. Fothergill started a small dispensary in his home for the treatment of poor people on certain mornings before his coachman, Joseph, called to take him on rounds throughout London and into the surrounding country. Writing to his brother Samuel, Dr. Fothergill described a day of professional duty lasting seventeen hours during which he had mounted at least fifty flights of stairs at no small distance from each other.

Two descriptions of his appearance in an eighteenth century sickroom have been found. Fanny Burney, author of *Evelina*, a best-selling novel of the day, described him with literary skill when he was sixty-five and she was a fashionable young lady of twenty-one. When Dr. Fothergill responded to a call from her father, Dr. Charles Burney, the celebrated London organist and musicologist, to attend his ailing wife, charming Fanny received the aging Quaker physician. Accustomed as she was to guests of the polite world who flocked to her father's hospitable house — musicians, actors, artists, travelers, and writers — she found Dr. Fothergill disconcerting because, by Quaker custom, he wore his broadbrimmed hat in the house and even in her presence. "He is an upright, stern old man," she wrote in her diary: "He is an old prig." But when Fanny herself fell ill with a sore throat, "the putrid kind," she had the grace to change her opinion. The doctor became her very good friend, she relates, "and that whether I would or no . . . and really has been . . . amazingly civil and polite to me . . . , as kind as he is skillful." "Dr. Fothergill makes his visits very seldom," Fanny wrote. "He says he always knows when his patients are really recovering by these signs; if men, he finds their beds covered with newspapers; if women, he sees them with new top-knots, or hears them exclaim, 'Dear me, what a figure I am!'"

When Dr. Fothergill made his last visit to the Burneys, Fanny reported his leave-taking. "After complaining of his fatigue and great business," he turned to her suddenly, took her hand, and gave this warning: "My dear, never marry a physician. If he has little to do, he may become distressed; if much, it is a very uncomfortable life for his companion."

A description of Dr. Fothergill's appearance, written by his great-nephew and namesake, John Fothergill of York, adds animation to what we observe in the stiffly posed figure of Gilbert Stuart's portrait of the Quaker doctor, painted posthumously for the Royal Academy Exhibition of 1781. Word picture and portrait alike depict Dr. Fothergill as slender and rather delicately built, with an alert face expressing great sensibility. His features are strongly marked, his forehead high and finely molded, his mouth determined. His eyes, "brilliant, acute and deeply penetrating," are light in color. His coat, waistcoat and breeches are made of superfine cloth, nearly white. The "coat, made without a collar, has large cuffs and several buttons." The ends of his cravat are tucked within his waistcoat. His stockings, John adds, "were silk, the color of his clothes, and his shoe-buckles small," presumably of silver. He always wore, as customary with Quakers, a large, low three-cornered hat, over "a medical wig with rows of small curls descending one under another from near the crown of his head almost to his shoulders."

Earlier in life when Dr. Fothergill was a newcomer to London, he wrote an amusing letter to his brother Joseph describing wealthy doctors he often observed lolling in their coaches as they were driven through the city streets. He idly wondered then: "Would not such a state mightily become me?" — but quickly scorned the notion as mere "vanity in the bud." Thirty years and more have passed. Dr. Fothergill has his coach, a daily necessity, and his coachman. Great-nephew John describes both in full detail:

His coach was dark green, with wheels of the same color; the horses were black ones with very short docked tails, after the old manner. His coachman . . . weighed at least sixteen stone; his livery was a plain cocked hat, a white wig, a light drab coat with a velvet collar the same color, and bright haycock buttons.

Commendation from Lord North, Prime Minister of England — expressed in a proposal which probably never came to the doctor's ears — was something he would never have expected. A letter, 10 September 1774, included by Sir John Fortescue in *The Correspondence of King George III*, seriously suggests Dr. Fothergill to fill a vacancy soon to occur in the King's staff of physicians.

Dr. Fothergill [he writes] is certainly as good a physician as any in the world, and is undoubtedly the man who has the greatest influence over the whole body of his Brethren. Lord North does not know whether he would wish for the appointment; nor has he considered what objections might be made, but . . . it occurred to him whether a compliment paid to him might not be attended with good consequences both in Great Britain and America.

As was to be expected, King George was not enthusiastic. He did not wish to propitiate the Pennsylvania Quakers. His Majesty did not object to Dr. Fothergill personally as one of his physicians, but could a Quaker hold an office that would require him to take an oath of loyalty? Lord North is however urged to find "whether the thing is practicable." Thus the appointment was shelved.

It is rather surprising that James Boswell, who seems to have known everybody of consequence in eighteenth century England, never mentions Dr. Fothergill. Not until 1799, in Edmund Malone's third edition of Boswell's inimitable biography, did the celebrated Quaker physician get even slight notice, and that merely because in conversation Dr. Johnson once testified to his respect for unnamed doctors who never change their religion to attract new patients. Dr. Charles Burney, who assisted in preparing this edition for publication, in a brief footnote clarifies Dr. Johnson's statement. "Fothergill, a Quaker, and Schomberg, a Jew, had the greatest practice of any two physicians of their time. B." Perhaps Dr. Fothergill never knew that he was living in the Age of Johnson.

IV. Botanical Friendships and a Garden

Dr. Fothergill's letters to his former teacher, Dr. Charles Alston, Professor of Botany in Edinburgh, picture the young physician when first thrown upon his own resources in London's medical world. He filled his letters with whatever botanical information was being circulated, commented on medical literature to which he now had access, and, at a time when water cures were much sought, revealed his plan to publish chemical analyses of springs near London.

In 1740 he recorded his pleasure in a new friendship with Peter Collinson, a well-to-do Quaker merchant trading principally with the American Colonies and the West Indies. Collinson's garden in Peckham (later moved to Mill Hill) was a treasury of rare imported plants and trees. He loved flowers, yet he described himself as "no Botanist." He confessed that he was too much concerned with the business of his counting house to bother about the Linnaean system of classification, holding the opinion that "the Science of Botany is too much perplexed already." After he was elected a Fellow of the Royal Society of London in 1728, he spoke frequently at the Society's meetings, often presenting the work of foreign scientists. He built up an extensive correspondence with naturalists in many parts of the world, and by this means became the acknowledged leader of an international circle which is one of the earliest examples of world-wide cooperation among scientific men for the dissemination of useful knowledge. It was undoubtedly Peter Collinson who arranged a meeting in 1748 between Dr. Fothergill and Sir Hans Sloane, president of the Royal Society.

From Dr. Alston, Peter Collinson, and Sir Hans Sloane, Dr. Fothergill received as it were a botanical laying on of hands. Like the older men, he found refreshment of spirit in his study of the life cycle of plants in a garden, established lasting friendships by correspondence with people in other countries who had similar interests, and in collecting botanical classics discovered an absorbing pursuit of intellectual and aesthetic value.

In 1762 Dr. Fothergill purchased an estate of some thirty acres at Upton in Essex. He was attracted to the property because of its accessibility to London, the seclusion it offered, and its fine trees — among them five Virginia cedars which he thought were undoubtedly some of the first of this kind ever brought to England. At Upton he created a botanic garden for the acclimatization of plants, shrubs, and trees imported from foreign countries — plants selected because of their beauty or utility. Through extensive correspondence with British colonists and wide acquaintance with sea captains, adventurous travelers, botanical explorers, and friends at work in foreign countries, he was soon receiving botanical rarities from all over the world.

From his country house at Upton, even during the winter Dr. Lettsom tells us, Dr. Fothergill could open glass doors and step directly into a "suite of hot and greenhouse apartments of nearly 260 feet in extent, containing upwards of 3400 distinct species of exotics, whose foliage wore a perpetual verdure, and formed a beautiful and striking contrast to the shrivelled natives of colder climates . . . [Here] the elegant proprietor sometimes retired for a few hours to contemplate the vegetable productions of the four quarters of the globe enclosed within his domain, where the sphere seemed transposed and the Arctic Circle joined to the Equator." In the outdoor garden there were eventually some three thousand distinct species of plants. A winding canal divided the planting almost equally, reflecting blooming exotic shrubs lining the paths along its course. When Sir Joseph Banks, in later years president of the Royal Society, visited Dr. Fothergill's country estate, he declared that no other garden he had seen in England, whether royally supported or in private ownership, had at that time so many rare and valuable plants.

Writing in 1772 to Humphry Marshall, Dr. Fothergill described a favorite part of his garden, in which he felt Marshall had a special share because of well-chosen contributions sent overseas:

Under a north wall I have a good border, made up of that kind of rich black turf-like soil mixed with some sand in which I find most part of the

American plants thrive best. It has a few hours of morning and evening sun; and is quite sheltered from mid-day heats. The plants are well supplied with water during summer, and the little shrubs and herbaceous plants have a good warm covering of dry fern, thrown over them when the Frosts set in. This is gradually removed when the spring advances, so that by never being frozen in the ground while the plants are young and tender I never lose any that come to me with any degree of life in them, and it is acknowledged by the ablest Botanists we have that there is not a richer bit of ground in curious American plants in Great Brittain; and for many of the most curious I am obliged to thy diligence and care. My garden is well sheltered, the soil is good, and I endeavor to mend it as occasion requires. I have an Umbrella Tree (the greatest Magnolia) about twenty feet high, that flowers with me abundantly every Spring. The small magnolia likewise flowers with me finely. I have a little wilderness, which when I bought the premises, was full of old yew trees, laurels, and weeds. I had it cleared, well dug, and took up many trees, but left others standing for shelter. Among these I have planted kalmias, azaleas, all the magnolias, and most other hardy American shrubs. It is not quite eight years since I made a beginning, so that my plants must be considered but as young ones. They are, however, extremely flourishing. The great magnolia has not yet flowered with me but grows exceedingly fast. I shelter his top in the winter; he gains from half a yard to two feet in height every summer; and will ere long, I doubt not, repay my care with his beauty and fragrance.

Flourishing contributions such as these from North America made Dr. Fothergill long for others. Writing again to Humphry Marshall, he made the following requests:

There is a kind of dogwood, whose calyx is its greatest beauty; it chiefly grows in Virginia, whether with you I know not. I want a few plants of it; and, indeed, it would be always agreeable to receive young well rooted plants of any kind. If they are taken up with a little earth and a good root early in the spring and the earth tyed close about them with strong paper and packthread; or if they are put into boxes, with moss only about their roots, and sent away in the spring, they would come very safe. The boxes should not be nailed so close but a little air may get in. Would it be possible to send one of those pretty little owls alive? I wish I could see one. Most of the Captains in the trade I believe would endeavour to take care of it; and a mocking bird, if they could easily be had; but it is best to keep these things alive with you all winter and send them in the spring.

As importations increased, Dr. Fothergill acquired several acres of adjoining property. These acquisitions enlarged his area for planting and yet left open stretches of greensward restful to the gaze, as advocated by the great landscape architects of the day. Tales of his botanical collections spread to the Continent. European visitors to the British Museum often sought entrance to his garden and as the result of continued demand for this privilege, tickets of admission (without charge) were issued upon application to a limited number of visitors on certain days.

By necessary orderly procedure, whenever botanical shipments reached the garden, new plants were registered by competent gardeners who recorded the origin of each addition, the name attached when sent and if necessary its historical equivalent, and the appropriate placement decided upon at Upton, whether in the open ground, in the "stove" (hothouse), or in a greenhouse of equable temperature. Sir Joseph Banks states that Dr. Fothergill "paid the best artist the country afforded" — later a number of young artists were employed — to draw each new plant as it came to perfection of growth, as a means of record in case it should be destroyed by accident or disease. Using the accumulated records, Dr. Lettsom was able to prepare for publication his scholarly *Hortus Uptonensis; or, A Catalogue of stove and green-house plants in Dr. Fothergill's garden at Upton, at the time of his decease* (London, 1781).

As the years passed, Dr. Fothergill found less time for personal supervision of the garden. It is said, however, that he was sometimes observed there in the dead of night, lantern in hand, viewing by its glimmer his botanical treasures. All recent contributions, recorded according to established custom, were still periodically inspected by him. Sir Joseph Banks reported one source of these rare plants as "those whose gratitude for restored health prompted them to do what was acceptable to their benefactor." Such patients were told that "presents of rare plants chiefly attracted his attention, and would be more acceptable than the most generous fees." Sir Joseph concludes, "How many unhappy men enervated by the hot climates where their connections had placed them found health on their return home at that cheap purchase!"

After the American war for independence broke out, shipment of botanical specimens became out of the question, and the constant flow of correspondence ceased between those happy few who had formed a botanical brotherhood.

V. Dr. Fothergill's Library

In the spring of 1781, Leigh and Sotheby of York Street, Covent Garden, announced their forthcoming sale of Dr. Fothergill's "entire and valuable library containing a fine collection in Physick, Natural History and Classicks, together with some good Prints, and an Excellent Collection of Drawings . . . by some of the most approved Masters." A catalogue of the sale can be seen today in the Library of The Society of Friends in London. Less than 1600 titles are listed, but a single title often covers several volumes; the series of *Mémoires de l'Académie Royale des Sciences depuis 1692 jusqu'à 1742* is credited with no less than 76 *tomes*; Pope's translations of the Iliad and the Odyssey with 11 volumes. Pamphlets devoted to special subjects were numerous.

Dr. Fothergill's medical books comprised a complete working library of the important medical and surgical texts of past centuries, combined with outstanding works of contemporary scholarship and books by his professional colleagues. Seventeenth century reprints were numerous, also some of the sixteenth century which were for the most part excellent Latin editions of the ancient, medieval, and Renaissance classics: Hippocrates and Galen; the biological works of Aristotle; the famous Boerhaave-Albinus edition of the great anatomical classic, *Corporis Humani Fabrica* of Vesalius; Latin versions of medical classics of Arabic scholarship — the *Medicina* of Haly Filius Abbas, the *De Re Medica* of Averrhoës, and the *Opera Medica* of Rhazes. He also possessed the famous *Regimen Sanitatis* of Italy's early Salernitan School, the important physiological works of Albrecht von Haller, and the pioneer pathological contributions of Morgagni in *De Causis et Sedibus Morborum*. Among anatomical atlases was that of his colleague William Hunter, *The Anatomy of the Gravid Uterus* — sumptuously published by the Baskerville Press and superbly illustrated by Jan van Rymsdyk.

The history of botany is traced from Theophrastus, the pupil of Aristotle, from Pliny the Elder and Dioscorides, through records of diligent search, extensive travel, and study by European and British scholars, to the accomplishments of Carolus Linnaeus of Sweden, who established the binomial classification of plants and created a great center of botanical investigation at Uppsala. Dr. Fothergill purchased every book Linnaeus produced as soon as his distinguished contemporary's work received publication.

Two pages of the Catalogue are filled with sets of classical authors, testifying to the owner's continued love of classical learning first acquired at Sedbergh Grammar School. Contemporary reference books include the two volumes of Samuel Johnson's *Dictionary of the English Language*, 1755; the three of Edinburgh's *Dictionary of Arts and Sciences*, 1771, from which the *Encyclopedia Britannica* developed; the four of *Biographia Britannica*, 1774; and fourteen volumes of Buffon's *Histoire Naturelle, avec grande nombre des figures*.

Dr. Fothergill had no novels; perhaps he never knew that his patient Fanny Burney had written a novel (*Evalina*), published anonymously, which gained great popularity. He had, however, many books of travel in all parts of the world.

Poetry was scantily represented; it included a set of Dryden's works in four volumes; six volumes of Spenser's poems; Abraham Cowley's poems; Steele's *Miscellanies* of 1727; John Gay's *Poems* of 1781 and his *Fables* in verse, 1750; a volume by Matthew Prior, dated 1718; the *Lyric Poems* of Isaac Watts, 1727; Alexander Pope's *Dunciad*, 1729; his *Essay on Man*, 1734, and his translations of the Iliad and the Odyssey already mentioned. Only Ovid, Catullus, and Vergil represent poetry among the sets of classics. We search in vain for Dante. Shakespeare's sonnets and his plays were neglected.

There was, however, a sizeable collection constituting a veritable history of religion in its infinite variety of allegiance — testifying to the liberality of mind which distinguished John Fothergill the physician, who was himself a loyal Quaker.

In conclusion, a list of books concerning the American Colonies is given here as entered in the 1781 Catalogue issued by Lee and Sotheby.

1. The American Physitian 1671
2. Josselyn, two Voyages to New England, 1674
3. Mather's History of New England, 1702
4. Francklin on Electricity, 1769; plates, elegant copy
5. Description Virgine et Marilan, 1701 (author unknown)
6. Colden, History of the Five Nations of Canada 1755
7. James Logan on Generation of Plants (no date given)
8. Causes of the Alienation of the Delaware and Shawanese Indians from the British Interest 1759
9. Smith, History of New Jersey, Burlington, N.J., 1765
10. Smith, History of Virginia (no date given)
11. Journal of Major Rogers in America, 1765
12. Morgan, Institution of Medical Schools in America, 1765
13. Pownall, On the Colonies, 1768
14. Lettres d'un Fermier de Pennsylvanie aux Habitans de l'Amerique Septentrionale, 1768 [Translation of John Dickinson, *Letters from a Farmer in Pennsylvania to the Inhabitants of the British Colonies*, 1768.]
15. Charter Laws and Catalogue of the Library Company of Philadelphia, 1757
16. Hutchinson, *History of the Massachusetts Bay Colony*, Boston, 1764
17. De la Population de l'Amerique, Amsterdam, 1767 (Author unknown)
18. Tennant, *On the epidemical diseases of Virginia*, 1742, a tract.
19. Votes and Proceedings of Pennsylvania, 1682–1752, 3 vols.; 1768, 1 vol.
20. An Historical Review of the Government and Laws of Pennsylvania, 1759

21. Washington's Journal sent to the Commandant of the Forces on the Ohio, with a map of the Country as far as the Mississippi; Williamsburg, 1754
22. Mark Catesby, Natural History of Carolina (Fr. and Eng.), finely coloured by himself, 1731
23. A Volume of above Three Hundred dried Plants, produced in North and South Carolina, collected, dried and coloured from the Life, in 1767, by William Young, jun.; 2 vols. [Priced at £3.10.0]
24. Storck's History of East Florida, 1769
25. Transactions of the American Philosophical Society, Vol. I, 1771. [A second volume was not issued until 1786]

VI. War and Peace

As a Quaker true to the principles of his religion, Dr. Fothergill could not condone strife between nations. As a resident of the British capital, however, he could not ignore what was happening in the rest of the world. He followed the struggles of the War of the Austrian Succession, and the lesser wars it bred, with apprehension. The possibility that shifts in the balance of power among nations might injure England made him fearful for her future. Toward France, England's chief rival in commerce and colonization, he developed an overmastering antipathy. As early as 1743, the year in which the London Yearly Meeting of the Society of Friends appointed him correspondent to the Philadelphia Yearly Meeting, France had become in his prejudiced view "a frothy, vainglorious, bullying nation." When in 1748 prospects of a European peace were circulated, he became aware of his own ambivalence. He feared a premature peace. Writing to his Quaker friend, Israel Pemberton of Philadelphia, he confessed, "for my own part I dread it as an Englishman, whilst as a Christian I sincerely wish another sword might never be drawn." England, if disarmed, might become "an easy prey" to attack. On the other hand, "by still pursuing the war with vigor, we may yet hope for a solid peace." The patriot and the Quaker were at variance within him.

In the 1750's Philadelphia Quakers, deeply troubled by governmental problems, sought Dr. Fothergill's advice. William Penn's colony was no longer the peaceable kingdom of its founder's idealistic conception. Thomas Penn, his father's successor, an absentee Proprietor who preferred London to Philadelphia, was a worldly man distrusted by the provincial Quakers. Indian raids upon defenseless settlers on Pennsylvania's borders led in 1755 to a Militia Act, which obligated all freemen aged twenty-one or older, Quakers excepted, to volunteer for service, form companies, elect officers, and hold military drill. At the same time, the assemblymen were considering a bill to raise £55,000 for defense. Thomas Penn, accused of evading his financial obligations as hereditary Proprietor of Pennsylvania by accepting exemption from taxation on his vast proprietary tracts, announced his contribution of £5000 for defense of Pennsylvania's frontier, and thereupon the Assembly voted the appropriation of £55,000. Work was started on the first of a chain of forts constructed and manned for protection of colonists hitherto defenseless on the borderlands of Pennsylvania.

Frequent complaints had made it obvious that a Quaker-controlled Assembly had not been prepared to cope with problems such as this. Averse by religious principle to bearing arms, reluctant to vote funds "for the King's Use" — being well aware of the sinister significance of this euphemism — strict Quakers had reached an untenable position. Dr. Fothergill frankly told his correspondent Israel Pemberton that the only solution to their predicament was for Quakers to resign their seats in the governmental Assembly and refuse to stand for re-election until conditions were stabilized. He was now willing to acknowledge that James Logan had been right in 1741 when, after forty years of personal participation in the colony's administration, he advised all Friends "who for conscience-sake cannot join in any law for self-defence [to] decline standing candidates at the ensuing election for representatives." By early November 1756, Benjamin Franklin was able to assure Peter Collinson of London that "Quakers have now pretty generally declined their seats in Assembly, very few remaining."

Henceforward, Dr. Fothergill was constantly reminding politically ambitious Pennsylvania Quakers that "your kingdom is not of this world." Release from political responsibilities would allow them to turn their energies into philanthropic channels. In such work he knew them to be singularly effective, notably in their management of the Pennsylvania Hospital, the first institution established in the American Colonies to offer properly organized medical care to the sick.

Philadelphia was indeed being transformed by increase in the city's population and by commercial prosperity. By 1750, Quakers constituted only 25 per cent of the city's inhabitants. Presbyterians, many of them Scots or Scotch-Irish, were becoming Philadelphia's foremost denomination, rivaling the Quakers in business and political success. The Church of England, under skilled leadership, with congregations made up of people of wealth and social prestige, was definitely the church of the gentry. Between 1740 and 1760, it has been estimated that Philadelphia's population mounted from 13,000 to 22,000 and by 1776 was pushing toward 40,000. The most astonishing phenomenon had been German immigration: thousands of displaced persons fleeing from religious persecution in their homelands — Moravians, Mennonites, Lutherans, Schwenkfelders — crossed the sea to take refuge in William Penn's haven of religious liberty.

It was no wonder that this heterogeneous colony developed serious problems. Dr. Fothergill's letters written during the restless decade 1755 to 1765 abound with references to a series of conflicts precipitated by the colony's rapid growth, development, and change. Indian outrages still persisted; dangers facing the colony were far beyond control by religious idealism. Sir William Johnson, Commissioner to the Six Nations and their allies, chose George Croghan, a well-known trader, and Conrad Weiser, called "the Provincial interpreter," to act as his deputies in dealing with the Delawares of Pennsylvania. Conrad Weiser, with his almost incredible familiarity with Indian dialects, became a prominent figure, trusted by all, in a series of meetings called Treaties, hopefully arranged to bring order out of discord. Scribes recorded the proceedings of these Indian Treaties, and each treaty transcript was inspected by one of the Indian agents and also by a member of the Governor's party. Franklin had these documents promptly printed at his press and dispatched as soon as possible to London for inspection by the Proprietaries, members of Parliament, Dr. Fothergill, and other prominent Quakers.

In 1757 the Pennsylvania Assembly, deeply troubled, asked Benjamin Franklin and Isaac Norris, Speaker of the House, to go to England for consultation upon various colonial administrative problems with the Proprietors, Thomas and Richard Penn. Benjamin Franklin accepted the part of Commissioner as a high honor, but Isaac Norris had to be excused because of poor health. Franklin reached London in September and soon afterwards sustained the respiratory ailment which kept him housed for several weeks under Dr. Fothergill's care and resulted in a long and valued friendship.

It was hard for Dr. Fothergill to abandon his eighteenth-century conception of the Indian as a noble savage, but he must have been forced to conclude that the Indians were children of Nature, guided by transient emotions rather than by reason. In any contest for territory which might arise between England and France, it was plain that the Indians, "either through fear or affection," would give allegiance to whichever nation seemed at the time most likely to win success and would be willing to pay a good price for assistance. The French and Indian warfare which beset the middle colonies was soon merged in the larger arenas of the Seven Years War (1756–1763) in which the chief contestants were openly Britain and France. Great Britain's ultimate hard-won

25

victory was glorious, but her war debt was appalling. To Parliament it seemed obvious that the American Colonies owed something more than gratitude to Great Britain for protection during years of desperate struggle. Colonial taxation was the price to be asked. A Stamp Act, placing a tax upon everyday necessities and transactions, was contemplated.

In the flood of publications appearing while the Stamp Act was under discussion, Dr. Fothergill's *Considerations Relative to the North American Colonies* (1765) remains outstanding. Though his little book reveals his romantic persuasion that America was a potential Utopia, it also emphasizes the practical values the Colonies had created for the extension of Britain's resources by their productive power. He registered a plea for Americans, "a free people descended from freeborn Englishmen, for the most part," who like their forebears looked upon oppressive power with "the same spirit of intolerance," and he finally put forward a proposal, far ahead of the thought of his time, for a closer relationship on a different scale, to ensure a more enduring tie with future generations:

If we promote scholarships for Americans in our Universities; give benefits in America to such Americans as have studied here, preferably to others; if the Government permits such youth as come to Europe on account of their studies to come over on the King's ships *gratis*, we shall unite them more firmly. The Americans by mixing with our own youth at the University will diffuse a spirit of inquiry into America and its affairs; they will cement friendships on both sides which will be of more lasting benefit than all the armies Britain can send thither.

In February 1765, Parliament, regardless of protest on both sides of the sea, passed the Stamp Act, designed to raise annually in the colonies £60,000, a sum claimed to be essential for maintaining continued colonial protection by British military forces. Colonial resentment was instantaneous and violent. Riotous outbreaks took place in every trading center of the Colonies, while British merchants predicted that the Stamp Act would ruin Britain's greatest commercial enterprise, her colonial trade. Such argument could not be neglected. In March 1766 Parliament repealed the Stamp Act.

In the excitement which prevailed at this time, the significance of a Declaratory Act passed later on the very same day seems to have been little noticed. This act asserted that Parliament had the right to make "laws binding" to the American Colonies "in all cases whatsoever." In 1767, Charles Townshend, original instigator of this Declaratory Act, took office as Chancellor of the Exchequer. Faced with grave financial responsibilities, he now framed a new revenue bill whereby American colonists would be taxed for importation of everyday necessities — glass, paints, lead, paper, and tea. To the colonists continuation of taxation at the insistence of Parliament still seemed utterly obnoxious. A cry of protest arose: "No taxation without representation!" Resentment developed into a movement for nonimportation of British goods. By the end of 1769 this policy had been adopted by every American colony except New Hampshire, which had not developed a maritime trade. Losses to merchants on both sides of the Atlantic were enormous, yet the American Colonies stood firm upon their resolution. Their industries flourished.

In 1770, Lord North proposed removal of all the Townshend duties except that on importation of tea in the American Colonies, and he also promised that no new taxes should be imposed upon the Colonies. Passage of this bill was unsatisfactory to the Americans, but it led to the end of nonimportation and to the resumption of Anglo-American trade.

Dr. Fothergill had actually proposed in 1769 that a peace conference between British and American political leaders might be the best way to solve the constantly recurring difficulties arising between kingdom and colony, but no such conference materialized. Doubt, uncertainty, distrust continued, and once again in 1774, while Dr. Fothergill was spending the summer in Cheshire, he wrote to James Pemberton urging a similar proposal. News had reached England that "a general Congress" would assemble in Philadelphia in September, to be attended by representatives from each colony. Could not "a few sensible sedate persons" be chosen immediately and sent to London for private consultations with individual members of both Houses of Parliament? Pleas made in person by men of reputation and authority, sent across the sea by the Congress, could not be summarily dismissed.

The only peace conference which Dr. Fothergill was ever able to arrange, however, took place in his own library in Harpur Street during the winter months of 1774–1775. Abnormal tension was moving from the threatening state of cold war into actual preparation for the outbreak of hostilities. Three anxious men, meeting periodically in the seclusion Harpur Street afforded, now attempted to formulate a plan to prevent the disaster of actual conflict. Working with full knowledge of the situation, and with unanimity of purpose, they hoped to find an acceptable basis for reconciliation. These three were Dr. Fothergill, his friend David Barclay, a vigorous Quaker merchant and banker and a man of seasoned judgment, and Benjamin Franklin of Philadelphia, shrewd, experienced statesman who had lived in London for ten years as accredited agent for several of the colonies.

Introduction

Just before the conferences began in Dr. Fothergill's library, Franklin accepted an invitation to play chess with Mistress Anna Howe at her home in Grafton Street. He was well aware of the distinguished service her three brothers had rendered in America during the Seven Years War: George, the eldest, had met with a hero's death at Ticonderoga, and the people of Massachusetts had raised funds to place a memorial tablet in Westminster Abbey to record his gallant deeds; William had risen to the rank of Major-General; Richard, now fourth viscount of his line, was a man of forty-eight at the height of his powers, having been promoted Rear-Admiral in 1770. In Grafton Street, Franklin found their sister a hostess socially at ease and accomplished at the chess board. She possessed, he said, what "is a little unusual in ladies . . . a good deal of mathematical knowledge" to direct her play. Franklin was invited for other evenings of chess. He was soon introduced to her brother, Lord Howe, and as the two men talked together, problems of politics with life-size figures succeeded the problems of pawns, knights, kings, and bishops on the chess-board.

Meantime, short meetings in Harpur Street, efficiently organized to save time for busy men and allow them to formulate decisions speedily, took place late in the afternoon, well before evening engagements. At the first session, Franklin was asked to chart briefly what terms he thought would suffice to reconcile the American colonists. If these terms could be brought to the attention of certain influential British political leaders, it was hoped Parliament might be influenced to grant the concessions necessary to preserve peace. At the next meeting, Franklin produced a list of seventeen points which he considered essential to any study of the situation — a list he thought might be entitled "Hints for Conversations that might probably Produce a Durable Union between Great Britain and the American Colonies." Beginning tactfully with acknowledgment that the tea thrown into Boston Harbor by masquerading "Indians" must be paid for — willingly by himself, he said, if funds were not promptly available elsewhere — he continued that it was not only desirable but necessary that the people of Massachusetts should be allowed to petition the King, stating their objections to a decree which had altered, without previous consultation, their form of government; that the Quebec Act allowing Canada extension of territory should be repealed; that no troops should be allowed to enter and quarter in any colony without consent of its legislature; that all duties from Acts regulating trade should be paid into colonial treasuries for the public good; that the Admiralty Courts should be locally regulated by the system used in England; that judges should be appointed and receive salaries in the colonies where they would hold office during good behavior; that Governors should be recompensed by voluntary grants as heretofore; and that the tax on tea should be abolished. These were the main points of the seventeen which now received discussion. Franklin, it is obvious, welcomed a chance to put on paper the convictions held by the majority of his countrymen, from whom he already knew there could be no eleventh-hour change of opinion to meet the single requirement heard at present everywhere in England — submission.

From early December to mid-March, the triumvirate of peacemakers met again and again in Harpur Street. From the first it was understood that when they had devised a plan considered suitable, a document would be prepared for circulation among certain Cabinet members chosen for their experience, discretion, and influence in Parliament. At Dr. Fothergill's request, David Barclay took upon himself final preparation of Franklin's points, somewhat revised for presentation, and now bearing a hopeful title, "A Plan Which 'Tis Believed Would Produce A Permanent Union Between Great Britain and Her Colonies." This "Plan" was duly presented to Dr. Fothergill's friend and patient, Lord Dartmouth, Secretary of State for the American colonies. It was also inspected by Barclay's friend, Lord Hyde, a highly respected elder statesman of firm principles, now Chancellor of the Duchy of Lancaster, who many years earlier had proposed and carried peace plans to the Continent during the War of the Austrian Succession. Lord Howe, taken informally into confidence after Franklin's chess games with his sister in Grafton Street engaged in consultation upon the project with Lord Hyde. It was known that through the influence of Lord Dartmouth, the document would certainly reach Lord North, the Prime Minister, although quite unofficially at this preliminary stage of proceedings.

After a period of study by their lordships, the document was sent back to the peacemakers of Harpur Street. The "Plan" was rejected. Some of its terms were indeed marked *Agreed*. Terms of the Declaratory Act (a discreet reference to the obnoxious tax on tea) would be reconsidered. The majority of the terms were, however, too hard to accept, or too high a price to pay for peace with the recalcitrant colonists.

Final rejection of Franklin's "Plan" occurred apparently before mid-March of 1775. He took ship at Portsmouth, accompanied by his grandson Temple Franklin, and reached Philadelphia on the evening of May 5, to learn, without surprise, that the long-dreaded war was actually under way.

Certain letters Dr. Fothergill wrote during this period reveal his increasing emotional reaction to situations in which his personal efforts failed to achieve results. A letter written in 1774 to Lieutenant-Colonel Ironside of the Bengal Army in Calcutta is filled with denunciation of British colonial policy, particularly in Massachusetts, and dread of its results. In scattered pages of an incomplete letter, probably sent in 1777 to Benjamin Franklin at the start of his diplomatic mission in Paris, Dr. Fothergill pours forth the vials of very un-Quakerish wrath upon "the one man in the kingdom . . . born for its destruction" — unnamed and unjustifiably condemned, since the causes of this conflict were varied and ran deep. The Quaker and the patriot were still at variance with one another, the peacemaker overwhelmed by catastrophe.

VII. The Society of Friends; Quaker Meetings

Because Dr. Fothergill came to be active and prominent as a member of the Society of Friends, a brief summary of its organization as it was in his time may be helpful. Quaker meetings for worship were held normally twice on first-day (Sunday) and also on a weekday morning. The local meeting was often referred to as a "particular meeting." In connection with each particular meeting, or group of such meetings, there was normally a meeting for church affairs known as a preparative meeting — Wensleydale Preparative Meeting comprised the local meetings of Countersett, Bainbridge, and Hawes. The preparative meeting was so called because it existed to prepare business for the monthly meeting, which was and is the principal administrative unit: it might be equated with an eighteenth century archdeaconry or with a rural deanery today. The monthly meeting was responsible for all matters of membership and discipline (as we have seen in the case of Alexander Fothergill), for finance and property, and for the regular answering of the queries, an exercise in corporate and personal self-examination. Monthly meetings were grouped in turn into quarterly meetings which were normally coextensive with a county or two counties. Quarterly meetings were in turn subordinate to the Yearly Meeting for the whole country.

This Yearly Meeting, held in London, usually started late in May and often extended into June. It was an important assemblage, attended by representatives from all over the country who during its sessions dealt with nation-wide problems of concern to the Society of Friends. In 1749, 1764, and 1779 Dr. Fothergill was appointed its Clerk, and in 1743 he was appointed its correspondent to Philadelphia Yearly Meeting. From the membership of London Yearly Meeting committees were chosen to take care of special problems. The principal committee, called the Meeting for Sufferings, was formed early in the history of the Society while Quakers were undergoing harsh persecution. When this unfortunate situation had changed, various opportunities to give relief within the Society or to the nation arose and the Meeting for Sufferings came to have larger scope. Its members, carefully chosen because of ability and experience, became the Executive Committee of London Yearly Meeting, allotting funds for many worthy causes. In the eighteenth century, the Meeting for Sufferings continued the work of the Kendal Fund, created in the seventeenth century by northern Friends to support Friends traveling in the ministry throughout Great Britain, to Holland, and especially to the American Colonies. In times of hardship or necessity, grants were made to individuals or to causes needing assistance. Improvement of Quaker education, which Dr. Fothergill fostered from an early period, was a project of utmost concern to this committee. The successful founding and operation of Ackworth School served as an incentive for the establishment of other Quaker boarding schools which flourish today throughout England. To the relief of suffering wherever it arises in the modern world from unexpected disasters, London's Meeting for Sufferings is today as responsive as the American Friends Service Committee, with which it shares deep personal concern for human welfare.

VIII. Foundation of Ackworth School

Dr. Fothergill's long campaign for the improvement of educational opportunities for Quaker children, particularly "for those whose parents are not in affluence," bore fruit at last in the foundation of a country boarding school for girls as well as boys. In 1777, he heard that some institutional buildings at Ackworth in his home county of Yorkshire would soon be put up for sale. London's Foundling Hospital had vacated this outpost of theirs because government support had been withdrawn. When Dr. Fothergill inspected the property, he was delighted to find commodious, dignified Georgian buildings, constructed from native stone, set in a wide expanse of green lawns. It gratified him to learn that the place had an adequate water supply installed under supervision of John Smeaton, the Quaker engineer famed for the construction of Eddystone Lighthouse on a reef outside Plymouth Harbor. This Yorkshire estate provided an ideal environment for growing children, he decided.

Because prompt action to acquire this property was necessary, and London Yearly Meeting would not be in session for months to vote money for the project, Dr. Fothergill approached David Barclay and other well-to-do Friends in order to place an option on the property. With such support, he could offer a purchase price of £7000. Since the original cost of land, buildings, and equipment had been three times as great a sum, this offer, if accepted, would be a bargain for the Society. In December 1777, a formal offer of this amount was made, and in the early spring of 1778, was accepted by the Governors of the Foundling Hospital.

In July 1779, while workmen were busy remodeling the interior, Dr. Fothergill and his sister came from their summer home, Lea Hall, to inspect the preparations. That autumn, Ackworth School received its first pupils, on October 18, 1779. Yearly Meeting entrusted government of the school to a General Meeting and management to two committees of twenty members each. The London Committee dealt mainly with financial matters and the admission of children; the Country Committee was responsible for the organization and running of the School. Ackworth was established on the principle that teachers and children together constituted "the family," thus helping to maintain a well-conducted combination of home and school. In October 1780, when Dr. Fothergill came again from Lea Hall, in company with his sister Ann, to attend a general meeting at the school, it had a full enrollment — 180 boys and 120 girls.

Ackworth School, now in the advancing years of its second century of successful operation, has a sister institution in the United States: Westtown School, not far from Philadelphia, was founded in 1794 by Quakers of Pennsylvania, New Jersey, and Delaware, who, with some modifications, took Ackworth School as their model. Both schools today have adapted their programs to twentieth century requirements and prepare their students for continued education in college.

IX. Last Days

Good weather seems to have favored Dr. Fothergill and his sister Ann on their autumn journey homeward to London in 1780, in the doctor's comfortable coach with his man Joseph skillfully directing the span of horses over roads that required careful driving. It took five days apparently to cover the more than two hundred miles, with a visit in Leeds to their favorite niece, Sally, now happily married to Dr. William Hird, to whom Dr. Fothergill thought at times he might turn over his practice.

Ever since Dr. John's serious illness late in 1778, which had confined him to bed for two or three weeks, his friends had noticed with concern his increasing frailty. He tired easily, but refused to give up his many activities. In June 1779, he had acted as clerk at London Yearly Meeting. For some months that same year he was actively engaged in correspondence with the Rev. Henry Zouch regarding reform measures in the counties of England, in which Yorkshire had taken the lead. In the late autumn of 1780, Dr. Fothergill was strongly advocating establishment of a system of public baths in London. He found his usual pleasure in corresponding with friends on subjects of public interest. On October 26, 1780, he wrote a spirited letter to Benjamin Franklin, then in Paris on an important diplomatic mission for his country. His last public appearance was made December 11, when he went to a meeting of the Medical Society (of Physicians). The next day symptoms of the urinary obstruction from which he had suffered severely two years earlier recurred and put him to bed. Again Percival Pott took charge, in consultation with Dr. Watson, Dr. Warren, and Dr. Reynolds. No remedy or skill of medical art then known could cure him or relieve his suffering, though he was given sedation. His friends David Barclay and Dr. Lettsom stayed with him at times to give him the comfort of their presence. On December 26, 1780, he died, mourned by all London. He was buried in the Friends' burial ground in Winchmore Hill, ten miles outside London, in a quiet, peaceful country setting such as he loved. More than seventy coaches and carriages of grieving Friends followed the hearse carrying him to his grave. His sister Ann soon thereafter left their home in Harpur Street for a small house, 68 Great Russell Street, where she outlived her brother by twenty-two years.

REFERENCES

The fullest modern account of Dr. Fothergill's career is the well documented work by R. Hingston Fox, M.D., *Dr. John Fothergill and His Friends: Chapters in Eighteenth Century Life* (London: Macmillan, 1919); the principal (and excellent) contemporary source is Dr. John Coakley Lettsom's three-volume compilation, *The Works of John Fothergill, M.D., with Some Account of His Life* (London: Dilly, 1783–84). Lettsom makes use of *An Affectionate Tribute to the Memory of the Late Dr. John Fothergill* (privately printed, 1781), by Dr. William Hird, Dr. Fothergill's nephew by marriage; of *Memoirs of the Life and a View of the Character of the Late Dr. John Fothergill* (1782), by Dr. Gilbert Thompson, a cousin of Fothergill's; and of material from many other associates. Lettsom's sources are supplemented by *A Sketch of the Life of John Fothergill, M.D., F.R.S.* (London: Harris, 1879), by James Hack Tuke, written for the centenary of Ackworth School. Tuke uses material from family archives, including manuscript records (1793) of John Fothergill of York. (*A Complete Collection of the Medical and Philosophical Works of John Fothergill, M.D. . . . with an account of his Life*, put together by John Elliot, M.D., London, 1781, is neither complete nor accurate.)
The direct quotation above from Dr. Withering comes from his *Account of the*

Introduction

Scarlet Fever and the Sore Throat (1793), quoted by Fox, p. 54. Fanny Burney is quoted from *The Early Diaries of Frances Burney, 1768–1778*, edited by Annie R. Ellis, in two volumes (London: Bell, 1907). The recommendation from Lord North to King George III and the King's reply are from *The Correspondence of King George the Third, from 1760 to December 1783*, 6 vols. (London: Macmillan, 1927–28), edited by John William Fortescue. The letters to Humphry Marshall (not included in this edition) are quoted from William Darlington, *Memorials of John Bartram and Humphry Marshall* (Philadelphia, 1849; facsimile reprint with introduction by Joseph Ewan, New York: Hafner, 1967). Sir Joseph Banks is quoted in Lettsom's memoir (*Works*, III); and Franklin on Mistress Howe comes from Franklin's account of the negotiations of 1774–75.

I
1735-1741

I am now thinking of spending the ensuing months in London, in one of the best shops there, or in one of the Hospitals, and am now only waiting for thy permission and assistance. . . . My stock is about a Guinea; and if thou thinks this agreeable and hast freedom in thy own mind, may order what thou pleases further.

To John Fothergill, Senior, 23.4.1735, O.S.

To John Fothergill, Sr., York, 23 June 1735

Edinburgh, 23.4.1735

Dear Father,

I hoped thou would get my last, ere thou left London.[1] I wished then I could have given a more certain account of what I should do; since then, about a week since, I had a letter from J.P.[2]: Informing me that the shop was let to another. I then thought I was at liberty to engage in my summer's work here, but was not permitted. I am now thinking of spending the three ensuing months at London, either in one of the best shops[3] there, or in one of the Hospitals, and am now only waiting for thy permission and assistance. I have nothing to urge for this speedy removal but a sort of an assurance of its being the pleasure of the same power I have been able to wait upon, upon some occasions. I had no thoughts of it, till one day last week, it darted with an unusual force into my mind. My Landlord[4] was then from home; when he returned, I acquainted him, and he thought it the most likely.

My Stock is about a Guinea,[5] and if thou thinks this agreeable and hast freedom in thy own mind, may order what thou pleases further. My kind Landlord will let me have what thou thinks necessary. I propose to go by sea. Here are good vessels go from here to London in about 6 or 8 days. My passage, I suppose, will cost about a Guinea. What I shall want when I come there I don't know. As I expect to return hither, I don't think of taking many books with me but leave them here. I propose when I get to London either to attend on Sil. Bevan's shop[6] or get to be an assistant in one of the Hospitals; but can't determine until I come there; but don't doubt but, as I have thus far been assisted, a watchful attendance upon the same hand will be my surest guide.

I dare hardly wish that thou should defer thy intended visit to this place till so far in the year as the 8th month, but if it would not be inconvenient, thou knows how grateful it would be to me. Our College sits down about the 16th of the 8th month,[7] so that I shall have near 3 months to spend. I hope this will meet thee at York and should be pleased to hear from thee from thence; here's a good vessel, and a person of good credit, with whom I am acquainted, designs to sail from Leith the next week. I should choose to go in it, but leave to thee to determine. I know my poor Mother[8] will be uneasy and very solicitous for my safety; gratitude obliges me to take notice and often remember her concern for my welfare. I know she desires my welfare every way, and is fearful lest either body or mind should suffer; I beg she'll not be uneasy, but hope, as we earnestly wish, to do nothing but in the will of the divine dispenser, these cares will not be in vain but will obtain a happy conclusion.

All here through mercy are pretty well; old William Miller[9] was with us last night and kindly remembered his love to thee, as likewise George (who, we expect, will be married ere long to Widow Bunting). My Landlord and Landlady desire their dear love to thee; William Miller, Jr. and his wife also. Give my dear love to tender Mother, Brother Alex, his wife and Friends that ask for me.

I am, in the nearest love,
thy very affectionate son
John Fothergill, Jr.

Ms. autograph letter, Fothergill family papers, Mr. Edward Fothergill, Edinburgh.

1. The elder John Fothergill (1675–1744/5) had been a representative of Yorkshire Quarterly Meeting at London Yearly Meeting of the Society of Friends, held between 26 May and 4 June. — Meeting Book for 1735, LSFL. The next session of Yorkshire Quarterly Meeting was scheduled to assemble in York late in June. This letter from John Fothergill, Jr., concerning his plans for the summer before his last term at the University, is the only surviving letter written by him in 1735.

2. Not identified.

3. Apothecary's shop.

4. Letters sent to John Fothergill, Jr., while in Scotland are addressed to the care of Thomas Areskine, Brewer, Edinburgh, undoubtedly his landlord.

5. British currency was worth at least eight to ten times as much as it is at present. — Bernhard Knollenberg, *Origin of the American Revolution, 1759–1766* (New York: Macmillan, 1960), 276.

6. Silvanus Bevan, a Welsh Quaker, established an apothecary's shop in London about 1715. He had many scientific interests and in 1725 was elected a Fellow of the Royal Society. He later admitted to partnership his younger brother Timothy, who is said to have studied "the art and mystery" of his trade in Leyden. Their shop was

in Plough Lane, off Lombard Street. — Arthur Raistrick, *Quakers in Science and Industry* (London: Bannisdale, 1950), 281–285, 289.

7. October 16, 1735.

8. That is, his stepmother, formerly Elizabeth Buck of Netherdale, "a woman of suitable age and deportment" who endeared herself to her stepchildren. — *Fothergill Genealogy,* below; R. Hingston Fox, *Dr. John Fothergill and His Friends: Chapters in Eighteenth Century Life* (London: Macmillan, 1919), 9.

9. The Millers were a Quaker family of gardeners and horticulturists. Old William (b. 1655) had charge of the garden at Holyrood Abbey for many years. George, his eldest son (b. 1682), worked for a time at Holyrood and later as gardener on the estate of the Duke of Hamilton. William, Jr. (1684–1757), rented the garden at Holyrood and carried on the business of a seedsman and nurseryman there. He was succeeded by his son, the third William, as gardener and nurseryman. — Raistrick, 244.

To Joseph Fothergill, Warrington, Lancashire, 8 June 1737

London, 8.4.1737

Dear Brother,[1]

Amidst a general hurry of business, in which I understand thou art engaged, steal a moment to think of thy absent Brother [2] who, secluded from the busy scenes of life is immured in his closet; thinks that the whole course of our time should not always be a continued hurry, but intermixed with seasons wherein we may take breath and consider what can really be the motive of such assiduity; what it is that can enable us with ease, nay with pleasure, to pursue so many schemes which we every day form and somewhere of every day fruitlessly vanish? Pardon me awhile in that unexpected thought — for such it really is. I hope to gain thy excuse for it!

If thou imagines that I would wish to see mankind proselyted to my way of thinking, thou wilt readily observe thy mistake. It is not any splenetic disorder that frowns upon the busy world excited by envy because I am not of their number. I confess my prospect might occasion such a gloom, was my mind as much cramped as my eye is confined by my neighbouring fabrics. (I am not in a garret, though these are generally esteemed the proper mansions of the Poorer Sons of Apollo, the patron of physick as well as poetry). Through the mercy of heaven, my mind often acquiesces with the dispensations of providence. I am really [happy] when I compare myself with the inhabitants of an hospital. It is not entirely vanity to say that I am sometimes not disposed to

39

change with princes, if my mind must change as well as external circumstances.

But it is not always so. I confess sometimes that I could not look upon an overgrown Doctor, wealthy at the expense of his fellow-citizens' lives, lolling in his chariot, without some envious emotion, and tacitly asking myself, if such a state would not mightily become me? The thought was pleasing, though vain. And it generally happens, through the goodness of my divine guard, that this vanity is quickly mortified; and the empty thing, from believing itself capable of becoming to advantage so much magnificence, dares scarcely lift up its head, being out-stripped in its first attack. My leisure gives me room to reflect on my behaviour. I confess that I am generally charitable enough to myself to censure easily. This, however, nips vanity in the bud, and keeps me within tolerable bounds. I don't say that thou ever had any ambitious visions; I dare not assert the contrary, but methinks we are something related in this, as well as otherwise. Suppose we should forever banish from our minds any hope of becoming conspicuous in the world, would this make us discharge our duty with less vigour? If it would, depend upon it, we are on a wrong footing, and it is really worth our while to consider to what purpose or end our ensigns are levelled. I am hindered from saying what I should say from want of time. I hear thy father [3] below waiting for me. I am ashamed to send it so abrupt, but if thou can fathom nothing else from it, let it evince that I think of thee and Sister, that I love you affectionately, and am with sincere tenderness

Your loving Brother,
J. Fothergill

My dear love to Brother Samuel of whose welfare and prosperity I am glad to hear by several friends, and when he is at leisure shall be pleased with a few lines from him. Remember me to S. Croudson. [4]

Ms. autograph letter, Port. 22/81, LSFL.

1. Joseph Fothergill (1713–1761), who had married Hannah Kelsall in 1735, was living and working in Warrington.

2. Dr. Fothergill was "walking the wards" at St. Thomas' Hospital, apparently living near by in lodgings, and very probably attending Gracechurch Street Meeting.

3. Joseph's father-in-law (—— Kelsall). His own father did not return until the following summer from his second religious visit to the American colonies.

4. A well-known Quaker woman preacher whose steadying influence on Samuel was welcomed by his family.

To Dr. Charles Alston, University of Edinburgh, 13 October 1737

Gracechurch Street, London 13.8.1737

Esteemed Doctor,[1]

The several testimonies of thy respect which I received whilst I was under thy instruction, make me believe that a tender of my assistance will be accepted as a mark of real gratitude; at least if it be presuming too far, it was only a desire to acknowledge the favours received, which was the motive and therefore I hope excusable.

I have sent in a Box of Professor Monro's,[2] a small quantity of a root which was lately imported, and which I imagine is going to be very much in vogue here. I can give but a very imperfect account of it, but a printed relation of its virtues etc., I hear, is going to be made public. It at present gets the name of Rattlesnake root, or Seneca Snakeroot.[3] It is used in some countries, and I suppose in those which lie along the Senegal (according to its name), as an antidote to the poison of some snakes. In those places, but more especially in the Spanish West Indies, peripneumonias are often very fatal to the blacks. A gentleman observing that those who were bit by the snake, and those who were seized with the peripneumony had several symptoms in common — it induced him to exhibit the same remedy in both disorders. The experiment proved successful, and saved the lives of multitudes of the poor objects (as the report is); 'tis now brought hither, what fate it may meet with, I know not. The root has a peculiar taste. I think as if the pyrethrum [4] and some neutral salt were combined and wrapped up in some mucilage! Its appearance very much resembles a piece of an intestine separated from the mesentery, and a little twisted. If the account is published, I shall endeavour to procure a little more of the root, and send it along with it. I likewise put up a drop or two of pure native *Sang. Draconis.*[5] I had it by me, and sent it as thinking it was not an improper specimen.

I shall always be glad to serve thee in anything of this nature, and should be extremely pleased could I merit thy correspondence. I also enclosed an account of some experiments made upon the human Stone, occasioned by the gentleman being relieved by a *Lithontriptic,*[6] which

41

of late has been made use of here. I design to make my business to enquire, and if it be acceptable, thou may command the account from thy

Obliged Friend

J. Fothergill

Please to direct for me at Robert Bell's in Gracechurch Street, London

Ms. autograph letter, Alston Collection, UEL.

1. Charles Alston (1683–1760) held the chair of Botany and Materia Medica, Edinburgh, for almost fifty years.

2. Alexander Monro (1697–1767), was Professor of Anatomy at Edinburgh, 1726–1760.

3. Seneca snakeroot, *Polygala senega*, indigenous to North America, was used as a remedy for snake bite by the Seneca Indians of New York. The resemblance of its long twisting root to a snake may have suggested the name as well as its value to the primitive medicine men who believed in the "doctrine of signatures." — Eric Stone, *Medicine among the American Indians* (New York: Hoeber, 1932), 31, 62, 69, 70.

4. *Anacyclus pyrethrum*, also called pellitory of Spain, having a pungent root (*radix pyrethri*) used medically.

5. Dragon's blood, a brilliant red gum or astringent resin exuding from certain tropical trees such as *Dracaena draco*.

6. A medicine supposed to break up accretions of stone in the bladder. The particular medicine mentioned here, a "discovery" by Joanna Stephens, is described in the next letter.

To Dr. Charles Alston, University of Edinburgh, 6 September 1738

Gracechurch Street, London 6.7.1738

Dear Doctor,

[*Short passage omitted.*] I yesterday returned from a journey I made into the North, having seen Scarborough [1] and some other places that I was desirous of seeing before I sit down to practice.

The Spaw there is entirely recovered, and affords a quality nothing inferior to former years; and according to experiments, and the account of intelligent persons who have attended several years, its virtues are in no way impaired. I was very much pleased on my return to meet with thy letter, acceptable on more accounts than I now have leisure to mention.

I shall await with impatience to see thy papers which I hope will not be refused to the public. I have now in my hands a short sketch of an ingenious person's sentiments on the same subject. I have not opportunity now to transcribe it (the bearer telling me he leaves town this evening), but I shall not omit sending it along with the Camerarius *Epistola de Sexu* [2] . . . if I can meet with it, by the first ship for Leith. The best sort of Labdanum [3] will, I am afraid, scarcely be met with, the 2nd and 3d sort which J. Miller [4] mentions are common. I have inquired already at several druggists' shops but find none. I accidentally mistook this morning a substance under the title of Labdan Liquid. No one in the shop could inform me what it was, whether it was imported so, or [if] it was strained. I looked upon it as a curiosity, and have sent a specimen, along with two small phials of *Bals. Gileadensi*,[5] the best I could find at present. I believe that the phial marked T.W. will prove the better of the two. My usual way of trying them is to let fall a drop upon a glass of water, and that which spreads the soonest, provided the scent, taste and colouring agree with the quick dispersion, to me it seems to discover something more than the different degrees of consistency, since 'tis a volatile, active principle that promotes its spreading on the surface of the water, and the more this prevails the more valuable the medicine. But I am only giving my Master an account of what I have learned from him. I disdain all other pretensions.

I look upon it as my duty to inform thee of a project I have lately formed, though I have communicated it to very few, as uncertain whether ever it may take place. I give thee full power to decide against it, if on consideration it may appear either prejudicial to thyself, derogatory in any respect to the credit which thou hast gained here, which I can assure thee without flattery is very considerable, very much superior to my abilities. I have had some thoughts of giving lectures on some parts of medicine, the materia medica will be the principal. The students of medicine here are generally unacquainted with the importance of medicines; the rest will be pretty much according to thy plan, and I shall then have an opportunity of doing justice to at least one of my preceptors. I have got together some of the officinal simples, and am proceeding to collect the rest. I had some thoughts likewise of making remarks on one of the most elegant modern *Pharmacopoeias*,[6] and of contenting myself with exhibiting the simples there mentioned. It will give me frequent opportunity to show my real esteem for the ingenious authors and point out their accuracy in prescription. When leisure prompts, please to favour me with thy sentiments on this scheme. I have some

43

thoughts of spending a few months in Holland this winter; if there be anything I can serve thee in, I shall be glad of the opportunity to show that I am

Thy faithful Pupil
John Fothergill

P.S. The *Lithontriptic* which I formerly mentioned is still upon trial. Several persons have been searched, the stone found, and are now taking medicine. She gives to the quantity of an ounce of soap at a time, disguised with some black powder, as of charcoal, and dissolved in some emolient decoction. She gives also a powder which some suppose is quicklime, exposed a little to the sun to make it less caustic.[7]

Ms. autograph letter, Alston Collection, UEL.

1. Scarborough and Bath were England's favorite watering places in the eighteenth century, possessing mineral springs used medicinally both for drinking and bathing. In 1732 Sarah, Duchess of Marlborough, described Scarborough as crowded, dirty, and disagreeable, but after taking the waters for a week, she admitted that the itching caused by her scurvy had almost stopped. She believed that she might be benefited by a longer stay. — Ms. letter quoted by Louis Kronenburger, *Marlborough's Duchess* (New York: Knopf, 1938), 283–287.

2. Rudolphus Jacobus Camerarius expounded a theory of sexual reproduction in plants in his book, *Epistola de Sexu Plantarum* (1694).

3. Labdanum, more commonly spelled ladanum (not to be confused with laudanum from the opium-containing poppy), was a medicine made from the gum resin exuding from plants of the genus *Cistus* (rock rose).

4. Joseph Miller, *Botanicum officinalis, or, A Compendious Herbal giving an account of all such plants as are now used in the practice of Physick, with their descriptions and virtues* (London, 1722).

5. A fragrant medicinal preparation, often called Balm of Gilead (reminiscent of the Bible verse, Jeremiah 8:22), of resin from *Commiphora* (Balsamodendron) *opobalsamum*, the Mecca myrhhtree.

6. *Pharmacopoeia Collegii Regii Medicorum Edinburgensis* (3d ed., 1735), prepared for publication by thirty physicians, including Dr. Alston and Dr. Andrew Plummer, another of Dr. Fothergill's teachers. This early pharmacopoeia, then considered a standard authority, listed medicines officially approved by the College and gave directions for their preparation, use, and proper dosage.

7. On 9 June 1739, the *London Gazette* announced an Act of Parliament proposing "a Reward of £5000 to Joanna Stephens upon a Discovery made by her, for the use of the Publick of some Medicines for the Cure of the Stone." To meet criticism against this decision, a body of Trustees undertook to investigate the situation. These included the Archbishop of Canterbury, the Lord High Chancellor, the Speaker of the House of Commons, the President of the Royal College of Physicians, and some of the Censors of the College; also William Cheselden, M.D., and other surgeons. Upon questioning, Joanna Stephens revealed that her remedy contained egg shells and snail shells "burnt to blackness," a variety of herbs, a quantity of strong Alicant soap from

Spain, and honey. Lye had been suspected as an ingredient, but was never acknowledged. The medicine was prepared in three forms: a decoction, a powder, and pills, all of which, Joanna insisted, must be used. Though distrusted by some physicians, her medicines were eagerly sought by the public.

The *London Gazette* on 18 March 1739/40, announced that Joanna Stephens had received the reward by decision of the Trustees, after a meeting and examination of her medicines "in the Princes' Chamber, adjoining the House of Lords." Four persons had appeared "on whom the medicines had been tried," with complete cure. All Trustees present had signed the certificate which accompanied the reward, except Dr. Thomas Pellett, President of the Royal College of Physicians, and Dr. Roger Nesbitt, one of the Censors. These two physicians presented separate certificates testifying to the cure of one individual. — *Joanna Stephens, Receipt for the Stone and Gravel, with Proper Observations and Explanations thereon* (London: published by the Trustees, 1739); Stephen Hales, *An Account of Some Experiments and Observations on Mrs. Stephens' Medicines for Dissolving the Stone* (London, 1739); *Pharmacopoeia of the Royal College of Physicians* (London, 1757), evidently reprinting entries from an earlier volume.

To Israel Pemberton, Jr., Philadelphia, 20 October 1738

London, 20.8.1738

Esteemed Friend,

Professions of respect and friendship from one whom I have no reason to expect anything but sincerity are too engaging not to merit the heartiest, the best return I can make. I am pleased that an acquaintance so short, and which I did not suspect would ever have been revived, should be so agreeably commenced, and which I hope on my part to continue as much as I can.[1] I may inform thee that my Father landed safe at Lancaster in 4th month last,[2] since which time I have been in the North to pay him a visit. His health and vigour have been wonderfully preserved. It surprised me to find that two years absence, attended with a great deal of fatigue and exercise of various kinds, has had no farther impression upon him. I met him at the Quarterly Meeting at York, where several things contributed to render the time agreeable to most, and to some a memorable season. As for my part, gratitude to the supreme being for restoring us a Father filled with peace and love, joy for seeing him once more among us, and emotions which could not be restrained upon the occasion affected me in a manner I need not mention; thou knows how to excuse me for dwelling so much on a subject in which I had so considerable a part. I have this day wrote to him and mentioned to him what thou requested.

I know not in what terms to acknowledge thy kind offers of assistance, but at present I have laid aside all thoughts of seeing America. This place seems to be it, where I must fix. I expect not a long series of years anywhere; my constitution forbids it. To discharge the part of a person in some degree useful to society, has of late been my wish, regardless where my sphere of action may be allotted, provided I may be happy as to be in it.

The box for W. Hird [3] shall be taken particular care of; I understand by Dr. Bond that the person who puts them up is an extraordinary Genius, and much employed by several virtuosi here.[4] I hope at one time or other to increase the number of his acquaintance by recommending him to the professor of Botany at Edinburgh,[5] an honest, ingenious, candid man. Whilst I was in the North this summer I called on my Friend W.H.; he still preserves his lust for books, though I hope his edge that way is rather abated. It is possible to read, as well as eat too much, though the consequences of the one are not regarded by the generality of mankind as much as the other. I believe that he knows very well that whatever knowledge [he] may acquire concerning the sublimest truths, will perish whenever the [holder] of that acquisition perishes; and that whenever we are deprived of this infinite variety of objects around us, if we have no acquaintance with some being that will offer itself as an object adequate to the [desire] of a mind disengaged from matter and material objects, his [condition], as well as that of all mankind under the same conditions will be as miserable as it is possible for a created existence to be which is [full] of an insatiable desire, unlimited, yet incapable of uniting with a[nother] adequate to it; our choice having been fixed already upon finite objects; the human mind being created to admire infinity above all.

Perhaps ere this arrives, a young man whom I have a particular re[gard] for, may be landed (his name is J. Hunt) and is coming to visit Friends in America.[6] I need not recommend him to thee. I believe thou will re[adily] discover so much in his conduct and appearance, as will engage thee to esteem and love him. Remember my dear love to him, and let him know that when I wrote this we were all much as he left us, anxious for his welfare and preservation through the difficulties he has to encounter. I must also request thee to do the same piece of service to Elias Bland [7] of whom I am pleased to hear a good account from several hands.

I have had some of Dr. Bond's company.[8] He is an intelligent person and has made considerable advances in the knowledge of his business. He intends I believe to leave England pretty soon; it has not been in my power to do him any considerable service; though I would readily do [so] both on thine and his own account. I have now only to request as thou hast generously begun this epistolary commerce, thou will please to continue it, if thou finds the remittance will any way repay thy trouble.

I am, thy respectful Friend,
J. Fothergill, Jun.

Ms. autograph letter, Gilbert Collection, II, 127, College of Physicians, Philadelphia; a letter difficult to decipher because of deterioration from age. Certain words have been supplied where the ms. was illegible.

1. Israel Pemberton, Jr. (1715–1779), like his grandfather, Phineas, and his father, Israel, Sr. (1688–1754), came in time to be known as "a weighty member" of the Society of Friends. With his brothers he profitably carried on the family export-import business and became one of Philadelphia's foremost citizens. He was prominent in the establishment of the Pennsylvania Hospital and long a member of its Board of Managers. He backed creation of a fire department, a fire insurance company, poor relief, improvement of racial relations with Indian tribes, and as early as 1739 became a member of the Library Company of Philadelphia, helping in 1742 to revise its charter. He ordered quantities of outstanding Quaker books, and sold them throughout the Colonies. Seven children were born to him and his first wife, Sarah Kirkbride. Greatly bereft by her death, he married in 1747 a widowed Quakeress, Mary Stansbury Jordan. After his father's retirement from politics, Israel, Jr., was elected to the Pennsylvania Assembly in 1751. He served as clerk of Philadelphia Yearly Meeting for some fifteen years and as clerk for the Quaker schools from 1743 until his death. His first of numerous visits to England was made in 1735. — Theodore Thayer, *Israel Pemberton, King of the Quakers* (Philadelphia: Historical Society of Pennsylvania, 1943).

2. John Fothergill, Sr., returned from his third and last visit to the American Colonies in June 1738.

3. William Hird of Woodhouse lived in the country near Bradford, Yorkshire. Hirds, Hustlers, Bartletts, and Horners were all Quaker families, closely connected by intermarriage. A short genealogical record of the Hird family is available in London in the Library of the Society of Friends.

4. John Bartram. See F. to Dr. Charles Alston, 11 November 1738.

5. Dr. Charles Alston.

6. John Hunt of London, an able Quaker merchant, was frequently in Philadelphia and became prominent in the tobacco trade which flourished between the American Colonies and England.

7. An English Quaker, engaged in Anglo-American trade as a factor, or commission merchant. — Frederick B. Tolles, *Meeting House and Counting House: The Quaker Merchants of Colonial Pennsylvania, 1682–1763* (Chapel Hill: University of North Carolina Press, 1948), 60.

8. Thomas Bond (1712–1784) is the first physician from the American Colonies whom Dr. Fothergill mentions. Born of Quaker parentage in Calvert County, Maryland, he served a medical apprenticeship in Annapolis, and then spent a year abroad visiting medical centers. Later, his younger brother Phineas (1718–1773) went abroad and received a medical degree in Rheims. The two brothers formed a partnership in Philadelphia, becoming leaders in their profession and in civic and cultural enterprises. To Thomas Bond belongs much of the credit for the inception of the Pennsylvania Hospital, chartered in 1752. There in 1766 he began a course of clinical lectures for medical students, an innovation ahead of his time, provocative of enthusiasm by all attending. — Records of Births, Friends Meeting, Herring Creek, Maryland; *The Papers of Benjamin Franklin*, ed. Leonard W. Labaree, and others, IV (New Haven: Yale University Press, 1961), 190; Elizabeth H. Thompson in the *Journal of Medical Education*, 23 (1958): 614–624; George W. Corner, Sr., *Two Centuries of Medicine: A History of the School of Medicine, University of Pennsylvania* (Philadelphia: Lippincott, 1965), 24, 25.

To Dr. Charles Alston, University of Edinburgh, 11 November 1738

Gracechurch Street, London 11.9.1738 O.S.

Dear Doctor,

At length after pretty much search, I have got a specimen which I think answers to Miller's description of Labdanum. I could only find another piece of about the same bigness of this which I have sent. Along with it I put up two other specimens of the second and third sort. They seem to be very good of the kind and to contain a pretty deal of the gum. I can't yet meet with Camerarius's *Epistola* etc., nor have I got the tin and iron ores. I have got a friend to write into Cornwall for a piece of the former, and to another part of the country for the other, and expect to have them ready to send down in the spring. I know not how far some experiments on the iron mine (as the ore is usually called in most parts of England), might assist us in forming a just judgment of Chalybeat waters,[1] but it don't look improbable but by combining it with some of those principles, or principles of the same nature as those which are usually combined with iron, into several of the mineral waters of most note, and macerating these in water in various proportion, one might easier become acquainted with any chalybeat waters that should be offered to our view than with any method hitherto in use. It is probable likewise that a better succedaneum might be procured from the *minera ferri* [2] than from some others of its preparations. I was led into thoughts of this kind from some observations I had the opportunity of making this summer at Scarborough. I intend to procure some quantity and satisfy my curiosity by some experiments upon it.

I send also inclosed a copy of a paper which I received not long ago from Philadelphia.[3] The author only gratifies his curiosity by inquiries of this nature as a relaxation from affairs of more consequence, he being till of late pretty much concerned in the Government of that province. He is an ingenious, learned man, and I question not very accurate in his experiments. I should like to know how your sentiments quadrate in this affair. I lately had occasion to write to him, and among other things gave him an account of the Society,[4] and also as much account of the paper thou entertained them with as I could collect from thy letter. I likewise engaged (pardon me if I was too rash) to procure thy thoughts upon his scheme as of one who I would with confidence assure him was a competent judge in matters of this nature. It is intended to be part of a much greater work, which the author is about, principally insisting upon the moral duties of mankind as they may be known from what is discoverable in nature and illustrated by these.[5]

I lately was presented with a very great curiosity from that place, viz., a piece of a root and the top of a plant which they call *Ginseng*, as perfectly agreeing with P. Du Kalde's description of that celebrated vegetable.[6] It is but lately discovered, and in a very small quantity. I hope, however, to procure next summer a specimen or two of the whole plant and root. If I can, thou may depend upon partaking with me of a curious (but not very useful) addition to thy collection. As far as I can discover . . . one might imitate it pretty nicely by a proper proportion of holly bark and liquorice, or the shavings of holly and the latter. I am informed also that they have in Pennsylvania a very celebrated natural botanist [7] who, without any learning but of his mother tongue, viz., English, has acquired a very extensive knowledge of the indigenous plants of those parts of America from autopsy. The *Ginseng* was discovered by him. If a correspondence with such a person would be of any manner of use to thee, please to let me know it, and I'll endeavour to find out some means to begin it.

I must, ere I conclude, request thy opinion of the scheme I mentioned in my last. Some few here to whom I have proposed it are inclinable to think it might answer. However I shall make no hasty steps without thy approbation. The situation I am in with regard to intelligence from several parts of the world is some encouragement to me, having sometimes the opportunity of settling a correspondence with men of judgment and veracity in most places where the English have commerce. I can't do it at once, but I find in time it will not be impossible.[8]

I fancy thou art very intent on thy annual labours. I heartily wish that the encouragement may in any respect be answerable to the address and application with which they are executed. I shall always remember the advantage I reaped from them with gratitude. I shall be pleased to have a few lines from thee when thy leisure will permit.

I am

Thy respectful friend,

J. Fothergill

Ms. autograph letter, Alston Collection, UEL.

1. Chalybeate waters impregnated with iron were recommended at the Spa in Buxton for people easily fatigued and suffering from poor health, a condition often arising from what is now known to be anemia. Drinking these waters, daily outdoor exercise, periods of rest, and a chance to enjoy programs of amusement provided by the Spa often produced an improvement in health.

2. Specimens of an ore high in iron content.

3. Probably a draft of James Logan's account in Latin of his experiments with Indian corn, *Experimenta et meletemata de plantarum generatione*, which was published in Leyden in 1739. James Logan (1674–1751), Quaker, political leader, and jurist, was the outstanding intellectual leader in the colony of Pennsylvania before Franklin inherited that leadership.

4. Professor Alston was almost certainly a member of the society which published five volumes of *Medical Essays and Observations* between 1731 and 1743 and in 1783 became the Royal Society of Edinburgh. Dr. Fothergill had belonged to a students' society founded in 1734 which in 1778 became the Royal Medical Society of Edinburgh. — Fox, 139–141.

5. Undoubtedly Logan's projected treatise on ethics, "The Duties of Man Deduced from Nature," which he never completed. See Frederick B. Tolles, *James Logan and the Culture of Provincial America* (Boston: Little, Brown, 1957).

6. Ginseng, once used medicinally, grows in regions as widely separated as northern China and the eastern United States of America. Both Chinese and American varieties (*Panax ginseng* and *P. quinquefolium*), though distinctive, have aromatic roots with a flavor like licorice. Dr. Fothergill's library catalogue lists a copy of P. du Kalde's *History of China*, 2 vols. (1738).

7. John Bartram (1699–1777), Quaker farmer and gardener living a few miles outside Philadelphia. He had been tutored in Latin, perhaps by James Logan, who lent him botanical books laden with Latin terminology and taught him how to use a microscope. He developed a successful business, sending plants and seeds to England to fill orders from nurserymen and supplying special orders from botanists and from noblemen who wanted American flowers, shrubs, and trees on their estates. Bartram became internationally known to botanists, and in later years was one of Dr. Fothergill's faithful correspondents. — Tolles, *James Logan*, 201–202, 213; Ernest Earnest,

John and William Bartram, Botanists and Explorers (Philadelphia: University of Pennsylvania Press, 1940), 2, 21–33, 68, 101, 102.

8. Pressure of medical work in the hospital, combined with attention to a few private patients, apparently occupied the young doctor so fully that he was unable to write the paper promised and intended as a tribute to the Pharmacopoeia recently prepared by Dr. Alston with the aid of associates in the University of Edinburgh.

To Susanna Fothergill, Warrington, Lancashire, 24 May 1739

London, 3rd Mo., 24th, 1739.

Perhaps this may come to thy hands sooner than brother gets home; if so, it may not be unpleasant to hear that we parted at Oxford on third day last.

I have been much pleased with his conduct, as well as his company, since he came to town; thou may be sure that my affection for him led me to observe him carefully, and I can only say, upon the whole, that I, as well as us all, have fresh occasion to be thankful that Providence has placed you together. I take notice, with pleasure, of an increase in solidity and prudent behaviour, since I last saw him at Warrington; and I doubt not but his affection will engage him to regard whatever thou shalt think he ought to do; for I cannot but believe that his quick and steady progress has been, and yet will be, greatly promoted by thy watchful, affectionate concern for him.[1] Gratitude, dear sister, calls for affection in return, for restoring us a brother, and in part making him what he is. The sensible part of Friends here have unity with him; the rest, who applaud or condemn, as mere fancy leads them, are not to be hearkened to.

J.F.

Excerpt printed by George Crosfield, *Memoirs of the Life and Gospel Labours of Samuel Fothergill* (Liverpool: D. Marples, 1843; New York: Collins, 1844), 75.

1. Samuel, Dr. Fothergill's brother, had recently married the woman preacher, Susanna Croudson, who was much older than he. The Society of Friends was at that time the only religious body "to allow a share in the management of its affairs to the Female Sex . . . we find them in every department . . . They have also their Meetings for Discipline, in which like care is taken of Female Youth and the good Order of their Sex, as is done for the Men of their own." — John Fothergill, M.D. (with the assistance of Samuel Fothergill), *A Brief Account of the People called Quakers, Their Doctrines and their Disciplines* (London, 1773).

To Dr. William Cuming, Dorchester in Dorset, 1740

London [Anno 1740]

[*Translation*]

Having examined several well-fortified cities of Flanders, we traveled through much of Brabant.[1] On the way from Ghent to Brussels, a spacious, splendid city, we passed through a little town called Assche, formerly fortified by a moat and wall, or rather an embankment of earth. This place is well known to the inhabitants of Brabant because Englishmen first got their hops from this locality, and learned there the methods of cultivation, to the great loss of the whole country roundabout, which hitherto was famous for that commodity. From Brussels we went on to Liege, called by the Germans Lüttich, and by the natives themselves Luich. From there, we went to the little town of Spa and to Aachen (Aix la Chapelle), places known all over the world. At the first, I gave special attention to the mineral waters, and at the latter to the hot springs. I drank the waters, and made experiments as best I could without having with me the proper apparatus. We next went to Maastricht, Sylvam Ducis (Bois le Duc),[2] Dordrecht, then to the famous city of Rotterdam, a commercial center, visiting also the city of Delft, the matchless village of The Hague, the cities of Leyden and Haarlem, and the noblest city of them all, Amsterdam. After making a thorough visit, we sailed through the straits commonly known as the Zuyder Zee to a town the Dutch call Worcum in Westfrisia, about twenty miles distant from Leeuwardia, the principal city of that province, a well-kept and well-fortified place.

From there, we traveled to Groningen, making our way through a sandy region, quite uncultivated, until we reached the city of Oldenburgh. Proceeding then through a number of widely separated places, we came finally to Bremen, a free city and a center of wealth. Here they display to travelers, in a crypt under their great Cathedral, some human bodies long preserved after death, hard and firm, dried entirely by natural processes, without use of preservatives of any kind, but merely by the drying anti-putrescent atmosphere of this crypt. The place is not very deep. It is exposed on one side to the wind, and has an exceedingly dry situation, since the whole countryside is sandy. Although there are many other crypts under this same church, and also under many other churches thereabouts, not one has been found which has the same property. We saw twelve such bodies — quite intact, one of which is estimated to be two hundred years old; another probably one hundred and fifty years in age; the rest of various ages and times.[3] All seem perfectly dry, lying there lightly — but so firm that by placing one's hand under the chin, the whole body may be lifted up without the least bending. The inhabitants of Bremen claim that the great quantity of nitre there is the cause of this phenomenon. Nitre is in fact so plentiful in this region that it may be dug up in abundance. Every pound weight of earth in this cavern is said to contain two ounces of the purest nitre.

These paragraphs are from a letter written in Latin by Dr. Fothergill to Dr. Cuming in 1740 and printed in *The Works of John Fothergill, M.D., with Some Account of His Life,* ed. J. C. Lettsom (London: Dilly, 1783–1784), III, pp. xvi–xx, with a translation in a long footnote. The original manuscript can no longer be found. The translation given here has been modernized by the senior editor, closely following Dr. Lettsom's earlier version. For the Latin text, see Appendix I, below.

William Cuming, the son of a prominent Edinburgh merchant, became John Fothergill's friend while both were medical students in the University of Edinburgh. Cuming took a leading part in forming the students' medical society the year before Fothergill entered the medical school. In 1735, Cuming left Edinburgh to continue medical studies on the Continent. In Leyden he attended lectures by Boerhaave and later he went to Rheims, where he took final examinations in Latin, successfully passing all subjects required for the medical degree. In 1739 Dr. Cuming returned to Great Britain, settled in Dorchester, and soon developed an extensive practice. Although urged later to move to London by Dr. Fothergill and others, he could never be induced to exchange residence in the charming town in Dorset for a city practice. In 1752 the University of Edinburgh recognized his merits by bestowing an M.D. *ad eundem* upon him. Soon after, he was elected Fellow by Edinburgh's Royal College of Physicians. — Fox, 125–127.

1. This letter gives the route of the only European journey Dr. Fothergill ever made. In 1740, before setting up his independent practice, he had a few weeks free for a holiday. Some Friends from Gracechurch Meeting went with him. The first city they visited was Ghent.

The young doctor's scientific interests led him to visit the ancient watering-places of Spa and Aachen (Aix-la-Chapelle), established long ago like Bath and Buxton in England by the Romans, and still thronged at this time. Later he paid a visit to Leyden, but apparently made no attempt to see the University's famous medical school, perhaps because it was the summer season. Boerhaave, largely responsible for the reputation the institution held, had died in 1738. The last city visited was Bremen in north Germany.

2. Hertogenbosch, not far from Dordrecht.

3. In the twentieth century, tourists from the United States have been shown these same gruesome anatomical exhibits in the Cathedral crypt, two hundred years after Dr. Fothergill's visit there.

To Dr. Charles Alston, University of Edinburgh, 19 February 1740/1

Gracechurch Street, London 19.12.1740/1

Dear Doctor,

[*Short passage omitted.*] About 2 or 3 weeks ago I gave a little parcel of seeds to Capt. Angus directed for thee. Some are for the Greenhouse, others for the open air, but those are marked. There is a small parcel of the seed of the Cranberry plant from New England; it's a native of bogs and mossy places, and may probably be cultivated in some such-like near Edinburgh. The fruit is much larger than ours, and I think excels them in every respect in that one grand use of furnishing materials for Tarts, so that if the species can be propagated perhaps the *utile* as well as the sweet of curiosity may be reaped.

Don't know whether I have mentioned in any of my former letters that I am obliged to a particular Friend for most of these seeds, as well as for many other favours, but gratitude I think obliges me to name him, and as I have frequently mentioned to him for whom I intended the favours he conferred on me in this way, I believe he would be very well pleased with a few lines from Dr. Alston. He has this morning sent me in a considerable number of seeds of different kinds which I intend to dispatch as soon as I can.

The Gentleman's name is Collinson, very well known amongst the Virtuosi here; he has a good collection of plants in his own garden, and has a settled correspondence with the curious in most parts of the world. By his means several things have appeared in the Royal Society's collections which would otherwise very probably have been lost. A letter addressed to Peter Collinson, Merchant, in Grace Church Street, London will come very safe.[1]

Whilst I was in Holland I had the opportunity of seeing Dr. Gronovius in Leyden.[2] He is very intimate with Dr. Linnaeus,[3] as my Friend Collinson is with both. I did not take it well that Linnaeus had made no mention of the Physick Garden in Edinburgh in his *Fundament. Botan*,[4] though he had taken notice of some that less deserved it.[5] The Gentleman who called upon me by thy orders gave me his own copy of the late edition of the *Collectio Plantarum qua in Hort. Edinb. etc.*[6] This I sent over to Gronovius some months ago; I dare say he'll be glad of it, and if there be a second edition of his book, justice will be done. But I am without a copy for myself or a friend; I'll say no more.

Along with the parcel of seeds which I shall next send, I intend to put a specimen or two of iron and tin ore with a piece of the *Cadmia fornaeum* from Goslar. In melting the copper ore, the back side of the furnace is covered with a strong metaline crust, as is also the front, which is only a thin stone yet capable of bearing a very intense heat. After the metal is in fusion and let out into the hole where it is suffered to harden, the workmen take out the crust from the back which is the *Cadmia fornaeum,* and serves in making brass, though more of this is required than of the *Cadmia fossilis* or *Calamine.* The crust on the forepart is zinc, and seems to differ from the former in that the blast of the bellows and alternate cooling, to which in some degree it is more exposed from the thinness of the stone, have made it more capable of fusion into a *metaline regulus.*

The native vitriol which I sent came out of the famous mines of Goslar.[7] Some of the caverns out of which the ore has been dug some time ago are beautifully covered with vitriolic icicles (if one may be allowed the term) which, by the assistance of the lamps we had with us, looked very pretty. I had got some genuine *Misy,*[8] but being obliged to send it by the way of Hamburgh, and home by sea, the moisture of the ship had dissolved almost all of it, otherwise a specimen should have attended these things.

If it is not using too much freedom, I would request the favour of a specimen of your copper and lead ores, and if it could easily be had, likewise of silver. A gentleman from Leipsic, whom I fell in with at Goslar, requested my assistance in procuring him specimens of some of our ores. I have sent him one little cargo of such as I had, and intend another shall go this spring. He promised me in return some specimens of the minerals of Saxony and some from Hungary, especially the minerals of quicksilver and antimony.

A Merchant who has been in the East Indies informed me the other day that most of the camphor which we have comes from China; that the Chinese buy up the camphor of Borneo etc., to which places they trade, at a very high price, but from 1 lb. of this genuine camphor they are capable of producing near 20 lbs. of the common saleable camphor. Whether they only mixed it, or sublimed it with some production of their own, he could not tell, but assured me the other was fact. I find

55

I have no need to write often. I can be of little help, being dull and insipid as I am prolix; but regard an intention well designed and believe me to be with a great deal of respect

Thy obliged Friend
J. Fothergill

P.S. I returned too late to make any further trial last year about the *Elaterium*,[9] but I hope to have a good opportunity the next season. — I want to know how the Society proceeds, and when we are to see any of its productions. I now hear nothing of what is doing at Edinburgh. — The design I mentioned some time ago seems to be at a very great distance from execution. I have not entirely dropped it, nor have I of late done much about it. Adieu.

Ms. autograph letter, Alston Collection, UEL.

1. Peter Collinson (1694–1769), a prosperous Quaker merchant principally engaged in trade with the American Colonies and the West Indies, was elected to the Royal Society of London in 1728. — See *Some Account of the Late Peter Collinson in a Letter to a Friend* (London, 1769), by Dr. John Fothergill, reprinted in *Works*, ed. Lettsom, II, 333–353.

2. Johannes Fredericus Gronovius (1686–1762) of Leyden, practicing physician and successively Senator, Sheriff, and Burgomaster of Leyden, is chiefly remembered for his close association with Carl Linnaeus (1707–1777) and as a botanical editor. While Linnaeus was at work in Holland, Gronovius helped his Swedish friend to arrange the publication in Leyden of *Systema Naturae* (1735). A short time later, Gronovius received, perhaps through Peter Collinson, an unusual collection of American plants with descriptions sent across the sea by a little-known clerk, John Clayton, of Gloucester County, Virginia. In sorting and classifying this collection, Gronovius was able to bring order out of chaos by using the Linnaean classification, then in its first stage. In 1739 (the year Linnaeus went back to Sweden), Clayton's work, *Flora Virginica*, was published by Gronovius under his own name. A second printing in 1741 and a completely revised edition in 1762 also bore the name of Gronovius, although the manuscript had been extensively corrected with help from well-known botanists in both America and England. Today this botanical classic at last is correctly ascribed to Clayton. — "Selections from the correspondence of Cadwallader Colden with Gronovius," ed. Asa Gray, *American Journal of Science*, 1st ser., 14:85–133 (1843); Brooke Hindle, *The Pursuit of Science in Revolutionary America, 1735–1789* (Chapel Hill: University of North Carolina Press, 1956), 18, 28–30.

3. In tribute to Gronovius, Linnaeus (1707–1777) named a plant *Gronovia*. It was "a creeper which embraces all other plants within reach . . . like . . . the man who has few equals as an embracer and collector of plants." — Knut Hagberg, *Carl Linnaeus*, trans. Alan Blair (London: Jonathan Cape, 1952), 104.

4. *Fundamenta Botanica* (Amsterdam, 1736).

5. The botanical garden of the University of Edinburgh was much extended and improved during Dr. Alston's tenure. — J. Reynolds Green, *A History of Botany in the United Kingdom* (London: Dent, 1914), 187.

6. Charles Alston, *Index Plantarum praecipuae officinalium quae in horto medico Edinburgensi . . . demonstrantur* (Edinburgh, 1740).

7. Evidently Dr. Fothergill had visited Goslar during his continental journey in the summer of 1740.

8. Misy, of which he collected a specimen, is now technically called copiapite, or yellow copperas. It is a silicate of iron.

9. Contemporary pharmacopeias listed *elaterium* as an accepted drug. A precipitate from the juice of the squirting cucumber, it was used as a purgative and emetic. Following directions from an old herb woman, Dr. Fothergill tried to make elaterium but failed. He believed that some secret had been withheld. — Letter to Dr. Alston 22.7.1739, UEL, not included here.

To Israel Pemberton, Jr., Philadelphia, 28 March 1741

London 28.1.1741

Dear Friend, I. Pemberton,

When I received thine of the third month last I little expected I should be so long in answering it. One circumstance which very probably thou may be unacquainted with will stand in my favour, otherwise I might justly acquiesce with the censure of being an ingrate.

Some agreeable company offering at the beginning of last summer, I concluded to make one of the party in a range through Flanders, Holland, and some parts of Germany. I did not so much look at the little reputation which the vulgar generally attribute to a Physician who is travelled, be it ever so little, as the use that I hoped would accrue from establishing an acquaintance with some ingenious people abroad, as well as thinking it one proper step to teach one to judge of other nations without prejudice, and assisting one in the tracing of the history of man with more exactness. I reflected that travellers were apt to characterize persons and things agreeable to the humours they themselves were in while amongst them, bad lodgings, cross landladies, uneasy vehicles and suchlike distasteful occurrences have, I believe, many times diminished beauty and virtue, and in the same proportions have magnified petty failures, peccadillos and painted them as gross enormities; as well as good usage has oft produced the contrary effect. This was a principal motive, and I have the satisfaction of discovering so much as to put me in a better condition of judging of persons and things. Wiser heads need no such help, but a person who is conscious of his defects may plead in defense of extraordinary steps of this kind the necessity he finds himself under to remedy them; and if I mistake not, the kind of Friend I am writing to did not cross the seas and risk his person for the sake of material interest alone; so if I did amiss in this respect, I hope not to be without good company.

We have heard pretty much of late a good deal of talk of some religious stirrings amongst some people in Germany.[1] Some of them have been in your parts (as well as in many others), where I question not but thou hast seen and conversed with them. From the relations I had received, I could not but be a little prejudiced in their favour and was far from being uneasy that a people not bearing our name, should have made such eminent advances in piety and virtue as the reports gave room to hope for. Whilst I was on the continent, I had several opportunities of being with some of them and conversing a little, but soon found they had apprehended more than they knew from experience, and that from their inward senses.[2] I could not but have a weighty sense of the favour of Heaven to our first Friends for ripening them so fully before they were led out to bear their testimony to the world. Another cause of thankfulness likewise occurred from observing the profuseness of compliments to one another and the servile adoration they mutually pay and receive, a conduct unbecoming rational beings, unworthy of honest men and nauseous in the greatest degree to a cautious observer. The Germans, as well as many of their neighbors, are as much slaves of ceremony as is possible. There seems to be no state of independence amongst them. 'Tis not easy to decide whether they exact a slavish obeisance from their inferiors, resent the want of it from their equals, or pay it to their superiors with more unmanliness; however this I think I am sure of, that the early lectures which they give their children on these heads, and the custom of everybody around them, breeds such a servile fear in their minds that they are never able afterwards to get quit of it. It seems to affect them so far as even to prevent them from using their understanding. Custom is their sovereign guide, and if the force of truth ever prevails so far as to make them suspect they may be in the wrong path, and even to persuade them to take some steps in the right one, yet whenever they meet with any opposition, or are likely to draw upon them displeasure of the great, they falter, let go their faith and submit. This made me applaud the fortitude of our early Friends, who showed the mark of a valour not easily to be matched in withstanding the same kind of folly which at the time they appeared prevailed very much here. And

I question whether that generous, open-hearted sincerity, for which the English are noted, had now been alive even so much as it is, had they not been led on to stem this impetuous tide, and persisted in it so firmly as they did. But their degenerate offspring, unacquainted with things of this nature, give up the cause their fathers had gained, and seem to rejoice in nothing more than in the prospect they have of the footsteps of this combat being in a likely way to be erased. All are not of this mind, and it's a shame that any should be, but some such there are. I am afraid I have now tired thee, but I have not yet done. If patience fails, lay it aside. Another minute will finish and perhaps with more pleasure in reading, though [I] am afraid the subject will yet be less agreeable.

My absence prevented me from having thine so soon as otherwise I should; though at my return I had it, and the box and snakes safely delivered. I found myself so embarrassed in several things at my coming home that to think of my absent friends was all I could do; and now and then look in, to see how the fire kept, and when the blaze of Friendship seemed less bright to add fresh fuel by calling to mind the several good qualities and valuable things that had first kindled that flame. This I frequently do, and not without success.

I question not but thou has been long since informed of the removal of our valuable friend Joseph Green and two of his sons.[3] He and his eldest son were two of my companions as far as Hamburg. There they left us, and returned, I am afraid too precipitately, being seized with a violent fever the day after their coming home, and both died the eleventh day after. About six weeks after, the youngest son, a hopeful manly child was seized at school, brought home and died in two days of a fever, though not of the same kind. The night he died, the only surviving son was also taken ill, but narrowly escaped through a dangerous fever to comfort his distressed mother. He was scarce got down stairs, when Nanny Green, the only daughter, a fine young woman of 18, was affected and narrowly escaped with her life. 'Tis impossible to relate the grief and affliction of that family; but those who are happy with agreeable companions and beloved offspring are capable of conceiving part of the distress that would follow such a separation. As an addition likewise to her grief, she has now the afflicting circumstance of our Friend Thomas Story's indisposition [4] to bear, for whom she has given proofs of an uncommon regard through the whole series of their acquaintance. He had not been well for some months. The loss of his dear Friend had shocked him very much. A few weeks ago he was seized with a slight shock of the palsy, though in a very affecting way; it having deprived him so far of his memory of the names of things as to make him almost unfit for conversation. Though I am afraid never to be the same T. S. exactly, I recommended to him some of the Rattlesnake wine,[5] and I think it has been of service, as a gracious cordial and restorative.

In thy next, be pleased to let me know how much I owe for it and I shall take the first opportunity I can to remit it. — Let not my late conduct have any influence upon thee, but as often as convenience will permit, show that thou remembers

Thy very respectful Friend
John Fothergill, Jr.

Ms. autograph letter, Gilbert Collection, College of Physicians, Philadelphia, II, 139–140.

1. Dr. Fothergill refers to the Moravians, an evangelical sect originating in the province of Moravia, now a part of Czechoslovakia. With the encouragement and financial backing of their protector, Count Zinzendorf, they developed the most important missionary organization of the eighteenth century. In 1735 Moravian missionaries emigrated to the American Colonies, establishing headquarters in Savannah, Georgia, where John and Charles Wesley as well as George Whitefield were already active. When the southern colonies were threatened by Spanish invasion, Whitefield took passage on a sloop for Philadelphia and Moravian missionaries accompanied him. Attracted by Whitefield's description of a tract he had acquired in the vain hope of establishing a school for Negroes, the Moravians agreed to purchase the 5,000 acres offered; there they hoped to organize a school and community to christianize the Delaware Indians.

In December 1741, Count Zinzendorf arrived from Europe to inspect the place where his followers were living, still under primitive conditions. On Christmas Eve, he conducted a religious ceremony for the little group and named their site Bethlehem. After much toil, communal life — with a church, a school, and living quarters — was gradually established in well-designed buildings of native stone. Many of these buildings still stand, bringing the charm of another age to what has grown into a great industrial center of the twentieth century as headquarters of the Bethlehem Steel Corporation, but still remains the musical center the Moravians made it two centuries ago. A Bach Festival held there annually in May attracts people from all over the world. — Henry Rimius, *A Candid Account of the Rise and Progress of the Herrnhüters, commonly known as Moravians* (Philadelphia, 1753); *Memorials of the Moravian Church*, ed. William C. Reichel (Philadelphia: Lippincott, 1870), 157–187; M. C. Brailsford, *A Tale of Two Brothers: John and Charles Wesley* (London: Oxford University Press, 1954), 70, 73, 109–115, 123–129.

2. The Moravians adorned their churches with sacred images and introduced instrumental music in their services, whereas Quakers and quietist sects believed that guidance came through silent worship in assemblies devoid of ritual.

3. The fatalities in the Green family cannot be explained. Before Dr. Fothergill returned from the Continent, Joseph Green, father of the family, died on 3 July 1740. He had held the office of recorder of births, marriages, and deaths among members of the Society of Friends in London. — Devonshire House Records, LSFL.

4. Thomas Story (1666–1742) of Westmoreland, England, a convinced Quaker, had been educated in London as a lawyer. He went to Philadelphia during the early years of settlement, rendered indispensable legal advice to William Penn, and proved his efficiency as Master of the Rolls, Keeper of the Seals, and Commissioner of Property. As a "Publick Friend," he traveled widely in the American Colonies to counsel and preach. In 1715 he returned to England where he devoted himself to the Quaker cause until the failure of his health prevented activity. — Tolles, *James Logan*, 18, 26, 210.

5. Rattlesnake wine must have been recommended medicinally because of an ancient belief that the flesh of snakes had curative powers. Israel Pemberton had promised to send some to Dr. Fothergill. Comments on these customs are made by Eric Stone, *Medicine among the American Indians*, 31.

To Elizabeth Bartlett, Bradford, Yorkshire, 13 August 1741

London, 13.6.1741

Dear Betty,[1]

Thy letter was no less acceptable than unexpected, for I had entirely given over the hopes which thy promise made me entertain; but be assured that I had charity enough to excuse thee, and am so far from looking upon thine as a debt that I esteem it as a favour, and can hardly forbear prophesying that as it is the *first* that thou wilt make it the *last* I must ever expect from thee. Women sometimes take a pleasure in disappointing us, and it's now, thou sees, in thy power to do it with respect to me.

Please to acquaint thy Father that J. Busby[2] charges 30 shillings for the hat and 2/6 for the box. I prevailed upon him to make another instead of the first which he has not, I believe, yet disposed of, and if thy Father knows of anybody that wants such an one, would be glad to send it — may also let Benne know at his return that I procured the instruments according to his order, and sent them by Godfrey Laycock[3] to Halifax.[4]

He has never been so kind as to let me have one line since he set out. I have assiduously courted his correspondence but without the success I could have wished for. And I am now resolved to be less lavish that way; he is mistaken if he thinks I can't live without scribbling.

61

I was last night at Spital Square; [5] the family there was well, only affected by the loss of poor Will Bridges, as Benne may perhaps have informed thee. T. Story still intends for the North, before winter, and is looking out everywhere for a horse. He is much in the same condition as when Father saw him at the Yearly Meeting. Thy friend and correspondent Julia has, they say, made some impressions on Sam Vandewal, but — 'tis a secret. They say, likewise, that "the Dr." pays his addresses there very earnestly, but I believe the report is not well grounded. The Dr. is content with having it in his power to be in the company of persons of sense of that sex, when he chooses to spend an hour that way, without any designs of making a prey of one more than another, or to act in the least to the disadvantage of anybody. He endeavours to have his heart as plain as his coat, at the same time to keep both as whole as he can; and when he thinks soberly cannot look upon any character more worthy of his pains to acquire than that of integrity, an undesigning simplicity and benevolence.

It will perhaps be some news to hear that at length I am in hopes of escaping out of purgatory, and getting into lodgings which I think will every way suit me. 'Tis at a watchmaker's in Whitehart Court, next door to the meeting house, but I shan't remove there, six weeks.

My disconsolate neighbor J. T—n is yet alive. 'Tis well he had the dismal story from his sister, for he kept continually teasing me about news from Bradford. I was forced to shun him for his own peace sake, and I could really so far sympathize with him as to say woe to the man who is born to be disappointed. — I don't now call to mind any remarkable change that has happened to any among thy acquaintance. P. Plumstead has been not well and in a great deal of danger, but is now quite well. My Landlord's intimacy there is on the decline. He has been at Spital Square several times of late but was very genteelly received; P. Elliot is very seldom there, and consequently J. Whitehead and the rest, as usual.[6] Excuse me for troubling thee with a very dull epistle. I am quite jaded and fatigued, incapable of anything but scribbling to a friend who I believe has good nature enough to accept of an intention to please. Don't forget to make my best respects acceptable to thy kind Father and Mother, and be assured that I shall always be glad to hear from thee and make the best return in my power for the favors thou may trust me with. I am, dear Betty, thy respectful friend

John Fothergill

Ms. autograph letter, Dimsdale Mss., LSFL.

1. Betty, the only daughter of Benjamin Bartlett (1678–1759), the apothecary of Bradford, had been known since her childhood to John Fothergill junior, who had been apprenticed to her father. "Benne," Betty's older brother, Benjamin Bartlett II (1714–1787), inherited his father's business and in 1766, by Dr. Fothergill's advice, moved to London. He was treasurer of the Society of Antiquaries for many years, wrote essays for publication, and was the author of a small book, highly praised by coin collectors: *The Episcopal Coins of Durham and the Monastic Coins of Reading.* — W. R. Hodgson, *The Society of Friends in Bradford* (Bradford, Yorkshire: privately printed, 1926), 31–37; Raistrick, 76, 282–283, 327.

2. Shopkeeper, location unknown.

3. Unidentified.

4. Halifax, Yorkshire, near Bradford.

5. A residential area near Spitalfields Market. The names of street and market are derived from an ancient hospital where travelers as well as the ill found refuge.

6. No attempt has been made to identify Betty's circle of London acquaintances.

II
1742-1744

I find that Friends of your [Philadelphia]
Yearly Meeting have thought proper to add me
to the number of their correspondents . . . 'Twas
before my inclination, 'tis now my duty; and it
will always be a sincere pleasure to be a part of
the channel of communication betwixt the two most
considerable parts of the Society.

To Israel Pemberton, 14.3.1743 O.S.

To Elizabeth Bartlett, Bradford, Yorkshire, 11 February 1741/2

London, 11.12.1741/2

Dear Betty,

I was no less surprised than pleased to have in my hands a letter from a person whom though I wished yet I durst not hope to retain in the little number of my correspondents. I was prevented by some little intervening affairs from acknowledging the receipt of thy acceptable present before this time; it came a few days after I had thy letter, very safe, very good and no less acceptable, though I confess more than I had the least cause to expect, as the services I did were so little that thy good-natured acceptance of them, such as they were, was a more than equal return. And 'twill be long before I think the debt I am in to your family anything like being paid.

I confess, Betty, I have no room to find fault with my new lodgings. We have no Bachelors in it besides me and one much younger, and I have this further inducement to alter my condition of seeing an instance of a very happy conjugal life every day before me. I have no dislike to the state in others. I look upon it in the most favourable light, but if I must be obliged to remain as I am, deal gently with me — and don't increase my misfortunes by adding the most disagreeable of titles to that of Dr. Fothergill, viz., that he willfully chose to be called an old Bachelor.

I believe 'tis very true what you hear about Nancy[1] having a great number of admirers, and which I cannot but look upon as a great piece of unhappiness. Not that it in any way affects me, because I am pretty certain that whenever I make any attempts there I shall unquestionably succeed, in spite of all the rivals I shall meet with! But as I know very few mortals who are proof against flattery (the most bare-faced of the kind being not always disgustful), I cannot but pity anyone who must never hear a syllable of truth to her face.

I have been very little at their house for several months; their acquaintance increases every day with people of a turn different from what I should wish to be acquainted with. I know of nobody that makes any advances, I mean regular ones. S. V-nd-w-l [2] was talked of, and I believe might have been caressed, but he did not care to engage with a person whom he might easily see would value him more for 50,000 pounds than anything else. She's unhappy in not having her Father's prudence to assist her at this critical juncture, and equally so in being insensible of any loss she has sustained by his death. We now and then talk 1/2 an hour away about our shells, but she's accustomed to richer sauces than my plain table will afford. I mean the brilliant conversation she every day shines among; and the continual incense of flattery renders plainness insipid, and I am resolved never to contribute to the happiness of any of the Sex I so much esteem by telling them they are either wiser or prettier than they really are. Yet I am always pleased when I have an opportunity of doing justice to their merits and amiable qualifications.

Be assured that a few lines will always be acceptable from thee. Yet I dare not expect that thou will ever favour me with another, so with as much philosophical indifference as I can, I subscribe myself

Thy respectful Friend
J. Fothergill, Junr.

Ms. autograph letter, Dimsdale Mss., LSFL.

1. Nancy or Nanny Green, whose father's unexplained illness and death have already been described (J. F. to I. Pemberton, 28 March 1741).

2. Probably to be identified with Samuel Vanderwall (1719–1761) "an eminent merchant" who in 1744 married Martha Neate. — Joseph J. Green, "Some Account of the . . . Family of Van de Walle," typescript in LSFL, 1902, pp. 66–69.

To Israel Pemberton, Jr., Philadelphia, 8 April 1742

London, 8.2.1742

My dear Friend,

I don't know how long it is since I received any letter from thee, but I know it is a great while, and though thou art one in my debt, yet I can't forbear sending another to solicit for my due and at the same time increase thy account. I think our Friendship is not of the ordinary kind, built upon formality and maintained only through complaisance. I am sure I feel a stronger engagement, and I have not the least doubt but that thou hast the same [opinion], however circumstances may have prevented thee from giving me such frequent assurances of its being so, as would have been in some sort necessary to maintain a less cordial warmth of affection than what I have in reality for thee.

Besides the little notices which one usually conveys to one's Friends by letters, there is one thing which I cannot omit to take notice of, which relates to the affairs of your Province. I doubt not but every circumstance is carefully conveyed to one Friend or other, but different ways of telling the same thing sometimes help to give lights, at least to explain, what in one may be less understood.

'Tis now several months since I received from my kind Friend, J. Logan, a copy of his printed paper sent to your Yearly Meeting,[1] at the reading of which I confess I was not a little troubled and surprised. Not that I believed it would be of so much weight as to occasion any considerable embarrassment among yourselves, only as it would be a public declaration of differing sentiments and a basis for your enemies to build a good deal of mischief upon, as I observe has since happened, and no doubt has been one motive for the petitioners to style some persons *prudent men*.[2] And I cannot forbear calling to mind on this occasion the fable of the Fox and the Crow — it looking so like the artful flattery of the first to deprive the poor Crow of her Cheese.

The sight of this paper induced me to inquire as carefully as I was able into the structure of your Province and the present condition of things there, in order to make some remarks upon the paper sent me, in an answer which I was to return to his letter. This inquiry almost insensibly interested me so much in your concerns as to make me very attentive to whatever passed relating to them, and though no way capable of assisting, yet I could not but be pleased to see others take a share and acting with vigour.

Our Meeting for Sufferings, upon reading the letter from your Yearly Meeting, very readily engaged in the business and proceeded so far as that a petition to the Board of Trade[3] was drawn up, requesting that a proper time be granted to make good your own cause against the unfair aspersions or false representations of your adversaries — signed by many

Friends and presented to the Lords of Trade in person. It had the effect that it lessened a prejudice against you, and made them so far equitable as to promise not to proceed in making a report to the Council, till we had petitioned that body in like manner, for a sufficient time. Some Friends had likewise an opportunity of acquainting the Board of Trade that several of their allegations were extremely unjust, and of convincing them that to the wisdom of the Proprietor and the equity of the succeeding administration of the laws, under providence, was owing the present happy and flourishing condition of that Province — and consequently — that the exclusion of any part or any set of men in the administration any otherwise than by the free voice of the people could not but be productive of numerous calamities. This happened no longer ago than yesterday.[4] I was hindered by my employ from being present, but I could not but be pleased with the success, and I question not but many of your Friends here will be very hearty in the cause.

I have not yet given J. Logan my sentiments on his paper. I had once thought to have entered into the merits of it, but weak arguments always strengthen an opponent in the good opinion of his own side of the question, I shall avoid that, and only show a just dislike for the whole. The argument entirely turns upon his assertion of all government being founded on force. If this is once heard and it is demonstrated that even supposing, though not allowing, that this is so, yet to prove his argument of any force in this case, he must make it plain that there is no difference in the degree of it, but that the force exercised in the correction of a child is the same as in cutting the throat of an enemy. I must confess that there are some remarks interspersed that I could not have expected from a person of J. Logan's penetration, had not I considered how difficult it is for great ability to obscure simple truth!

I looked over several messages and votes of your house of representatives for the year (I think) 1740, and if I may be permitted to give my opinion of the management of your controversy with the Governor,[5] I can scarcely on the whole forbear to take his side. Your cause is undoubtedly good, but I am afraid you discover a little more warmth than is quite consistent with the moderation we profess. The provocations, I confess, are great and more than flesh and blood can well sustain, but there is a Rock which many of you know where to seek — but to which he discovers himself a perfect stranger. The arguments made use of by the Assembly are strong and cogent, but he justly accuses you of too much acrimony. Truth never appears more agreeable than when dressed with mildness of temper, and though I cannot just now lay my hand upon any particular circumstance (the papers not being in my possession), yet I wish I knew how to recommend some sort of observance on this hand. I am but a poor politician I own, yet I think I could readily adopt your first governor's system and method of conduct. If yours is agreeable to his, it will not be in the power of the present to do you the injury he seems to intend. And, my dear Friend, be pleased to remember that a deference is due to a magistrate in some sense — though a wicked one — and in every step of opposition to his measures, plainness and inoffensive simplicity are the principal arms we can manage.

As to the present condition of public affairs, our papers give a better account than I can pretend to. They will show the general condition of Europe — the effects of French perfidy and corruption, the extreme poverty and extreme pride of this last; our own commotions and renversements. Scenes of confusion, villany, cruelty and the products of ambition appear everywhere, and not the least glimpse of their conclusion. Heaven only knows the consequences of this universal uproar! We are hitherto the least affected by the general calamity and the least thankful, I am afraid, for the mercy. May his tender visitations at last make us submit to his will in all things and constantly regard him in faith as our protector. Here, and here only, will be quietness and an uninterrupted assurance. And, oh! may it be our happy lot to enjoy it. — Farewell, my dear Friend. Remember my love to my Father's Friends, and accept the unfeigned offer of it from thy

John Fothergill, Junior

P.S. I thought to put an end to a tedious epistle before but I had forgot to mention T. Story who got down as far as Carlisle several months ago; pretty hardy in every respect but in his memory of words which still continues defective. He is busy in planting and building. Active dispositions, we see, contract such habits of industry that it's not in the power of old age to break it! I dare hardly mention Michael Lightfoot [6] because I know not that I ever saw a much greater man — and here I must stop. He left London some weeks ago, very well. He was here in a very seasonable time and helped us to several necessary pieces of information [illegible].

Ms. autograph letter, Pemberton Papers, II, 2, HSP.

1. James Logan (1674–1751), secretary to William Penn, member of the Provincial

Council of Pennsylvania 1702–1747 and its president 1736–1738, chief justice of the Supreme Court 1731–1739, though a leading member of the Society of Friends had become convinced that Indian attacks on Pennsylvania's borders called for armed resistance. In September 1741, shortly before the annual elections to the Assembly, he sent to the Philadelphia Yearly Meeting a strong letter declaring that "civil government . . . is founded on force" and therefore "Friends as such in the strictness of their principles ought not to engage in it." Warning that continued opposition to voting funds for proper defense would alienate Parliament and perhaps result in withdrawal of the charter granted to William Penn, he urged that the Yearly Meeting encourage Friends "who for conscience-sake cannot join in any law for self-defense [to] decline standing candidates at the ensuing election for representatives." — Tolles, *James Logan*, 154–156, 218n. The letter was referred to a committee which laid it on the table, stating that it concerned only "matters military and geographical." Logan thereupon had thirty copies of his letter printed "with a design to send them to his Friends in England," but apparently distributed only a few of the copies. From one of these the letter is reprinted in the *Pennsylvania Magazine of History and Biography*, 6 (1882): 402–411. Logan's urging had little immediate effect; the Quakers continued to hold a majority in the Assembly.

2. The petitioners mentioned were "divers merchants and other inhabitants of Pennsylvania," whose petition "setting forth the defenceless condition of said province, occasioned by the opposition of the Quakers" had been received by the Privy Council and on 18 January 1742 had been referred to a committee which on 19 February referred it to the Board of Trade. — *Acts of the Privy Council of England (Colonial Series)*, vol. III:1720–1745 (London: H.M.S.O., 1910).

3. The Board of Trade (the Lords commissioners of Trade and Plantations) was a committee of eight active members, with others attending ex officio, which supervised colonial activities. This Board reviewed colonial petitions and acts prepared by royal colonies and the proprietary colony of Pennsylvania. — Knollenberg, 47.

4. On Wednesday, 7 April 1742, "several Quakers . . . presented a petition subscribed by them on behalf of their friends, inhabitants of the province of Pennsylvania [in opposition to the petition noted above]." — See *Journal of the Commissioners for Trade and Plantations* from January 1741/2 to December 1749 (London: H.M.S.O., 1931), in which the history of both petitions can be followed.

5. The Pennsylvania Assembly during this period was almost continuously and bitterly opposed to the policies of the Deputy Governor, Colonel George Thomas, concerning "defense, pacifism, authority, taxation, and currency." Thomas complained repeatedly in letters to the Board of Trade of "the defenceless state of the province" and of the Assembly's antagonistic attitude. — Thayer, *Israel Pemberton*, p. 41; *Pennsylvania Archives*, 8 ser. III, IV (1931); entries beginning 14 January 1741, in *Journal of the Commissioners for Trade and Plantations . . . 1734/5 to December 1741* (London: H.M.S.O., 1930).

6. Michael Lightfoot (1683/4–1754), a Quaker minister of Irish birth, emigrated to Pennsylvania in 1712. Having won a reputation for "honour and integrity," he was appointed treasurer of the province in 1743, an office which he held for eleven years, until his death at the age of seventy. — *A Collection of Memorials Concerning Divers Deceased Ministers and Others of the People called Quakers in Pennsylvania, New-Jersey and Parts Adjacent* (Philadelphia, 1787), 423–425.

To Israel Pemberton, Jr., Philadelphia, 12–14 May 1743

London, 14.3.1743

Respected Friend,

I could not omit the opportunity of my friend Dr. Bond's return [1] to throw a few lines in thy way; as I believe it is only due to a multiplicity of engagements that I don't hear more frequently from thee; I don't scrupulously keep to a formal correspondence, but write on as leisure permits or opportunity or matter offer.

I was prevented by indisposition from being present with many friends, last night, at the arguing of your Assembly cause before the Privy Council.[2] I should have been glad upon a double account, both to have heard your cause asserted with so much force of eloquence and sound reasoning as gained the applause of the audience in general, as well as to have been able to have given thee some account of what was urged on both sides. The case was argued with much warmth on both sides near three hours. But one of the counsel for the Assembly, I am told, in everybody's opinion urged his cause inimitably well. What decision will be come to is yet unknown; but it's expected to be as favourable as possible.[3] I imagine they are unwilling on one hand to reflect any blame upon the Governor; [4] yet the capital part of intermeddling with the constituents of a free people, where nothing has been acted but what is agreeable to a large majority of their electors, is so tender that very probably it will be dropped.

I think Friends in Pennsylvania can hardly quite clear themselves of some blame in not furnishing either your agent or the Meeting for Sufferings, with some authentic proofs of what was alleged on your behalf. None of which that I know of have come to hand. When the petition that Friends here had laid before the Council [5] came to be mentioned, I was in some pain about it. We requested time. We have had a whole year, and in all that time have not been furnished with any new circumstances, or anything corroborative of what had been alleged by us as a foundation for council to plead upon. It's much if you don't hear of this from other quarters. I don't mention it as a reflection, but that I may be furnished with something to answer this objection. I find that some have letters in town which mention a kind of contention betwixt the Governor and Assembly, which, if it is on a sound footing,

73

I shall be much pleased with. A prudent suspicion of each other's conduct is sometimes necessary, when those that are at the head of affairs may possibly have different interest in view, but open altercations I believe very rarely do good. The public affairs in these parts of the world are yet in an unhappy condition. We have thrown such a weight into the Queen of Hungary's scale, both by money and men, that France I believe will not be able to counterpoise.[6] And if the news that has been handed about with us this day or two be fact, viz., that the Austrians have killed and taken prisoner 7000 Bavarians with their General Zuckendorff[7] himself, the poor old titular Emperor must quit his country in his old age, and perhaps be obliged to take refuge in France.[8] One cannot without the deepest concern look over the miseries which the distressed Bavarians must have felt; one [into] which they have been dragooned by their polite auxiliaries the French. The Austrians have in their turn treated it as an enemy's country; these have given place to the French again, who like the locusts eat up every green thing; and now both are contriving who shall share what remains of the unhappy Bavarians. I am very little attentive to news or politics, but everything of this sort cannot but be acceptable to a person of thy acquaintance with public affairs. The French seem to lose their credit almost everywhere, and I know of none else who could have kept theirs so long upon so rotten a bottom as they have. Their impudence is consummate, and their perfidy matchless. A frothy, vainglorious, bullying nation capable of sacrificing whatever they would be thought to deem the most sacred to their interests; wretched, poor and wretchedly proud; but enough of this.

Since the above was wrote, I am informed that the Privy Council have come to a resolution as favourable to the Assembly as could have been expected; all that will be done will be to order the Governor to take what care he can of the province, but without any particular directions. But R.P.[9] will be able to give you the best account of this affair.

Our annual assembly [10] begins in little more than a week. I had some hopes of seeing my Father here, but now I find I am likely to be disappointed. He has his health in general pretty well, except in one respect, which is so much the more affecting to me as it will be a means of preventing me from seeing him so often as I should desire. Upon any little riding, however gentle, he is apt to be troubled with the strangury, and sometimes makes bloody water. I think it may probably arise from his frequent and assiduous or rather diligent travelling on horseback, which has so affected those parts as to render them liable to this disorder. I have hitherto only been able to palliate it, and have sometimes helped him to go a journey with more ease; to cure it entirely I am afraid is not practicable at his years.

My neighbour John Bell[11] in Leonard Street married his third wife yesterday. She is a daughter of Thomas Zacchary, and had been married to one Owen who has been dead some years. Priscilla Plumstead was married a few weeks ago to a young man from Birmingham. Nanny Greene has thrown herself away upon a person not of our Society, and is likely to be much disappointed in the only thing she married for, viz., to show away, as 'tis called, herself. He gratified her vanity a few months; she shone at all public places of diversion; displayed her jewels and fine clothing upon every occasion; visited in her chariot, two footmen etc.; and now I find is obliged to hear the unpleasant account of the necessity of retrenching and submitting to learn the duties of a wife. Her husband is a gay man, above forty, has some estate, and has sense enough to be unwilling to spend it *all*, as he has done, a part. I pity her on the account of the mortification she must undergo of spending a great part of her time in a way she has no taste for, yet her growing fondness of herself made it necessary, even for her own sake.

I find that Friends of your Yearly Meeting have thought proper to add me to the number of their correspondents; I place this mark of their respect, to the kindness they still retain for my dear Father and perhaps to some intimations of thine, more favourable than I deserve. A person of more authority and experience would have had it in his power to have done you more service; but as far as my ability will permit, I hope never to be wanting to discharge the trust reposed in me. 'Twas before my inclination, 'tis now my duty; and it will always be a sincere pleasure to be a part of the canal of communication betwixt the two most considerable parts of the Society; I mean not only in respect of numbers; but of that part wherein our very essence and union consists. I now must close, and with dear love to M. Lightfoot, thy Father, and spouse (though unknown), I am thy affectionate Friend

J. Fothergill

Ms. autograph letter, Pemberton Papers, XXXIV, 4, HSP.

1. Dr. Phineas Bond returned from England to join his older brother, Dr. Thomas Bond, in practice. Much respected for his civic interest, he was a member of the

Governor's Council for many years. With other prominent citizens, including Richard Peters, he took an active part in planning for the expansion of the city's Academy into the College of Philadelphia (now the University of Pennsylvania) and was elected to its first Board of Trustees. — Thomas G. Morton and Frank Woodbury, *History of the Pennsylvania Hospital*, 2d ed. (Philadelphia: Times Printing Office, 1895), 488.

2. During the colonial period, the Privy Council, through the agency of its Committee for Hearing Appeals, remained the final judicial court of appeal for settling cases in all the American Colonies, whether royal, proprietary, or corporate. — Knollenberg, 46, 47.

3. On 11 May 1743, the Privy Council, after hearing arguments on both sides of the continuing controversy between the Deputy Governor and the Proprietors on one hand and the Quaker-dominated Assembly on the other, "concluded only that instructions should be sent to Governor Thomas to lay before the King what he considered necessary for the security of the Province."— Mabel P. Wolff, *The Colonial Agency of Pennsylvania, 1712–1757* (Philadelphia: the author, 1933), p. 106.

4. George Thomas (b. Antigua, B.W.I., *ca.* 1695, d. London 1774), Deputy-Governor of Pennsylvania and the Lower Counties 1738–1747, though unpopular with the Pennsylvania Assembly dealt tactfully with the Indian tribes. With the aid of Conrad Weiser, the Indian Agent, he was able to come to terms with the Iroquois, thus making possible settlement of the back country by newcomers from Europe.

5. On 7 April 1742; see letter of 8 April 1742, above.

6. The War of the Austrian Succession (1740–1748) was devastating Europe in a prolonged struggle for power. Maria Theresa, Archduchess of Austria, Queen of Hungary and of Bohemia, was supported by Great Britain in her claim to the Hapsburg lands under the Pragmatic Sanction arranged by her father, Emperor Charles VI. The disputing claimant, Charles Albert of Bavaria, was supported by Prussia, Spain, Sardinia, and especially, by Britain's ancient rival, France. After a series of victories, Charles Albert proclaimed himself king of Bohemia, and in 1742 he won election to the crown of the Holy Roman Empire as Charles VII. In the same year Prussia withdrew from the war. Up to that time Great Britain had not taken an active part in the conflict, but British soldiers had been stationed at certain Dutch ports to prevent hostile access to the Channel. Early in 1743, King George II had personally taken charge of the Pragmatic Army of British, Hanoverian, and Prussian soldiers. At Dettingen, in Bavaria, on 27 June 1743, only a few weeks after the date of Dr. Fothergill's letter, they achieved a notable victory over the French. — *The New Cambridge Modern History*, VII (Cambridge University Press, 1957), 200–204, 397, 408, 416, 428, 437–439.

7. Zuckendorff is probably a mistaken rendering of Seckendorff. Count Friedrich Heinrich von Seckendorff was a distinguished commander in the Bavarian service. No account of the disaster Dr. Fothergill mentions has been found. — *NCMH*, VII.

8. Without backing from France, Charles Albert found himself the helpless leader of a lost cause. While settlements were under discussion for the Treaty of Hanau (1743), John Carteret, who had crossed the Channel with King George II as His Majesty's diplomatic secretary, saw to it that the "old titular Emperor" received due consideration. By the terms of this treaty, Charles Albert's hereditary dominions were restored to him, with promises of further assistance from Great Britain. Rallying a few devoted followers, Charles Albert returned to Bavaria. Worn out by fruitless struggle, he died in 1745. — *NCMH*, VII, 425, 431.

9. Richard Partridge (1681–1759), son of a prosperous merchant of Portsmouth, New Hampshire, had lived in London since 1701, first as agent for his father and

later as agent, from time to time, of several of the colonies and of other colonial interests. He was also for some time parliamentary agent for the London Meeting for Sufferings. In 1740 he had been appointed agent of Pennsylvania by vote of the Assembly. One of Governor Thomas' complaints was that this appointment was illegal. See Wolff, *Colonial Agency*, 83–106; *DAB*.

10. London Yearly Meeting, which in this year designated Dr. John Fothergill its correspondent to Philadelphia Yearly Meeting.

11. John Bell of London collected data commemorating the lives and services of Quaker ministers. His biographical accounts were published in a series of volumes entitled *Piety Promoted*. This work continued for years, with a change of editors when necessary. — LSFL.

To Israel Pemberton, Jr., Philadelphia, 12 September 1743

London, 12.7.1743

Dear Friend,

I must take time to acquaint thee that I was much pleased to hear by E. Bland [1] of thy welfare and that, though leisure will not permit thee to tell me so, yet thou art sometimes pleased to remember me. I should be unjust if I did not accept the utmost remarks of thy respect for me as they are intended. Leisure to write and a proper disposition for it don't always occur at the same time to men of business, and because they do not, to omit any opportunity in our power to oblige a friend is a little unkind.

I was favoured with an opportunity of seeing my friends in the North this summer. I spent some days with the best of Fathers; I had heard he was indisposed and though his disorder I fear admits of no cure, yet I contributed a little to his relief; and believe me that I know not that I ever felt so sensible a pleasure as when I found that the good old man's heart seemed rejoiced because I had thought it my duty to see him. Thou knows what it is better than I do, as heaven has put it more in thy power to enjoy the secret pleasure every day of doing some kind thing to a virtuous, sensible parent. Their fears, their cares are inexpressible; sometimes methinks I feel some part of the load they bear on our accounts. A stranger that merited one half so much at our hands would be almost adored as a prodigy of Liberality. Nor do they deserve less grateful return. But I need not mention these things to thee, but rather ask excuse for suffering a concern of my own to become so much the subject of what ought to be devoted to thy entertainment.

I am much pleased to hear that your domestic feuds are a little hushed.

77

May the truce be lasting, and its consequences happy! In Europe affairs seem to be extremely perplexed. We are all ruining each other to the utmost of our power. The French would be soon reduced to terms, were not the allies afraid of a storm breaking out on the side of Prussia. The French have found means to insinuate themselves into the good graces of that prince. If they found him disposed to promote arts and sciences, some of these immediately offered their service.[2] They have perfectly studied him, and are in a fair way to become his masters.

I am afraid we shall soon begin to feel in a pressing manner the effects of a long continued, fruitless, expensive war. I see some symptoms appear which look threatening; I wish my apprehensions may have magnified them. Indeed heaven has thus far favoured us with excessive plenty of grain, and the manufactures in various parts are in a very flourishing condition. This I apprehend is partly owing to the great drain of men which the French have endured, and many of these their artisans. Some scruple not to say that they have lost above 100,000 men, besides those now in arms. A nation must be rich indeed that finds no inconvenience arising from such a loss.

I spent a few days about Leeds. What are left of our Friends in that part of the country are well. Poor Tabby[3] and I talked of thee not a little; as well as in many other places, thou was the subject of our conversation. The loss which that family has sustained in the loss of the father and son quite sunk my spirits. But we must be all called away at one time after another. I wish with ardour that I may get ready for another country, and if heaven sees meet to spare my father the grief of burying a son that he has some little value for, I should not then care how soon I am going. I don't think it an happiness sometimes that I have none of those endearing bonds of wife and children, but if I am without them, my exit will be of the less consequence. My profession obliges me sometimes to be present at such scenes that though I am amply convinced that the most consummate happiness that mortals can attain to has been tasted; yet alas my very soul has been racked to see it in a moment dissolved, and one party left inconsolable. But no more of this; I can't relate it.

I oft pay an imaginary visit to thy spouse and self and see you extremely happy; I partake of the satisfaction with you and wish you an increase. Don't rob her of it by an extreme application to business. Heaven will never permit the virtuous to want; why then should a moment be lost that might be better employed in tasting the solid satisfaction that the present time affords, rather than to be painfully solicitous about what may never happen?

Before I conclude I'll just tell thee what darts into my thoughts upon reviewing what I have wrote. I have sometimes wondered why I had not a line from thee, but I see mine are so trifling they are not worth it. I'll trouble thee, I think, no more; excuse what has passed and believe that I shall always remain, with sincere good wishes for thy solid happiness,

Thy affectionate Friend
J. Fothergill junr.

Be pleased to remember my dear love to the worthy Michael Lightfoot.

Manuscript autograph letter, Pemberton Papers, XXXIV, 5, HSP.

1. Elias Bland, the son of an English Quaker merchant, was sent by his father from London to Philadelphia to be trained in the counting house of John Reynell. After five years of apprenticeship, Elias Bland returned to London in 1743 to carry on export-import trade with the American Colonies as a commission merchant. — Tolles, *Meeting House and Counting House*, 88, 90n, 93, 94, 95n.

2. Frederick II of Prussia (1712–1786), a brilliant man devoted in his youth to literature, philosophy, and music, was at this time enjoying the dangerous game of power politics. He had withdrawn from the war in 1742, but renewed his alliance with France and Bavaria in 1744.

3. "Tabby" is undoubtedly Tabitha Horner, of Leeds, Yorkshire. She greatly admired the preaching of John Fothergill senior, and corresponded occasionally with his son, Dr. John (see his letters to her, 1745 and 1745/6, below), upon whom she depended for medical advice. She attended London Yearly Meeting whenever possible, and probably had first met Israel Pemberton during a session of this annual assemblage. He was always a welcome visitor to the English Friends, bringing news of colonial affairs which letters could not report in full detail.

To Dr. Charles Alston, University of Edinburgh, 14 September 1743

London, 14.7.1743

Dear Doctor,

A young man who has been recommended to me as a sober, studious person, and who intends to apply himself to Physick, though educated with other views, desiring a few lines to some of the Professors at Edinburgh, prevailed upon me to give you this trouble. As he is quite unacquainted with medicine, I advised him to get into some Shop in Edinburgh, to attend the Materia Medica and Anatomy the first winter, and to go through a course of Experimental Philosophy.[1] As the study of medicine is his choice, I am in hopes he will prove industrious and endeavour to deserve the countenance which from experience I know Dr. Alston is disposed to afford to industrious strangers.

I have desired him to put into thy hands a specimen of the Persian Manna; [2] it's described by Rauwolf in Ray's *Travels*,[3] and seems to be a very pleasant sweet. It came to me by the way of Petersburgh, or rather to my Friend P. Collinson who gave it me. I intend to make trial of its effects, having 2 or 3 ounces of it; and to give the result, with a description of it from the thing itself, Rauwolf's account, and the Arabian's to the Royal Society.[4]

I have lately been turning over a pompous performance lately printed in Germany by Sendelius. It's a description of Amber containing insects etc. in the King of Poland's collection at Dresden. He has a large digression *De Generatione Succinorum*,[5] and endeavours to prove it a bitumen, which he thinks is hardened by a vitriolic acid. He thinks that whilst the Amber was in its fluid state from some accidental rupture of the mountains, insects etc. were carried into the veins by the wind. But from a careful consideration of his description of the Amber vein, and collating it with Hartmann's, I am fully of the opinion that Amber in its origin is a vegetable resin, indurated and changed into the form in which we now see it by a mineral acid, the *acidum vagum fodinarum*. I have drawn up an abridgement of Sendelius's whole book of 320 pages in folio, in about 12 sheets, to which I have subjoined notes referring to the facts he gives us, and endeavouring to demonstrate how much easier the several phenomena are explicable from the supposition I advance than any other. I yesterday put this into the hand of an ingenious physician. If he approves it, this must also go to the Royal Society. It would have given me a singular pleasure to have run over the thing with a person so well versed in these affairs as thyself, but I am debarred that privilege at present. If I offer it to the Society, and they think fit to print it,[6] I'll beg thy acceptance of a copy. If not, I'll some way or other send the Ms. down. I have some experiments to advance on behalf of my hypothesis, but I think not to offer them yet. I am in hopes that the materials which Sendelius has afforded me will be sufficient; if not I'll produce all the evidence I can.

I begin to despair of ever meriting thy correspondence as it has been thus far so little to thy advantage; but I shall take every opportunity of this kind that offers, to testify the sincerest regard which I constantly pay to those who have contributed their utmost to make me what I am, till I find that it proves disagreeable. This tribute I think is due, and beg that it may be candidly accepted from

Thy obliged, respectful Friend

J. Fothergill

Ms. autograph letter, Alston Collection, UEL.

1. A course in general science — elementary physics and chemistry — requiring observation of natural objects and phenomena, with some chance to make simple experiments. John Aubrey (1625–1697) writes amusingly from Oxford, the home of classical learning, about early seventeenth-century distrust of "an inventive and enquiring Witt" probing into the secrets of nature: "Till about the year 1649, when Experimental Philosophy was first cultivated by a Club at Oxford, 'twas held a strange presumption for a Man to attempt an Innovation in Learnings; and not to be good Manners to be more knowing than his Neighbours and Forefathers. 'Twas held a Sin to make a Scrutinie into the Waies of Nature; Whereas it is certainly a profound part of Religion to glorify God in his Workes; and to take no notice at all of what is dayly offered before our Eyes is grosse Stupidity." — *Aubrey's Brief Lives*, ed. Oliver L. Dick (London: Secker and Warburg, 1950), xliii.

2. Exudate of a Levantine plant of the genus *Alhagi*, mentioned by Avicenna (A.D. 980–1037) as used by Arabian physicians, but apparently unfamiliar in Great Britain in Dr. Fothergill's time.

3. John Ray (1627–1705) devoted the first volume of his *Curious Collection of Travels* (1693) to a translation of Rauwolf's Old German text: *Aigentliche Beschreibung der Raise so er vor dieser Zeit gegen Auffgang inn die Mörgenländer* (1582, 1583). Ray added a catalogue of plants which Rauwolf mentioned, together with lists of his own collecting in Egypt and Crete. — Charles E. Raven, *John Ray, Naturalist: His Life and Works* (Cambridge: Cambridge University Press, 1950), 274–277; Agnes Arber, *Herbals: Their Origin and Evolution* (Cambridge: Cambridge University Press, 1953), 280.

4. Dr. Fothergill carried out his projected study, as he reported to Dr. Alston on 19 September 1744 (below, see especially note 3).

5. Nathaniel Sendelius, *Historica Succinorum Corpore Aliena Involventium et Naturae Opera: Pictorum et Caelatorum; Ex Regis Augustorum Cimelis Dresdae Conditis; Aerie Insculptorum; Conscripta a Nathanele Sendelio, D. Medico et Physico, Elbingensi Ordinario* (Leipzig, 1743). Sendelius may well have paid personally for publication of this sumptuous volume.

6. "An Essay on the Origin of Amber," read before the Royal Society of London 1 March 1743/4. — *Phil. Trans. R.S.*, 43:21–25 (1744/5); extract in *Works*, ed. Lettsom, I, 251–256.

To Alexander Fothergill, Carr End, Wensleydale, Yorkshire, 28 January 1743/4

London, 28.11.1743/4

Dear Brother,[1]

I received thy acceptable letter of 28/9, and at the same time one from dear Father and from Brother Samuel which pleased me not a little. Thy expressions of affection and kindness were not unobserved or forgot, though I delayed writing longer than I first intended. I own I almost promised Justice Metcalf [2] a letter, but upon second thought I knew not how to send anything worthy of his perusal.

I spend the morning until ten over a book; till one I visit my patients and do what other business abroad I have occasion for. I then dine and take up my book or pen, except I have company calls. I then go out for an hour or two; sometimes I spend an evening at a friend's house, if not, alone with a book. This is my general course. I now and then read the papers of the day, but not constantly. Judge then for thyself, how unable I am to furnish a person so knowing in public affairs with any account worth his reading. Gratitude indeed frequently prompts me to make some acknowledgements for his constant kindness and regard to my honored Father and his offspring — if I take my pen in hand I could say nothing else; besides I fancy he is by this time at York where I know not how to direct him.

I could not but be desirous when I was in the country to see thee and thine at Carr End once more; I was glad I did so and though the little opportunity we were together was so uncivilly interrupted by so much company, which I could not avoid sensibly regretting; yet as we neither could help it, it could only be submitted to.

I mentioned to thee that I should be glad if thou could procure me a little piece or two of hung beef; and likewise to send with it any curious stones or fossil shells that come thy way. I fancy some of thy acquaintance in Swaledale would be able to get some things from the miners there that would be acceptable, as different sorts of lead ore, spars, etc.[3] If it fall in thy way, please to engage somebody to collect a few; and if they can come at it, what quantity of metal is generally produced from such and such kind of ore, and the name of the place. I should wish to have a pretty large lump of a sort, a pound or two in weight or more rather than less. In return only let me know what would be acceptable to thee from hence, and I'll not be unmindful to discharge my debt. Only one thing I must bar against — and that is Law. I own I dread the consequence of thy application to it. The people about thee don't deserve it at thy hands.[4]

Dear Brother, suffer me to give my opinion without a fee, and accept it with the affection it is offered in. An ignorant, ungrateful race will be always working upon thy goodnature until they have served their own ends and injured thee irreparably, both in the loss of time which ought to be devoted to provide for a rising family, and which is of worse consequence, almost have estranged thee from thy own breast and the glimmering of that light which only promotes the happiness of men.

Farewell, and believe me thine and wife's

Affectionate Brother

J. Fothergill

Ms. autograph letter, Fothergill Family Papers, Wallis Collection.

1. Alexander Fothergill (1709–1788), farming the family homestead, in 1733 had married Jane Blakey, who died in 1735 leaving an infant daughter. In 1737 Alexander married Margaret Thistlethwaite. — Fothergill Genealogy, below.

2. Thomas Metcalf, Justice of the Peace, employed Alexander Fothergill as clerk and assistant. (See Introduction, above.) After studying law in London, Metcalf had returned to live in his ancestral home, Nappa Hall, near Askrigg, completed in 1495 by his ancestor James Metcalf. — Marie Hartley and Joan Ingilby, *Yorkshire Village* (London: Dent, 1953), 51, 52; W. C. Metcalfe and G. Metcalfe, *Records of the Metcalfe Family, formerly of Nappa Hall . . . in Wensleydale* (London: privately published, 1891).

3. In the eighteenth century, Swaledale, "thirty miles of dale stretching from Tailbrig on the west to Richmond on the east" (and immediately to the north of Wensleydale, to which it runs parallel), had productive lead mines which provided occupation and livelihood to most families in this neighborhood. — Marie Hartley and Joan Ingilby, *The Yorkshire Dales* (London: Dent, 1956), 250–255.

4. Dr. Fothergill is protesting against Alexander's attention to legal affairs in the Wensleydale villages of Yorkshire.

To John Bartram, Philadelphia, 22 February 1743/4

London, 22.12.1743/4

Esteemed Friend J. Bartram,

I think myself highly obliged in the first place to my friend Dr. Bond for his favourable description of me, and in the next to thyself for thy acceptable present which came safe, and yet more for thy generous offer of assisting me in procuring such material productions as your country affords.[1] I must own it was what I had long wanted, and must have intruded myself into the number of thy correspondents, had not my friend P. Collinson frequently communicated whatever he could spare me. I always admired thy industry and exactness as well as the surprising progress thou has made in the knowledge of plants, a branch of my profession which I have just applied myself to so as to be able to know the principal officinals of our own country, and to collect the best accounts I could meet with of their genuine effects. I claim this acquaintance with them by now and then taking a walk to Peckham [2] or Chelsea,[3] but cannot prevail upon myself to launch far into a study which would rob me of more time to cultivate with success than my present situation will admit of.

The fossil productions have always suited my inclinations most, but I have made but little progress. I don't so much collect with a view to have a great number of odd things together as to have so many productions of different kinds, natures, compositions, figures, and so forth, as when laid together may assist me in forming some general idea of the production of several of their kinds of substances, more consistent with the nature of things than I have yet met with from others. This is the entertainment of leisure hours, and is a structure which can only be executed from a multitude of materials which time perhaps may supply me with, and the kindness of my friends. The *Amianthus*, or cotton stone, was very acceptable. E. Bland had sent me a very little bit, which was the only specimen I had till thine came to hand. The fossil shells were likewise very acceptable. Whatever of this kind comes to hand will always be welcome. Elias likewise sent me a little bit or two of Bolar earth; I should be glad to know whether you have it in plenty, and to have a pound weight or two sent for experiment. He sent me likewise a small square black pyrites. Have you these in plenty? If you have, please to send a few of them. Crystals, spars, ores, sulphurous matters, as liquid or solid bitumens; if you have any marcasites, very singular earths, stones, and fossil shells will be agreeable.

But there is another affair of more consequence than these in which I should be glad of thy assistance. 'Tis possible I may now and then have occasion to prescribe for persons in your country. I should be glad to be informed of what helps I might expect which are peculiar to your country. In the first class of which I must mention mineral waters. Have you any of considerable note? And near the inhabited parts? Hot or cold? chalybeat, sulphurous, or not manifest either, but salt and purgative? Tincture of galls, oak bark, or green tea leaves [laid] in water will discover the first. If sulphurous, the smell will discover it, and its changing silver black; if salt, the taste will manifest it. After I am informed of these circumstances, I can easily give thee direction how to acquire a still more accurate knowledge of their nature and effects.

The next thing I should be glad to be informed about is, what simples of considerable efficacy, peculiar to your clime, at least indigenous, are in use among your practitioners, or even celebrated among the vulgar. I should be glad of some specimens of such, whether roots, leaves, fruits or what else, not barely as specimens to know the plant by, but an handful or two of each, carefully dried for experiments, with the names they are commonly known by.

I am told that the sassafras tree when in bloom casts a most delightful fragrance around it. Pray, has ever any trial been made to procure a distilled water from the flowers? I fancy they would afford a grateful and efficacious one, unless the odoriferous particles are extremely fugitive indeed. I think, if the experiment has not been made, it would be worth while to have some gathered at the proper season and distilled — some with water alone, some with the addition of a third part of rum, molasses spirit or some other spirit, if you have any clean and cheaper. I should be glad to have a few dried flowers sent over, and some put into a quart bottle when fresh gathered, and some molasses spirit or rum poured upon them, and then close corked.

Thus thou sees, my good Friend, that thy generous offer is like to be followed with not a little trouble and some expense, but whatever of this kind happens shall be thankfully repaid, and thy trouble acknowledged in the best manner I can.

I am,
                                    thy obliged Friend
                                    John Fothergill, junior

Whatever figured stones as spars, crystals, talcs, pyrites, and so forth come in thy way, with any other remarkable fossils that occur, will be very acceptable. It just now occurs to my thoughts . . . that a collection of several natural productions of your colony would be a fine addition to your Public Library.[4] No one is fitter for the undertaking than J. Bartram, and some means ought to be considered to make it worth his while. This hint may at least be so far useful as to induce thee to keep a part by thee of everything curious, lest thou should be called upon for that purpose. Farewell —

J.F.

Ms. autograph letter, Bartram Papers, IV, 15, HSP; also published in William Darlington, *Memorials of John Bartram and Humphry Marshall* (Philadelphia: Lindsay, 1849), 333–337.

1. This is Dr. Fothergill's first letter to Bartram, of whom, apparently, he had first heard through Dr. Thomas Bond.
2. Location of Peter Collinson's garden at this period.
3. The Apothecary's Company established Chelsea Physic Garden in 1673.
4. The Library Company of Philadelphia, organized in 1730/31 by Benjamin Franklin, who raised funds from fifty subscribers, was the first subscription library established for public use in the United States. After 1740, the Library Company had its quarters in a room at the State House, now Independence Hall. Any "civil gentleman" was welcome to read the books there, but only subscribers could withdraw volumes. — *Franklin Papers*, ed. Labaree, III, 49.

To John Toft, Leek, Staffordshire, 31 March 1744

London, 31.1.1744

Respected Friend,[1]

Though I have been prevented from sending thee the receipt longer than I intended, I do not omit observing thy request to get it with all expedition. If I can at any time be of any little service, use me freely without an apology! The people at the office demanded no more than what is mentioned in the receipt, and I paid no more.

The city has been in much flurry today on account of the Declaration of War against France [2] which was performed at noon with the usual formalities. Unthinking heads are pleased with the show, little considering the unhappy consequences which must unavoidably ensue to thousands of our own species, equally sensible of hardships with ourselves. Providence has signally protected this nation, and even lately. May the Hand that averted the stroke never be forgot! Please to remember my dear Love to thy Brother Joshua, thy wife and son, and give my kind respects to Dr. Key.

I am, thy affectionate Friend,
John Fothergill, Junior

Ms. autograph letter, Port. 22/90, LSFL.

1. John Toft (1713–1768) was the brother of Joshua Toft, a well-known Quaker minister in Staffordshire.

2. To check the rising power of France, Britain had considered support of Maria Theresa's cause in the War of the Austrian Succession "a glorious undertaking," necessary to preserve the balance of power in Europe. France, eager to prevent further expansion of British commerce, declared war on England 15 March 1744. Britain's official response, a declaration of war against France, when announced 31 March 1744 in London and Westminster, was received amidst the loudest acclamations ever expressed on a like occasion. — Samuel Boyse, *An Historical Review of the Transactions of Europe from the Commencement of the War with Spain in 1739 to the Insurrection in Scotland in 1745* (London, 1746), 11–13; *A Compleat View of the Present Politics, in a Letter from a German Nobleman* (London, 1743).

To Joseph Fothergill, Warrington, Lancashire, 23 June 1744

London, 23.4.1744

Dear Brother,

'Tis almost unnecessary to tell thee that I was glad to hear of thy safe return and that thou found all well at home. The little accommodations I could give thee don't deserve mentioning again; if they had been better, it was my duty to make thee as welcome as myself to whatever I had in that respect.

As I would willingly stand fair with my Friends everywhere and cannot be unconcerned where my profession is involved though ever so slightly, thou may be sure it gave me not a little surprise to find from thy letter that I had been so extremely ill used. Thou requested me to furnish thee with material to vindicate my character, and 'twas the part of a Brother and a Friend to do so.[1] But with regard to the Minute which seems to be the principal cause of complaint, I need say very little; the Minute is the act of the Yearly Meeting; and why should I or anyone else be called upon to vindicate that assembly? 'Tis unreasonable to expect it from me, and those who are not content with the Minute ought not to exclaim against me but that body. That is all the justification that any person is entitled to from me upon this head, but there are two other points in the charge which affect me singly.

I'll endeavour to give thee or any other thinking person all the satisfaction I can. The first is a most uncharitable reflection upon my integrity that the little share I had in that affair was owing to interested views. I abhor such a conduct from my soul, but as nothing will work upon people who are accustomed to follow no other motive in their conduct but interest, to believe any are free from the same bias and capable of acting upon any other principle, I despair of being believed, whatever I may say. The principal sticklers against the present Minute therefore take this method to black my reputation by paying as great a compliment to my abilities as they detract from my integrity, but they are equally mistaken . . . I give thee authority to assure them in the first place that the person of all others I am most intimate with in London, and who has it more within his power to affect my interest than all the rest taken together on the side of the question I appeared with, was in his sentiments directly contrary to my way of thinking. In the next place, both personal friendship, a great many obligations, a prospect of more, would have certainly induced me to think as he did, if a careful and mature consideration of the arguments on both sides had not inclined the scale the other way. I have nothing to hope for, I have nothing to expect. Will this declaration satisfy? If not, be assured that nothing will, and that no Christian spirit can in this case activate the promoters of the calumny.

I know that in cases of this nature, numbers are led into things unawares, from want of knowing both sides of the affair. They have no opportunity of informing themselves of the whole truth but from persons who have declared themselves party, and are suffering disappointment by traducing an innocent person.

The next charge, I observe, is that . . . I rudely interrupted others, and prevented them from delivering their intentions. 'Tis possible I might stand up when another did. I was served so more than once. A youthful ardor might perhaps prompt me to do something contrary to the rules of good order which I might not then perceive. And supposing this to be the case is it just, is it reasonable, is it becoming to men of understanding to suppose that even this absurd behavior of mine could have weight with the Meeting to have fallen in with my sentiments, if they had not carried some sort of conviction with them? A youth, a stripling unaccustomed to speak in large assemblies, throws out in haste a few remarks in a broken hesitating manner; they appear just to the Meeting and the affair is issued. Those who happened to lose their favourite point immediately dress him up in a bearskin, and then make an outcry. And thus I have commenced as an advocate for the city of

London, to gain the esteem of some who can do me very little service and to displease those who are my best friends. But I scorn to be a tool to any party, and 'tis ungenerous, nay wicked, to raise such an insinuation.

But the whole of my crime is this: I prevented the Minute as it now stands from being rendered absolutely preposterous. It consists of three parts. The first directs what shall be done when the party's inclinations are known. The second describes in what condition they stand, if they proceed to accomplish their intentions, and in general prescribes what is necessary to be done by the Society. I say, in general, because as this was the tender point, those who drew up the Minute were cautious of tying down Monthly Meetings by any particular direction when and how far the offenders should be dealt with, only that something should be done.

Then comes the concluding part which directs their absolute disunion in case what has been done proves of no effect. If the Minute is read over carefully, this must appear to be the plain state of it. The mighty outcry against me is because I prevented the third paragraph from being placed where the second is, and the second to have come last, which I take the liberty once more to assert would have made the Minute absolutely preposterous, without gaining one grain of weight in their scale who would have the parties cut off without any dealing at all.[2]

This is the short of the case, and I dare appeal to every person not biased and of common understanding for a justification of my conduct in this respect. But the case was too plain to admit of any debate, except by two or three whom I was amazed to see so inconsiderate. The Meeting acquiesced with the explanation I gave them, and the thing was presently concluded. I am really sorry to find any Friends so pleased as they seem to be with the distinction of London and the County Friends. As for my part I know not that we have any other than one interest, and I speak my opinion for the good of the whole, as far as I know. But since the Friends of our County are disposed to be of a different opinion, I must request thee to acquaint those Friends, who once thought I might serve them in the capacity of a representative, that I must beg to be excused from engaging in it, since I can never submit to serve those who have not as good an opinion of my honesty as my abilities.

Through an unexpected engagement, thy box was not sent till last fifth day. The certificates came in S. Clark's parcel. I have taken some care about the poor woman's letter; when I hear what is done, I'll let thee know. Excuse me for detaining thee with such a long detail of circumstances. Use them as thou pleases; let me know the worst.

And believe me, with dear love to Sister, relations, and self,

Thy affectionate Brother

J. Fothergill, Jun.

Ms. autograph letter, Port. 22/89, LSFL.

1. The Society of Friends had become exercised because many younger members were marrying non-Quakers in ceremonies conducted by "priests." The Society feared its membership would be decreased by such marriages. Some Friends believed strong measures should be adopted to discourage "marrying out." During the discussion reported in this letter, many Friends thought that Dr. Fothergill's attitude was too liberal.

2. Part I of the Minute of 1744 earnestly advised, as hitherto, that Friends should endeavor to prevent young members from "marrying out" by priests. Part II, placed in this position by Dr. Fothergill's proposal, stated that "When any do marry by the Priest, or in any other manner contrary to the Established Rules of our Society, they shall be dealt with in a Spirit of Christian Love and tenderness agreeable to our known Discipline . . . after the Commission of such Offense and during such Dealing, their Collection shall not be received, nor shall they be relieved in the manner of Poor Friends, nor be admitted to sit in Meetings of Discipline until they are restored in Unity with the Monthly Meeting to which they belong."

Part III (placed last, by Dr. Fothergill's advice) reads: "And we earnestly advise all Friends that you watch diligently over One another for Good, and that you deal in due time with such Offenders and all others that walk disorderly, Endeavouring to Reclaim and Restore them by brotherly Admonition and Counsel . . . But when after patient waiting, you find that your continued Labour of Love hath not its desired Effect, That you neglect not to testify against and Disown such persons; thereby preventing the Reproach and Dishonor which might be brought upon our Holy Profession through their misconduct, and that the End and Design of Friends in settling a wholesome Discipline amongst us may be answered: which is substituted in Lieu of the Minute made in 1741, respecting Marriage by Priests." — Minutes of London Yearly Meeting, no. 9, pp. 233–234.

To Dr. Charles Alston, University of Edinburgh, 19 September 1744

Gracechurch Street, London 19.7.1744

Dear Doctor,

I have several times intended to acknowledge the receipt of thy obliging letter in answer to several of mine, but have been and still am prevented. I was in hopes to do it now, but time will not permit, so that

I can only acknowledge the obligation I am under and at the same time contract a fresh one by recommending a gentleman who brings this to your notice. His name is North Vigor. He intends to apply himself closely to the study of medicine, and has been initiated into some parts of it in the country. I was consulted about the place where he might expect to receive the most information, and I think justly gave the preference to Edinburgh. I imagined he might have this farther advantage there of being introduced to some of the gentlemen who teach. I have therefore used this freedom to request this privilege for him from thee. His sobriety and application I hope will render him not unworthy of the favour.[1]

I have been doing little this summer but looking after two or three patients, and preparing myself for some examinations, which I have lately undergone at our College in order to be admitted as a Licentiate. I can't be a Fellow as I am not a graduate in either of our English Universities. I might have deferred it some years longer, but I was advised to offer myself and have gone through the requisite trials for that purpose.[2]

The gentleman who gave me the Persian Manna requested my sentiments on it. I looked into such of the writers as I had by me, extracted the opinions of some of them, and added my own conjectures that this must be the *Tereniabin* of the ancient Arabians. He carried my papers to the Royal Society where they were read. But there are few in that body any way solicitous about those affairs. Whether they will be published or not, I can't tell.[3]

In the paper on Neutral Salts which is in the *Medical Essays*,[4] there is one paragraph so darkly expressed that no one can so much as guess at the true meaning of it. I had some thoughts of explaining it in a subsequent volume, but happened to mention it too late. What kind of performances or from what persons (whether the respective members solely or not) your new Society [5] accepts of I know not, but I should be glad of some opportunity of mentioning my sentiments more at large and presenting the public with a necessary hint or two on that affair — which in short amounts to this: That the principal difference betwixt Alkaline salts arises from the Neutral they contain; that in prescribing the anti-emetic mixture of Rivière,[6] 'tis difficult to order such an exact proportion of acid and alkali as to have an exactly neutral fluid; that *Sal Tart.*, which is frequently used for the *Sal Abs.*, fraudulently contains very little neutral salt. If it is neutral 1 scruple will saturate 1/2 ounce of *suc. Lim.* But genuine *Sal Abs.*, if the ashes in making it are thoroughly washed, contains near a third of the neutral salt, which as it has no effect upon the acid, if the usual proportion of 1 scruple to the 1/2 ounce be used, will leave the mixture strongly acescent. I tried 6 different parcels of what I met with in 6 different places for *Sal. Abs.* Two of the parcels which I know were genuine required — one, grains 28; the other, 32, to saturate 1/2 ounce. Had I a suitable opportunity of correcting that passage, I would not only say what I there intended to say but add a few experiments to prove these hints, which in this place I am satisfied are necessary. I should likewise propose that the cheapest alkali to be met with should be used upon these occasions, if it appeared from experiment to be alike useful, in order to prevent the common abuse of substituting one for another of them.

But to keep myself in employ I have been laying out a plan for a more important affair, and which if I can succeed in it, I almost flatter myself will be of some service to the Faculty here. It is to give some account of the mineral waters in the neighborhood of this place. I should not go to work as Dr. Short [7] has done and tire the public with a number of dry experiments. My design is to make the exactest trials I can, and only to publish the result of them. I would give an account in the introduction of my proceeding in general, and why I deemed such a water to be of this or that class, and in short the rationale of those experiments we make to discover the virtues of mineral waters. Though we have a considerable number, yet they might be reduced to a very narrow compass, and when ranged according to their virtues and quality might easily be consulted by those who are disposed to use or recommend them. But this is only in embryo — and may be work of years if I live . . . Permit me to assure thee that I am

Thy respectful obliged Friend
John Fothergill

Ms. autograph letter, Alston Collection, UEL.

1. North Vigor completed his medical studies satisfactorily in the University of Edinburgh. His thesis, *Dissertatio medica inauguralis de diabete* (Edinburgh, 1747), is dedicated with expressions of deep gratitude to his uncles *Guglielmo et Benjamini Vigor, Mercatoribus Russiensibus*, whose generosity had made possible his medical education.

2. In the eighteenth century, a license to practice medicine in London and within seven miles adjacent to the city was only obtainable by passing a strict examination

set by the Censors of the Royal College of Physicians. One of the requirements was ability to translate at sight passages of Latin selected from the writings of ancient medical authors. — Fox, 144. Fellowship in the Royal College of Physicians, founded in 1518 by Henry VIII, was restricted to holders of medical degrees from Oxford or Cambridge. The College excluded from its ranks physicians of alien birth, those who held foreign degrees, Roman Catholics, members of certain dissenting sects, "irregular" practitioners, surgeons, apothecaries, and practitioners of midwifery. — Lloyd G. Stevenson, "The Siege of Warwick Lane," *Journal of the History of Medicine and Allied Sciences*, 7 (1952): 105–121. John Fothergill, Jr., M.D., was admitted Licentiate of the Royal College of Physicians on 16 October 1744. — Exact date obtained by the kindness of Dr. Kenneth Robson, Registrar, Royal College of Physicians.

3. The specimen of *Manna Persicum* received from Peter Collinson (see letter to Dr. Alston, 14 September 1743) was a "dirty reddish brown-coloured mass," within which Dr. Fothergill found, embedded in earth, numerous "globules hard as sugar-candy and as pleasing to the taste," together with "sticks, leaves, and long reddish pods" which held "from 1 to 6 or 7 . . . somewhat kidney-shaped seeds." Under his personal care these seeds produced little plants such as Rauwolf must have found on his travels in 1582–83. Dr. Fothergill identified this *Manna Persicum* with the *Tereniabin* of the ancient Arabian physicians, reported by Rauwolf as derived from the camel's thorn (*Alhagi*), and described by Joseph Pitton de Tourneforte (1656–1708) as mentioned by Avicenna. — John Fothergill, M.D., "Observations on the Manna Persicum," *Phil. Trans. R.S.*, 43:86–94 (1744/5); *Works*, ed. Lettsom, I, 257–263.

4. John Fothergill, M.D., "Remarks on the neutral salts of plants and on Terra Foliata Tartari," *Medical Essays and Observations*, V (1742), 177–183.

5. The new society — soon to be known as the Philosophical Society (of Edinburgh) — had absorbed the group which since 1731 had been compiling *Medical Essays and Observations*. — Fox, 137.

6. Lazare Rivière (1589–1625), a French physician who combined citric acid with bicarbonate of soda to make an effervescing potion.

7. Dr. Thomas Short (1690–1772), a Scottish physician residing at Sheffield, had published a volume of 359 pages entitled *The Natural, Experimental and Medicinal Waters of Derbyshire, Lancashire and Yorkshire, particularly those of Scarborough, wherein they are carefully examined and compared . . . together with the natural history of the earths, minerals and fossils through which the chief of them pass . . . a methodical abstract of all the treatises hitherto published on these waters, with many observations and experiments* (London, 1743). The volume included four copper plates representing the crystals and the salts of thirty-four of these waters.

To Dr. Robert Key, Leek, Staffordshire, 6 October 1744

London, 6.8.1744

Dear Doctor,[1]

Since I wrote to thee by S. Lucas I have had a further opportunity of enquiring about the price of Cowper's *Anatomy*,[2] and believe, if it be not disposed of, that I can get 5 Guineas for it of a neighbouring surgeon, supposing the book is clean and in good order. As I thought this information might be of some use to the person who has it, I have given thee the trouble of this letter chiefly on that account.

I wrote everything by that opportunity which occurred to my thoughts in the least worth thy notice. Since then scarcely anything material has cast up. I am lately returned from an excursion I made to Bath to see my Father who has been indisposed. He was on a visit to some places about Bristol and Bath. I advised him to make trial of the Lyncomb water, and paid him a visit whilst there, stayed with him about 2 days, and returned with all the expedition I could. Dr. Hillary[3] was well; he has pretty good business, but it's a place that I should choose to reside in the last of all others. The people are accustomed to behave well to everybody while present, but more than that they don't seem to think is expected or necessary.

I made no acquisitions in my progress — my time would not allow any searches after fossils etc. I just took a transient view of the remains of the celebrated ancient temple at Avebury[4] on Marlborough Downs, which, if it was what Dr. Stukeley[5] says it was, has been a most astonishing performance, and by what appears it seems not unlikely. I have no literary news from abroad. Monro is at work on comparative anatomy.[6] He has laid down a very extensive plan and works hard to complete it. And now, with as good a grace as I can, I must intreat thee to remember thy promises; be so good as to favour me with a copy of thy notes as soon as convenience will permit. I want to get the affair out of my hands, but I don't intend to look into it again until I have thy assistance. Pray how did the case proceed which thou mentioned in thy last?

P. Collinson has frequent letters from Dr. Gronovius, who is well, and closely employed as usual in natural history. The little searches I have made that way have, I think, been useful to me, that having applied the little I know in chemistry and natural history of fossils together, I think I am master, as I have hitherto suggested, of a better plan for a general account of mineral waters than most of what have yet appeared in our language. Neither Drs. Short nor Shaw were sufficiently acquainted with both these parts. Dr. Shaw is a chemist, no natural historian. Dr. Short seems to be little of either. Yet the one has written a tract for writers on this subject to follow; the other, one would think from the size of his book, had exhausted Nature.[7] Short's talent is industry — and I wish he could impart some to me, and I was going to say to *Somebody Else*, but this I'll lay down as gently as I can!

I have heard lately from Joshua Plot of Newcastle who I find is an acquaintance of thine; he has promised me some fossils from their part of the country which I fancy must afford some good ones — but I must give over this empty scrawl, and with tenders of my kind respects, conclude myself

Thy affectionate Friend
John Fothergill

Ms. autograph letter, Toft Mss., no. 42, LSFL.

1. Dr. Robert Key of Leek, Staffordshire, is portrayed as a devoted and estimable Friend, loved and respected for his uncommon worth. — "Dr. Key's Character Attempted," Toft Mss. II/72, eulogy by J. Swan, M.D., LSFL.

2. William Cowper (1666–1709), *The Anatomy of Humane Bodies* (Oxford, 1697), illustrated with figures drawn from life by some of the best masters in 114 copper plates; a later English edition, 1737; Latin Edition, 1739. A foreign publisher gave Cowper the copper plates used earlier to illustrate Godfried Bidloo's anatomical text *Anatomia Corporis Humani* (Amsterdam, 1685), which had only a limited sale. Without asking permission, Cowper illustrated his book with these same plates; Bidloo accused Cowper of plagiarism and a heated controversy followed. — Ludwig Choulant, *The History and Bibliography of Anatomical Illustration*, ed. Mortimer Frank (Chicago: University of Chicago Press, 1920), 250–253.

3. William Hillary (1697–1763), the son of Wensleydale Quakers, was born in Birkrigg near Hawes. He was apprenticed to the Bradford apothecary, Benjamin Bartlett, and studied medicine in Leyden. In 1722 he set up practice in Ripon; in 1734 he moved to Bath. — C. C. Booth, "William Hillary, a pupil of Boerhaave," *Medical History*, 7 (1963), 297.

4. In 1694 John Aubrey discovered Avebury's ancient monuments while hunting on the Marlborough Downs. To him "These Downes . . . Sow'n with great Stones, very thick . . . in a dusky evening . . . look like a flock of Sheep . . . One might fancy [the village] to have been the Scene where the Giants fought with Stones against the Gods . . . I was wonderfully surprised at the sight of these vast Stones of which I had never heard before." The archeological significance of this region had in fact been completely overlooked heretofore. The "great Stones" had been used by the countryfolk for building materials. — *Aubrey's Brief Lives*, ed. Dick, xliii.

5. Dr. William Stukeley (1687–1765), trained in medicine and theology, was also celebrated for drollery, absurdity, ingenuity, and superstition. He delighted in long antiquarian tours. Two of his books, *Stonehenge: A Temple Restored to the Druids* (1740) and *Abury: A Temple of the Ancient Druids* (1743), are listed in the catalogue of Dr. Fothergill's library.

6. Alexander Monro, Primus, *An Essay on Comparative Anatomy* (London, 1744).

7. In 1743 Peter Shaw, M.D., published a translation of Fredericus Hoffman's *New Experiments upon Mineral Waters*, to which he added his own study of Scarborough's "spaw water," together with directions for analyses of various other mineral waters. For Dr. Short, see letter of 19 September, above.

To Joshua Toft, Leek, Staffordshire, 6 November 1744

London, 6.9.1744

Dear Friend,[1]

An accidental mislaying of my papers is the reason why I have been so long in answering thy request with regard to the proposal sent down for printing J. Besse's account of Sufferings. Joseph Besse acquainted the Yearly Meeting that the remaining part of his account of Friends Sufferings was nearly ready for the press, and that it would probably take up about five volumes more in octavo of the size with those printed already. He at the same time acquainted the Meeting, that upon considering the work and conferring with the printer, he found that to print the remaining five volumes would cost almost as much to the subscribers as to have the three former volumes reprinted, with what was now ready, in two volumes in folio. He alleged that besides putting the whole account into a better method, leaving out, for new modelling, the tables and indexes, he should by this means have an opportunity of correcting several mistakes that happened in the former volumes.[2]

It was observed upon this representation that the three former volumes would be then wholly useless; it was proposed to print the remaining part in octavo and have a folio edition of the whole likewise. But to this it was answered that two editions of the same work would not be taken off, and that the printer would not undertake it etc. After a good deal of time spent in considering the affair (for I very well remember the debate upon it), the Meeting at last concluded to order the whole to be got ready for the press, and to be printed in folio, as it is now proposed.

So that notwithstanding it appears hard that those who have the three first volumes should be obliged to purchase them again, yet the Meeting upon considering that it would cost as much to have the remaining five volumes as it would to have the whole work amended, methodized and published together, agreed to order it to be done as is now proposed.

The Meeting for Sufferings have ordered a committee to inspect J. Besse's papers, revise them with him, and it was in consequence of the Yearly Meeting's orders that they sent down those proposals, and are taking what care they can that the work may be carefully completed.

96

If any further information is wanted, I'll endeavour to procure it; and am with dear love to Brother's family and thyself,

thy affectionate Friend

John Fothergill, Jun.

P.S. Please to tell Dr. Key that I am in expectation of a letter from him, almost every post.

Ms. autograph letter, Port. 22/92, LSFL.

1. Joshua Toft (1689–1769), a successful Quaker merchant of Leek, Staffordshire, served the Society of Friends for forty-eight years as a minister. During the last fourteen years of his life he was blind, but bravely kept at work. — Crosfield, 114.

2. Joseph Besse (1683?–1757) had been employed from 1729 in preparing for the press an abridgment of the records of sufferings and the first three volumes of *An Abstract of the Sufferings of the People call'd Quakers* were published in octavo, 1733–1738. In 1741 five more volumes were ready for the printer and it was at this Yearly Meeting that Besse had proposed that this method of publication be abandoned in favor of a differently organized two-volume folio edition. This was agreed and Besse reported to Yearly Meeting 1744 completion of the revised manuscript, and Meeting for Sufferings was then asked to send down to the counties proposals for printing it by subscription. Response was slow and it was not until 1753 that the two volumes were printed as that classic work, *A Collection of the Sufferings of the People Called Quakers.*

III
1745-1754

I am happy in an employment that suits my
disposition, that has thus far suported me
decently, and preserves me in great degree
independent, and respected among my
acquaintance.

To Samuel Fothergill, 28.12.1746 O.S.

To Ann Fothergill, Knaresborough, Yorkshire, 2 February 1744/5

London, 12th Mo., 2d, 1744/5.

I can say nothing to thee upon the present distressing occasion [1] but what thy own prudence will suggest to thee; we both feel that our loss is great, yet we don't know it to the full; our best friend, protector, and counsellor is no more; it would be unnatural not to grieve. But still we must remember that he is only gone before to that possession where we shall at last arrive, if we tread in his steps; to excite and encourage one another in this race, oh, may it be our constant employ.

Through his care, and the blessing of kind Providence upon his earnest wishes and prayers, I am at present in a way of life, that both affords me what I have occasion for, and seems not unlikely to continue so; and whilst it is, neither be afraid of wanting thyself, nor think thou art obliged to me. In this part, while I am able, I will be a father, thy friend and brother; I should not say I will be these things; it is that good hand that blesses my endeavours, for that dear good man's sake and thine. Brother Samuel has written to me, but very short hints of every thing. Do, dear Sister, take the first opportunity of acquainting me as fully as thou canst with all that has passed since he began to decline, and if any memorable expressions dropped from him in his illness, please to let me know.

. . . I find Brother has collected most of his papers; the rest I shall be glad to have, in order that, from those I have in my hands, and the rest, I may be able to finish that account which dear Father had begun, partly at my request.

J.F.

Excerpt printed in Crosfield, *Memoirs*, 107.

1. John Fothergill, senior, had died 13 January 1744/5, in Knaresborough, York-shire, where he had lived in retirement for some time with his daughter Ann (1718–1802) as homemaker and devoted nurse.

To Israel Pemberton, Jr., Philadelphia, 11 February 1745

London, 11.12.1744/5

Dear Friend,

I could not well longer forbear throwing a few lines in thy way to revive in some respect a correspondence which though frequently inter-rupted I dare say is not omitted designedly on either side. I heard with great concern of the accident which happened to thee,[1] and with much pleasure I have been informed by several of thy almost total recovery . . .

I doubt not but thou wilt by the time this comes to thy hand be informed of the great loss I have sustained in the removal of my dear and honoured Father. But I am stripped of the best of parents, the kindest friend, my ornament and protector, and even more than I can yet be fully sensible of; the certainty of his happiness and the honourable esteem which survives him in the minds of all who knew him, together with the sympathizing regard of many Friends, at the time they give some ease, yet make the sense of my loss still greater. But through mercy I have never murmured nor repined, but have been kept pretty still, and sometimes in a sort of pleasing pain. He had not long since begun some short hints respecting the early part of his life and travels, partly at my request, partly from a secret drawing in his own mind but had proceeded a very little way. And it has been my unhappiness in some respects to be absent from him so great a part of my life that many of those incidents which he could not but sometimes impart to his family have quite escaped me. I was taken from under his care, to be placed with my mother's relations, when about two[2] years old; and from that time till now, adding all the little sojournings together, I have not been ten months under his roof. I speak it with regret, but the course of my education prevented me from enjoying his company. It was, I know not how, very early implanted in my mind that I could not enjoy any share of my dear Father's affection unless I behaved in such a manner as he recommended, both by precept and example. This often struck me in the midst of my diversions, and was one means of preserving me less culpable than otherwise I should have been. The few papers that he has left I intend to transcribe and show them to some friends here, and if they are not printed (which I am afraid they are too imperfect to be), I'll send thee a copy, but it will be sometime before I can have leisure to sit down to the task. But I prosecute my business not with that satisfaction I used to do; I have lost him for whom I could have laboured with more pleasure than for myself. I valued reputation as I knew it would be agreeable to him, and wished for success, as to see me in an easy situation would make him so. He lessened every care and heightened every enjoyment; allow me then to lament a loss which is not to be repaired.

Your worthy Friends, E. Shipley [3] and White, have been with us, but were much indisposed most of the time. They got better before they left the city, and I hear keep on pretty well.

I was just going to desire thee to remember my love to my dear Father's friends with you, but this is too extensive; a few were intimately beloved by him and he by them; thy worthy Father I know was one, thyself, and both families; to these please to give my dear love, and when it is in my power I hope not to forget their kindness to him. Farewell, dear Friend, and once more be assured that I am

affectionately thine
J. Fothergill

Ms. autograph letter, Pemberton Papers, XXXIV, 9, HSP.

1. Elections in 1742 had been marred by contention and violence in Philadelphia. A sailors' mob had terrorized the city, attacking those "with a plain coat and a broad hat" and Germans from back-country farms, who like the Quakers were conscientious objectors. During the riot many were injured, including Israel Pemberton, who received a severe blow on the head. — Richard Peters, Letterbook, 1737–1750, HSP: letter of 17 November 1742 addressed to Honoured Proprietors; Thayer, *Israel Pemberton*, 48, 49.

2. In the original letter the word *two* is unmistakable. Perhaps this is merely a slip of the pen. John Fothergill, senior, did not make his second journey to America until 1721, when John junior was not yet ten.

3. Elizabeth Shipley (1690–1777) was born in Springfield, Chester County, Pennsylvania. She was the daughter of Samuel Levis, began to preach in young womanhood, and went with Jane Penn on a religious visit to Barbados in 1724–25. In 1728 she married William Shipley and lived in Wilmington, Delaware, for a time. In 1743 she went to England with Esther White on a mission for the Society of Friends, and in 1760 "travelled in the ministry with Hannah Foster in New England." — *The Journal of John Woolman*, ed. Amelia M. Gummere (New York: Scribner, 1922), 539–540.

To William Logan, Philadelphia, 5 March 1744/5

London, 5.1.1744/5

Dear Friend,[1]

I receive thy letters with that cordial satisfaction which I believe thou wishes I should do; they come from the worthy Son of a wise and good Father and must, were it for that reason only, be acceptable, but they are so on their own account. They come from a mind sensible of friendship, and disposed to maintain it with those who it apprehends are like itself, industrious, benevolent, and willing to fill up the duties of this life with credit to themselves and advantage to others: yet regarding other motives, and acting from other principles than either ease or the applauses of men.

With such as these it is my great satisfaction to converse. Their letters help now and then to revive becoming thoughtfulness, and suspend that attachment to things of small importance which I am too prone to slide into, partly from a naturally active disposition, partly from the example, and in this respect, the evil influence of those about me.

But it's time that I take some notice of the agreeable presents which thou sent and intended for me. I received the ms. copy of your last Treaty,[2] which I was pleased with, and am afraid I can only repay the uncommon care and pains thou took upon that occasion by keeping it by me as a monument of thy pleasure in obliging thy Friends. I have likewise received the printed copy which thou sent me of the same Treaty which was very acceptable. My intention in procuring the former Treaty to be reprinted here, was to inform several people here, that the Indians were not despicable, ignorant, stupid brutes, which many persons conceive all those must be who bear the name of Indians; and in the next place to show with what prudence, moderation, and equity they had been and still were treated by the Government of Pennsylvania, and how capable the Indians were of resenting a contrary behaviour. At present I have no thoughts of doing any thing more in that way; but shall be glad of seeing a copy of any future Indian treaties, or any remarkable productions of your press upon any other subject.

I am in great hopes that the rattlesnakes which thou was so kind as to provide for me, are yet safe and well in Philadelphia, and may yet live to come over. I need not mention to thee, how long animals of that kind will live without any visible subsistance, and yet retain a good deal of vigor. Had they been sent at the end of the year, the cold would unavoidably have killed them, either before they left your country, or before they had got into my hands. I believe the properest time to send anything of that kind is in the spring, and then they arrive here in full vigor, in the summer.

I must desire thy acceptance of a little trifling present which I know not whether it will be either useful or agreeable. 'Tis a candlestick to be used in reading or writing. I have put up a pair, one for thyself, another for thy Brother James. They save the eyes very much, and make either reading or writing by candlelight much more easy. I thought one of them would be of some advantage to thy Brother and perhaps not unacceptable to thyself. [Passage omitted.]

I have deferred as long as I can, mentioning a circumstance which I know will give thee pain, but hard as it is I must not omit it. My dear and honourable Father is removed from us. I have sent to thy worthy Father a larger account of it than it would be pleasant for me to write or for thee to receive from me.[3] I can only say at present that I am glad I was not ignorant of his worth before I lost him, and that at least I had resolved to afford him all the satisfaction I could, and make some returns of gratitude for his abundant care of me, for sometime before he was taken from me. I can say no more at present, but that I am with kind respects . . .

thy affectionate Friend
John Fothergill

The original letter was once in the possession of Dr. R. Hingston Fox of London; a typescript copy is in Port. 38/82, LSFL.

1. William Logan (1718–1776), son of James and Sarah (Read) Logan, after attending school in Bristol, England, under the supervision of his uncle, Dr. William Logan, returned to Philadelphia for training in the counting house of another uncle, his mother's brother-in-law, Israel Pemberton senior, whose first wife was Rachel Read. William Logan became an able merchant, active in public affairs, holding office as provincial councilor from 1747 to 1775. Upon his father's death in 1751, he inherited Stenton, the family mansion, where he lived the rest of his life, devoting much time to improvement of the agricultural resources of this vast estate. — *Hannah Logan's Courtship*, ed. A. C. Myers (Philadelphia: Ferris and Leach, 1904), 156.

2. Representatives from Pennsylvania, Maryland, and Virginia met in Lancaster with chiefs of the Six Nations in 1744. Pennsylvania's Governor Thomas persuaded the southern provinces to come to terms with the Indians in disputes over territory. The Iroquois made overtures to the Catawbas, who promised to maintain neutrality. By agreements of this treaty, protection of Pennsylvania's borders seemed for a time to be assured. — Tolles, *James Logan*, 183, 184.

3. This account sent to James Logan has not been located in Philadelphia.

To Tabitha Horner, Leeds, Yorkshire, 19 October 1745

London, 19.8.1745

Dear Friend,

When I received thy very acceptable letter of the 21st Inst., I did not intend to let it lie by me so long unanswered, but so it has happened, and I have only to intreat thy usual indulgence to me. It gave me and thy Friends here a sensible pleasure to hear of thy safe return home and with so much reason to be satisfied with thy journey — but it was scarce possible that it should have been otherwise.[1]

If thy indisposition is not entirely carried off but that now and then some returns of pain are felt, I should recommend the use of Limewater made from burnt oyster shells: one pound of the burnt shells will require about 10 pints of water to be poured upon them. As soon as the boiling is over, put one ounce of Sassafras bark, 2 of Stick liquorice, 2 of Juniper berries, and half an ounce of either sweet fennel, cassia or annis seeds, as most suits thy palate. Let stand 24 hours, run the liquor through a cloth and bottle it for use. Betwixt 1/4 and 1/2 a pint may be taken twice a day, at the most convenient times; and if a quarter of a pint with half as much warm milk put to it, could be taken every morning before rising, I think it would be of service.[2] In some very obstinate cases of this sort, I have met with great success from this method which I was induced to fall into upon considering the nature and effects of Bristol Water.[3] If any return of thy disorder makes trial of it necessary, be pleased to inform me of its success.

I believe it is very true what thou asks me about Dr. Clark. M. Weston has been his friend and managed his affairs for him. She has recently been dangerously ill, but is recovering, and as soon as she is able to go abroad, I suppose they will proceed. 'Tis of consequence, I find, in the interest of the order. N. Tillotson and the Dr. Bean are strong instances. Yet there is something to me extremely dangerous in such conduct. Should either of their wives tell the offending person: I am not so happy as I expected, or as thou hast desired me — what remorse it would occasion or might it to occasion, at least.[4] But I must leave a subject which people in our situation are oftener more fond of speaking than acting in — and turn to one of a more serious nature.

I don't doubt but that it has been a very trying, afflicting time with you in the county upon many accounts. The apprehension of approaching danger, on one hand; [5] a fear of doing anything which might not have good effects among ourselves; a desire of promoting the public safety, so far as could be done, on the other, have, I question not, occasioned thee many anxious painful inquiries. Many will consult their fears more than their duty, [6] and embarrass themselves, and bring difficulties upon others. It may probably be some satisfaction to know what is done here. I'll transcribe a Minute which was agreed upon yesterday at the Meeting for Sufferings, which will introduce and explain my sentiments pretty clearly.

[*Most of this Minute is omitted, its conciliatory tone being well summarized in the following paragraph.*]

As we are conscious of our firm regard and affection to our rightfull Sovereign, King George and sensible of the obligations we are under of fidelity and chearfull submission to his mild and just government, so we trust that our principle against bearing arms is so well known to all that our not joining in such associations and subscriptions will be attributed to no other cause than a conscientious adherence to our Christian belief and persuasion.

The Great Council of the Nation are now met. Let us now cheerfully comply with their decisions for the public safety. We are then acting the part of good Subjects, and if we promote a true regard for the King's Honour and security among ourselves to the utmost of our power, we shall not be charged with ingratitude — threatening as the present Rebellion is. I am almost as concerned at what may be the consequences of this general Vigour. If the Chiefs are not rewarded as they expect, they will perhaps be as clamourous as they are now cordial.

But I am called away; please to send a copy of the Minute to B.B. [7] Give my dear love to the family, and be assured that I am

Thy affectionate Friend,

J. Fothergill

Ms. autograph letter, Port. 22/95, LSFL.

1. Tabitha Horner (1693/4–1746), described as "portly, but very agreeable and of an upright, majestic appearance, of an affable and generous conduct, with nobility of mind," had distinguished herself throughout England as a Quaker preacher, and especially during a long journey undertaken alone which took her into remote parts of England and into Wales, covering 2,200 miles on horseback during an absence of many months from her home in Leeds. — Thomas Lancaster's Testimony, Horner Mss., LSFL.

2. If Tabitha Horner's disorder was the result of hyperacidity, the homemade limewater Dr. Fothergill recommended would have been helpful. The herbal ingredients suggested were to provide pleasant flavoring. Homemade medicines were fre-

quently in use at a time when chemists' shops dispensing drugs were not numerous.

3. Presumably bottled water obtained from springs near Bristol, where Clifton, a district at the west end of the city, was a favorite watering place in the eighteenth century.

4. No information has been found elsewhere confirming this gossip about itinerant gospel teams.

5. Residents of the North of England were greatly alarmed by the threat of a French invasion led by the Young Pretender, Charles Edward Stuart. Actually, Charles Edward with only a few friends had landed in the Hebrides in early August, crossed Scotland, gathering an army of Highlanders as he went, occupied Edinburgh, defeated a British force at Preston Pans on the Firth of Forth on 21 September and was proceeding southward.

6. The Society of Friends found practical means to aid British soldiers on their march through the northern counties of England. Several of the most prominent Quakers of London volunteered to provide warm woolen garments designed to fit under the soldiers' uniforms to protect them from the bitter weather they would encounter on their northward march. When the purveyors of General Wade's army arrived in Darlington (County Durham), they asked help from all the bakers and butchers in town, urging them to have supplies of food ready in quantity when troops on the march to Newcastle arrived. Throughout the North of England, response to the needs of the soldiers was general, especially from Quakers realizing the need for defense of their loved country. — W. Hylton Dyer Langstaffe, F.S.A., *The History of the Parish of Darlington in the Bishopric of Durham* (Darlington: The Proprietors of the Darlington and Stockton Times, 1849), 158, 159; also published by Henry Parker, 377 Strand, London, in 1854.

7. Benjamin Bartlett of Bradford.

To Alexander Fothergill, Carr End, Wensleydale, Yorkshire, 4 January 1746

London, 4.11.1745/6

Dear Brother,

I received thine of 5 October in due course which was very acceptable. When it came to hand I proposed to have wrote to thee very shortly but have been delayed by several unexpected affairs. — As I doubt not but thou has some method of getting a sight of the public papers, thou sees everything there that I can inform thee of with respect to the national concerns. I interest myself in news as little as possible, since it commonly happens that the lie of one day begets one for the succeeding. Since the peace concluded between the Empire, Prussia and Poland, we have in general been very easy, both with regard to the Rebellion at home and the threatened invasion from France. I mean with regard to their consequences. It will be doubtless the interest of France to support the Rebellion to the utmost of their power, as it will detain our forces at home and dispirit our allies. It may possibly even be kept up all winter, as ships may continually slip in during the long winter nights, in spite of the utmost vigilance of our admirals. But as so strong a force is sent against them, Carlisle taken, the people in Scotland arming for the Government, and France in fear of a powerful diversion, the Rebellion must be crushed.[1] The King and Parliament are unanimous, therefore set that lie to the account of the Jacobites.

Admiral Vernon [2] has struck his flag. This will be worked up against the Government. But the reluctance with which he obeyed any rules or orders whatever, made it, I am told, quite necessary to recall him. If thou reads the *Gentleman's Magazine,* in that for December thou will see a letter (I have forgot the page) addressed to the good people of England, and showing them what reasons they have to hope well, and how little to fear — wrote by a near relation of thine. It was printed and reprinted in one of our daily papers, and taken into the magazine for the public encouragement.[3] It was the first political essay he ever published — and I fancy it will be the last. — The author will prove mistaken in one point. He apprehended that the D. of C.[4] would not have stopped at Carlisle, but would have followed the rebels till they had passed the opulent city of Glasgow, which by his staying at Carlisle they now are plundering. However he had doubtless his reasons for it which at this distance it is impossible to know. — The people believed a long time that we had got the younger son caged in the Tower, but that belief now loses ground; and he is sunk into Derwentwater's son.[5]

I shall be obliged to thee for the bone thou mentions, and with it what other curiosities of that nature have occurred to thee. I hear thou has some thought of seeing Warrington ere long with J.R.[6] — I have wrote to Sister this evening and have given in to her opinion. I should be glad to know the terms proposed, and how 100 pounds might be best settled to her advantage, that she might always command the produce of that sum or the capital itself in case of emergencies, for I think it in some sort my duty to make her a present of so much, as dear Father had not in his power to provide so well for her as I could wish.

Remember my dear love to Sister and relations, and accept the same from

Thy affectionate Brother
J. Fothergill

To Alexander Fothergill, January 4, 1746

Ms. autograph letter, Fothergill Family Papers, Wallis Collection.

1. In the fall, Charles Edward had invaded England, taken Carlisle, and moved on through Lancashire toward London. English Jacobites and Lowland Scots, however, gave him small support, and although by 4 December he had pushed south as far as Derby, he came to recognize the hopelessness of conquering England with his small army and fell back to Glasgow. He was decisively defeated at Culloden in April 1746.

2. Sir Edward Vernon (1684–1757) had had a stormy but distinguished career in the Royal Navy. In April 1745 he had been promoted to be Admiral of the White and assigned to command in the North Sea — an important post because of the threat of a French invasion in support of the Young Pretender. Angered because he was not appointed to supreme command of the British naval forces, he complained of his treatment and in December 1745 asked to "quit a command" where he had been "contemptuously used." News of this action appeared 4 January 1746 in the *London Daily Advertiser.*

3. Dr. Fothergill's letter to the *Gentleman's Magazine* has not been identified among several others, unsigned, dealing with the same subject. Alexander Fothergill's personal papers contain an account of an unusual adventure, 17 December 1745, when he rode out from Carr End with a party of neighbors to Clifton Moors near Penrith. They witnessed a minor engagement in which Loyalist soldiers were put to rout by the Rebels. In the confusion which followed, Alexander's horse was seized by some soldiers, and he lost sight of his companions. While wandering on the moors, he attracted attention because of his dalesman's garb and consequently was questioned as to why he was there. Once he actually talked to General Oglethorpe. Luckily he found a deserted cottage where he spent the night with other refugees. Next morning he went to headquarters bringing with him weapons found on the moors and in return received his stolen horse.
Alexander's opinions on the conduct of the war agree with Dr. Fothergill's views. — "A Quaker Critic of an Engagement in the Forty-five," *Army Quarterly* (London), 11 (1940): 329–335.

4. William Augustus, Duke of Cumberland, who led the British Army in quelling the Rebellion of 1745/6.

5. Newspapers had reported a mystery when H.M.S. *Sheerness* captured a French privateer, the *Soleil,* bound from Dunkirk to Montrose, Scotland. In addition to a considerable number of soldiers on board, there were civilian passengers, including "a Mr. Radcliffe with a young gentleman he calls his son." Rumors started that this youth was Henry Stuart, Charles Edward's younger brother. Later investigation proved that Mr. Radcliffe was actually Charles Radcliffe, fifth titular Earl of Derwentwater, who had been associated with the Stuart cause in Paris and in Rome. As soon as he was identified, he was taken off the *Soleil* together with the "young gentleman," who really was his son, James Bartholomew Radcliffe. Both prisoners were transferred to the Tower of London, where Charles Radcliffe was condemned to death and beheaded as a traitor. Young James, after long delay, was released from prison under pardon because of his youth. He remained in England, eventually married, and became the third Earl of Newburgh. — *Horace Walpole's Correspondence with Sir Horace Mann,* edited by W. S. Lewis and others (New Haven: Yale University Press, 1954, The Yale Edition of Horace Walpole's Correspondence, v. 17), 172, 173, 180, 181.
To appreciate Dr. Fothergill's play on words — "sunk into Derwentwater's son" —

one must know that the Radcliffes had chosen the designation Derwentwater for their earldom from the lovely lake of that name in Cumberland. Their family mansion stood on one of Derwentwater's larger islands.

6. Ann Fothergill's unidentified suitor; possibly John Routh of Manchester. Whoever he was, Ann remained a spinster all her life.

To Samuel Fothergill, Warrington, Lancashire, 30 January 1746

London, 30.11.1745/6

Dear Brother,

I received thy acceptable letter by last post and thou'll excuse me for sending to thee so soon and before I can inform thee what is said to thy account, having yet had no opportunity of showing it to anyone. I wrote the earlier that I might not occasion any disappointment in regard to money, and to assure thee that I cannot at present command 5 guineas. I have 120 pounds in two Friends' hands here from whom I cannot yet demand it; 20 pounds I lately remitted to T. Areskine; 50 pounds I paid to J. Hunt on Brother Joseph's account, and this with some little trifling sums is my all. But as I know now where it will be acceptable, if ever I should be master of more, thy own security will be all I shall expect.

Brother Alexander writes to me that there is 60 pounds due me out of the Carr End estate, and requests that it may lie awhile in his hands, for which he'll give me security. I propose to give this to Sister Ann as part of 100 pounds I intend hers, so that if she is satisfied with having it there, I am quite so, and therefore Uncle Hough if he pleases may reconvey the estate at Carr End to Brother Alexander.

I am in more pain about Brother Joseph than I know how to express. I write to him by this post with a mixture of grief and compassion. Shall I write to Uncle Hough or his father Kelsal? [1] What can be done? Something must, and the sooner the better; 'tis no trifling now.

I am sorry the horse came lame. He was quite sound when he went hence and in very good condition. I shall be obliged to thee for thy care about a horse; I have yet seen none to please me. I need not tell thee that he must be broke to the road. If anything should come in my way I'll acquaint thee first post, so that unless necessity urges thee to conclude the bargain instantly, delay it and let me know. I paid thy last

111

bill for M. Kinsey at sight, to save any further trouble and before I received thy advice on it.

I am obliged to go to Kingston, about 12 miles off, almost every other day at present to see a patient. He has been frequently and severely afflicted with an uncommon disorder, and is at length committed to my care. What success I may meet with I know not, if it's answerable to my wishes I shall be an instrument of helping the only son of a very opulent family to enjoy without misery the fruits of his parents' industry.[2] This takes up a good deal of my time which seems to be still more and more divided and employed amongst the sick; though not in the most lucrative manner, yet to my solid content and often exciting thankful addresses to the great supporter of his[3] creatures. Farewell, dear Samuel, and let us not forget amid public confusion or private anxiety that it is to him we owe our all, and that he is worthy of our first, our latest cares. I commit you all to his protection and am

Your afflicted, affectionate Brother
J. Fothergill

Ms. autograph letter, Port. 22/101, LSFL.

1. Joseph's father-in-law. Joseph was apparently in financial straits.
2. The patient was the young son of a wealthy Quaker merchant, Thomas Barnard of Fenchurch Street, who retired from business at the age of seventy-one to live in Kingston-upon-Thames. — Records of Surrey and Sutton Births and Burials, LSFL.
3. Dr. Fothergill does not capitalize such references to deity.

To Tabitha Horner, Leeds, Yorkshire, 20 February 1746

London, 20.12.1745/6

Dear Friend,

I often think it is a great advantage to have a Friend to converse with who is willing to take up with a very slender entertainment. I am sure of late I have been in no condition to afford any other. But I am wearied of complaining of myself, and yet perceive that it will be an inexhaustible topic! I own thy letters often do me good, and I can't but endeavour to procure as frequent returns as I can, if thou art still kind enough to accept of the trifles I send as one kind of payment. Thy concern on my Sister's account is becoming thy regard for us all; I'm afraid she'll give way; her affections have become a party against her. Early friendships often produce nearer alliances; and love for one's native soil is strongly implanted in many. I am happy that it's indifferent to me; but I fancy this, though a secret yet, is one strong inducement. I wrote her immediately upon receiving thine, and once more put her in mind of our dear Father's opinion of the whole affair, but J.R.[1] is now over, and I imagine the thing will be agreed upon. Sammie knows my sentiments; his tenderness to her may have induced him to give way, but he is not hearty. Alexander is his strongest advocate; and interest, the prospect of his family's situation, and the estate that may center in hers, is his bait. May not I know the person who had affection enough for my Sister to wish her this? I shall esteem him as a Friend, though I fear I must not call him Brother, a title which I can't at first very cordially apply elsewhere.

Alas! I see little effects from all the visits we have been favoured with. B. Kidd[2] alone is like himself, a true Gospel minister. During the time he was with us, I was obliged to be out of town at Kingston very frequently so that I had scarcely half an hour of his company. There are none besides thyself and him to whom I can unbosom myself with the utmost freedom, and when I miss an opportunity of confessing to him, I'm like an honest Catholic burthened for want of absolution. Twice I was with him at a meeting, and much to my satisfaction. As to the rest, I have found little but noise. I scratched out *we* lest I should do anybody injustice. Ed. Peckover[3] is with us, — and *semper idem*. He may be honest, may think it his duty; he is esteemed, admired . . . but my hapless soul meets with nothing but pompous sound. But I lament poor Isaac Sharpless,[4] with unfeigned pain. He copies, and that's the ready way to lose the original. He was sometimes hard put to it to find words to clothe very incoherent matter; and this will be forever the case with people who will be great preachers, cost what it will. I have long paid him a just regard, and [he] so deserved esteem that it is with the utmost pain that I see him in tracks that lead to a fatal precipice. He is removing to Hitchin which will not contribute to his real advantage, I fear, whatever it may do to his interest.

Mary Smith[5] and her companion are yet with us. The first is less tart [in her remarks] than she used to be; full of commendations to the hopeful youth and prophetic raptures upon their excellencies. But she deals so much in dictionary words and unintelligible jargon, and never fails to display such gross affectation and conceit that she has quite lost my attention. She does not spare them in her addresses to the supreme

113

being: *Generalissimo* appeared two or three times in a prayer for the Duke of Cumberland. *Sanctum Sanctorum* is familiar. *Coeval, coeternal, coessential, essentiality, specious ideas,* and a multitude of such terms which she throws out at random would make a person of any degree of common sense quite sick of the poor conceited enthusiast. But T. W-te-d [6] and some others are rapt into the third heaven the moment she opens her lips. The very sound of her voice, when they know not a word she says, sets them on fire — and they are companions of angels immediately. But it's a melancholy case, and not to be sported with. It's in vain to think of a remedy where neither the parties themselves nor those they converse with apprehend any disease.

I believe the affair of E.G. with G.D.'s nephew is entirely a mistake; [7] at least I never saw any room to suspect it, and I believe that E.G. would inform her father of it the moment she perceived any designs of that kind; he will leave the place and go abroad as soon as any opportunity offers. The other business is just as it was, if anything rather upon the decline.

I was surprised last night by a letter from Brother Samuel with an account of my Mother's unexpected decease.[8] It is one of those events which humanity obliges us to be affected at, yet silently to acquiesce under. I am glad she received the little marks of the regard I owed her, and which had she lived, should have sometimes been repeated.

I am obliged to thee for thy care, but I have not yet paid William Hodgson,[9] which is chiefly owing to confinement from a stroke upon my ankle, but I hope to be at liberty in a few days more to go about as usual.

A. Purver [10] has published two numbers of his translation of the Old Testament, with large notes. The numbers are one shilling each, and he computes the whole will come to about three Guineas. I think both he and the work deserve encouragement. Shall I order a few numbers to be sent down? Perhaps some Friends as well as others would subscribe, had they an opportunity of seeing the specimens. The publication, I believe, will be continued once in three weeks or a month, as he has leisure. But I am wearied, and shall tire thee. Give my dear love to thy Mother and Christy,[11] whose indisposition I am sorry for, but I hear she is going to follow the way of the world and make a Friend in Boar Lane happy. Whether my information be true or not, I wish her happy — and will assert that we may be so, even single! Please write to me soon and be assured it will be very acceptable to

Thy respectful Friend,

J. Fothergill

Ms. autograph letter, Port. 22/96, LSFL.

1. Ann's suitor has not been identified.

2. Benjamin Kidd, a Yorkshireman, who had been a preacher all his life and traveled as a Publick Friend, finally settled in Oxfordshire, where he died in 1759. — *Piety Promoted*, VIII (1775), 59.

3. Edmund Peckover belonged to a Quaker family of Bradford, active in the woolen industry. — Raistrick, p. 29.

4. Isaac Sharpless (1702–1784), of Lancashire, was for sixty years a Quaker preacher. — *Piety Promoted*, IX (1796), 81.

5. No estimate of Mary Smith's importance as a preacher is made in *Piety Promoted*.

6. Thomas Whitehead, of Peel Meeting, a Quaker preacher, spent two months in the American colonies. — Ms. "Testimony Concerning Ministers," 377, LSFL.

7. Circumstances unknown.

8. Elizabeth Buck Fothergill, Dr. John's stepmother, survived her husband only a year.

9. Unidentified.

10. Anthony Purver (1702–1777), an obscure Quaker schoolmaster of Andover in Hampshire, had taught himself Hebrew, Greek, and Latin in order to make a new translation of the Bible in everyday language. He worked at this task for thirty years. — Raistrick, 296. The completed translation was published in 1764.

11. Tabitha's sister Christiana. — Horner Mss., LSFL.

To Elizabeth Bartlett, Bradford, Yorkshire, 16 August 1746

London, 16.6.1746

Dear Betty,

The marks of friendship which I received from several persons at Scarborough make me believe that they will not be displeased to hear that I am arrived safe at London; and I could not think of anyone who would be less displeased with the expense of a letter than thyself. We spent the forenoon after we left Scarborough very agreeably at Castle Howard.[1] The beauties and grandeurs of the place quite exceeded our expectations. Everything there does not merit our applause, but there is sufficient entertainment for three or four hours in a most agreeable and pleasing variety. Friend Barnard[2] was struck with the Mausoleum which is at once a fine repository for the dead and a beautiful august structure.

115

We spent the next day in dull, inactive York, and got to Ripon on the seventh day evening. My company went next morning to see Studley Park,[3] and I embraced that opportunity to ride over to Knaresborough. I stayed [through] the meeting, and went in the afternoon to visit the place where my dear deceased Father's remains were deposited. This I had wished for before I left London, but despaired of it till accident, or I would rather say the same kind Providence which has protected me singularly in this journey led me to the place. Filial affection paid the tribute due to a Father's memory; the grief was pleasing. The only sorrow I felt was to see myself so unlike him. I begged that I might never lose sight of his virtues. — My company was ignorant of the motives of my leaving them; I could not tell them till a few days had given me command enough to do it without discovering my weakness. They joined me in the evening. We called at Harrogate the next day, and got to Leeds in the evening.

I longed to see Bradford once more, but in vain. Our route was fixed, and I could not alter it without giving uneasiness. We arrived at Doncaster on the third day night, and came from thence by easy journeys home.

Friend Barnard has often mentioned thee with great respect which always gave me pleasure; for though I should not choose in all things to follow her example, nor wholly admit of her taste, yet as she has seen a great deal [of] life, she is in some measure a judge of what is coming. — Tommy held his journey very well, and grew daily heartier, which gave her not a little satisfaction.

We passed Lord Lovat [4] several times upon the road. We first met him at Burrow-bridge where I had a very full view of him as he got out of the coach. At Nottingham we overtook him again. We lodged at the same house in Leicester, where I found means of procuring Friend Barnard and her companion to be admitted into his room. At Northampton I saw him again, and yesterday for the last time I believe, as they were conducting him to the Tower.[5] — Before this letter comes to thy hand, 2 of the 3 condemned Lords will probably have suffered. 'Tis amazing how eager people are to see the shocking spectacle.[6] Scaffolds and stands are erecting all about Tower Hill, and half a guinea per head given for places, such is the barbarous curiosity of multitudes! As for my own part, though I have a place offered to see the procession, I believe I shall not accept it; to see the execution I could not be hired.

J. Rhodes is at Hackney, I have not seen him; I don't hear that S.F.[7] and he are yet engaged. Jenny Bevan [8] is in town, and a young person from Exeter said to be a 60,000£ fortune, viz., Dr. Dicker's daughter.[9]

Nothing material has happened amongst my acquaintances since I left London. I have been very little wanted, and have the pleasure of receiving a hearty welcome from my Friends. I am once more hid amongst this mass of mankind, enveloped in smoke and dirt; but with all its disadvantages, I think it my home, and it would be folly not to think it agreeable. I can here spend an hour by myself, with a friend or my book; or talk to my Friends at a distance. This relieves some uneasy moments, and if my Friends don't flatter me too much, gives pleasure to them.

[*Passage omitted.*] My writing I fear is scarcely legible; the subjects I mention are thrown together very oddly. Every circumstance makes it seem almost improper to send it to thee; but as I have had the satisfaction of placing myself in thy company whilst I wrote it, I shall venture to let it go . . . I believe I need not tell thee that a letter from thee will be very acceptable to

Thy respectful Friend
J. Fothergill

Ms. autograph letter, Dimsdale Mss., LSFL.

1. Dr. Fothergill's admiration of Castle Howard near Malton, Yorkshire, was shared by Horace Walpole (1717–1797), who described his delight and surprise when seeing "at one view, a palace, a tower, a fortified city; temples on high places; woods each worthy of being a metropolis of Druids; the noblest lawn in the world, fenced by half the horizon; and a Mausoleum that would tempt one to be buried alive; in fact, I have seen gigantic palaces before but never a sublime one." — "Horace Walpole's Journals of Visits to Country Seats," *The Sixteenth Volume of the Walpole Society* (Oxford, 1928), 72–74.

2. Friend Barnard was traveling with her son Tommy who is mentioned earlier as Dr. Fothergill's patient, the only son of opulent parents (F. to Samuel Fothergill, 30 January 1745/6, above).

3. This park, surrounding the mansion, Studley Royal, is situated about four miles from Ripon (Yorkshire), and not far from Fountains Abbey.

4. Simon Fraser (ca. 1667–1747), 12th Baron Lovat, a Scottish peer, played a double game of intrigue with Jacobites and non-Jacobites. After the final defeat of the Young Pretender at Culloden (16 April 1746), Lord Lovat took refuge on an island in Loch Morar. Discovered there months later, he was ordered to the Tower of London for trial. On account of his age, he was taken down from Scotland under heavy guard, traveling by easy stages with time allowed for rest. Friend Barnard wished to offer him religious consolation while he was at Leicester. Events of these months are summarized by Boyse, *An Historical Review*, II, 172.

5. London newspapers reported that Lord Lovat was driven to the Tower in an open landau drawn by six horses, and escorted by a detachment of Ligonier's Horseguards. — *London Daily Advertiser*, 11 August 1746.

6. On Monday, 18 August 1746, William Boyd, eighth Earl of Kilmarnock, and Arthur Elphinstone, sixth Baron Balmerino, were executed for treason as active participants in the Rebellion. A third Lord, George Mackenzie, third Earl of Cromarty, had his sentence stayed by the clemency of the King, who had been influenced by the pleas of his pregnant wife, already the mother of eight children. Lord Cromarty remained a prisoner until pardoned in 1749. — Lord Lovat was executed in 1747. Archibald McKay, *A History of Kilmarnock, including biographical notices* (Kilmarnock, Scotland: M. Wilson, 1848), 62–82; Sir William Fraser, *The Elphinstone Family Book of the Lords Elphinstone, Balmerino and Coupar* (Edinburgh: Constable, 1897), II, 128; "A Particular Account of the Manner of Execution of the Earl of Kilmarnock and Lord Balmerino . . . and their Behaviour . . . ," *Gentleman's Magazine*, August 1746, 391–394; *State Trials*, comp. T. B. Howell (London: Longman, 1813), XVII, no. 52, pp. 442–503.

7. J. Rhodes, evidently a Friend, may have been the J.R. who was Ann Fothergill's discarded suitor; S.F. cannot be identified.

8. Jenny Bevan was probably a relative of the London Bevans, well-known apothecaries.

9. Dr. Michael Lee Dicker (1695–1754), a Quaker physician, received his medical degree at Leyden in 1718 and was admitted Extra-Licentiate of the Royal College of Physicians the same year. He settled in Exeter and gave devoted service to the Devon and Exeter Hospital. His portrait was placed in the Hospital Board Room. — William Munk, *Roll of the Royal College of Physicians of London* (London: The College, 1878), II, 58, 59.

To Alexander Fothergill, Carr End, Wensleydale, Yorkshire, 11 September 1746

London, 11.7.1746

Dear Brother,

I met with thy kind letter at my return from Scarborough relating to Dr. Hillary's intended voyage, and now sit down to acquaint thee what I know of it. As S. Bevan did not write to him I had no occasion to say much, and indeed I could not till I knew from the Doctor himself his principal reasons.[1]

He set out from hence to Bath on second day last. During his stay in town he conferred several times with S. Bevan and several persons of note who mostly discouraged him from going thither so that all thoughts of going to that place are laid aside. Whilst he was here, news arrived of the death of the only physician at Barbados. I procured him an interview with a person who gave him an exact account of the affairs in that island. He likewise spoke with several others who jointly recommended the place as much preferable to Jamaica. His relations I doubt not will be averse to his leaving England at any rate, but as his situation at Bath is not the most agreeable nor the prospect very pleasing, and at the same time one-half of life may perhaps be over whilst he sees himself stripped of what might have rendered the remaining part pleasant, can one avoid listening to any proposals that may tend to remove this inconveniency?

I was always averse to Jamaica. At Barbados there are several Meetings, the island pleasant and healthy, the people much more humane and polite than anywhere else, with a prospect of good employ. I have been far from urging him to go to either, yet was I in the like situation, I own I should be strongly drawn to this last place; and if he should apply to his relations for their consent, I think they should not too positively refuse him. The galling situation he is in at present I see renders life a burthen to him; but this betwixt ourselves.

I got home about the middle of last month, and found my absence had not been of much disadvantage, but was cordially received by my Friends.

My dear love attends Sister and thyself,

from thy affectionate Brother,
J. Fothergill

Ms. autograph letter, Fothergill Family Papers, Wallis Collection.

1. Dr. William Hillary apparently had been considering going to Jamaica. Subsequently, for eleven years, 1748–1759, he practiced at Bridgetown, Barbados. This experience made possible an important contribution to medical literature, his *Observations on the Changes of the Air and Concomitant Epidemical Diseases in the Island of Barbados; to which is added a Treatise on the putrid Bilious Fever, commonly called the Yellow Fever; and such other Diseases as are indigenous or endemical in the West Indies or in the Torrid Zone* (London: C. Hitch and L. Hawes, 1759). The section on tropical diseases contains accounts of lead colic and also of infectious hepatitis, then unrecognized and hence unnamed, and also gives the first known description of what is now called tropical sprue. Dr. Benjamin Rush of Phildelphia found this book valuable enough fifty-two years later to publish an American edition (Philadelphia, 1811). — Christopher C. Booth, "William Hillary, Pupil of Boerhaave," *Medical History*, 7 (1963): 297–315; *The Letters of Benjamin Rush*, ed. Lyman H. Butterfield (Princeton University Press, 1951), II, 698.

To Alexander Fothergill, Carr End, Wensleydale, Yorkshire, 24 January 1747

24.11.1746/7

Dear Brother,

[*Passage omitted.*] With respect to the collection for Sufferers by the Rebellion, it is not till very lately that we could inform the country about it.[1] The Quarterly Meeting of Cumberland was so dilatory that we had it not in our power to acquaint you. The sum of losses will not amount to £400, including Scotland, so that I should think your Quarterly Meeting might order them a sum and raise it in your next general collection. Subscriptions have come in slowly, though I doubt not but there will be more. And as the overplus will be melted down into the National Stock, Friends need not be afraid of a surplus. — So much for public concerns.

Brother Samuel would very probably tell you that I am likely to commence housekeeper in a little time. At the next Quarter my Landlord quits the house where I now lodge, and I have taken it upon myself. Thus far it seems easy to me, though the expenses I shall draw upon myself will be greatly increased. I hope however to be enabled to support them. I have no near views of altering my condition, nor has any person yet cast up in my way that I can easily think the one allotted me. However I am through best help, I hope, kept pretty easy under my circumstances; and daily wish to learn in this, as well as in every other condition or situation, to be resigned and content with my lot, be it what it may. My business does not lessen, and I hope the regard which my Friends have all along treated me with here does not cool. I don't much abound, but through Mercy I never wanted what was necessary or convenient for me.

I am glad that Dr. Hillary's relations were satisfied with the part I acted in his affair. I hope they will none of them have reason to complain of my want of willingness to serve them. I'll endeavour to save some leisure hour to write to Justice Metcalfe, but this is my circumstance: I can't be up in a morning before 7; the family is not stirring; I rise about that time or 8 — as I have gone to bed early or late; I get breakfast, dress me; and one or other calls on me about business of one sort or another till near 10. I then go to see my patients which take up my time as they are in number or live at a distance, till one or two; and I have often visits to pay and business to do for persons in the country till evening. When meetings or committees don't take up my time, sometimes I have a friend to visit me; at other times I am out, and necessarily on the same occasion. About seven or eight I come home and often extremely wearied, too much exhausted to write or read anything that requires attention.

Thou will ask what business I have to do exclusive of my employ. I have now two manuscripts to revise — one will make 2 volumes in quarto; another I have the care of in the press; a third lies before me to correct; and I now [must] patch up a little paper for myself, as the others are for persons I can't refuse. Judge what leisure, what freedom from avocations I have, yet I must submit to these things for awhile.

I hope not, however, to be prevented from giving thee now and then a few lines, and cementing that affection which ought to subsist amongst us. We may perhaps be sometimes instrumental in recalling one another to our duty and prompting to watchfulness. If we expend our strength and vigour in the service of the world, though mankind should liberally reward us, yet at last we shall think it of small import. Let us then dear Brother, study how to secure that one thing needful, and pray continually that we may not be led into temptation. — Remember my love to Sister and thy young family, and be assured of the affectionate regard of thy brother

J. Fothergill

Ms. autograph letter, Fothergill Family Papers, Wallis Collection.

1. Quarterly Meetings, organized in the counties, were custodians of relief funds collected from members of the Society of Friends in the smaller meetings of each area. Dr. Fothergill apparently expected a prompt response from Yorkshire, less affected by hardships of "the 45" than Cumberland and Scotland. If more money than expected were raised, the surplus would be paid into the National Stock, the central fund for special needs and services, which was controlled and administered by the Meeting for Sufferings, the executive council of London Yearly Meeting. — Information by courtesy of Mrs. A. E. Wallis.

To Samuel Fothergill, Warrington, Lancashire, 28 February 1747

London, 28.12.1746/7

Dear Brother,

When I last wrote to thee I did not think of paying thee a literary visit so soon, but the occasion is new as it's necessary, at least it has cast up in my thoughts since I wrote to thee. Thou knows I must soon commence housekeeper; next month I must be left in the house I now lodge in. A multitude of things will be wanting, and amongst the rest household linen of various kinds. Perhaps thou may procure some part as good in its kind and as cheap as I can, and I request thou will please to do it. I am told Irish linen will do very well for the table; and that I must have a half dozen tablecloths and a dozen or two of napkins. Thou knows my way, that I would have what's good and neat and becoming the situation I am cast into, but am no judge here what is so. Please to consult Sister about the quantity necessary, get it to me as soon as thou can and draw for the charge. If a pretty good piece of cloth for shirts casts up, please to send it with the rest. — Bed linen, I am told, is best of Russia linen, and this I shall get from my acquaintance here.

Thou will smile at my singularity when I tell thee that I am determined to know as little of housekeeping as possible. If I can, I'll get a trusty servant; if not, I'll be cheated rather than be confined to marketing and have to do with bartering and cooking. Through mercy I have enjoyed my health this winter very well. I am lavish in coach here, but it contributes to my ease and affords me the same pleasure as others find on horseback.

Thou wants to know what progress I make towards matrimony. None at all but advancing years. I hinted once that an overture had been obliquely made. I thought about it a good deal carefully. I did not trust myself in her company till accident threw us together at a Meeting. Her behaviour there determined my resolution — not to think about her any more in that light. — Oh! that P.[1] was what I wish her, and that it was destined we were to be one and happy. She knows not that I wish it, nor very few besides thyself. — I shall wait sometime longer with great calmness, and only wish that everything may happen that is for the best, whether it is agreeable to my inclination or not. — I am happy in an employment that suits my disposition, that has thus far supported me

122

decently, and preserves me in great degree independent, and respected amongst my acquaintance. For this I am thankful. I pray to be more so, and to live as becomes such favours best. Sometimes I am helped to repose a secret confidence in the kind hand that thus blesses under distressing prospects, and humbly to acquiesce with every dispensation. Solitary, absent from my nearest relations, weak and contemptible, I am kept from repining at anything that occurs to me. I know thou wants to hear what and how I am. I tell thee abruptly but as truly as I can.

If thou thinks that I had better have any other linen than Irish, or that it will be inconvenient for thee in any shape to procure what I mentioned above, please to let me know as soon as thou canst. — Accept the nearest regard of

Thy affectionate Brother
John Fothergill

[*Written in Dr. John's hand, a list of household linen appears on the back of the last page of this letter.*]

2 Tablecloths 3   yards wide, 3 1/2 long Damask
2   "   2   yards wide, 2 1/2 long $\left.\right\}$ Diaper [2]
2   "   1 1/2 yards wide 2   long
1 doz. damask napkins
1 doz. diaper   "
1 doz. small tea napkins
1 piece Holland linen @ 4/ and 5/
4 pr. sheets @ 2/8d
2 pr. sheets @ 2/   and 2/6d
4 pr. sheets @ 1/   or   1/3 for the servants
4 pairs pillow cases a full yard wide

If any of these are improper for thee to send, let me have the rest without them. I can easily have the smaller matters here.

Ms. autograph letter, Port 22/102, LSFL.

1. Miss Ursula Somervell of Cambridge, England, suggests that the mysterious "P." is Martha Hudson, nicknamed Patty, the daughter of John Hudson of Bush Hill, Enfield. In 1749 Patty married David Barclay, Dr. Fothergill's close friend. Miss Somervell bases her conjecture upon "A Letter of Advice to a Young Patient," signed J.F., which is among the Barclay Mss. This letter, professional yet almost paternal in tone, is published by Fox, Appendix I, 413–415.

2. A linen fabric, with a small geometrical or conventional pattern woven into the cloth.

To Samuel Fothergill, Waterford, Ireland, 7 March 1747

7.1.1746/7

Dear Brother,

Thy readiness to assist me is very obliging. I have spoke with some of my acquaintances here who think the choices you have made for me very judicious. If Sister will undertake the trouble of cutting them out, it will be an additional favour as perhaps some dexterity may be required in it; if none is required by whatever seamstress known, order what thou buys up to London directly.

I received thy former letter and the bill enclosed which was duly paid. I have now more money in my hands than I shall immediately want, and I hope almost as much as I shall want for some months, so that I can at any time allow thee [some upon] a month or two's warning at least. The money in thy hands on dear Father's account may remain there to replace what thou expends for me.

I am in hopes ere long to sit down to dear Father's papers. I only wish that thou would let me have every memorable circumstance of his conduct that thou canst recollect as many may have come to thy knowledge that I am ignorant of. If thou will undertake the whole, I'll send the papers.

I have long been unfit, but if I can get leisure, I hope it will be of use to me to place [on record] that good and great example so strongly, repeatedly in my view. Yes, Brother, I'll undertake it, and may gracious, condescending goodness guide my pen.

I'll say nothing about thy health now. Write to me at thy return. I shall not omit to make use of Joseph's presence in town to help him if I can. I am glad that I have not given him any cause to dread me by being severe. My affairs fall easily and pleasantly on.

The servant maid who was in the family when thou was with us chooses to stay with me. She's sober, honest and concerned for my interest. Harry will live with me as long as I please, so that I am fixed for servants. Who must be the Mistress is unknown! What if it be P., at last? I am not indifferent to her. I dare say no more on this subject.

Don't find fault with me for unloosing my heart to thee in the simplest manner possible. Are not my letters only my own history, poor as it is? And why should thou be under any uneasiness about balancing our correspondence? Do the same by me. If thou had not a wife to unbosom thyself to, thou would. As I have none, and love nobody more than thyself, allow me the liberty to make thee of my counsel at least. — But I forget that thou art surrounded with noise, tumult and intolerable din of the scolding contentious W-lch.[1] Happy thou that thou canst bear it! Happy I that I am not doomed to it. — Farewell, and believe me

Thy affectionate Brother

J. Fothergill

Ms. autograph letter, Port. 22/103 LSFL.

1. This baffling statement may only mean that Samuel and Susannah were employing noisy Welsh servants. Susannah was constantly at work in the dry goods shop they kept in Warrington. Samuel was often away from home preaching wherever sought. A correspondent has suggested that the statement may be a comment upon a visiting delegation of Welsh Quakers always feeling the need for recognition by the parent Society of Friends in London.

To Alexander Fothergill, Carr End, Wensleydale, Yorkshire, 12 March 1748

London, 12.1.1747/8

Dear Brother,

[*Passage omitted.*] I am very sorry to hear that the distemper amongst cattle is broke out in Yorkshire;[1] it will be ruinous to particulars, and of the worst consequence to the public. It is really infectious, and is communicated not only by infected cattle amongst those that are not so; but even men may carry the venom in their clothes and communicate it to the sound cattle. Horses, dogs, swine, nay fowls may carry it from one place to another. In short you have no way left to stop its progress but by keeping your cattle wholly within yourselves, suffering no fresh cattle, however sound to appearance, to come amongst them, no butchers or others that are conversant with cattle to be admitted into your stocks on any account. When the disease comes near, and whilst it is at a distance the only way to keep it so, is for the neighbourhood to agree not to buy in any new stock, not to drive any cattle to market, for perhaps the cow that stands next her may be infected; to keep those that are fat by themselves; and either to kill her at home, and send the meat to market, or suffer the butcher to see none else. But if the magistrats of particular districts would agree to meet once a week to direct the orders

125

of council to be put in execution strictly without favor or affection, it would secure you the most effectually. Promote this as much as possible. Persuade people not to run to distant places to buy cattle for half price and bring them home to their own neighbour's ruin. Let fairs and markets be suppressed, and the present loss will soon be amply recompensed.

I am forced to write abruptly, having several letters to dispatch by this post . . .

Thy affectionate Brother — and ready to serve thee —
John Fothergill

Pray give my very kind respects to Justice Metcalfe.

Ms. autograph letter, Fothergill Family Papers, Wallis Collection.

1. Spread of the cattle plague threatened farmers in the North of England with loss of livelihood. Despair deepened with the news that casualties in the Low Countries, also afflicted with this disease, had mounted to 300,000. Dr. Richard Brocklesby (1722–1797) described the disease in his first published paper, *An Essay Concerning the Casualties among Horned Cattle* (London, 1746). It included a dry cough, shivering, insatiable thirst, refusal of fodder, diarrhea, frothy discharge from the mouth, purulent discharge from the nostrils, pustules on neck and foreparts, and swollen glands of the head. Pathological examination showed extreme inflammation of the stomach, less of the intestines, and extensive "peripneumony." It now seems evident that the cattle plague must have been contagious pleuro-pneumonia. This disease is caused by a special micro-organism intermediate in size between the bacteria and the viruses, first isolated more than a century later in the Pasteur Institute, Paris, by Nocard. — H. J. Morowitz and M. E. Tourtelotte, "The Smallest Cells," *Scientific American*, 206 (1962): 117–126.

To Israel Pemberton, Jr., Philadelphia, 25 April 1748

London, 25.2.1748

Dear Friend,

Though writing of late has become more a task to me, than ever it did since I knew how to use my pen, and for this reason I have easily excused myself from it, yet I am glad that necessity in some measure at present compels me to renew our correspondence. J. Hunt [1] and myself received a letter from thee and J. Kinsey [2] desiring us to find out some proper person to send over as a schoolmaster.[3] We have made inquiry, but without the success we could desire; the young man who brings this, we hope, under the prudent directions of the managers will in time give satisfaction. As is mentioned in the letter to J. Kinsey and thyself, he was judged a tolerable proficient when at school; he was afterwards placed as an apprentice to a wholesale dealer; but not liking the business and having a turn for study, his master gave way to it, and he went down to Edinburgh. He studied there, but for want of sufficient support, he was obliged I believe to begin practice sooner than was convenient, and whatever genius he might have, his manner and address not being the most taking, he has not succeeded in his business to much advantage. I apprehend that an education less confined than happens to the generality of schoolmasters, might enable him to supply to advantage the want of practice in teaching. I have urged him to turn his thoughts to this, and to make himself master of the different methods in use in our schools. I believe he is untainted by any vicious habits; he is naturally a little overbearing and impatient of contradiction, easily offended and soon reconciled, but under all, honest and well meaning. I must entreat thy care over him, and I hope he will not fail to pay a just regard to thy judgement. This I have recommended to him as earnestly as possible, and have only to wish he may behave so as to merit thy notice.[4]

I believe thou would now and then have heard from me last summer had I not been engaged in an affair I little expected. Not matrimony, for this is yet to come — if it ever happens — but in building. I literally pulled an old house over my head, and have been busy in repairing it, and at length made it a commodious habitation. To a person accustomed to reading and the business of attending the sick, this was an unpleasant employ, but I hope it is done for life and this makes me forget the fatigue it cost me with more ease. I heard by I. Greenleaf[5] thou was just upon a second engagement which I heartily wish may be a happy one as possible.[6] I am somehow or other placed in such a situation as not easily to meet with a person every way suitable to it. I am therefore yet forced to continue single; 'tis not the life I choose, but I sit down with remembering the old maxim that whatever is, is best; and if I can't be as happy as I *would* be, endeavour to be as much so as I can.

We are amused today with the report of approaching peace and that the preliminaries are already signed; as for my own part, I dread it as an Englishman, whilst as a Christian I sincerely wish another sword might never be drawn. By pursuing the war with vigour we may yet hope for a solid peace in time; by accepting peace such as a perfidious enemy will condescend to give us, we suffer ourselves to be disarmed and

127

must soon become an easy prey; yet for ourselves I wish for peace that an end may be put to those animosities and contentions which your situation gives rise to.[7]

Accept my warmest wishes for thy health and happiness; favour me sometime or other with a few lines. Don't let us suffer the fire to go wholly out, nor the chain [8] to grow rusty but as little as we can. Farewell, dear Friend, and be assured that I am

Thy affectionate Friend
John Fothergill

Ms. autograph letter, Pemberton Papers, IV, 108, HSP.

1. John Hunt (1712–1780) was a London merchant active in the Society of Friends. He had vsited America in 1738.

2. John Kinsey (1696–1750), also a Quaker, was Attorney-General of Pennsylvania 1739–1743, Chief Justice 1743–1750, and Speaker of the Pennsylvania Assembly 1739–1750. After his death, his house was made into a temporary hospital while the Pennsylvania Hospital was under construction. — Morton and Woodbury, *Pennsylvania Hospital*, 28, 32, 113.

3. From 1743 until his death in 1779, Israel Pemberton served as clerk for the Quaker schools. — Thayer, *Israel Pemberton*, 33.

4. The young man was Robert Willan, a Yorkshireman who had started medical practice in Scarborough, a health resort already well supplied with experienced physicians. In 1746, according to *Munk's Roll*, he published "a sensible Essay on the King's Evil." The Overseers of Friends Grammar School (Penn Charter) in Philadelphia provided him with passage money from England and a salary of £150 per annum "to teach Latin, Greek, and other parts of learning." The Minute Book of Philadelphia Monthly Meeting (28th. 6mo. 1748) records his arrival in the city. He produced "the customary certificate" from the meeting he had attended in Scarborough, necessary to transfer his membership to Philadelphia's Society of Friends. — Thomas Woody, *Early Education in Philadelphia* (New York: Columbia University Press, 1920), 38; *Munk's Roll*, II, 350 (in an account of his son, Dr. Robert Willan, 1757–1812).

5. Isaac Greenleaf was John Hunt's junior partner.

6. On 27 December 1747, Israel Pemberton married, as his second wife, Mary Jordan, *née* Stansbury, already twice widowed and eleven years his senior. Thayer, *Israel Pemberton*, 26.

7. The Treaty of Aix-la-Chapelle, finally agreed upon 1 October 1748, made little change in the status quo except to guarantee possession of Silesia to Frederick II of Prussia. Trade between England and Spain was not regulated, although disagreement on that score had originally set off the conflict. — NCMH, 436–439.

8. The chain of friendship, a metaphor used by contemporary translators in recording testimony from Indians at treaty sessions.

To Alexander Fothergill, Carr End, Wensleydale, Yorkshire, 27 August 1748

London, 27.6.1748

Dear Brother,

I received thy affectionate and very acceptable letter in due course. I am glad to find our inclinations mutually disposed to cultivate that nearness and regard which is so becoming and often helpful.

One reason of my taking my pen in hand at this time is to acquaint thee that I am making use of the leisure I now have to transcribe and digest the few papers I have relating to dear Father. At my request, and in consequence of his long intended resolution, he had begun the account of his own life and had brought it to his return from his first voyage to America in the year 1707. I have a few short notes of some others of his travels but chiefly consisting of times, places and persons; things that might [slip] his memory, whilst the many instructive observations he made, and which no time could efface, were laid up in his own breast and are gone with him. As thou was more with him than any of us and hast heard him mention many of the circumstances of his life, and was a witness to his exemplary conduct and conversation, I must intreat thee to set down such hints as occur to thee as soon as thou can. With respect to style, or order, or any circumstance of that kind, don't be solicitous. To look back upon the many instances of his pious care, his zeal, his circumspect behavior in all things must give thee satisfaction and, I doubt not, help. I am sure the perusal of his papers has helped me — which makes me hope I am neither putting thee upon a painful nor useless employment. If any more copies of letters, either to your Monthly Meeting, Quarterly Meeting, or remains of journals cast up, please to let me have all and as soon as thou canst. [*Passage omitted.*]

I am obliged to thee for mentioning thy family; I wanted to know some little about ye. Whether I may ever see my native country again, I know not. But I shall never cease to remember it, and those who are there whilst I can remember anything. Give my kind love to our cousins at Countersett, to the Hillary and Robinson families,[1] and to that good old man, R. Alderson,[2] whose good desires for me I know are strong and are justly valued by me. Give my respects, if thou pleases, to that worthy magistrate and friend to our Father's family, Justice Metcalfe. Often have I thought of writing to him and as often been deterred by

129

having nothing material to communicate worthy of his perusal or worth his expense.

Thou will doubtless see sometimes in the papers accounts of the locusts that have of late been found in these parts. I have some of them by me that were catched in this city; I have some likewise from the East Indies, and one from Gibraltar. They are all of the same species, but ours is a less size than the former, about 2 1/2 inches long. They are the same that are now ravaging Transylvania etc. Those we have here are in too small numbers to be mischievous and seem only to be straggling parties of a larger army which I hope perished in the Western Ocean. A sailor told me this day that he met with some of them ten leagues off at sea, and this is often their fate. If they continue to advance and our seasons are not too rigorous, they will in a few years, I am afraid, commit great depredations upon us. But the uncertain seasons may defend us.

I have only room to bid thee farewell, and assure thee that I am

Thy affectionate Brother

J.F.

Ms. autograph letter from the papers of Dr. Crichton Fothergill of Darlington, County Durham, England.

1. The Hillary and Robinson families were prominent members of Countersett Meeting. Richard Robinson's daughter Mary married John Hillary of Birkrigg in 1692. Their eldest son, Isaac, living in Burtersett, was a friend of Alexander Fothergill. Their second son was Dr. William Hillary. — Quaker records consulted in local Minute Books, Yorkshire.

2. The Aldersons were a family of dalesmen once owning much property in Wensleydale. Fields in the vicinity of Askrigg village are still known as Alderson Lands. — Hartley and Ingilby, *Yorkshire Village*, 103.

To Dr. William Cuming, Dorchester in Dorset, 7 February 1749

London, 7.12.1748/9

Dear Doctor,

Before this arrives I hope that the reason of my silence will appear; which indeed was no other than a close application to the subject of the essay on the sore throat, a copy of which I sent to Hilches [1] some weeks ago. I could not however dispense with myself from taking notice of thy very affectionate letter which yesterday's post brought me, though

I believe the cause of every painful apprehension will have ceased ere this.

From the moment I determined to write upon the subject, every leisure hour was necessarily devoted to this task; when I had finished it, I was so much exhausted that I could not with pleasure take pen in hand almost on any affair, and this alone hindered me from giving thee an earlier account of my engagement in it; — 500 copies were printed off,[2] and the bookseller tells me this afternoon that there are not above 20 left in his hands; so that I am looking over it again, and shall be glad of my friend's assistance in making it less faulty than it is. If anything appears obscure; if the diction can anywhere be altered for the better; if anything appears useless, or wanting, in short if the tract can be altered for the better, as I doubt not it may, be so good as to act the part of a friend, and let me know it as speedily as possible. I won't promise to be so humble as to acknowledge the favour in print, but I shall receive any corrections with pleasure and return the favour when I can with gratitude.

I would have sent a copy to Dr. Jacobs,[3] but I knew not how; and I hope he'll attribute the seeming neglect to no other cause. — I have had the satisfaction of seeing it better received by the faculty [4] here than I expected. Dr. Edward Hulse [5] has been pleased to mention it favourably as have some others. This gives me the more pleasure as I hope my friends and intimate acquaintances will have the less pain on my account; and as it is a proof that those who endeavour to deserve well of the public have no reason to despond of a candid reception, let their performance be never so trifling.

I shall expect a long list of *Corrigenda*, in a post or two, or I shall be afraid my late behaviour is not totally forgiven.

Adieu, my worthy Friend, and believe me to be

Thy affectionate Friend
J. Fothergill

Ms. autograph letter, Charles Roberts Autograph Collection, Haverford College, Pennsylvania.

1. Although the manuscript has been read "Hilches," this name is probably Hitch; C. Hitch was a London bookseller, and the London publisher of several medical books by Dr. Fothergill's friend Dr. William Hillary.
2. *An Account of the Sore Throat attended with Ulcers* (1748) established Dr. Fothergill in the esteem of professional colleagues and the general public by reason

of its timeliness and its recommendation of a moderate and practical plan of treatment (see Introduction, above).

3. Dr. Jacobs, not listed in *Munk's Roll,* was probably a dissenter who received his M.D. from a continental school.

4. London's medical profession.

5. Sir Edward Hulse (1682–1759) was educated at the University of Cambridge and received his M.D. in 1717. Elected Fellow of the Royal College of Physicians in 1718, he served the College as Censor in 1720, 1721, and 1735, and as Consilarius in 1750, 1751, and 1753. Physician in the royal household to both Queen Anne and George I, he was created baronet in 1730. He practiced medicine in London for forty years, with reputation and success. — *Munk's Roll,* II, 62, 63.

To Alexander Fothergill, Carr End, Wensleydale, Yorkshire, 24 June 1749

London, 24.4.1749

Dear Brother,

This time it was me who was in fault; I owed thee a letter, and was only waiting to inform thee of an affair of some little consequence to myself before I gave thee an answer. However thine was not the less acceptable because unexpected. Though I have not always the leisure I could wish, yet I am glad to have it in my power to assure thee that thy letters are more and more engaging and cement that affection which ought to subsist between us more strongly.

When H. Thornton[1] called upon me to take his leave, I had not leisure to procure any other token of my regardful remembrance of thy children than a little piece of money which thou must distribute as justice requires. The two books were intended for thyself and Justice Metcalfe, for whose friendly regard I have the most grateful esteem, and I request thou will remember me to him when it falls in thy way.

The weather has been no less seasonable with us, than it has been with you. We had a severe frost, about the same time it affected you which destroyed all our apples in the bloom, and even killed some trees. Two weeks in the beginning of this month were colder than a great part of December last. It affected France and the neighbouring countries as well as us, and killed several trees with them which survived the severity with us. — This is the first day that has felt like summer for these three weeks.

I am sorry to hear that this distemper amongst the cattle creeps so near.[2] If it is possible, let nobody come near them, except thy own

132

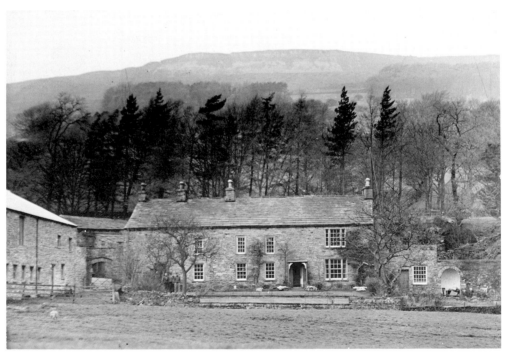

Carr End, Wensleydale, Yorkshire

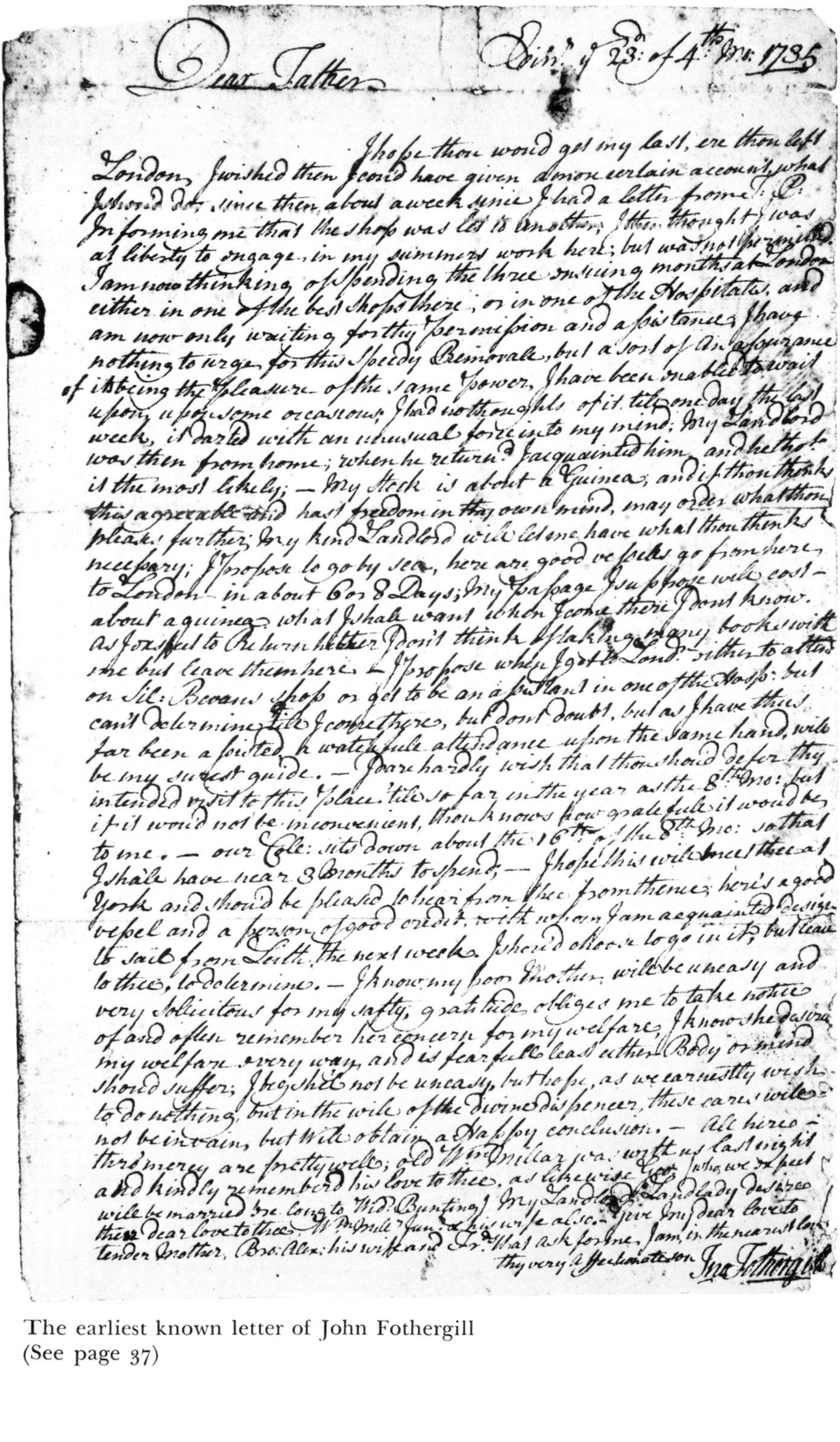

Dear Father — Edinr. ye 23: of 4th Mo: 1735

I hope thou would get my last, ere thou left
London, I wished then I could have given a more certain account what
I should do, since then, about a week since I had a letter from [illegible]
Informing me that the shop was let to another, I then thought I was
at liberty to engage, in my summers work here; but was not [illegible]
I am now thinking of spending the three ensuing months at London
either in one of the best shops there, or in one of the Hospitalls, and
am now only waiting for thy permission and assistance. I have
nothing to urge for this speedy Removall, but a sort of an assurance
of its being the pleasure of the same power, I have been enabled to wait
upon, upon some occasions; I had no thoughts of it till one day the last
week, it darted with an unusual force into my mind; my Landlord
was then from home; when he returnd I acquainted him, and he thot.
it the most likely; — My stock is about a Guinea; and if thou thinks
this agreeable and hast freedom in thy own mind, may order what thou
pleases further; my kind Landlord will let me have what thou thinks
necessary; I propose to go by sea, here are good vessels go from here
to London in about 6 or 8 Days; my passage I suppose will cost
about a guinea, what I shall want when I come there I dont know.
as I expect to Return hither I don't think of taking many books with
me but leave them here. I propose when I get to Lond: either to attend
on Sil: Bevans shop or get to be an assistant in one of the Hosp: but
can't determine till I come there, but dont doubt, but as I have thus
far been assisted, a watchfull attendance upon the same hand, will
be my surest guide. — I dare hardly wish that thou should defer thy
intended visit to this place till so far in the year as the 8th Mo: but
if it would not be inconvenient, thou knows how gratefull it would be
to me. — our Coll: sits down about the 16th of the 8th Mo: so that
I shall have near 3 months to spend; — I hope this will meet thee at
York and should be pleased to hear from thee from thence; here's a good
vessel and a person of good credit, with whom I am acquainted design
to sail from Leith the next week. I should choose to go in it, but leave
to thee, to determine. — I know my poor Mother will be uneasy and
very sollicitous for my safty, gratitude obliges me to take notice
of and often remember her concern for my welfare, I know she desires
my welfare every way, and is fearfull least either Body or mind
should suffer; I beg she'll not be uneasy, but hope, as we earnestly wish
to do nothing, but in the will of the divine dispencer, these cares will
not be in vain, but will obtain a Happy conclusion. — All here
thro' mercy are pretty well; old Wm. Millar sen: with us last night
and kindly remembred his love to thee, as likewise [illegible] who we expect
will be married ere long to Wid: Bunting] My Landlord & Landlady desires
their dear love to thee, Wm. Millar Jun: & his wife also. — give my dear love to
tender Mother, Bro: Alex: his wife and Fr: that ask for me, I am, in the nearest love

thy very affectionate son Jno Fothergill

The earliest known letter of John Fothergill
(See page 37)

family; keep away all butchers especially. And if it could any way be done, keep but a few together, that if one parcel is seized, another may have some chance to escape. If one beast is seized, take it immediately from the rest, and kill it as the late order directs; or else make some little hut in the remotest part of the grounds and keep it there, not permitting the person who attends it to come near the rest. Don't bleed the beast that is seized, but though the creature seems very hot, give very warm and cordial drenches frequently, such as a pint of warm ale with an ounce of anise seeds, an ounce of cummin seeds, 1/4 of an ounce of ginger every six hours with three or four spoonfuls of vinegar. When the scouring or purging comes on, give an ounce of *Bole Armenium* and half an ounce of Millindate twice a day in the same liquor, or oftener if the discharge is frequent and the beast in great pain; and give them as much gruel and mashes as possible.

I think it will not be amiss to call upon T. Areskine, but if it does not suit him to pay, don't press him by any means.

I have made some distant overtures in relation to altering my condition to a person at some distance from this place. I have as yet received no answer, so that I am altogether uncertain with regard to the employment of this summer. I was waiting to know the issue of my proposal before I wrote to thee, but as I have not yet the account, I chose not to delay writing to thee longer, nor at the same time to conceal from thee the situation I am in; but this must remain a secret — even to thyself if possible.[3]

I heartily wish your assembly may be favoured with the extending of divine regard, that you may be strengthened and renewed to every good word and work. I salute thee in much love, and am

thy affectionate Brother

J. Fothergill

Ms. autograph letter, Fothergill Family Papers, Wallis Collection.

1. Not identified.

2. The cattle plague, described by Dr. Richard Brocklesby in 1746, and mentioned in Dr. Fothergill's letter of 12 March 1746/7 to his brother Alexander, had broken out again. Brocklesby's method of treatment employed heavy bleeding, dosing with soothing liquid medicines, setons in the neck, ointment of hog's lard and Swedish tar, drenching with a camphor-honey-saltpetre solution, or one of valerian and snakeroot with salad oil or with Venice treacle. Bodies of casualties had to be burned at once, with immediate burial of the remains eight to ten feet deep in earth. — Brocklesby, *Essay Concerning the Mortality among Horned Cattle*; current discussion in *The Gentleman's Magazine*, London; *Munk's Roll*, II, 201–204; Edward Hughes,

North Country Life in the Eighteenth Century (London: Oxford University Press, 1952), 145–150; for "Venice Treacle," see George W. Corner, "Mithridatium and Theriac, the most famous remedies of old medicine," *Johns Hopkins Hospital Bulletin*, 26 (1915): 222–226.

3. Two months later, Dr. Fothergill's letter dated 22.6.1749 (Port. 22/104 LSFL, not included in this book) reported to his brother Samuel: "I am still in the dark with regard to J.D.'s family, having not received any answer to a letter I sent to them near 3 months ago." Nothing came of Dr. Fothergill's proposal of marriage to J.D., whose identity remains a puzzle.

To Peter Collinson? London, 1 November 1749

London, 1.9.1749

Dear Friend,

Agreeable to thy request when we parted, I send this little scrawl [1] to inform thee of my health. I wish I could say that my indisposition was at all abated; in the daytime I am almost exactly as when thou saw me; at night every symptom increases, so as to make the fore part very tiresome. By dint of bleeding, blisters and a long use of bolus,[2] draughts and other pharmaceutical artillery, I think it daily becomes more plainly intermittent; and if those who have the care of me are of the same opinion, I intend to call in the assistance of my good old friend, the Bark,[3] tomorrow morning. I can look over the misery I must endure tonight with less uneasiness, as my hopes are not a little sanguine that it will be the last. However, in this I shall endeavor to be resigned to superior direction. My best wishes attend the whole family from thy affectionate Friend

J. Fothergill

Ms. autograph letter, lacking name of correspondent and without cover, found in a notebook of Peter Collinson's at the Linnean Society, London.

1. This letter was probably to Peter Collinson. No other bit has been found of correspondence between these two men, who were often together in London, during almost thirty years of friendship.

2. Bolus (defined as a large, soft pill) is used by Dr. Fothergill as a collective noun; the modern plural is boluses. Such pills are used today only in veterinary practice.

3. A medicine first made from the powdered bark of cinchona trees of the tropical forests in South America. First used in Peru, and exported by the Jesuits, it was often called Peruvian or Jesuits Bark. Its use is said to have been introduced in England by Dr. Thomas Sydenham (1624–1689). Until nineteenth-century chemists isolated pure alkaloidal quinine from the bark, the crude powdered form was a greatly favored remedy for chills and fever. — John Gray, "An Account of the

Peruvian or Jesuits Bark," *Phil. Trans. R.S.*, 40:81–86 (1737). Norman Taylor, *Cinchona in Java* (New York: Greenberg, 1945), 28–34.

To Dr. Charles Alston, University of Edinburgh, 18 April 1750

Gracechurch Street, London 18..2.1750

Dear Doctor,

I take the opportunity of the bearer's return to Edinburgh to send a few packets of seeds which I received from my friend and fellow-student, G. Cleghorn.[1] They were collected in Minorca the season before the last, and seem to be still in good condition. I should have sent them earlier in the spring, but waited for a proper opportunity which did not occur until the present. Those which have *Indig.* wrote upon them are indigenous to Minorca, the rest are brought from other places and cultivated there for use or pleasure.

I dare not look back to the time when our correspondence ceased with any hopes of seeing it revived, as I am so much in fault. But the cause I'll beg leave to mention. It was an answer to several of mine! It required a long and accurate answer, and gave a larger commission to execute than I could find time at once to do. I thought of it in some respects as boys do a task — and no wonder then that I suffered slight occasions to set my design aside! I believe, however, my indolence would now and then conquer a short epistle; and I am sure it would be a strong inducement to it, could I do anything to oblige Dr. Alston.

At present we have nothing material on the carpet here in the medical way. We have shorter ways to fame and opulence than through the mirey track of study, and it's enough for a young Physician here if he can obtain a smattering of every kind of knowledge but that of his business — provided he has friends.

I have just been turning over a part of the 1st Vol. of *Histoire Naturelle*,[2] lately printed at Paris. It will, I doubt not, be a very valuable work, as those concerned in it will have every advantage they can wish for. Buffon lashes Burnet,[3] Whiston[4] and Woodward[5] very hard, and this last, I think sometimes undeservedly. Their schemes are doubtless faulty and in many things absurd; but I think our author is not one bit behindhand with them. For after having treated Burnet's theory as a

135

romance, Whiston's as little better than presumptuous and wicked, Woodward's as absurd and improbable, he condescends to acquaint us that this Ball of earth and the planets were at different times knocked off from the Sun, by a comet's striking it obliquely; that the matter thus struck off was vitrified, and the scum of this vitrification, together with some of the glassy mass itself, have by mutual attrition formed a great part of the body we call earth, sand etc. Notwithstanding the use which our author has made of them, he has collected a great many facts, and has some new and curious remarks.

We now begin to receive considerable quantities of *Ginseng* from America. It is not yet much used, but I have one very singular instance of its good effects in a case of impotency, which after a long and fruitless trial of very efficacious medicines, and a considerable discontuance of them, proved effectual. — I have given some persons directions to gather and cure it in the same manner as it's said the Chinese do; not that this will add to its virtue, but it may probably render it no inconsiderable article in trade to that part of the world.

If my past behavior has not made me unworthy, and it should once again be put in my power to retrieve my character, I think I should take some pains to do it; and assure thee that I am

Thy respectful Friend,
John Fothergill

Ms. autograph letter, Alston Collection, UEL.

1. George Cleghorn (1716–1789), Fothergill's friend of student days in Edinburgh, went to Minorca in 1736 as an army surgeon.

2. The great work of Georges Louis Leclerc, Comte de Buffon (1707–1778). Volume 1 (1749) challenged current orthodox thought based upon Biblical narrative. Buffon himself traced "a primitive and general design" of cosmic evolution through vast ages of the earth to explain natural phenomena. — *NCMH*, VII, 86–90; Loren Eiseley, *Darwin's Century: Evolution and the Men Who Discovered It* (Garden City, N.Y.: Doubleday, 1958), 40–45.

3. Thomas Burnet (1635–1713), Fellow of Christ's College, Master of Charterhouse, author of *Telluris Theoria Sacra* (1681). He likened the earth to a monstrous egg, the shell of which had been crushed by the Deluge until internal waters had burst forth. Fragments of this displaced shell were supposed to have formed the mountains. The equator by his theory had been diverted from its original coincidence with the ecliptic by the force of the cataclysm. John Ray (1627–1707) was stimulated by differences of opinion to write *Miscellaneous Discourses concerning the Dissolution and Changes of the World* (1692). — Raven, 430–431.

4. William Whiston (1667–1728), Isaac Newton's successor as Lucasian Professor at Cambridge, was the author of *The New Theory of the Earth from its Original to the Consummation of All Things, Wherein the Creation of the World in Six Days*

. . . As Laid down in the Holy Scriptures are shewn to be perfectly agreeable to Reason and Philosophy (1696). He thought that the Deluge had been caused by collision between the earth and a comet dragging after it by attraction the great water courses which were increased by condensation of the comet's tail. — Raven, 434, *passim.*

5. John Woodward (1665–1728), physician and geologist, founder of the Woodwardian Collection at the University of Cambridge, was the author of *An Essay Towards a Natural History of the Earth . . . With an Account of the Universal Deluge and of the Effects it had upon the Earth* (1695). He believed that because an overwhelming deluge had churned up the earth's contents, the marine creatures and shells had been deposited in layers by gravitation. — Raven, 434–437, 449–451; Eiseley, 75, 76.

To James Logan, Philadelphia, 4 May 1750

London, 4.3.1750

Esteemed Friend,[1]

I am more obliged to thy generosity than I can easily express for still remembering me after such strong appearances against me as might in a less equitable mind have wholly extinguished regard. Want of health at some times, unavoidable engagements at others, have defeated both inclination and duty. The only time I can set apart for writing is late in the evenings, and this is not always certain. Sometimes the thoughts of a day have made me incapable of doing it, and this is the reason why physicians are worse correspondents than others. We cannot like tradesmen reserve proper times for proper business, but must go when and where we are called.

In respect to J. Martin,[2] I looked over the translation of his letter to Voltaire, and don't find the quotation mentioned in it.[3] I have not the book now at hand, and cannot be so certain as I would wish. In the latter part of his life he was very remiss and inattentive, and I don't at all wonder if he suffered egregious mistakes to escape him. He had been under the necessity of subsisting on his books in a great measure for some years, and had sold several at different times so that he had no more left than were sold for betwixt 3 and 400 £ at most.

I am still of the same opinion in regard to the origin of Amber that I formerly mentioned.[4] I am obliged to thee for pointing out a passage that would not otherwise have fallen within the compass of my reading; but I hope to explain the affair in such a manner as to obviate every difficulty. It is agreed on all hands that the facts contained in the *Essay on the Generation of Plants* are curious and well conducted; in regard to the theory built upon them, people doubt whether it will hold good. In some of the Latin academical dissertations printed lately at Upsal, I see the *Experiments* are oftener than once quoted, which makes me think it is well received by the botanists of that country, Sweden, who are at present the most industrious of any in Europe.[5]

I have sent by Jonah Thompson, a Friend in the ministry of good repute amongst us, and I think well worthy of regard, Knight's *Discourses*,[6] a number of the *Philosophical Transactions* which contains the only copy I have of an *Account of Siberia*,[7] and a little tract upon a medical subject which I laboured hard at the winter before last.[8] The disease of which it treats has committed great ravages in some places where a different method of managing it was pursued; it is not yet wholly extinct, but seldom proves of fatal consequence. As I hope this spring to get more leisure to answer some of thy unmerited favours, more particularly than at present I can, I'll only beg leave to assure thee that as I am perfectly sensible of thy regard for me and the honour I receive from such correspondence as well as advantage, so it gives me great uneasiness when the leisure I had devoted to make the best returns in my power is snatched away from me by some unexpected avocation. Accept my best wishes for the preservation of thy health and continuance amongst thy Friends, and believe that I am

thine, with gratitude and sincerity,

J. Fothergill

P.S. Please give my very kind respects to thy son William. It is a very great pain to me that I cannot write to him by the present opportunity, but I hope to do it soon. J.F.

Ms. autograph letter, Maria Dickinson Logan Family Papers, HSP.

1. James Logan, after nearly half a century of public service in Pennsylvania, had retired from the Provincial Council in 1747. Despite partial paralysis and a general arthritis constantly increasing in severity, he remained mentally active, and continued to add to his remarkable library. After 1749, his health seriously failed, and by the time Dr. Fothergill's letter reached him he was becoming incapacitated. He died 31 October 1751. — Tolles, *James Logan*.

2. James Logan had asked Dr. Fothergill to clear up some questions provoked by Josiah Martin's volume, *A Letter from One of the People Called Quakers to Francis de Voltaire, occasioned by his Remarks on that People in his Letters concerning the English Nation* (London, 1741; reprinted more than once, and translated into French

in 1745). Martin devoted many pages to criticism of Voltaire's appraisal of the Quakers, accusing him of "facetious levity" and advising him, "Devote thy pen and the talent that God gives thee to the Service of Truth."

3. To this particular query Logan apparently found an answer, as disclosed in a letter dated 2.4.1750, dictated to an amanuensis. The name of the person addressed is not given and the letter, left unsigned, was naturally never mailed. It has been found by chance among James Logan's miscellaneous papers. — Society Collections, HSP.

4. "An Essay on the Origin of Amber," *Phil. Trans. R.S.*, 43:21–25 (1744/5). See also letter to Dr. Alston, 14 September 1743, above.

5. James Logan's account of his experiments on Indian corn (see letter to Dr. Alston, 11 November 1738, above) was published in 1739 at Leyden through the courtesy of Gronovius. Dr. Fothergill prepared an English translation for a second edition (1747), which contains, on opposite pages, Logan's original Latin text and Fothergill's English version. The impressive title page of this volume carries the full Latin title and authorship: *Experimenta et Meletemata de Plantarum Generatione, Autore Jacobo Logan, Judico Supremo et Praeside Concili, Provinciae Pennsylvaniensis.* A short appraisal of Logan's accomplishment in botanical science is given by Frederick B. Tolles in "America's First Scientist," *Isis*, 47 (1956–57): 20. In his Uppsala dissertation, *Sponsalia plantarum* (Stockholm, 1747), Johann Gustavus Wahlbohm, a pupil of Linnaeus, says of Logan's work on maize: "I do not mention ZEA [Indian corn], whose [sexual] reproduction Siegesbeck and others deny because of the position of the anthers and the pistils; for the experiments made by Mr. Logan at Philadelphia in Pennsylvania are conclusive." (ZEAM non loquor, cuius generationem Siegesbeckius et alii negant, ex antherum et pistillorum situ; sufficant enim experimenta Domini Logani in Philadelphia, Pennsylvaniae, capta. vid. Log. exp. de Plant. gen., 45.) Wahlbohm's dissertation appeared later in Linnaeus, *Amoenitates Academicae* (Leyden, 1749), I, 61–109. The fact that Linnaeus heavily edited dissertations prepared by his students and later claimed them as his own work is disclosed by William T. Stearn, *Carl Linnaeus, Species Plantarum: A Facsimile of the First Edition*, 2 vols. (London: Quaritch, 1957–59), I, 51–55.

6. Dr. Gowin Knight, Fellow of the Royal Society of London, received its Copley Medal in 1747. An able investigator, his *Discourses* mentioned here were probably included among those he published in *A Collection of Some Papers . . . Relating to the Use of Dr. Knight's Magnetical Bars* (London, 1758).

7. " 'An Account of Some Observations and Experiments in Siberia,' extracted from . . . *Flora Sibirica, sive Historia Plantarum* etc., Auct. D. Gmelin, Chem. et Nat. Hist. Prof., vol. I (Petropoli, 1747)," read before the Royal Society, 11 Feb. 1747/8 and published in *Phil. Trans. R.S.*, 45:248–262 (1756). *Works*, ed. Lettsom, I, 317–322.

8. *An Account of the Sore-Throat attended with Ulcers*, mentioned in the letter to Dr. Cuming, 7 February 1748/9, above.

To Alexander Fothergill, Carr End, Wensleydale, Yorkshire, 5 January 1750/1

London, 5.11.1750/1

Dear Brother,

It is difficult at this distance to propose anything that can be of much use to prevent a repetition of the like calamity that has deprived thee and Sister of so amiable a child.[1] To give them a gentle purgative once or twice a week will be the most proper means to render the disease favourable in case they should be seized with it. A little senna tea, with the liquor of a few shived prunes will be the most safe and easily procured medicine for this purpose. In case the disease has already appeared on them, to keep them moderately warm, and well supplied with liquids as gruel, weak sage or baume tea, milk and water, or thin milk pottage will be both food and physic. Let them have as much as they will, but force or urge none upon them. Small amounts of white wine whey may be given if they seem low or faint; otherwise keep them wholly to the other liquors. This in respect to regimen is all I can think of at present necessary to be communicated; and as to medicines perhaps few or none will be necessary, except a little *Syrup of Diacodium* to be given at bedtime in case they don't rest. But this should not be used until they begin to complain of soreness and seem to want for sleep only from that cause; a moderate common spoonful in a little warm water or gruel will be full enough for the eldest, a smaller quantity will do for the rest.

But if the kind of smallpox about you is a very bad one, and proves generally mortal, I should earnestly advise inoculation.[2] 'Tis an operation easily to be performed, and in the manner I am going to direct it, seldom is attended with any ill effects. In common, those who have it this way, get through it with the least danger.

A common sewing thread of moderate thickness may be drawn through a ripe pock, in such a manner as that some part of the thread may be a little moistened or wetted with the matter, this may be dried a little, put into a dry vial or little box and sent to thee. Purge the children twice or thrice as above directed, then with the point of a needle make a small scratch in the skin, a little below the knee, either inside or out; cut off a short bit of the moistened part of the thread, which may be known by its colour, for instance the eighth part of an inch or less in length; lay this on the little bleeding scratch; cover it with any kind of

140

sticking plaster — and the whole is done. About the eighth day or seventh at night, the children will begin to be hot, with headache, sickness and the other usual symptoms. If these seem to be violent, let some blood be taken away; if not, let everything alone. Keep them in bed or in a warm room. The pocks will appear in the usual time, commonly in a very small number.[3]

After the matter is applied as above, they should be kept within doors, eat no salt meat nor much cheese or butter; their usual breakfast, a light pudding at dinner, milk at supper as is common.

As I am clearly convinced that procuring the disease in this slight manner will be of great advantage, so I cannot but warmly recommend it to all who have numerous families of small issue, and have paternal regard enough to wish their offspring safe through a most loathsome disease at a time they are on all accounts best suited to endure it.

Sister [4] joins me in sincere remembrance to you and sympathy in your affliction, and with dear love to both, conclude —

I am thy loving Brother
J. Fothergill

Ms. autograph letter, Fothergill Family Papers, Wallis Collection.

1. Alexander, Jr. (born in 1738), a boy of exceptional promise, had been sent when about ten years old to David Hall's school in Skipton. In 1750 he fell ill from smallpox of the most virulent kind and died before his parents could reach the school. — Fothergill Family Papers in possession of Mr. Edward Fothergill of Edinburgh.

2. Inoculation had first been promoted in London three decades earlier by Lady Mary Wortley Montague upon return from Turkey where her husband had served for two years as British Ambassador. Their six-year old son had been inoculated in Constantinople, and made a perfect recovery in a week's time. General acceptance of the practice had been retarded in England because of fear of the disease and opposition by the clergy, many of whom considered it interference with the will of God. Many physicians remained unconvinced of its value.

3. Dr. Fothergill provided his brother with simple, practical directions for protecting his family against smallpox, which was widespread in England during the eighteenth century. It was not until 1798 that inoculation was superseded by vaccination, discovered by Dr. Edward Jenner.

4. Ann Fothergill, who had come for a visit to her brother in 1749, and for the rest of his life made her home with him.

To Alexander Fothergill, Carr End, Wensleydale, Yorkshire, 26 January 1751

London, 26.11.1750/1

Dear Brother,

I have put on board the Batchelor, Capt. Milner, Master, for Stockton,[1] this afternoon a small bag of acorns and a cargo of some hundred young elms, as well secured as possible, directed for thee. I give thee this early notice, that thou may get some person to inquire for them, and convey them to thee as soon after they arrive as possible. I did not pay the charge of freight, but I'll be answerable for all expenses, if thou will be at the trouble of planting them. As there are a considerable number, I think it will be best to plant the largest out where they will remain; some in the hedges on low ground, others in more exposed places, and here and there little knots, as they bear transplanting pretty well. If the acorns are sown where they are intended to grow, it will be best; the ground must be dug, and now and then weeded as they come up.

I shall leave it to thee where to put them, and if anything further occurs to me I shall take the liberty to recommend it to thy care, and I hope it will be to thy benefit. I wrote a few weeks ago, and should have been very glad to know how thy family fares. Sister joins me in tenders of sincere affection to thee and thine — from

Thy loving Brother
J. Fothergill

Ms. autograph letter, Fothergill Family Papers, Wallis Collection.

1. Stockton-on-Tees in County Durham, from whence the shipment would be transported by cart to its destination.

To Dr. William Cuming, Dorchester in Dorset, 18 May 1751

London, 18.3.1751

Dear Doctor,

I had fully intended to have sent a copy of our Friend George Cleghorn's Epidemics of Minorca [1] to C. Hitch last night, but some unexpected avocations prevented it. He has been in town several months, very busy in compiling this account. We perused it together, and I have had a considerable share in correcting the press.[2] I must say nothing of the performance itself. I send it with his service, as a compliment from our Friend. He has been attending Hunter's course [3] with the assiduity of a young anatomist, and is now working upon Smellie,[4] with no less application. He is the same cheerfully industrious, plodding mortal as usual, and is laying up a fund of knowledge which I hope he will soon find a proper place to employ, with honor to himself and advantage to others. The regiment is in Ireland. He proposes to fix at Dublin, and if he sees the coast clear and things easy, to teach anatomy at that place.

Along with this treatise, I proposed to send a tract upon Electricity, wrote by a Gentleman with whom I have corresponded and who I think has said more sensible things on the subject, and let us see more into the nature of this delicate affair, than all the other writers put together. I send it, therefore, as a valuable tract of the kind, and as a proof that laziness has not hindered me from answering thy most obliging and Friendly letters, as this little work was published under my care and, so far as related to the press, my correction.[5] The proposal I had of sending one or both these pieces a long time ago prevented me from answering thy letters till it has become impossible to excuse myself and wipe off the appearance of disrespect. Let these, then, serve as a peace offering, and judge of my disposition when I acquaint thee that I had not resolution to open thy last for some time, the consciousness of my omission and the room I had given for just reproaches intimidating me more than I can ever remember on such an occasion. One or two little essays in the *Magazine* [6] are all that I have had time to do — and these at a year's distance — on Inoculation. I remember to have mentioned the principal circumstances contained in both in a letter I wrote long ago, when the smallpox broke out in Dorchester. — But for all this, I am not idle. My time is filled up with doing one thing or other all the day long. The evening is the only time I have for writing, and I need not say how irksome this sometimes is, though to a bosom Friend, after a day of moderate fatigue and to a person of no large share of strength or spirits.

I'll send Dr. Mead's late performance.[7] If it be not acceptable, please to return it. — I am glad to hear Dr. Glass [8] is engaged in a subject he is fitted for, and doubt [not] but this will confirm the reputation his first performance produced. The unavoidable engagements that have succeeded each other have hitherto prevented me from seeing Dr. Templeman.[9] Whilst G. Cleghorn stays my leisure will be less than afterwards. In about a month, the town will be thinner and business less. I will then wait upon him and confer with him upon the subject.

I dare not attempt to cancel the remembrance of my omissions by large promises of more punctuality, but it would be doing thy Friendship for me great injustice not to acknowledge the sincere and tender respect which thine discover, and which I'll endeavor to return as well as I can with the affection they deserve, and whatever delay a busy scene of life occasions me to make, yet a person who favors me with so disinterested regard will never be forgot. It is not the business of my profession that engages me altogether, but a number of little offices that are to be discharged on one account or another, and which often leave me little leisure.

Accept my best wishes, imitate a better example than mine. Let me know if I may send my packet by the means of Hitch, and be assured that I am

Thy affectionate Friend,

J. Fothergill

Ms. autograph letter, Richmond Academy of Medicine, Richmond, Virginia.

1. Dr. George Cleghorn had been a student at Edinburgh when Cuming and Fothergill were there. His *Observations on Epidemical Diseases of Minorca* (London, 1751) is an authoritative account assembled from notes made during years of practice in the Balearic Isles. Seven chapters, devoted to diseases afflicting both British soldiers and natives in Minorca, give clear accounts of "enteric fever, when complicated with tertian ague, with dysentery, with pneumonia," etc. His lucid descriptions of these cases, studied under conditions prevailing in the Mediterranean area, throw light upon many statements hitherto unexplainable in the Hippocratic writings. — "British Science" (unsigned), *Dawson Catalogue*, no. 142 (London, 1962), 142.

2. Proof sheets.

3. William Hunter (1718–1783), anatomist and obstetrician, conducted a private school of anatomy which gave superior training in this basic discipline of medicine. Hunter's school, first located in the Great Piazza, Covent Garden, was removed in 1767 to Great Windmill Street. — George C. Peachey, *A Memoir of John and William Hunter* (Plymouth, Eng.: Brandon, 1924); B. C. Corner, *William Shippen, Jr.: Pioneer in American Medical Education* (Philadelphia: American Philosophical Society, 1951), 69–73.

4. William Smellie (1697–1763), a well-known "man-midwife" in London, is said to have been the first to insist on pelvimetry in obstetrics. — R. W. Johnstone, *William Smellie: The Master of British Midwifery* (Edinburgh: Livingstone, 1952).

144

5. The Boston Public Library possesses one of Benjamin Franklin's personal copies of his *Experiments and Observations on Electricity Made at Philadelphia in America* (London, 1751), containing corrections and a table of contents in Franklin's own handwriting, and his own penciled shelf-mark. Franklin also added the name of the man who wrote the unsigned preface: Dr. Fothergill. — Edwin Wolf, 2d, "A Key to the Identification of Franklin's Books," *Pennsylvania Magazine of History and Biography*, 80 (1956): 407–409.

6. The essays to which J.F. refers here are presumably two brief anonymous articles, in his style (but not listed by the contemporary editors of his complete works) printed about this time in *The Gentleman's Magazine:* "Remarks on the Practice of Inoculating for the Smallpox," 20:147–148 (April 1750) and "Further Remarks on the Practice of Inoculation," 21:123–125 (March 1751).

7. *Monita et Praecepta Medica* (London, 1751), by Dr. Richard Mead (1673–1754). An English translation became available later in the year.

8. Dr. Thomas Glass (d. 1786) was preparing *An Account of the Antient Baths and Their Use in Physick*, published in 1752. In the same year, his earlier book, *Commentarii . . . de febribus ad Hippocratis Disciplinarium* (London, 1742), was published in translation.

9. Peter Templeman (1711–1769) took his medical degree at Leyden. He settled in London but never practiced, preferring a life of scholarly pursuits. In the 1750's, he asked for Dr. Fothergill's help in starting a quarterly journal of abstracts from important European and scientific journals; the venture failed from lack of subscribers. In 1758, when the British Museum was established, Templeman was chosen Keeper of Printed Books. In 1760, he left this post to become Secretary of the newly formed Society for the Encouragement of Arts, Commerce, and Manufactures, a position which required careful study and wide correspondence. In 1762 the Académie Royale des Sciences of Paris elected him to membership in recognition of his accomplishments in furthering scientific knowledge. — John Nichols, *Biographical and Literary Anecdotes of William Bowyer* (London, 1782), 275–276.

To Alexander Fothergill, Carr End, Wensleydale, Yorkshire, 18 June 1752

London, 18.4.1752

Dear Brother:

I received thine of the eleventh and thy former relating to dear Father which was acceptable.[1] In answer to thy last, I am sorry 'tis not in my power to be of much service to the young man; his case seems to be a confirmed consumption [2] and little chance for his recovery. However, I have ordered some little affairs on the other side which may be made use of, though I am afraid to little other purpose than not to have it said that I could not ease him.

145

A mild diet almost altogether will be proper, and no meat except the very lightest and that in small quantities must be allowed; thin broth, gruel, rice, sago and such like with milk may be allowed. He must keep warm, ride out in moderate weather and sheltered places, as his strength may permit, and avoid doing anything that would fatigue or expose him to fresh cold. A calf's foot baked in moderate heat in two quarts of water and one of milk, with a little cinnamon, would make a pleasant nourishment for him. Please to give my respects to the family, and assure them of my readiness to serve them, though in the present case I fear 'twill be without success.

As to thy Friend Whaley,[3] I know not well what to advise; I think little journeys, long continued, would be of most use; and if he could bear a journey to London, though an expensive yet would be a beneficial remedy. A proper season is approaching when he may expect both good company and good roads. I have ordered some pills that will prevent his being restive if they are regularly continued for some time.[4]

I had little expectations of the young trees, as the weather set in; I am glad however that the box came safe.[5] I had ordered the carriage to be paid, but my servant neglected or forgot my order to him. Had I always a proper opportunity of sending, I should not scruple any expense to furnish thee with things of this nature, as I am very certain that in time they will amply repay both the trouble and expense to thyself, besides the pleasure of seeing a naked country daily covered, with shelter to thy cattle, fuel, and timber. I must therefore request thee to take care of this sort of nursery with some assiduity and to fill up every vacant or proper spot as full as possible. I wish thou would get some poplar cuttings from Cheshire, stick 'em into hedgerows near the water, and they'd grow without care and soon be fit for various uses. I propose to send some osier plants, with directions to manage them, at the end of the summer if I am well; if these are planted near the water's edge, in a year or two they'd afford a fine crop and make the ground firm at the same time.

I have scarce left room to tell thee that we are through mercy well, and I continue to have some little employ. We had some expectations thou would have seen us this spring but from thy silence we conclude it will not be so. Thy employment on the road we fear will keep thee from home, but don't unnecessarily make it more. Remember thy lonely companion who claims all thy regard and will do all in her power to keep alive in thee as well as in herself a due sensibility and dependence.

Farewell, and believe us affectionately thine,

J. Fothergill

Ms. autograph letter, Fothergill Family Papers, Wallis Collection.

1. Alexander evidently sent some information relating to their father for Dr. Fothergill to use in the memorial volume he was preparing.

2. Phthisis pulmonaris, or tuberculosis.

3. Friend Whaley cannot be distinguished from many others bearing that surname in Yorkshire. He was evidently psychically disturbed and needed a change of scene and slight medication.

4. The placebos written on the other side as prescriptions to impress the patient have not been included here.

5. In an earlier letter, not included here, Dr. Fothergill had promised to send by carrier "a small parcel of little elms in hopes that they may grow, and a parcel of acorns to be thrown into some sheltered spot defended from the cattle. Sow 'em not over thick, and let them take care of themselves."

To John Smith, Philadelphia, 20 August 1753

London, 20.8.1753

Esteemed Friend,[1]

I have long thought myself under various obligations to thee for transmitting useful productions of your press. The acknowledgment that accompanies this is at present the only one I can make, and which I hope will not be unacceptable. I received thy kind letter by Dr. Willan whose precipitate return from the province made such an introduction necessary, for as I had some share in procuring him the place, I considered myself in some respects answerable for it, and to those under whose direction he had undertaken to act.[2] If the School is again well supplied, I shall rejoice. If not, as it's a thing of great consequence, and [if] my reputation [is] not quite forfeited, I shall readily do all in my power to assist you, and am not without hopes but I might prevail upon a young man I have in view to come over, though as yet he has not been spoke to about it. Though I am not personally acquainted with thyself and wife, yet I have been so much accustomed to hear you both spoke of with great respect that I cannot but esteem you, and wish that you may long continue happy in each other and ornaments to your profession — for a conscientious attention to the duties it prescribes will be the best ground for mutual affection to flourish in.

I am with, true regard,
Your assured Friend
John Fothergill

Ms. autograph letter, Watson Annals, I, 298, HSP.

1. John Smith (1722–1771), of Burlington, New Jersey, a descendant of Yorkshire Quakers, operated a line of packets sailing regularly between Philadelphia and Liverpool and conducted an export-import trade. He was a member of the first Board of Managers of the Pennsylvania Hospital and treasurer of the Philadelphia Contributionship, the first fire insurance company in America. In 1748 he married James Logan's daughter Hannah. In 1751 he succeeded Israel Pemberton as Clerk of the Philadelphia Quarterly Meeting and became Overseer of the Friends Grammar School. He was elected to the Provincial Assembly in 1750 and again in 1751. In 1756 he retired from business in Philadelphia and returned to Burlington. That same year, Hannah Smith became a minister of the Burlington Meeting and sought "to shut out from her mind all worldly vanities." She died in 1762 at the age of forty-two. John Smith died nine years later at the age of forty-nine. Four children survived them. — R. Morris Smith, *The Burlington Smiths* (Philadelphia: Privately printed, 1877); *Hannah Logan's Courtship*; Nicholas Wainwright, *The Philadelphia Contributionship* (Philadelphia: privately printed, 1952).

2. Robert Willan, M.D., had been recommended for the post of schoolmaster in a letter to Israel Pemberton, 25 April 1748 (above). The reason for his sudden return to England is unknown. In December 1749, James Logan, writing to Dr. Fothergill, had reported: "Robert Willan, who brought me the last letter I have had from thee, recommends himself more and more amongst Friends, and appears now to be in a way that he may depend upon for a small living. Friends have lately built a handsome and commodious School-House in several apartments, where he teaches Latin in one ground floor." — James Logan Letter-Book, p. 30, letter of 12.14.1749 (uncatalogued), HSP. After his return to Yorkshire, Robert Willan established a successful medical practice in the region of Sedbergh, living nearby in the family homestead, The Hill, where his son and namesake was born in 1757. This son received an Edinburgh M.D. in 1780 and became a famous dermatologist. — *Munk's Roll*, II, 350–353.

To Alexander Fothergill, Carr End, Wensleydale, Yorkshire, 12 January 1754

London, 12.1.1754

Dear Brother,

Sheltered in a warm abode and screened from many an inclement blast that you endure, we often look towards you and with some share of commiseration. You are accustomed to it from year to year and feel it less, yet you do feel it and so do we, with all the guard we can procure.

If you are well and contented you are happy. Kings can have no more, and myriads depart the stage without enjoying even this. But enough of these reflections — they show we remember you as we doubt not you do us, and a few minutes respite being allowed, I embrace it to give thee some account of us.

My time is much less my own than ever, and if I live must still be less so for a season. My business is not the most gainful. Many, very many I attend as a duty which costs me labour and some thought; yet all my business is not of this kind. I have greater income than ever I expected, but my expenses are likewise large, and as it is but very lately that I was fairly upon a [financial] level, so it will be long, if I live, ere I get so much as to maintain me with less labour. I generally go out at nine and am traversing the streets till two or past. I then come home to dinner, and if not called out before, I begin about 4 o'clock and have something to do till between 7 and 8, now and then till 9. It would perhaps surprise thee to hear that last year afforded me not less than 18000 [1] pounds and that I spent not much less than 1000 pounds, yet this is not far from the truth. I imagine that my business is greatly magnified, but so intimate a friend, so near a relative ought to be better informed.

When I consider my beginning, progress and present condition: a youth, a stranger, with little money, without friends, being utterly unknown in the place — and that from thence in the space of about 17 years, two of which were wholly spent in improvement here, I should be favoured so far, it raises many a serious and sometimes grateful consideration and acknowledgement to a power whose great name I am not worthy to mention.

Thy son, I hope, will be taken suitable care of at Coz. Gilbert's.[2] The expense I shall cheerfully defray. Sister Ann has had some care and thought at least on Jane's account,[3] and has been thinking of some means of enabling her to get a better subsistence than by service only; if what she proposes is practicable, I shall do my part towards executing it, and do it with pleasure in order to convince thee of the unfeigned affection I bear thee as my Brother and my Father's son, as well as to excite thee to a diligent application to thy own immediate concerns for the benefit of thy family. For as by nature and duty thy children are more thy own care than they are of mine, so if thou waste on the affairs of others that precious time which ought to be employed in the first place in overseeing their nurture, and in the next in providing for their present and future subsistence, I am afraid the account will at one time or other prove very painful and dissatisfactory to thyself. — I should perhaps give pain was I to enter into particulars, but this I don't intend. I am not perfect, and have no reason to take up the stone. Yet, in brotherly love, permit me to intreat that as much as possible thou wilt refuse every unnecessary appointment, and not suffer a good understanding and very valuable qualifications to be made a sacrifice to knaves and fools, while thy own may want and justly demand the whole of thy attention.

The kind presents at length came safe and were acceptable. I shall discharge thy obligation to Sister Ann for the sum of 10 pounds as desired. She proposes to write soon. — One word more and I must conclude: remember planting, the time is at hand. And as firs grow with so much expedition, put them down everywhere when while young they may be defended and under their covert every other species of timber. Farewell, accept our dear love to thyself and family, and be assured that I am

Thy affectionate Brother
J. Fothergill

Pray remember me to the Worthy Justice.[4]

Ms. autograph letter, Fothergill Family Papers, Wallis Collection.

1. £18,000 as written in the original letter seems a relatively large sum for a young physician practicing in London.

2. Alexander's son John was to attend a school in Penketh, Lancashire, conducted by Gilbert Thompson II. This Quaker school, founded in 1687 by Gilbert Thompson I, remained in family charge for three generations. Pupils coming from places outside Penketh were boarded in the homes of local Friends. — Crosfield, *Memoirs,* 493, 494; Fox, 127, 128.

3. Jane Fothergill (1735–1820), only surviving child of Alexander Fothergill's first marriage. — Fothergill Genealogy, below.

4. Thomas Metcalf.

To Israel Pemberton, Jr., Philadelphia, 11 November 1754

London, 11.11.1754

Much esteemed Friend,

I must commit to thy care the enclosed packet for my Brother and Catherine Payton.[1] The former may perhaps have left you ere this; C.P. and her companion [2] may probably be with you or near you when this arrives. We have yet had no account of my Brother's arrival with you,[3] but I have little doubt that all is well as the season was so favourable and the cause he is engaged in of the best. Thy kind and pressing invitation of him to thy house is an obligation upon me. In return, when thou once more visits England, if I have a house, make it thy home. It would give me I think as much satisfaction as anything I know to see you [in Philadelphia] but this cannot, must not be. I am fettered to this spot, I believe for life, but my mind visits you, and my warmest wishes for your good, your steady progress in that way which heaven has cast up for you, not indeed devoid of trial and of the deepest kind, but a way that he can and will enable you to persevere in, if it is chosen preferable to any other.

Wise and great are the chiefs among you. Some of them have left solid and lasting memorials in this Island; if they met with opposition, they met also with unity and love, as well as admiration of the goodness of the great master in keeping such to preserve wisdom in the earth.

Though I have had notice some days of Capt. Hargraves sailing, yet I have been prevented from writing till the evening before his departure, and have several things to say, if I am not interrupted to one or another. I have written a long letter to B. Franklin [4] on a subject that lately occurred to my thoughts in respect to thy present situation. How far my opinion is right I submit to thyself and other judges. Your colony has always been on a different and better footing with the Indians than the rest. You have spoke peace and observed it. — Would it not be prudent to invite as many Indians as possible to retire into your province for the present; and even to engage the most intelligent of them to go amongst the several tribes they know, not their allies tributaries or dependents only, and to offer them in your name support and assistance in their wants, if they retire amongst you, and subsistence to their wives and children during the present troubles? — What will be the consequence? Many will come and be a certain expense to you, but will not their being amongst you cement an indelible regard for you, and will they suffer your province to be invaded whilst you provide for their families? Are not you by this means preventing the French from forcing them to molest you, and pointing out to their own confederate Indians a place of security, for their members will be their own and your security? You consider the expense? It will be great, and you are able. And will you not have all hearts and hands concuring in furnishing cheerfully so consistent a supply? Will ye not by this means increase your consequence with the whole Indian name, on all future occasions, and be the umpires betwixt them and the other colonies in all their disputes? The Government here are in earnest in supporting in their manner the British rights, and will not suffer either fraud, flattery or force to deter them from asserting their rights. — But you have a different trait, yet at the same time may effectually serve the common cause.[5] By lessening their expense in subsisting the Indians who will rather [on the other hand] be imitated by the more corrupt example of the people in the other colonies than in yours. Think of it, if it appears reasonable, and I know there is little doubt if thou engages in it but many others will be of the same opinion. — I write in great haste, and I fear scarce intelligibly, but guess at my meaning and excuse me if I judge wrongly. — Please to remember me to J. Churchman and William Brown,[6] to Mr. Lightfoot, thy Brothers,[7] and accept the cordial friendship of

J. Fothergill

If Brother Samuel is not in Philadelphia please to pass the enclosed to him, put it under a cover and send it to him; only mention nothing that I had ever entertained a thought of coming over for this cannot be and would appear so romantic perhaps as to lessen the credit of the writer.[8]

Ms. autograph letter, Pemberton Papers, Etting Collection, I, 98, HSP.

1. Catherine Payton (1726–1794), the daughter of well-placed parents, received the gift of the ministry when she was only twenty-two, and thereafter made many religious visits throughout Great Britain during forty-six years of service. — *The Memoirs and Life of Catherine Payton* (Philadelphia, 1797).

2. Mary Peisley, the "endeared Friend" of Catherine Payton, also a Quaker minister and often Catherine's traveling companion. In 1757 Mary Peisley married Samuel Neale, a Quaker preacher, but unfortunately was soon thereafter "removed from mutability" and greatly mourned. Her husband, Samuel Neale, wrote a book commemorating their years of service as Quaker ministers. — *Ibid.*, 157.

3. On 2 August 1754, when Samuel Fothergill left his home in Warrington to sail for the American Colonies, he was accompanied by his wife and a party of thirty Friends as far as Leek, where he took passage on a stagecoach for London. At St. Albans, his sister met him. In London, Samuel stayed with John Churchman (1705–1755), a Quaker minister from Chester County, Pennsylvania, who was to sail with him on the *Carolina*, Capt. Stephen Mesnard. They took ship at Gravesend to Margate, but bad weather kept them in the Downs from 11 August to 18 August. The *Carolina* reached the "Capes of the Delaware River" on 23 September. A pilot came aboard to direct the ship "120 miles up the river above Wilmington," where, upon landing, they found Churchman's kinsman William Brown (d. 1786), another minister from Chester County, awaiting them. Although Brown had sailed from London three

weeks earlier, he had arrived only that day. Samuel Fothergill and Churchman hired horses and rode to Philadelphia that evening. They lodged at Israel Pemberton's house, where they met with a warm welcome. — Crosfield *Memoirs*, 150–151.

4. Not located. Franklin at this time was the recognized leader of the Pennsylvania Assembly; Dr. Fothergill had corresponded with him intermittently for some years, and had written the preface for his *Experiments . . . on Electricity* in 1751.

5. No satisfactory plans for helping the Indians to help themselves were made until very much later. They were very uneasy because of the presence of the French in the Ohio Valley, and their relations with the British colonists were precarious. During the winter of 1754–55, loyal Indians were supported at a fort west of Harris Ferry (now Harrisburg). In the spring they joined General Braddock's army on his march toward Fort Duquesne.

6. Both Churchman and Brown were returning from religious visits of four years' duration in Holland and England.

7. John and James Pemberton, brothers of Israel, Jr., and partners in the family mercantile business.

8. As requested, the "enclosed" was undoubtedly forwarded to Samuel. The undated scrap of paper containing this request and the few lines which follow was found among the Pemberton Papers (HSP), not definitely attached to any particular letter. Since both handwriting and color of ink match perfectly the script of this letter dated 11.11.1754, the message is placed here where it seems to belong.

IV
1755-1764

I think myself not a little fortunate that
at the time of life when my faculties (such
as they are) are at their most favourable
state, I have more frequent opportunities of
observation than many others of the profession;
. . . I would willingly be ever attentive to
the voice of nature as far as it is discernible
by observation.

To Cadwallader Colden, October 23, 1755

To Alexander Fothergill, Carr End, Wensleydale, Yorkshire, 2 March 1755

London, 2.3.1755

Dear Brother,

The post after thou left us brought the inclosed,[1] which according to thy request is sent thee by the first opportunity. — Two days ago I received another affectionate letter from Brother Samuel dated at Charles Town, South Carolina, 15th.2d mo., which left him very well, easy and thankful for many preservations through a long, long journey of upwards of 2000 miles in a wilderness country. He intended to set out the day after he wrote for Georgia, and proposes to reach Philadelphia by the end of this month, at which place I hope he will receive thine, and a number of other letters from Europe which his rapid progress has hindered him from receiving in other places. — He writes cheerfully with respect to himself, and fully satisfied in his place. His health has been uninterrupted, and secret strength afforded for every service to his content.

Sister Ann is still poorly, though I hope a little recruiting. This morning she sent me word she had a better night than any since she went into the country, and yesterday I thought her somewhat better, so that I hope she will soon be restored to her usual if not better health, and be long my Sister, my companion, my Friend and my example. — This I hope will meet thee got home in safety, and happy in thy family. Remember me to them affectionately, and endeavour to be to them what our Father was to us; so will providence bless thy care, and make them a blessing to thee in thy old age. Thou knows my wishes, my views, and let me say, my hopes that thou will withstand to the utmost of thy power, the seduction that lies near and, I confess, to us both. But greater

157

will be the triumph if with capacities to please, we rather choose to follow the dictates of simple unpleasing truth, and thus become fools for Christ's sake. — The hardest of all lessons to many. — With respect to public affairs, all is at present quiet. I wish well to my country, but if providence sees much to provide for our security by any other means than in bloodshed, it would give me double satisfaction.

I could not tell how to put up the inclosed, without some little intimation of an affectionate remembrance, and in haste have thus thrown out the sentiments of brotherly regard.

J. Fothergill

Ms. autograph letter, Fothergill Family Papers, Wallis Collection.

1. Probably a letter from their brother Samuel, still absent on a religious visit to the American Colonies.

To Israel Pemberton, Jr., Philadelphia, 8 July 1755

London, 8.7.1755

Dear Friend,

[*Passage omitted.*] Thy letter respecting your present public concerns came very seasonably, and I hope will tend, with some other intelligence of the like nature, to check the torrent of perfidious reflections that are poured out and propagated industriously by a set of men who, because they have once used us extremely ill, think the best way to prove that in making martyrs of some of our ancestors they did right is to continue the inveterate enemy, in secret at least, of those they have so evilly mistreated through every generation.[1] The judicious, pathetic Epistle from your Quarterly Meeting to the Meeting for Sufferings was read in this Meeting last 6th day.[2] Lest the members should not so generally attend as so important an affair required, the correspondents found means to have notice given to each one, so that the meeting was as full as could at the season be expected. The Epistle, I believe, gave general satisfaction, and had one or two expressions respecting the Proprietary's views been a little softened, not omitted, I think it would have been unexceptionable. [*Passage omitted.*]

And here I must in part take blame upon myself for advising R.P. to present the Assembly's address as early as he did.[3] A violent clamour was then raised through the nation by that scandalous invective, and I was in no doubt but your agent would have been furnished with ample material to vindicate your conduct and by a judicial determination stem the torrent of abuse we were subjected to on your account. But this happened not to be the case. The cause was debated before persons not inclined to favour you, and a determination framed as much to the defenders' wishes as the most sanguine favour of Despotism could desire. — The committee[4] were called upon last week by R.P. to have their opinion what further steps to take in the affair. It was advised to lie still at present. The popular odium against you is not fully subsided; but I have not much doubt but it will be in your power at length to subdue all groundless prejudice and create in the minds of some here more favourable sentiments towards you. Nothing will be lost we think by this delay, should it be necessary to bring the affair before a superior board.[5] Your agents will have more ample material; and . . . they will probably come before judges less prepossessed against them. This was the advice given, and here at present the cause will probably rest. — A few Friends some months ago waited upon the Proprietor respecting this affair, and acquainted him that it gave the Society great concern to see things carried to such lengths that the Society here could not long remain unaffected spectators; that we esteemed the Proprietary family, had always endeavored to manifest it, and should ever cheerfully embrace the like opportunity. But that as you and we were part of the same body, we could not see your liberties and privileges at stake, your characters impeached, and measures pursued that seemed oppressive without endeavouring to lend you assistance. [*Passage omitted.*] We were heard patiently, and in return were obliged to hear many things which at that time we had not materials to contradict sufficiently. We parted however in tolerably good terms, but without any success in our application which was to recommend a reconciliation.

The Proprietor is reserved, tenacious and inflexible, yet there is one person who I believe can influence him. I believe it will be proposed to the committee that this one person may be waited on by one or two persons whom he has some esteem for, and the state of the country in general and of the Society in particular, as contained in your Epistle, fully explained to him. The person I mean is the President of the Privy Council.[6] He is acquainted already with every particular on the Proprietor's side and with some on the other, and I think has so much moderation as well as good sense as to see from the whole that his kinsman's interest must suffer greatly if the contest is not soon and amicably adjusted. If impressions of this nature can be made on this nobleman, the rest of the work I think will not be difficult, and however it turns out, we may probably learn from such a conversation what success the cause may gain if carried up to the Council, for . . . from his knowledge as well as by authority, he has very great sway in that place . . . [Without] some such influence I fear that neither the entreaty of [the Proprietor's] friends, the voice of reason nor the demands of interest will bend a most determined resolution to pursue the same passionate measures.

There are two sets of people, one here, another both with you and everywhere, who I imagine are secretly strengthening the Proprietor's mistakes, and both with very different views. If I am not greatly mistaken, here are some very active and powerful people near the head of plantation affairs, who would be very glad to crush every appearance of liberty abroad, and are pleased that in a country like yours, so favourable a pretext is offering itself to make you an example. A temper like this is not likely to promote the most friendly sentiments concerning an Assembly so tenacious of their rights, but will rather stir up the flame. [*Passage omitted.*] I wish I may be mistaken in my opinion, but it cannot be amiss for any concerned in legislation on your side to look a little this way, and in every future message or resolution to leave out as much personal acrimony as possible, whatever room may be offered for it.

The other party who I suspect are promoting secretly and unweariedly the dissensions amongst you are the Presbyterians.⁷ No disagreeable circumstance happens but it is immediately sent to the party here; who besides employing it to give us pain are making use of it for other purposes. If they can so far imitate those in power here as to induce them to exclude us altogether from legislation, I mean in Pennsylvania, they gain a most important point, and this I cannot but think they aim at. What must be done under all these difficulties? Just what the wisest and best among you seem to be doing — acting faithfully and uprightly in your stations, and redoubling your care to be found in the way that is well pleasing to him who rules the universe.

It is not without very sensible regret that I see myself in such a situation as at present hinders me from keeping up such a correspondence with many as I believe would be to my benefit. I can employ no deputy, no assistant — the whole is to be done with one pair of hands, supported by none of the strongest constitutions. I am often engaged in the duties of my profession from morning to night with scarce sufficient rest, yet without being able to foresee in what manner I may with satisfaction be set free from it. At present it seems to be my duty; when it is otherwise I hope to drop anchor; hitherto neither the love of wealth nor fame are my principal inducements.

When leisure permits, write to me, and when I can I'll reply.

John Fothergill

Ms. autograph letter, Pemberton Papers, Etting Collection, II, 3. HSP.

1. Bitter feeling against the Quakers had been stirred up in England as well as in America by reports in the press of renewed controversy between the Pennsylvania Assembly and the Proprietary government over money, Indian affairs, and questions of defense. In January 1755 the Assembly, in which the Quakers were still a majority, had dispatched an address to the Crown, protesting vehemently the veto by Governor Morris in December 1754 of a bill granting £20,000 "to the King's use." The address implied that the responsibility for the veto lay with the Proprietors, and prayed for redress.

2. The Epistle, dated on 5 May 1755, set forth the difficulties distressing the Pennsylvania Friends — including disagreement among the Friends themselves — resulting from the political controversy. Quakers were willing, they wrote, to give up their Assembly seats provided that non-Quakers could serve the Province with equal devotion; but this they doubted. As long as they were evidently trusted by the majority of their fellow citizens, Friends were unwilling to relinquish their share in legislation. The Epistle asked the London Friends to intervene with the Proprietors "to obviate an apprehension that we are unwilling to allow the Propy's their just Rights . . . & would promote a change of Government by obliging them to resign it to the King." — See Wolff, *Colonial Agency*, 170–171, and Thayer, *Israel Pemberton*, 78. A copy of the Epistle is to be found in the University of Pennsylvania library; another, certified by Israel Pemberton, in the Library of Congress.

3. On the advice of influential Friends, Richard Partridge, agent for the Assembly, had approached the Proprietors directly in the hope of resolving the difficulty, but Thomas Penn insisted that the address take its due course. Accordingly, it was presented, referred from the Privy Council to the Board of Trade in April, and in May argued hotly before that board. On 30 May the petition was rejected, with a strong reprimand to the Assembly.

4. The Committee of the Board of Trade to which the address of the Pennsylvania Assembly had been referred.

5. The Privy Council.

6. John Carteret (1690–1763), first Earl Granville (1744), was President of the Privy Council from 1751 until his death. In 1744 he had married Lady Sophia Fermor, daughter of the Earl of Pomfret and older sister of Lady Juliana Fermor who in 1751 became the wife of Thomas Penn.

7. The Presbyterians, rivals of the Quakers in business and ambitious for political power, were realistically demanding military protection of the province from Indian attacks.

To Thomas Penn, Braywick near Maidenhead, Berkshire, 15 July 1755

London, July 15, 1755

Esteemed Friend,[1]

Though by the last account I received I thought there was just reason to hope for Lady Juliana's speedy recovery; and as I have received no intimation to the contrary, my hopes are the more confirmed, yet it would give me pleasure to know from thyself that everything proceeds agreeably. My solicitude for her welfare will plead my excuse for asking it, and had either the distance been less, or my engagements here would have permitted, I should ere this time once more have waited upon her. If she is so far recovered as to be safely left a day or two, and business calls thee to town, it would give me great satisfaction to be indulged with half an hour's conversation upon a subject I hope not altogether disagreeable. I have commonly something upon the table a little before 3 o'clock, and if it is convenient to be in the city about that time any day, be pleased to favour me with thy company.

The city has been in great and somewhat joyous agitation today, on account of an express arrived from Admiral Boscawen.[2] Two of the French men of war have fallen into our hands, a third struck, but escaped in the fog. It is said that the engagement was betwixt 3 and 3 of a side and that the French exceeded in point of metal about 30 guns, and men in proportion.

The flame of war is now inevitably kindled, in those parts of the world where it must in all probability terminate in our favour, provided no weight is unhappily cast into the opposite scale on this side of the ocean.

Accept my best wishes for Lady Juliana's happy recovery, and believe me that I am,

thy obliged respectful Friend
John Fothergill

Ms. autograph letter, Penn Papers, Private Correspondence, IV, 196, HSP.

1. Thomas Penn (1702–1775), son of William Penn and his second wife, Hannah Callowhill, had succeeded to his father's duties as Propietor of Pennsylvania, assisted by his brother Richard. In 1751 Thomas Penn married Lady Juliana Fermor, youngest daughter of the Earl of Pomfret. William Penn's descendants gradually drifted away from the Society of Friends. Secular dating of this letter by Dr. Fothergill

seems to indicate that Thomas Penn had already adopted worldly customs and, like his wife was now a member of the Church of England. — Howard M. Jenkins, *The Family of William Penn, Founder of Pennsylvania* (Philadelphia, The author; London, Hadley Brothers, 1899), 129–152.

2. Rear-admiral Edward Boscawen (1711–1761) had been given command of a squadron bound for North America, with orders to attack French ships wherever encountered. Overtaking the *Alcide*, the *Lye*, and the *Dauphin*, Boscawen captured the first two while fog aided the escape of the *Dauphin*. Because a violent fever was spreading among his seamen, Boscawen made port in Halifax to get medical assistance before starting back for England. On the return voyage, the casualties of his fleet totaled more than 2,000 before he reached Spithead. — NCMH, VII, 36, 46.

To Thomas Penn, Braywick near Maidenhead, Berkshire, 31 July 1755

London, July 31, 1755

Esteemed Friend,

Had leisure seconded my inclination, I should probably ere this have requested another night's lodging at Braywick; in the first place to have paid my respects to Lady Juliana and inquired after her health, and in the next to have known thy sentiments on the letter, a copy of which I took the liberty to put into thy hands when we were last together.[1]

Perhaps in taking this step, was it to be known, I might be deemed imprudent; but I thought it was so authentic a declaration of the sentiments of the cooler and best part of the Society in Pennsylvania in the favour of the interest which I wish well to, I mean the Proprietary family, that I thought it might assist thee in forming a judgement of the whole, by hearing this part of the body speak for themselves.

Pursuant to their pressing request to the Meeting for Sufferings, five or six persons are by them nominated to wait again upon thee, and to promote, if possibly they can, that harmony which cannot but be mutually desirable and beneficial.

Amongst those who are appointed are Thomas Jackson,[2] John Hanbury[3] and myself; the others I don't just now recollect. If for any reason I can apprehend any of the rest of our associates are improper and unacceptable, they will be prevented from attending a conference which it is hoped may be productive of mutual benefit.

Thomas Jackson is finally recovered, yet not so well as to go from place to place without some difficulty. If therefore it will be agreeable

163

to give the Friends appointed a meeting and at his house, it would be a great ease to him. The time is submitted wholly to thyself, and if I may be assured of it the day before, I'll endeavour to give proper notice.

It is neither from an opinion of my own fitness to engage in things of this nature, nor from a presumption upon the favourable regard I have always received from the Proprietary family in the way of my profession, that I have submitted to be one in this appointment; but purely with a wish from the most disinterested esteem, to join in removing every obstacle to that reciprocal confidence which alone can perpetuate under Providence the felicity which the people now enjoy, and in their happiness establish the Proprietary's interest on the most lasting foundation.

Was I in the least equal to the task, I know of no difficulty that would discourage me in so laudable an attempt, but if I can do nothing else, I hope always to be able to manifest an upright intention, at least, of faithfully contributing to this reciprocal confidence and by this, as well as every other part of my conduct, assuring thee that I am with great gratitude and respect

Thy sincere Friend,
J. Fothergill

Arranged
August 3 for
Thursday 4 o'clock, Thomas Jackson's
[*Added in another hand.*]

Ms. autograph letter, Penn Papers, Private Correspondence, IV, 198, HSP.

1. The Epistle from the Philadelphia Quarterly Meeting referred to in letter of 8 July above.

2. Thomas Jackson, proprietor of a medicinal warehouse in Fleet Market, held "the Royal Patent for medicine for Rheumatism and Stone, and supplied Country Shopkeepers . . . with most medicines in publick use, such as Bateman's and Stoughton's Drops." — Thomas Mortimer, *The Universal Directory* (London, 1763), London's first business directory.

3. John Hanbury of Tower Street (d. 1759), head of the Virginia Company, made his fortune from the tobacco trade. He was a member of an important Quaker family with numerous branches. Among Virginia planters trading with the Hanburys were Carters, Byrds, the Washington and Custis families. — Amy Audrey Locke, *The Hanbury Family*, II (London: Humphries, 1916), 299; Douglas Southall Freeman, *George Washington, A Biography* (New York: Scribners, 1948), I, 160–169; II, 264, 300–302.

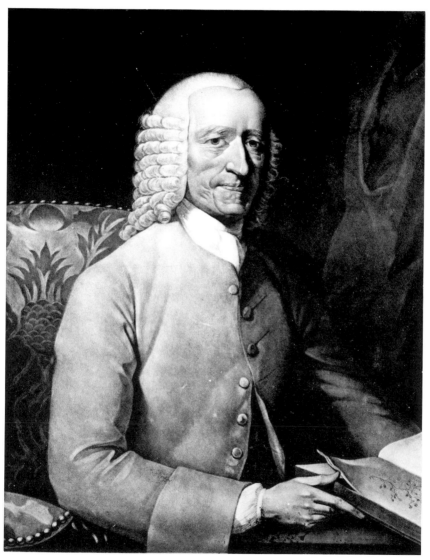

John Fothergill, M.D., F.R.S.
Engraved by Valentine Green, after the posthumous portrait by Gilbert Stuart

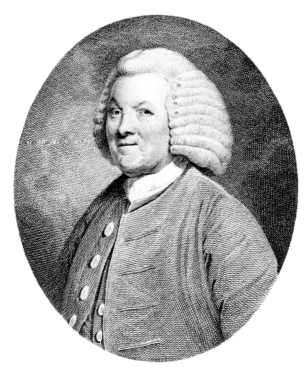

William Cuming, M.D.
Dr. Fothergill's friend from student days

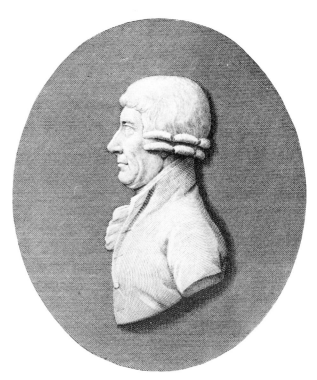

John Coakley Lettsom, M.D.
Dr. Fothergill's protégé and biographer

To Israel Pemberton, Jr., Philadelphia, 18 August 1755

London, 18.8.1755

Dear Friend,

· [*Short passage omitted.*]

I believe I may say that the Epistle from your Quarterly Meeting to the Meeting for Sufferings [1] fully answered your intent in sending it. It convinced many who doubted of the justice and propriety of divers parts of your conduct that had been otherwise represented, and induced them unanimously to coincide with your request that the Proprietaries here might be treated with on your behalf in the manner you request. And here I must request as I have done repeatedly in a former, that what I say, may be only to thyself, as probably I may otherwise incur deserved blame for what I intended for your benefit. — As I am employed in the Proprietary Family, and have been for some years and am treated by them with respect, I took the liberty to put a copy of your Epistle into his hands (T.P.),[2] in order to give him the most authentic proof of the just and becoming sentiments of Friends towards him. I have seen him since, and he has both it and the friendly remonstrances of divers of the Society here, who waited upon him, under his consideration; and I am not without some hope that some milder measures may at length be pursued.[3] And here give me leave to observe that we meet with no inconsiderable difficulty from the warmth with which he has been treated by some members of the Assembly, and particularly in the answer of the committee to his letter inserted in the votes.[4] I would by no means enter into a consideration of their propriety. Those who drew up and those who confirmed the report had doubtless just reason in their apprehension for what they did. But I would just take leave to observe, and that with the utmost deference, that a good cause may suffer by too passionate a vindication; and as there are many persons among you of very quick parts and great fire, so there ought to be a careful lookout not to suffer anything unnecessarily poignant to escape you. The tame and servile is doubtless as contemptible as the keen and vindictive are provoking; the happy mean is that mild and manly spirit which solid religion inspires, and I think one need only to ask how we would like to be treated by those who differ from us to know how we should treat others.

I would not be understood to censure what has passed. I only wish that

165

for your sake, for ours, who wish heartily to serve you, that at the same time you endeavor steadily to preserve your liberties, all acrimony may be kept down, as this only widens the breach between you. As the Proprietors have the whole state of the affair before them, and a deputation appointed to confer with them, they have no dislike to and have promised an answer speedily; it will not I think be long ere you hear further from us; and I heartily wish that harmony and peace may be once more restored.

We seem to be just at the eve of a bloody war though neither side have yet declared. This day two French prizes have been sent into the Downs [5] by a ship of war, and the first that have been sent in. But whether they are brought under pretense of their being spies, or on what other account, the public is yet uncertain. Great harmony, uncommon vigilance, impenetrable secrecy, aided by a few wise and experienced heads, seem to prevail in our councils, which both confounds our enemies and procures the Regency the confidence and approbation of the public. The French are angry to the last degree, uncertain what measures to take, sure of a dreadful havoc to their commerce by sea, should they declare war; and very doubtful of obtaining any advantages by land, should they vent their rage upon our confederates. To add to their difficulties, they are not without some vexatious embarrassments at home, and yet under all cannot condescend to do us the justice we require. Accounts are brought today that St. Johns [6] in Fundy Bay is taken, also 2 more men of war and some merchant ships, all of which are carried to Halifax.[7]

[*Short passage omitted.*]

You are all too partial in my favour. I can do but little to serve you, but you have always my wishes for the good and happiness of the Province.

J. Fothergill

Ms. autograph letter, Pemberton Papers, Etting Collection, II, 4, HSP.

1. See letter of 8 July 1755.
2. Thomas Penn.
3. The Proprietary faction in Pennsylvania was attempting to secure Parliamentary action excluding Quakers from the legislature. — Wolff, *Colonial Agency*, 171.
4. See the Assembly's address to the Proprietors (23 August 1751), the Proprietors' reply (23 May 1753), and the report of the committee of the Assembly which laid it before that body (11 September 1753). These documents were printed in the votes of the Assembly for the session of 1754–55, and laid before the Board of Trade by

Thomas Penn on 7 May 1755. — *Pennsylvania Archives*, 8 ser., V, 3808–3827; *Journal of the Board of Trade*, 1754–1758.

5. The Downs — that part of the sea between the shoals of the Goodwin Sands and the east coast of Kent, off Ramsgate and Margate, where ships could ride at anchor.

6. Properly St. John; St. John's is the capital of Newfoundland.

7. Halifax, the principal port of Nova Scotia, was named after Lord Halifax, President of the Board of Trade, 1748–1761. Nova Scotia, ceded to England by the Peace of Utrecht in 1713, had been a neglected outpost until its geographical importance became evident, after France developed Louisbourg, some two hundred miles northwest, into a great fortress and opened the region to settlement by French fishermen. To offset their rival's advantage, the British government transported 3,000 British subjects to Halifax in 1749, appointing General Edward Cornwallis Governor of the new colony. With its excellent harbor, Halifax made an ideal military base and remained the chief station of the British Army and Navy in North America until 1905. — *NCMH*, VII, 529–530, 533–534.

To Israel Pemberton, Jr., Philadelphia, 4 October 1755 (I)

London, 4.10.1755

Dear Friend,

Though I have had sufficient notice of this vessel's departure, yet such have been the unavoidable succession of engagements that I have only leisure left before the letters are called for to give thee some proof that I do not forget my Friends. The inclosed epistle to your Quarterly Meeting was yesterday committed to my care to forward.[1] I hope nothing contained in it will give offence, and if it be considered that it was one part of the Friends' intention who were drawing it up that the Proprietaries might receive some hints from it (for to one of them it has been sent), it will account for all of it. I believe T.P. fully intends to come over in a few months,[2] and I am afraid your vexations will not be lessened by his arrival at first. Afterwards perhaps they may, when he is out of the hands of those whose sentiments here influence him to his prejudice.

One of your Gazettes containing some messages between the Governor and Assembly relating to the bill for raising £50,000 is arrived here by the way of Boston.[3] I have not yet seen it, neither I believe has the Proprietor. I mentioned it to him — told him I was informed the Governor refused it on account of its taxing the proprietary estate. I hoped he would consider in what light such conduct at such a time must appear. However, if I might offer my opinion, I think nothing would so effec-

167

tually secure the Assembly the unanimous approbation of the people here as yielding to the dissent or exemption the Governor insists on, saving to themselves, nevertheless, a right of inquiry into the justice of such an exemption hereafter.

The people here are generally and justly incensed at the General's conduct, and the whole blame must be thrown upon him, as he neither wanted for proper caution on this or on the other side of the water.[4] — In this country we seem very sanguine for war. Whether there will be one or not is very uncertain. The French do everything but what they ought to do to prevent one, and our people seem to do everything they can to bring one on. It is certain that their trade has already suffered greatly; they had just begun to insure amongst themselves and all concerned in it are undone. Their finances are squandered by a luxurious court, and the disputes between the Parliament and the Clergy yet subsist. Those who have the principal hand in conducting affairs here are sensible of all this, and will not be cajoled into a precarious agreement for the present till our opponents have recovered enough to repay the injuries received. Time forbids me to add more than the tenders of sincere affection to thyself and family, in which my sister joins.

Thy affectionate Friend

J. Fothergill

Ms. autograph letter Pemberton Papers, Etting Collection, II, 5, HSP.

1. In reply to that acknowledged in the letter of 8 July 1755, above.

2. Thomas Penn did not visit the province as planned.

3. A bill for raising £50,000 for defense against Indian attacks was under consideration for several months before the Assembly and Governor Robert Hunter Morris could reach agreement upon how to raise this sum. Details are given in a letter (2 August 1756, n. 4, below).

4. General Edward Braddock (1695–1755) had been totally defeated 9 July 1755, and died a few days later of wounds received in an attempt to reach and capture the French stronghold of Fort Duquesne (now Pittsburgh) on the Ohio. His campaign had from the first been poorly planned. Landing British troops in Virginia (instead of a northern port) prolonged their trek. Necessary construction of a new road through the mountains delayed their start. Scarcity and inadequacy of transportation had harrassed the expedition, in spite of the fact that Benjamin Franklin came to the rescue in Pennsylvania, providing wagons and horses. Braddock's failure to establish base camps ahead of time hampered both the advance and later the retreat of his troops. Lack of enough Indians loyal to the British to guide soldiers who were used only to the terrain of Great Britain and the Continent resulted in confusion. General Braddock's reliance upon line-fire of regiment against regiment in combat left him wholly unprepared for fighting in a heavily wooded country where Indians in ambuscade fired from the shelter of trees or boulders. Young George Washington,

whom General Braddock had chosen as aide-de-camp in May 1755, distinguished himself for bravery during combat and in retreat, but had the duty of burying his commander in the wilderness. — Freeman, *Washington*, II, 15, 20, 23–26, 45–54, 64–84; *NCMH*, VII, 537.

To Israel Pemberton, Jr., Philadelphia, 4 October 1755 (II)

London, 4.10.1755

Dear Friend,

Since the packet was sent away which comes by the same conveyance, a circumstance has happened which to me appears of some moment, and I hope will prove favourable to your Province. The Proprietor was pleased to call upon me, and to acquaint me in general with the orders he now sends to your side the water. I hope they will prove grateful to the people in general; but if they should not be altogether so, yet let them be considered as the beginnings of more peaceful times, and I should rejoice if the Assembly have not just cause to dislike them.

I imagine that his disposition is such at present that a respectful application from the Assembly to him would avail greatly to the mutual quiet of both, and might pave the way to a better understanding. I dare not presume to say much as I am less acquainted with the matters in dispute than those who are immediate parties. But as I think there are many people who may be led and cannot be drove by force, so I think we have one on this side who may be so influenced to the benefit of his country and himself.

If thou thinks these hints, thrown out in the utmost hurry, are of any consequence, impart them to any thou pleases. I dislike servile obsequiousness but a respectful condescension to those to whom in the course of providence we are connected in some degree of subordination is by no means unbecoming. Soft words turn away wrath very often, both in public communities as well as among particular relations. — As I think the Proprietor's disposition at present is such as may by a generous confidence be worked upon to your mutual advantage in every respect, I wish, if so it seems proper to those who have the principal share in the management of things amongst you, that the present occasion may not escape, but if the offers he makes are in any way proper, as I hope they are, the most agreeable returns may be made. — I am not prompted by him or anyone to say these things. My wishes for a better understanding between the Proprietors and the people, in order to promote their general happiness is my only aim, and for this to the utmost of my capacity, a warm and honest heart to both sides would induce me to labour diligently. 'Tis late, I can only add farewell, and may best wisdom direct your conduct. I am thy affectionate Friend

J. Fothergill

Ms. autograph letter, Pemberton Papers, Etting Collection, II, 6, HSP.

To Dr. Cadwallader Colden, New York, 23 October 1755

London, October 23, 1755

Dear Friend,[1]

When I received thy obliging and instructive letter of a date I am ashamed to mention, I did not intend it should lie by me so long unanswered. But so it has been to my great uneasiness whenever I reflected on it which has not been seldom. I can earnestly plead that my silence has by no means been owing to intended neglect.

The account of the rise, progress and treatment of the ulcerated sore throat was extremely acceptable, and so likewise was the ingenious Hypothesis respecting the different series of vessels and the juices they contained being the parent or the source of different diseases. The thought was in a great measure new to me, but seemed highly worthy of attention; and if it should not at present lead to a more successful practice, which I don't despair of, may at least contribute to enable us to account more satisfactorily to ourselves for various appearances of whose origin we yet know but little. I think myself not a little fortunate that at the time of life when my faculties (such as they are) are at their most favourable state, I have more frequent opportunities of observation than many others of the profession; and though I despair of doing much, yet would willingly keep out of the Routine, except where it is confessedly good, and be ever attentive to the voice of nature so far as it is discoverable by observation.

I was so much pleased with thy instructive account that I could not forbear producing it in the medical society[2] lately formed here for revising and publishing such essays as may seem conducive to the improvement of medicine. It was received with unanimous approbation, and only waits for thy permission to have it published in the first volume of our transactions which is now ready for the press and contains some valuable papers from America.[3] Many here long regretted the want of some such repository for medical papers only, and thought it a dishonor to the nation that a place which abounded with so many opportunities of observation; that was closely connected with so many and such distant parts of the universe; that was the common center of intelligence to them all, as well as to the greatest part of Europe; that circumstanced as we are in these respects, nothing more beneficial to the art in general, more honorable to our country, more useful to our distant colonies could well be contrived than the establishing of a society, which from time to time should communicate to all the intelligence they received from particulars; should select the instructive and the true from the trifling and the doubtful, and by this means at the expense of a little labour and time do a signal favour to the present as well as to future ages. This, a few have attempted. Their first volume is ready for the press. Dr. Colden's letter has been carefully perused and unanimously agreed deserves publication (if the Doctor permits), and this I hope he will cheerfully grant and be kind enough to favour the infant design when leisure from a multiplicity of engagements, all of them rendered more important by the present distressing situation of affairs, will give leave.

The hint respecting inoculation[4] was very interesting and merits farther inquiry. We have lately been told that it is not practiced so frequently in Georgia and Eurasia as at first was reported, but that in all probability the operation was brought from Ethiopia together with the slaves and by them here and there propagated in Asia, as opportunity offered. It gains ground in this city considerably, though it still meets with a zealous opposition from some; and the surgeons who take upon them the whole management of the patients, insisting on pretty high terms, discourage others not hindered by persuasions of a different kind from giving in to it. I know the present cannot be a time for much reading, or I should have sent some little pieces that have lately appeared here on this subject. If we live to see peace once again restored, it will give me pleasure to contribute everything in my power to testify to the grateful sense I have of thy obliging condescension, and to assure thee that

I am, thy respectful friend
John Fothergill

Ms. autograph letter, Simon Gratz Collection, Case 12, Box 20, HSP.

1. Cadwallader Colden (1688–1776) was the son of a Presbyterian minister from Scotland who had charge of a parish in County Wexford, Ireland, for several years. Young Colden received an M.A. from the University of Edinburgh in 1705. Exactly where and when he received his medical training is uncertain. In 1710 he went to Philadelphia, practiced a few years, then returned to Great Britain. Going back to the American Colonies in 1718, he accepted in 1721 a political appointment as Surveyor General of New York. His work sent him north, where the acquaintance he gained with native Indian tribes provided material for *The History of the Five Indian Nations depending on the Province of New-York in America* (New York: William Bradford, 1727). This work went through a number of editions, with changes, including changes of title; *The . . . Five Indian Nations of Canada, which are . . . the Barrier between the English and the French in that Part of the World*, London: T. Osborne, 1747. Continuing in political life, he acquired a large estate (near the present Newburgh), where he developed an extensive garden on scientific principles. He was soon included among the international group of botanists who exchanged specimens and data, and is credited with introducing the Linnaean system into America. In his botanical work he was joined by his daughter Jane, whose skill in botanical illustration drew praise from European savants.

Colden was elected to the American Philosophical Society in 1744. He became Lieutenant-Governor of New York in 1761, and continued in office until 1775 when, because of his well-known Tory principles, he was ousted. He died on Long Island in the following year. — Saul Jarcho, "Biographical and Bibliographical Notes on Cadwallader Colden," *Bulletin of the History of Medicine* (Baltimore), 32 (1958): 322–334; "Selections from the Letters of Cadwallader Colden," ed. Asa Gray, *American Journal of Science*, 44 (1843); 85–103; *A Catalogue of the Graduates in the Faculties of Art, Divinity, and Law* (Edinburgh, 1858), 177.

2. In 1752 Dr. Fothergill had been a founding member of a medical society never officially named, but often referred to as the Society of Physicians. At its start, this was a group of only seven doctors — six of them members of the Royal Society — who met on alternate Monday nights, presumably at the Mitre Tavern, Fleet Street. Between 1757 and 1784 this group, gradually enlarging, published six volumes of *Medical Observations and Inquiries*. Dr. Fothergill held the presidency of the society at the time of his death in 1780. — Fox, 141, 142.

3. Among twenty-nine papers contributed to the first volume of *Medical Observations and Inquiries* (London, 1757), four were by prominent physicians in the American colonies: IX, "An account of a worm bred in the liver," by Thomas Bond (Philadelphia), pp. 68–80, describing a guinea worm, found at post-mortem examination; XI, "A relation of a cure performed by electricity," by Cadwallader Evans (Philadelphia), pp. 83–87 (a young woman suffering from convulsions, given electrical shocks under the supervision of Benjamin Franklin); XII, "Of the Opisthotonus and Tetanus," by Lionel Chalmers (Charleston, S.C.), pp. 87–110; XIX, "Extract of a letter to Dr. Fothergill, concerning the Throat Distemper," by Cadwallader Colden

172

(New York), pp. 211–229. Two papers, xxv and xxvi, are by Dr. Fothergill: "Of the use of Cortex Peruvianus in scrofulous disorders," pp. 303–322, and "Concerning an astringent gum brought from Africa," pp. 358–364.

4. Inoculation was actually a simple procedure, requiring, however, hygienic precautions by the operator. As described previously by Dr. Fothergill in his letter to his brother, 5 January 1750/1, introduction of the virus of smallpox into the body by puncture of the skin produced in most people a light case of the disease, rendering the person so treated immune if exposed thereafter to smallpox. Recent studies in Chinese medicine claim that inoculation was first practiced in China, and was carried by traders and travelers to Turkey and thence to Great Britain and the Continent. According to Norman G. Brett-James, *The Life of Peter Collinson* (London: Dunstan and Friends Bookshop [1926]), p. 159, "It was Colden who first told Dr. Fothergill of the habits of the Indians with regard to inoculation."

To Israel Pemberton, Jr., Philadelphia, 16 March 1756

London, 16.3.1756

Dear Friend,

[*Short passage omitted.*] The accounts, sent by those in your Province who are no friends to the Assembly of the past and present state of things amongst you, having never on the Assembly's part been denied or refuted, have in general obtained credit in this country. Few there are who seem willing, and fewer yet have been able to vindicate the Assembly. When I speak of the Assembly in general, I would be understood to mean the conduct of Friends in general, for though I and many others know that the Assembly is in no way connected with the Society, nor is the Society answerable for their behaviour, yet the multitude here knows no better and therefore throws all the blame, whether just or unjust, that proceeds from any part of the administration in your Province entirely upon us as a Society.

This has been done with so much steadiness, management and success as to raise the most popular dislike to us as a people that we have ever laboured under from the Restoration, and such is the prepossession that has occupied the minds of most here, high and low and of all parties, that they seem not intent upon anything more than how to manifest their dislike in the most signal manner. A few, a very few moderate persons, and happily for us, some of them in very high stations, think more favourably, though at the same time they seem resolved to exclude those of our Society in your Province from any share in the legislation. [*Passage omitted.*]

173

So far the clamours of your adversaries had succeeded that in a bill lately passed for raising some thousand Germans in your Province for its defense, after charging the Assembly as the cause of all the mischiefs that have happened in the back settlements, it was intended to be enacted that henceforth no person who refused taking the oath to the Government should be eligible into any Assembly in America.[1]

A person of great eminence [2] was pleased so far to interpose as to have this part struck out, yet it is evident enough that a great chasm is left in it from which this intended stroke was erased. — Here we were in hopes that all was ended; but we were soon informed that in consequence of the petitions received from great numbers in your Province, setting forth the defenceless state, the ravages committed by the Indians etc., the inability or the neglect of the Assembly to provide for the public safety, some steps must necessarily be taken; and that as the people in general seemed both able and willing to defend themselves, would the Quakers permit them, it remained only to dissolve the present Assembly, call a new one, to prevent any [Quaker] from being chosen again, by imposing an oath, by Act of Parliament here.[3] A bill for this purpose is now actually drawn up, and may be every day expected to be brought into the House.

How far it will be agreeable to Friends in general on your side of the water, or to the country in general to have such a law passed you know best. But the Society here thought that such an inroad upon your constitution deserved their most serious attention, and that they ought if possible to prevent it. In consequence of their opinion a committee appointed by the Meeting for Sufferings have taken all the pains they could for this purpose, and have personally represented in the strongest manner they could, to persons of the greatest weight in the management of public affairs, the apprehension the Society here were under that a measure so manifestly violating the fundamentals of your constitution, would not only affect you very painfully, but likewise excite great disgust in the minds of all who were your friends, which appeared to us to be the majority of persons of influence in your Province. [*Passage omitted.*]

The point upon which all rested was: You are unfit for government. You accept of a public trust which at the same time you acknowledge you cannot discharge. You owe the people protection and yet withhold them from protecting themselves. Will not all the blood that is spilt lie

174

at your doors? And can we, say they, sit still and see the Province in danger of being given up to a merciless enemy, without endeavouring its rescue? And this assistance cannot be effectual unless the Province unites with our views and cooperates to the best of their ability; but this they cannot do whilst you Friends have the majority in the Assembly, and as you are both numerous and wealthy, you will be sure of a majority unless you are totally excluded. It may be deemed an infraction of the Charter indeed, but what is a Charter compared with the desolation that must inevitably ensue if such men are still chosen and such measures pursued as have been of late years? This in short is the language of all we apply to — and what answer can we give?

A person of high rank, a steady friend to the Society, and very intimate with a Friend of ours who has a great share of his esteem, was desirous of communicating his opinion and advice to the Society on the present situation of your affairs; [4] a deputation accordingly waited upon him consisting of the following Friends, viz., J. Hanbury, Silvanus Bevan, Peter Collinson, Thomas How, John Hunt, myself, with Peter Andrews and Edmund Peckover, who both happened to be then in town.[5]

He told us that he discovered a general prepossession against us as a people both here and in America, that many seemed disposed to give in to the most violent counsels, that even some in considerable stations who had been our friends on many occasions were either wavering, or had joined in the popular cry, and that no measures could be proposed to either House so disadvantageous to us but what would probably be passed, or at least be strenuously supported.

[He said] that nevertheless himself and a few more, from motives of justice and regard to those who had been the principal means of raising the colony to its present flourishing condition, were in some hopes that this torrent of violence might be a little [abated?] and that they would much rather that we ourselves if possible should apply a remedy than that those should do it who seemed inclined to the severest [actions.]

That as it seemed much more eligible, our Friends should at present decline accepting seats in the Assembly of their own accord [rather] than be totally excluded forever from a possibility of sitting there, which would certainly be the case was there a majority of our profession in the next assembly. [*Passage omitted.*]

It was our unanimous opinion that the advice was the best that then occurred, and undertook to present the state of affairs to you in the strongest light we could, and in some respects took upon us to answer for your compliance, who we imagined were by this time sufficiently weary of your stations on various accounts. [*Long passage omitted.*]

We took the earliest opportunities to wait upon other persons in power; [6] represented the confusion it would occasion in the country to break through the fundamental principles of your constitution, and the injustice of those of our Society to be excluded a share in the management of that colony which they had been a powerful means of raising to its present flourishing condition. [*Passage omitted.*]

I need not now advise how to act. I may be mistaken in thinking so, but I apprehend it is not only the Society but the Province itself are obliged to us, and to those who have powerfully assisted us, in preventing a fatal blow to your constitution, which ends only in fixing one point which has been matter of debate, but not an essential. Remember that our credit is pledged for you. We are daily told we shall repent of the pains we have taken — it's in your breasts whether we shall or not.

One word more — your correspondent delivered the address to the Proprietors. They received it favourably, promised it due attention and might perhaps send an answer. T.P. called upon me the other day and desired me to acquaint Friends that he had been prevented by a multiplicity of affairs from returning a proper acknowledgment for the address, but that he soon intends it. [7] In the meantime he desired me to let them know he kindly accepted their respectful remembrance of his family and himself, that he was desirous of maintaining a good correspondence with them, that if he differed with them in one particular point, meaning provision for defense, it was not through dislike to them but because it seemed to be both his duty and for their interest — or to this effect.

He cheerfully told me I had great faith in becoming bound for my Friends. I told him I thought I knew the sentiments of many on your side the water so well that I could answer for them as I could for myself; that if the country in general thought such measures were necessary that I could not be concerned in, I would tell them so, and refuse any post they might offer me. [*Passage omitted.*]

J. Fothergill

P.S. London, the 19th

Since the above was wrote, I find the sentiments of the Administration are divided — some being of opinion that either somewhat more should be done than dissolving the Assembly, or nothing at all; so that I am almost of opinion that nothing will be done this session, and this is in a great measure through our application, on which account I must here do justice to our friend J. Hanbury who has exerted himself with great zest on this occasion with several people of the first rank. By the following postscript which P. Collinson wrote on the paper after he had perused it at home, thou will easily see in what condition we shall be if you do not for your own sakes as well as ours withdraw from an administration in which all that happens amiss will be charged to you and us, whatever is right will be overlooked. You will have a military Governor sent over; who he is to be is not, I believe determined. I had a good deal of converse yesterday with T.P.; the occasion must be the subject of another. Farewell. Please to acquaint I. Norris[8] and B. Franklin with the contents of the postscript relative to the present dubious state of their existence.

[*In another hand at the bottom of the page*]

This day Doctor Chandler,[9] an eminent Presbyterian parson, said to me, you have been very bold in that you have engaged for your Friends not being a majority in next Assembly — it's my opinion, says the Doctor, that they'll never comply with it.

P.C.

Ms. autograph letter, Pemberton Papers, Etting Collection, II, 10, HSP. Dr. Fothergill's concern about the important matter discussed in this very long letter led him, as he himself said, to "repeat the circumstances over and over". The editors have omitted a number of passages, totaling almost one-third of the letter, which although they reflect the writer's anxiety, do not add significantly to his message.

1. The bill referred to had been instigated by Lord Barrington, Secretary at War in the British Cabinet, who had proposed to protect Pennsylvania's borders by raising a regiment from His Majesty's foreign and other Protestant subjects residing in the colonies. A Royal American Regiment, in charge of British and German officers, did indeed have a brief existence in the summer of 1756, but its ranks attracted very few colonists. The regiment was largely made up of drifters described as "the refuse of the Army in Ireland." Early in 1756, Barrington came to the conclusion that colonial opinion must be a controlling factor in making plans for defense. As Dr. Fothergill goes on to say, the provision that would have excluded Quakers from the Assembly was eliminated from this bill. — See Stanley M. Pargellis, *Lord Loudon in North America* (New Haven: Yale University Press, 1933), 61–66, 111, 112; copy of a letter from Lord Barrington, 16 January 1756, to Richard Partridge, Franklin Papers, APS.

2. Lord Granville, President of the Privy Council. He had a personal interest in

the Colonies since he had inherited vast property holdings in North Carolina, granted to his father by the Crown. — Knollenberg, 48.

3. Quakers interpreted literally the Biblical injunction, "Swear not at all" (Matthew 5:31). An Affirmation Act passed by Parliament in 1772 made legal a statement still in use: "I, A B, do solemnly, sincerely and truly declare and affirm that . . ." — Elfrida Vipont, *The Story of Quakerism* (London: Bannisdale, 1955), 135.

4. The "person of high rank" was undoubtedly Peter Collinson's intimate friend Thomas Villiers (1709–1786), M.P. from Tamworth, a son of the second Earl of Jersey. Villiers, who had held several diplomatic posts in Europe, was shortly to become the first Baron Hyde and subsequently Earl of Clarendon. Edmund Burke described him later in the century as "a quiet, rather indolent man," not likely to make much stir when appointed Chancellor of the Duchy of Lancaster. — *The Letters of Edmund Burke*, edited by Lucy S. Sutherland (University of Chicago Press, 1960), II, 219.

5. John Hanbury was head of the Virginia Company; Silvanus Bevan, Peter Collinson, and Dr. Fothergill were Fellows of the Royal Society; Hunt and How were London Quakers, and Andrews and Peckover were Friends from the counties — a sensible and well-assorted group.

6. The Committee from the London Meeting for Sufferings interviewed Lord Halifax, President of the Board of Trade, and the Duke of Newcastle (Thomas Pelham-Holles), First Lord of the Treasury. Newcastle had greater knowledge of the colonial situation than any other cabinet member, having served during twenty-four years, 1724–1748, as Secretary of State for the Southern Department, which dealt with problems in the American Colonies. Throughout his career he advocated proper defense of the colonies and avoidance of harsh Parliamentary measures which might create friction and injure trade. — Knollenberg (on Halifax), 34, 35, 47; (on Newcastle), 12–15.

7. The address referred to is recorded in the Minutes of the Friends' Monthly Meeting, Philadelphia, 29th of 10th month, 1756. Thomas Penn's reply for the Proprietors follows immediately, on pages 260–262 of the Minute Book. — Archives Department of the Religious Society of Friends, Philadelphia.

8. Isaac Norris (1701–1766), an early leader of the Quakers in Pennsylvania and currently Speaker of the House of Assembly. He is best remembered today for having suggested the inscription for the Liberty Bell: "Proclaim liberty throughout all the land unto all the inhabitants thereof" (Leviticus XXV:10).

9. The Rev. Samuel Chandler, D.D., founder of a society in London to raise funds for the education of Germans in the American Colonies.

To Israel Pemberton, Jr., Philadelphia, 3 April 1756

London, 3.4.1756

Dear Friend,

[*Short passage omitted.*] I told thee in my last that the scurrilous invectives, transmitted in every shape from your Province hither, had raised such a general indignation against you that no measures so violent

could have been proposed but many of all parties, persuasions and interests here would have joined in supporting them. Charters, privileges,
immunities under the strongest sanction would have availed nothing.
Had it not been for Lord Granville's interposition [1] . . . you would ere
this time have been incapacitated (I mean Friends) from ever sitting in
any Assembly in America. This Nobleman very early communicated
to our Friend John Hanbury the temper of the people in power, the
views they seemed to entertain, the endeavours he has used to prevent
so violent a remedy, and gave him his opinion what seemed most proper
to be done under the present circumstances and repeated it to several
Friends who at J. Hanbury's request waited upon him on this occasion.
The purport was that he thought it much better for us, and for the
colony likewise, that those of our Society for the present should decline
sitting in the Assembly, rather than be forced out by an Act of Parliament from hence, which was already framed and would be carried, if
endeavours were not used by application to persons in power. [*Passage
omitted.*]

But fresh accounts of your danger arriving; the insufficiency of your
money bill and military law being insisted on; it was determined . . . to
dissolve the present Assembly immediately, yet this in the least disgustful manner. This, however, has been delayed, and we believe will not
again be taken up this session. So that as Lord Halifax told a Friend this
day, everything was left to you, in hopes that you would do that of your
own accord what they otherwise shall be obliged to do; and not so much
perhaps to your satisfaction.[2]

We are actually applying to such persons as may be proper to come
over to you, in order still to prevail upon you to coincide with the
favourable views of those here, who wish to preserve your constitution
from receiving some dangerous wounds. [*Passage omitted.*]

I am informed this evening by my worthy Friend J. Hanbury, that
——— Pownall Esq., a gentleman well known to many amongst you, is
actually appointed your Governor, and to come over as speedily as
possible.[3] He had it from himself, and from many others today with
whom he dined on a public occasion, and from persons who could not
but know. — The Proprietor had made an offer of the choice to the
Duke of Cumberland in expectation that a military man would have
been chosen your governor in these troublesome times. Many thought
that such a person should have been the last to have been sent to a

Province like yours.[4] A person to whom you are more obliged both as a Province and as a Society than you can ever know,[5] thought of the gentleman above mentioned as the most proper person, a person well acquainted with American affairs, with the nature of your late disputes and of your government, who has done the Society great justice in his conversation with the great, and represented you in a very different light from what some others have done. This gentleman is prevailed upon, and will soon probably be with you, not fettered by any painful instructions, fully bent on putting an end to private animosities, and unite all in their respective stations in one common concern for the common good. [*Passage omitted.*]

Many here scruple not to assert that Friends will never relinquish their seats in Assembly on any account; others think they will do it cheerfully whenever their country is of opinion that others can serve them better, or that the constitution of their country will be in danger from their persisting to keep them; of this last number I am one, and believe I shall not be disappointed . . .

John Fothergill [6]

Ms. autograph letter, Pemberton Papers, Etting Collection, II, 11, HSP.

1. See letter of 16 March 1756, above, at note 2.
2. Although Lord Halifax (George Montague Dunk) was often called "the Father of the colonies," he was a strict father who wished for firm control. He advocated Parliamentary taxation of the American provinces as early as 1755–56 and appointment of English bishops for each colonial diocese. — Knollenberg, 34, 35.
3. Thomas Pownall (1722–1805) already understood the problems of colonial administration in America. He had first gone to America in 1753 to become secretary to Sir Danvers Osborn, Governor of New York. Two days after Pownall's arrival, Governor Osborn, who had been severely depressed, committed suicide. Pownall thereafter remained in the colonies without official connection, but traveled as an observer to collect information for Lord Halifax and the Board of Trade. In 1755 he was given a temporary appointment as Lieutenant-Governor of New Jersey, from which he was released in 1756 to return to England.
4. William Augustus, Duke of Cumberland, hardened by campaigns of the War of the Austrian Succession and command of the British forces during "the Forty-five," was a soldier of distinction, but not a diplomat.
5. Possibly Thomas Villiers (soon to be Lord Hyde), previously mentioned as an intimate friend of Peter Collinson who kept him well informed on affairs in the American Colonies.
6. A postscript of two paragraphs written the next day has been omitted here because it merely reports rumors later proved to be without foundation.

To Israel Pemberton, Jr., Philadelphia, 8 May 1756

London, 8.5.1756

Dear Friend,

Though I am afraid I have so often contradicted my own intelligence that my credit is reduced to a low ebb, yet I once more sit down to mention what has since my last been in agitation. — I told thee that T. Pownall was appointed your Governor, and with satisfaction, as his character was such as gave me reason to believe he would have been very acceptable. He was nominated, accepted the station, but — when he found he should not be at liberty to do all that he wished to have done, he rather chose to decline it, and leave the place for some other.

A Military person is at length fixed upon,[1] and will perhaps very soon embark for your Province; he has hitherto held no very distinguished rank, but is thought by those who know him best to be a worthy, moderate, sensible man, and rather more fit for civil than military life, and is I believe for this among other reasons prefixed to your government. His name, I think, is ——— Denny; and I hope he will come over somewhat less fettered than some of his predecessors, inasmuch as it is no longer a secret to several in high stations that your Governors have not always been perfectly their own masters. T. Pownall goes over speedily, with Lord Loudon[2] as agent general, and will be Governor of New England, for which place his commission is now preparing. I believe he will be at all times disposed to serve the colony heartily, and I hope endeavours will be used to cultivate his friendliness. We are looking out still for proper persons to come over, and a letter is now drawing up to be sent by them. Those who take the part of Friends with you have a difficult task. We are told of your thirst of power, ambition, and what not. Some of us think we know you better, and that everything we ask and everything we have promised will be complied with. One thing is urged strongly against us which is your total silence in respect to your present situation, and your neither making any reply to the invidious libel published against you, nor furnishing any person here with the requisite material. — You have indeed sent over newspapers and the votes of your Assembly to a few, but these have not been sufficient, and I would request that some proper persons may immediately be set to work, and draw up a concise state of your late disputes and your present situation, without rancour or the least unbecoming warmth. If

181

this be done, under some such title as a *Review of the Publick Transactions in the Province of Pennsylvania during the Government of R.H.M.*,[3] and containing a regular recital of the several incidents of moment, you may do yourselves justice and inform the publick.

An answer, and I hope not an unsatisfactory one, to your address to the Proprietor is prepared, and will be sent by the first opportunity. It was sent to me late this evening, but as the other correspondents were not at hand, I rather chose to delay it a while longer, than to send it without their concurrence; it is still in the Proprietor's hand, but I shall get it as early as I can. [*Passage omitted.*]

Enclosed I have sent a newspaper [4] in which is contained an article that should not be altogether unknown to you. I am informed that the original from which this is printed is in the handwriting of one ——— Smith who is in some station in your Academy.[5] Was I to enter into the sentiments of many concerning it, I should take up more time than I can now spare. We are not less anxious to send two Friends over to reconcile you if possible to yourselves and one another than to urge your compliance with the request of the Government. — You may be assured that many of us are in no little pain about you, and that such invidious defamatory libels accumulated through every part of the nation are not very pleasant. — If thou knows the person who is supposed to be the author, I mean ——— Smith — it may not be amiss to inform him of it, and that I may perhaps apply both to the Proprietors and your new Governor on the occasion, and endeavour to convince them that such an incendiary is as far from being a good subject as a good Christian.

J. Fothergill

Ms. autograph letter, Pemberton Papers, Etting Collection, II, 13, HSP.

1. Captain William Denny.
2. The new commander of British troops in North America needed Pownall's services as adviser. John Campbell, fourth Earl of Loudon (1705–1782), appointed in 1756 to succeed General Braddock, had had no previous experience in the American colonies. In New York, Pownall, as secretary-extraordinary, was for a year a member of an intimate circle which made up Lord Loudon's household. Lord Loudon, a fellow of the Royal Society since 1738, a veteran field officer, and a major-general in the British Army, found problems of the American command too difficult to solve by methods based on his European experience. In 1757 he was recalled to England. He later regained military reputation by service on the Continent, and was promoted General in 1770. — Pargellis, 167, 266–270, and *passim*. In 1757 Pownall was appointed Governor of Massachusetts.

3. It was not until 1759 that such an account was issued, under Benjamin Franklin's auspices. See letter of 9 April 1759, below.

4. The *London Evening Advertiser*, 20 April 1756, according to p. 152 of Ketcham (cited below; see letter of 2 August 1756, n. 7).

5. The Rev. William Smith (1727–1803), relatively a newcomer to Philadelphia, a bitter opponent of the Quakers. His anonymous pamphlet, *A Brief State of the Province of Pennsylvania, in which the conduct of their Assemblies for several years past is impartially examined* (London, 1755), was one of the most potent in the flood of anti-Quaker literature. His letters printed in Philadelphia newspapers were sent to London for reprinting there. Born in Aberdeen, Scotland, he had been educated by the Society for the Education of Parochial Teachers and later studied in Aberdeen without receiving a degree. In 1751 he went to New York to tutor Colonel Josiah Martin's two sons, and in 1753 he published *A General Idea of the College of Mirania*, in which he outlined what he considered an ideal program of instruction for a college in the American Colonies. This publication interested Benjamin Franklin, who encouraged him to settle in Philadelphia. After a journey to England for ordination by the Bishop of London, he was elected in 1754 Rector of Philadelphia's Academy, and when it was rechartered the following year as the College, Academy, and Charitable School of Philadelphia, he was named Provost. — See Thomas H. Montgomery, *A History of the University of Pennsylvania* (Philadelphia: Jacobs, 1900), 184–208.

To Israel Pemberton, Jr., Philadelphia, 2 August 1756

London, 2.8.1756

Dear Friend,

I received thy kind letter by Captain Mesnard the 21st of last month, and was pleased with it on divers accounts. Brother Samuel arrived safe at Dublin the 9th of the same month, but was detained there by contrary winds, and we have not yet heard of his getting home, though as the wind has been favourable some days, he must by this time, I think, be at his own habitation once more, to the great satisfaction of all his relations in particular and many others in various parts of the nation. John Hunt and Christopher Wilson [1] were gone to Bristol in order to embark for Philadelphia when I received the account; as I thought it would be satisfactory to them, I found means of informing them of it before they set sail.

From the purport of some former letters thou will apprehend on what occasion they are coming . . . As the two Friends above mentioned not only found themselves easy to accept of the commission, but likewise under some drawings to visit you in particular on some other accounts, and as they were persons well acquainted with the business they are engaged in, not strangers to you and yet esteemed by us, we

183

were glad to find they were so engaged. I am in hopes they may be so far favoured as to arrive long before this, but lest through any accident they should be delayed and the business they come upon be in any measure retarded thereby, the Meeting for Sufferings have ordered duplicates of the papers they have with them to be sent by the first opportunity to thy hands — to be opened and the proper use made of the contents, which is to request Friends in general to decline accepting seats in the Assembly, agreeable to our engagement on your behalf. — The Province, and the Society, is greatly indebted to the author of the *Brief Account* and the sequel,[2] together with some other insinuations of the like nature, for this unmerited resentment. How the Assembly can overlook such treatment, I know not, but if one can be suffered to revile and abuse the whole provincial Assembly, subject the country in general to base insinuations, be almost the means of subverting your constitution, and with impunity, I must think very highly of their forbearance, or their fear, for I cannot fully attribute it to the spirit of meekness and forgiveness.

I have hitherto said little respecting the letter of advice given by some Friends in Pennsylvania. I sent thee a printed copy of it with Parson Smith's introduction.[3] It has occasioned not much less uneasiness amongst ourselves than it has added to the publick discontent against us here, and I wish its effects may have ceased among you. The Friends will have an eye to this, I believe, and will prudently endeavour to remove, so far as they find freedom, all occasions of misunderstanding on this account. There were divers who wanted not inclination to have sent a very explicit censure against it, and to have loaded the author with blame to the utmost of their power. Some private reasons operated in a few, but to justify ourselves from the imputation of refusing to pay taxes was the pretense. Many however thought it not safe to censure men of known wisdom, steadiness and experience, nor becoming, at any rate, to do it unheard. This therefore is quietly waived, and we hope will likewise produce no bad effects among you. — To me it appeared in this light to those who signed it. Friends have ever refused to be actively concerned in moderate military services and appointments and have scrupled to pay taxes directly for this end. — Yet there are some under our name who have imposed a tax on their Brethren for this very end, and have gone so far as to make those who have the distribution of it answerable to themselves, so that it was not altogether the payment of the tax, but that the tax should be raised, directed, and the use allowed by an Assembly, the major part whereof were of our profession, that gave the offense. — Had an Assembly of persons not of our profession passed such an act as this for raising £55,000,[4] I don't at present see how payment could have been refused and we in England justified in the payment of the land tax and so forth. Here I think the mistake lay: all were convinced of the inconsistency of the thing, and all thought some just dislike should be shown to it. But instead of advising against this payment, and thereby revolting against the judgement of the provincial representative, would it not have been more proper to have desired the Monthly Meetings, to which the several voting members belonged, to have dealt with these members for acting so inconsistently with their profession? This, as the affair appears to me at present, would have been the safest and most consistent method of proceeding with persons who had acted a part their profession did not altogether warrant. A clamour would doubtless have been raised against you on this score, but you might have vindicated yourselves with more ease, and the peace of society in full as well preserved.

[*Passage omitted.*] I offer this only as my opinion, and heartily wish the whole business may quietly subside.

I am much obliged to thee for sending me the minutes of your conferences with the Indians.[5] Various copies came over at the same time and by some means have been laid before the public. The Governor's friends [6] were obliging enough to ascribe the whole merit of the affair to him in one public paper; this was thought by some to be depriving those who set it on foot of their just due and accordingly placed their transaction in its proper light. I don't know who published the conferences but it's plain he is no enemy. [*Passage omitted.*]

I see by one of your prints . . . that Parson Smith has brought tumult into a disagreeable situation.[7]

As the time of the Assembly dissolution draws near, a new Governor daily expected, I think had I been in the Assembly, I should have continued there, had nothing immediately cogent occurred till its conclusion, endeavouring to have stayed free from blame if possible.

I have inclosed the Proprietor's answer to the address of your Monthly Meeting.[8] It has been in my hands longer than I intended.

I have seen and spoke with Tench Francis [9] several times. He has kept himself very private here, but is friendly and kind. He thinks both sides are wrong and carry things to much greater lengths than they ought.

He is very apprehensive that if the new Assembly does not consist of very moderate people, some severe militia law will be enacted, as much with a view to oppress you as to give the country service, but as these hints are passed in private conversation, I think it would not be proper to make any mention of his sentiments, or that we had much acquaintance. I hope your new Governor [10] is arrived by this time, and that you have forgiven me for sending you a mistaken account. T.P.[11] was actually appointed, accepted of it, but declined when he was farther appraised of the terms. The Present comes under less restraint, and as he is allowed to be a person of prudence and moderation, I hope he will give peace to the colony and restore unanimity among yourselves. One thing give me leave to mention, and I care not how many hear it, provided they will make proper use of it. Prosperity, ease and independence have given almost the notion of subordination among you. There is a proper medium between servility and a state that knows no superior. — Perhaps none have been more culpable than ourselves in some biting provocations. They have hurt you greatly here, and have almost gained the style of insolence. An honest plainness is becoming; quickness and repartee hurt one's cause which is that of patience and forbearance. Urge some care in this respect, especially among the younger part. Your climate disposes to vivacity, but religion would correct havoc and restrain constitution.

John Fothergill

By this day's post I have received the agreeable news that Brother Samuel arrived in good health at his habitation, the 31st Ult.

Ms. autograph letter, Pemberton Papers, Etting Collection, II, 16, HSP.

1. Christopher Wilson (1704–1761), son of John Wilson of Graysothern, Cumberland, traveled in the ministry on both sides of the Atlantic. In 1756 London's Meeting for Sufferings sent him with John Hunt to Philadelphia to confer with Quakers who were being accused of unreasonable pacifism while Indian attacks on Pennsylvania's borders were alarming the populace. — *John Woolman*, ed. Gummere, 511, 512.

2. William Smith's pamphlet, *A Brief State of the Province of Pennsylvania*, was followed by *A Brief View of the Conduct of Pennsylvania for the Year 1755 so far as it affected the general service of the British Colonies, particularly the expedition under General Braddock* (London, 1756). Copies of the *Brief View* were on sale in Philadelphia in May 1756.

3. The letter of advice has not been located; therefore the reference to "Parson Smith's introduction" is obscure.

4. After Braddock's disastrous defeat in July 1755, depredations by the Indians threatened to increase, and the Assembly resolved that an appropriation of £50,000

was necessary for proper protection of the colony. A committee of six, including Benjamin Franklin, drafted a bill proposing to tax all estates, both real and personal, including the vast, largely undeveloped holdings of the Penn family. Governor Morris returned this bill, proposing amendments to exempt the Proprietors from such taxation. A bitter controversy ensued, delaying appropriation of necessary funds for months while the dangers grew. It was not until 22 November 1755 that a letter arrived from Thomas Penn announcing his contribution of £5,000 toward proper defense of the colony. Disputes thereafter came suddenly to an end. The Assembly, after due consideration, voted that because of Thomas Penn's gift, "it would not be reasonable nor just at this time to impose a tax upon proprietary lands." A new money bill was therefore drawn to raise £55,000 in bills of credit, in addition to Penn's gift of £5,000. Approved by the Governor, this bill became law on 27 November 1755. — *Franklin Papers*, ed. Labaree, VI, 129, 130, 257.

5. During treaty conferences with the Indians, interpreters were always at work. Minutes were carefully prepared. Manuscript copies were circulated until Benjamin Franklin had prepared a text suitable to print. — See Julian P. Boyd, ed., *Indian Treaties, Printed by Benjamin Franklin, 1736–1762* (Philadelphia, 1938). The minutes acknowledged by Dr. Fothergill were those of earlier conferences. As he was writing, Israel Pemberton was bending all his effort toward renewing peace with the Indians, and a new conference was about to assemble at Easton, in Pennsylvania.

6. Thomas Penn himself was one of those influenced by information sent by Governor Morris.

7. William Smith's attacks had not ceased with his second pamphlet. — See Ralph Ketcham, "Benjamin Franklin and William Smith: New Light on an Old Philadelphia Quarrel," *Pennsylvania Magazine of History and Biography*, 88 (1964): 142–163.

8. The Proprietor's reply has not been located.

9. Tench Francis (d. 1758), son of the Rev. John Francis, Dean of the Lismore Cathedral of the Church of England, received a legal education and emigrated to Talbot County, Maryland, where he married Elizabeth Turbott. In 1739, seeking greater opportunity for advancement, he moved to Philadelphia, and from 1741 to 1755 he was Attorney General of Pennsylvania. In later life he spent much time in England, supposedly as an agent for the proprietary family. — *Hannah Logan's Courtship*, 278, n. 1.

10. William Denny (1709–1765), the new Governor, was an Oxford graduate who chose a soldier's career. Recommended by the Duke of Cumberland as a good man for wartime duty, Denny was promoted Colonel, for North American service only. Richard Peters, provincial secretary for the Proprietors and member of the Provincial Council, met him in New York and conducted him to Philadelphia where he was welcomed by festivities including a dinner given by the Assembly at which Benjamin Franklin made the principal address. Franklin, canny enough to avoid opposition, relates that between Denny and himself "no enmity arose; he was a man of letters who had seen much of the world; and was very pleasing and entertaining in conversation." Peter Collinson had written from London that he considered Denny "a mild, moderate man determined to heal all differences." — Carl Van Doren, *Benjamin Franklin's Autobiographical Writings* (New York: Viking, 1945), 752–753; Darlington, *Memorials*, 308.

11. Thomas Pownall.

To Israel Pemberton, Jr., Philadelphia, 21 February 1757

London 21.2.1757

Dear Friend,

About ten days ago I received thy acceptable letter of November 22 last, together with a copy of your late Treaty for which I think myself greatly indebted to thee.[1] Nevertheless I wait with some impatience for thy further account of this transaction. You are still subjected to the most outrageous representation. All that is said against you is believed and the little, the very little, alleged in your defense utterly discredited. — It is already asserted that J.H. and C.W.[2] met the Indians beforehand and tampered with them to speak as they did, and therefore so far are you from deserving commendation that your conduct is highly culpable. This representation is sent over to this country; it is propagated with success, and I mention it that you may both see with what malicious attention you are watched and that you may clear yourselves from an imputation I believe altogether unjust. But this is not all. — You are taxed with using your utmost endeavours to carry the late election in the favour of Friends and their partisans. A letter from a person of eminence in your city has been sent to another of no less note in the neighborhood of this, charging Friends with the most unwearied artful endeavours to get themselves elected; or at least to get those elected who were under their immediate influence. I want not to widen the barriers between you; but I think it necessary to say that this letter came from one eminent Presbyterian to another,[3] and that it was shown with great diligence to most of the people in high station here, and not with a view to your advantage. [*Passage omitted.*]

In the meantime I should be glad that your Meeting for Sufferings would send us ... ample accounts of whatever concerns them ... Your enemies send accounts which we cannot always contradict ... It is more than six months since we received any account from Friends in your Province, though you are daily the subject of our care and endeavours. [*Passage omitted.*]

A season of anxiety seems approaching which may possibly have some good effects. We are in a lethargy, and some sharp stimulant seems necessary. People of all conditions seem to have forgotten him on whom they ought to daily depend ... The highest forget that they owe their inferiors a good example; the lowest are too far gone in corruption to think at all — the middle are too much divided between the preceding ranks.

This is wrote after a day of exceeding fatigue. — The hasty thoughts of a hurried mind, but the bearer, a Friend from your parts, telling me that he sets out tomorrow prompts me ... to renew the appearance of my affectionate regard.

J. Fothergill

Ms. autograph letter, Pemberton Papers, Etting Collection, II, 20, HSP.

1. An important conference ("treaty") had taken place at Easton, Pennsylvania 8–17 November 1756, between Governor Denny and representatives of the Delaware Indians. The Governor presided: members of his Council were present, also Indian Commissioners of the Province, also a party of Quakers including Israel Pemberton and Charles Thomson, and certain other important citizens, notably William Logan. It was at this time that Teedyuscung, King of the Delawares, made his accusation of land frauds. A deed of 1686 had originally conveyed to William Penn as much land west of the Delaware River and north to Tohiccon Creek "as far as a man can walk in a day and a half." For generations, however, Indians kept complaining of unjust seizure of land which was theirs by inheritance. To appease them, in 1737 James Logan and Thomas Penn (succeeding his father as Proprietor of the province) decided to stage another Walking Purchase and hired three athletic young men to repeat the walk. In preparation for this event, the path was cleared of underbrush and forest growth. Two Indian observers were then engaged to watch the progress of the walkers. The Indian scouts, claiming that the white men ran instead of walking, soon withdrew. The young athletes, going at a steady dogtrot, got well past Tohiccon Creek by the end of the first day, but one of them gave out from exhaustion at this point. The following day, after the Kittatinny Mountains were passed, the second young man collapsed; the third, continuing for a few miles, came into rocky, barren country undesirable for settlement. The Proprietary Agent accordingly set his boundaries at the mountains, and in addition laid claims to valuable land reaching the Forks of the Delaware, including Easton, a region already settled to considerable extent by the British. While relating this story at the Easton meeting in November 1756, Teedyuscung became much agitated and told Governor Denny on 13 November: "This very ground under me [striking it with his foot] was my Land and my Inheritance, and is taken from me by Fraud; when I say *Ground*, I mean all the Land lying between Tohiccon Creek and the River Susquehannah." Governor Denny, having listened attentively, thanked Teedyuscung for the freedom and openness of his information, and was inclined to promise redress of these wrongs; but the Indian Commissioners advised that the Governor's evident official approbation was all that was needed, and proposed putting an end to the discussion as soon as possible. Accordingly, a distribution of valuable goods was made at a farewell party on 15 November. Useful gifts to the value of at least £400 had been sent by various inhabitants of Philadelphia, and a special lot by members of the Society of Friends. Business of the treaty was transacted the next day, and after a short session on 17 November, the conference was brought to a conclusion, with promise of adjustments during the following summer. The copy of the treaty sent to Dr. Fothergill must have been in manuscript, since printed copies were not available

in Philadelphia until 10 March 1757. — *Franklin Papers*, ed. Labaree, VII, 111, 112; Anthony F. C. Wallace, *King of the Delawares: Teedyuscung* (Philadelphia: University of Pennsylvania Press, 1949), 17–19, 124–136; Paul A. Wallace, *Conrad Weiser* (Philadelphia: University of Pennsylvania Press, 1945), 459–465; Nicholas B. Wainwright, *George Croghan, Wilderness Diplomat* (Chapel Hill: University of North Carolina Press, 1959), 524; Boyd, *Indian Treaties*, 150–156; Tolles, *James Logan*, 178–183.

2. John Hunt and Christopher Wilson, sent from London as intermediaries between the dissident factions in the Society of Friends.

3. Probably from William Allen, Chief Justice of Pennsylvania (1750–1774), to the Rev. Samuel Chandler, D.D., of London.

To Samuel Fothergill, Warrington, Lancashire, 31 March 1757

London, 3d Mo., 31st, 1757.

Yesterday I received an agreeable account from cousin Charles Chorley of thy recovery. As soon as thy strength, the weather, and the roads permit, the easy motion of a carriage will, perhaps, be beneficial; be very careful, however, of the first cold, for this may plunge thee again into great difficulties.

... This, I hope, will find thee fast recruiting, and if not yet able to write thyself, yet let us hear from thee through some channel, as often as possible. I must leave to our sister, for a while, the management of a correspondence which is one of the principal pleasures I enjoy. But I am almost oppressed at present, though, I trust, it will not be of long continuance; and I write this after having mounted not less than fifty single pairs of stairs today, and some of them at no small distance from each other; but whilst I have any sense left remaining, whether I am able to express it or not, I shall always remain thy affectionate brother,

J. Fothergill

Excerpt printed in Crosfield, *Memoirs*, 303–304.

To Samuel Fothergill, Warrington, Lancashire, 1 August 1757

Scarborough, 1.8.1757

Dear Brother,

Through mercy I am arrived safe at this place, and am easy under an apprehension that it may be beneficial to me.[1] Though I came down in the least fatiguing manner, and with much less exercise than I daily sustain, yet I found myself more debilitated than I expected and am the more confirmed that a recess was necessary. This night I enter upon lodgings that I think will be agreeable. I have met with very few who know me, and avoid as much as possible contracting any new acquaintance. I am early at the Spaw,[2] get home by the time many are going thither; I intend in a few days to get out a little on horseback, and to do the best I can to answer the end of my coming to this place. I propose to leave it as this day month, to come easily by Knaresboro to Leeds and Bradford and to fill up the week in and about these places. I shall then come towards you as expeditiously as I can and propose to stay till over the first day following, and then to set out homewards.

Unless thou find some particular inclination to meet me in Yorkshire, I think I would rather choose to meet thee about Manchester, nearer home, as I shall be a good deal engaged among my Friends at Bradford and thereabouts, and would sometimes part with thy company for theirs, or at least share myself more than may be pleasant. T. Collinson[3] leaves me tomorrow and will take a circuit through the Northwest of Yorkshire, to Durham, Newcastle, perhaps Edinburgh, Glasgow, and to Carlisle, Cockermouth, Kendal, Lancaster, and will meet me in about 5 weeks at Warrington to return with me home.

Thus far I had proceeded last night, having half an hour's leisure, and deferred the conclusion till today, expecting that I might hear from Sister Ann and inform thee of her welfare. The account she gives me is very satisfactory. I have been little wanted since I left home, and most seem pleased that I have done myself this piece of justice. Thou will probably hear from me again ere long, when strength and spirits are a little more recruited. Farewell, dear Brother — and be assured of the affectionate remembrance of

Thy loving Brother
J. Fothergill

191

Ms. autograph letter, Port. 20/36, LSFL.

1. When this letter was written Dr. Fothergill himself was taking the water-cure which he had recommended to many patients.

2. The spelling "Spaw" (for Spa) probably represents the eighteenth-century pronunciation of the word.

3. Thomas Collinson, Peter Collinson's nephew, was on circuit duty as a Quaker minister. Thomas Collinson later married the daughter of the Quaker banker Hinton Brown, and eventually became a member of the banking house of Brown, Collinson, and Tritton. — Raistrick, 324.

To Samuel Fothergill, Warrington, Lancashire, 30 March 1758

London, 30.3.1758

Dear Brother,

I had sooner acknowledged the receipt of thy last if proper leisure and disposition had concurred. I now write that I may not seem to forget thee long together; forget thee I cannot. I have passed a laborious winter, unpleasant to myself in some respects, but I hope not altogether unprofitable; I mean not only with respect to temporal advantage, of this I might have as much as one in a private station ought to look for, but I gladly encourage the rising question, to what end? And I hope, in one respect or another, I am kept duly mindful in degree of the winding up of all things.

Since John Hunt has returned he has been much engaged in divers affairs respecting Friends in America,[1] and I hope has been instrumental to their good with some people in considerable station here, as well as with the Proprietaries. He seems to have kept his place steadily, and together with his worthy companion to have been preserved steady, wise and diligent in their service. We are forming a plan for an honest trade with the Indians, and trying to settle the heads of a bill with the Proprietaries for this purpose, to be passed in the Assembly of Pennsylvania. If it succeeds, we are in hopes it will secure the Indians resolutely to the British interest.[2]

It has been this afternoon agreed to propose to the Meeting for Sufferings tomorrow that an intimation may be given to the several Quarterly Meetings, to recommend it to their members to advise Friends at present to decline accepting the office of constable. For a Militia Act will very probably be passed and not very much unlike the former, and this officer will be so much concerned in carrying the Act into execution that it is thought no Friend can easily, if at all, discharge it without acting contrary to his principles,[3] nor is there any prospect of obtaining relief in this respect in the Act itself. If the Meeting should think it a point in which they cannot safely interfere, yet I think private persons should at least suggest to their Friends the hazard they are exposed to, and for this reason I mention it to thee, and have wrote to York to the same import that no amicable application should be omitted that might save our Friends from the difficulties which holding this office will unavoidably expose them to. I have not yet looked into the inclosed,[4] but I imagine it is to request thy Friendly assistance to the writer. I believe him a person of integrity, drawn from his proper sphere by his wife, and to satisfy her ambition forced to another way of [life] to which his capacity is equal, but is not the least of all others dangerous to a person who is not at all times covered with the armour of life and stability.

Could I by unwearied application get myself more at liberty a few weeks hence to sit down with my Friends at our ensuing Solemnity here,[5] I should be glad. But of this I have not so much as the faintest hope. I shall see you now and then as a traveller, but if I can keep so far alive as to rejoice when the will of heaven is done, I shall be satisfied, if nothing more is permitted to be my portion.

I have seen thy neighbor P. Bold[6] several times on account of his health, and hope I have been of some little service to him on this account. I rather shun than court employment of this kind, but if it may be the means of rendering him accessible in emergencies where his interposition might be useful, I shall be pleased.

Brother Joseph perhaps has acquainted thee that Coz John F. is likely to be placed with him.[7] I should like it, if my nephew and his Friends have no objection to it, that he should be inoculated before he is bound. If this be consented to, I would desire that before the summer comes on, Dr. Pemberton[8] might be desired to take care of him. Let a proper lodging and a nurse be provided, and the same care taken of him as of your own, but at neither of your houses.

With tender and affectionate remembrances, Sister, Peggy[9] and myself salute you. I am as much as ever

thy J. Fothergill

Ms. autograph letter, Port. 22/105, LSFL.

1. John Hunt and Christopher Wilson had returned from their visit as mediators between Philadelphia Quakers and the provincial government in dealings with native Indian tribes.

2. For more about trade with the Indians, see the next letter.

3. Members of the Society of Friends excused in England from military service could not consistently take part in the conscription of soldiers.

4. No enclosure has been preserved; circumstances unknown.

5. The London Yearly Meeting.

6. Not identified.

7. Alexander Fothergill's son John, aged fifteen, was to be apprenticed to his uncle Joseph, engaged in the iron industry at Warrington. Apparently John had not received inoculation after the death of his brother from smallpox in 1751.

8. Dr. Thomas Pemberton of Warrington, Samuel's physician.

9. Peggy, one of Joseph Fothergill's daughters, was visiting her uncle and aunt in London.

To Israel Pemberton, Jr., Philadelphia, 12 June 1758

London, 12.6.1758

Dear Friend,

I am indebted to thee for a great many letters and divers papers relating to your affairs. Thy last is of April 6 last, which came to hand a week or two after our Yearly Meeting which fell earlier this year than usual.

Nothing but the want of time has prevented me from being as punctual and diligent a correspondent as thou could desire, but in the midst of a populous city, with Friends not a few in various parts of the world, and a disposition to cultivate a friendship with the virtuous and the good, I am banished from human society. This is my situation at present, and how to extricate myself I cannot yet see; neither the love of money, popularity nor any pleasure I have particularly in my business more than as duty to the public, urges me to undergo as laborious an employ as I can ill sustain. Not a day, not an hour is exempt from calls, not easily to be denied, and even this short account of myself is wrote after a day of fatigue, and I mention it as a proper excuse for the abruptness of my expression, endeavoring to say as much as I can in the little time allotted me.

I received the several letters and papers thou was so kind as to send me from Easton [1] with the proceedings relative to the important treaty held at that place. I endeavoured to make the best use of them I could, first to satisfy all amongst ourselves who seemed to have any doubt about the propriety of your conduct, and in the next to put the necessary extract into the hands of such persons who might have it in their power to make proper use of them.

But still we are heard with difficulty, the first prejudices raised by the *Brief Account*[2] still remain, and there is nothing can yet be heard that will convince the generality of the wickedness and falsehood of that representation. It is still believed that we influence the conduct of public affairs in your Province, and that we have as much influence in them as if we actually composed the majority in Assembly.[3] This however ought not to give us any anxiety, it is enough that we are innocent (this can sweeten any sufferings), and bear with composure the unjust imputations of the ignorant whether of the great or little vulgar. For in reality there is as much of that self-sufficiency which is the fruit of ignorance; as much credulity and pertinacity in error amongst the great as the little, nay somewhat more, as the first are oft much above being taught, whereas the last most commonly want instructors.

It is owing to this unhappy prepossession that B. Franklin has not yet been able to make much progress in his affairs.[4] Reason is heard with fear, the fairest representations are considered as the effects of superior art; and his reputation as a man, a philosopher and a statesman, only serve to render his station more difficult and perplexing. Such is the unhappy turn of mind of most of those who constitute the world of influence in this country. You must allow him time and without repining. He is equally able and solicitous to serve the Province, but his obstructions are next to insurmountable. Great pains had been taken, and very successfully, to render him odious and his integrity suspected to those very persons to whom he must first apply. These suspicions can only be worn off by time and prudence.

The letter published by his son soon after his arrival here had a very good effect in regard to us.[5] It silenced those who were determined not to be convinced that we had been abused; it staggered those who were less resolute, and brought over those who wished to find us innocent. It was generally allowed to be well wrote by all, but I know not whether it did not serve to render the PP.[6] more inflexible.

John Hunt, I imagine, has informed thee that divers of us are willing to contribute what we can towards settling a just and equitable trade with the Indians.[7] If the Association [8] are of opinion that the method we have pointed out is practicable and will avail to the purposes intended, and likewise that themselves are willing to second our intentions cordially, a small number of us who think justly and favourably of your endeavours, who earnestly wish that you may deserve that confidence which your ancestors have acquired for you, will readily join in any measures that may be thought prudent and conducive to the end proposed. Some of the Friends engaged in this affair were about when the letter was sent, and through the haste and inattention of the copier we fear in some parts it will scarcely be intelligible.[9] From the same causes it happened not to be addressed to the Society but it is intended to be laid before the Association for Regaining and Preserving Peace with the Indians.[10] We are about 6 in number; more would join us were it necessary, but we think the business here may be better transacted by a few who are acquainted with your affairs than by a larger number of such who cannot see for themselves. A letter relative to this affair may either be directed to me or J. Hunt, and will be properly regarded. Considering the present temper of those to whom we must apply for any legal protection, we rather think it will be more prudent to trade with the Indians in the manner allowed by the present laws rather than to wait till any other can be obtained. Besides we imagine that unless some very unforeseen disasters befall you, the Indians will have more prudence under the present position of affairs than to break with the Province immediately; since if the French power is lessened, they have reason to fear some chastisement for their cruelties. But I hope the love of justice will not cease when power to elude that justice may be obtained. The English can get nothing by making and keeping the Indians their enemies. They may gain a great deal by acquiring their friendship, and this I hope Friends will be able to effect; this they will have the consciousness of deserving, and if the merit is not ascribed to them by others, their usefulness is not diminished.

Public affairs here wear a more favourable aspect. We have a Ministry who seem to act with equal prudence and resolution. We have a formidable armament actually arrived on the coast of France; our confederates in Germany successful. The French everywhere on the defensive. Yesterday an account came that the principal settlement they had on the river Senegal was taken.[11] We are daily in expectation of hearing the same of Louisbourg.[12] Domestic concord is restored, plenty is promised and trade flourishes; a change within little more than a year, scarce to be credited, and this, under the favour of providence, brought about by the virtue of a few. So far for general affairs — our last Yearly Meeting was large, and I think the business of it conducted with wisdom. Several things which were expected to have brought on pretty warm debates were either prudently composed or treated with such steadiness and conviction as to prevent much disputing. Nevertheless it must be owned that a manifest loss appeared in the removal of many worthy ancients, which seemed to dishearten many and gave those who had more forwardness than discretion too frequent opportunities to impose on assemblies who could have wished for less interruption of this sort.

In the vessel by which this is intended to be sent I apprehend will arrive Mary James of your Province and Mary Kirby, a public Friend from this country.[13] Nobody doubts of her being an honest well meaning woman, and we believe she may have had some service. We would by no means shut up her way, being rather desirous to help than otherwise, yet we believe it would have been a satisfaction to divers if she could easily have stayed at home. [*Passage omitted.*]

If I am not so punctual a correspondent as either of us could wish yet don't omit acquainting me from time to time with anything that may occur that concerns you; for though I am prevented by a multiplicity of affairs from writing so oft as I could wish, yet I endeavour to make a suitable use of the intelligence I receive by mentioning it where it may be useful.

I have not seen Benjamin Franklin some weeks; we have both been engaged. Moore and Smith's case [14] was referred to the Attorney and Solicitor General to hear and make report. The Assembly were treated with more abuse by the Council than can easily be expressed, some of which will doubtless stick close to the report, though some unprejudiced by slanders thought that the Assembly's counsel as much exceeded their opponents in argument and clearness as the others in Billingsgate. — Whether the report is yet made to council I have not yet learned.

I have sent a public paper printed here which I think contains the most material transactions in a little compass, with some other occasional papers I have omitted hitherto, only as thinking thou was better supplied by other hands, but I shall be very glad to continue this kind of barter and should be glad to have likewise any original pamphlets, books, maps and so forth that may be printed with you relative to

America, or if they are informing upon any other subject. Thou will see T. Corbyn's [15] name in the copy of our letter to the Association, and not in the letter itself. I thought I might add it in the copy as he would have done to the original had he been in town, but it was sent by a vessel that departed sooner than was expected and just at the close of the Yearly Meeting when we were all in a hurry. This must account for the inaccuracy of the letter itself and the omission of it being properly addressed. But we shall soon get into better method, keep some short minutes of our proceedings, and if anything occurs, transmit some account of them to you.

My brother Samuel and C. Payton were with us and well. They both left us for their respective habitations, soon after the Meeting. M. Yarnall [16] is visiting the Eastern counties, and we hear is very well and his labours acceptable and edifying. [*Passage omitted.*]

I am, thy affectionate Friend,

J. Fothergill

Ms. autograph letter, Pemberton Papers, Etting Collection, II, 32, HSP.

1. The treaty held at Easton 8–17 November 1756, was followed as promised by another at Easton, 25 July–7 August 1757. Teedyuscung was determined at this time to secure a reservation for his people in the Wyoming Valley. At the opening session of the treaty, he demanded that the original deeds of early land transactions, which had been the subject of discussion in November 1756, be produced. While a messenger went to Philadelphia to get the documents, Teedyuscung demanded a personal secretary to examine the deeds and make copies which should be sent to King George III of England for final judgment, and Charles Thomson was appointed.

When the deeds were finally brought from Philadelphia, Israel Pemberton wanted to have them examined and thoroughly discussed, but the Indians wished now to leave, being quite satisfied by promises of resettlement. Teedyuscung, after being plied with liquor for days by the anti-Quaker party, was in a thoroughly complaisant mood. He called dramatically for the peace belts which, according to Indian custom, were brought into the council-ring for exchange between the Indian chieftains and colonial leaders while solemn pledges to maintain everlasting peace and ties of brotherhood were spoken. This Treaty of July 1757 achieved a basis for improved racial relations. The Pennsylvania Assembly responded to the recommendations of the conference by promptly appropriating funds to build cabins and a protective stockade for the Delawares in the valley of the Wyoming, and carpenters under military escort arrived that autumn to start construction. — Thayer, *Israel Pemberton*, 138–149; Boyd, *Indian Treaties*, 191–212; Wainwright, *George Croghan*, 127–135.

2. Dr. Fothergill's reference — he almost always calls it "Brief Account" — is to *A Brief State of the Province of Pennsylvania*, the Rev. William Smith's indictment of Penn's "Holy Experiment" of government under present conditions.

3. In June 1756, six of the most conservative Quakers, including James Pemberton, had resigned their seats in the Assembly, and four more had resigned after election in the fall. — Thayer, *Israel Pemberton*, 119, 120.

4. Benjamin Franklin arrived in London on 27 July 1757, to begin his work as colonial agent for the Pennsylvania Assembly. His early conferences with Thomas Penn revealed how greatly their opinions differed. A confidential letter Franklin wrote to Isaac Norris on this subject unfortunately got into circulation in Philadelphia, after having been taken to the Assembly for consideration. Richard Peters, known as "the Proprietary watch-dog," took advantage of this situation by sending a copy of this letter to Thomas Penn. Since Franklin had expressed utter contempt of Penn, their relationship deteriorated beyond repair. An extract of the original letter (which cannot now be found) appears in *Benjamin Franklin's Autobiographical Writings*, ed. Van Doren, 110, 111, reprinted from Thomas Balch, *Letters and Papers relating chiefly to the History of Pennsylvania* (Philadelphia: Crissy, 1855).

5. William Franklin, assisting his father in London, wrote a letter to refute prevalent British criticism of Pennsylvania's government. Benjamin Franklin paid a guinea to have the letter published on 16 September 1757, by the *Citizen, or General Advertiser*. The *London Chronicle* reprinted this letter immediately in its issue of 17-20 September, and it was featured in the *Gentleman's Magazine*, 27:417, 418 (September 1757). — Crane, *Franklin's Letters to the Press*, xlvi, xlvii. The letter was reprinted in the *Pennsylvania Gazette*, 8 December 1757.

6. The Proprietors, Thomas and Richard Penn.

7. The project mentioned in the preceding letter, to S. Fothergill, 30 March 1758.

8. See note 10 below.

9. As indicated in the last paragraph but one of this letter, Dr. Fothergill here refers to the letter describing the London Quakers' offer to help with promoting the Indian trade.

10. This Association, founded in 1756 by Israel Pemberton and other idealistic Quakers, was endeavoring to further trade with the Indians as a means of preserving peace. Since assistance from British Quakers would prove obnoxious to government officials in Pennsylvania, Dr. Fothergill and his friends felt it best to remain inconspicuous. The efforts of the Quakers to promote peace with the Indians were described, for the Association, in an account by Charles Thomson and sent to Friends in England, but not published until 1759. See letter of 9 April 1759. The Association, having to some extent accomplished its purpose, came quietly to an end with the ending of the French and Indian War in 1763. — Thayer, *Israel Pemberton*, 190, 191.

11. Capture of Saint-Louis, headquarters of the French in Senegal, opened the rich resources of West Africa's Gold Coast to British commercial enterprise. — *NCMH*, VII, 570, 571, 574.

12. Within a few weeks, on 26 July 1758, Louisbourg, the great fortress erected by France on the Île Royale (now Cape Breton Island), was captured by British amphibious forces under command of Admiral Boscawen and General James Wolfe. — *New Cambridge Modern History*, VII, 538.

13. No record of Mary James has been found. John Woolman records in his *Journal* meeting "Mary Kirby of England," a native of Southrepps, Norfolk, who made frequent religious visits during thirty years of her ministry. She died in 1799 at the age of ninety. — Ms. testimony, Devonshire House, London.

14. Judge William Moore of Chester County, Pa., and the Rev. William Smith, Provost of the College of Philadelphia, had been jailed early in 1758 for promoting and publishing a "libelous attack" upon the Assembly. Appeals for release to Chief Justice William Allen and Governor Denny brought no action, from fear that intervention "might endanger the entire province." Meantime Provost Smith's loyal

students were allowed to come to the jail to continue their classes. In September the Supreme Court freed Judge Moore and soon after, when the Assembly adjourned, the Provost also was released. In October, when the legislators again assembled, a new writ imprisoned Smith, but late in November he disappeared, and subsequently it was learned that he had sailed on 1 December for England to seek justice in British courts of law. — *Pennsylvania Archives*, 8 ser. (Harrisburg, 1931–1935), V. 4099, 4117, 4173; *Minutes of the Provincial Council of Pennsylvania* (Harrisburg, 1851), VII, 764–768, 777–779, 781–783; Horace Wemyss Smith, *Life and Correspondence of the Rev. William Smith, D.D.* (Philadelphia: Ferguson Bros., 1880).

15. Thomas Corbyn (1711–1791) was a Quaker apothecary in London. — Woolman, *Journal*, ed. Gummere, 571.

16. Mordecai Yarnell (1705–1771), a Quaker preacher who traveled widely in the ministry, made his home in Willstown, Chester County, until 1747, when he moved to Philadelphia. — Woolman, *Journal*, ed. Gummere, 586.

To Israel Pemberton, Jr., Philadelphia, 25 September 1758

London, 25.9.1758

Dear Friend,

[*Passage omitted.*] I borrow a few minutes at this time to revive our connection . . . as I have a convenient opportunity of sending by my Friend Robert Proud,[1] who is the bearer of this and whom I must recommend to thy friendly notice and advice.

He is descended from respectable Friends in the North, bred up a scholar, and after having officiated some time as an Usher [2] in the country, came up to town and has been several years in our Friend Silvanus Bevan's family instructing his Brother Timothy's sons [3] who have profited greatly by his tuition in every respect. But his situation in that family of late not having been altogether to his satisfaction, and having entertained some thoughts of seeing America, he obtained his dismission, leaves them on very friendly terms and with their good wishes, and comes over to seek employ in any capacity he may be thought fit for.

I own I part with him with regret, as I think him better qualified for the business of instructing youth than most of that employment he leaves behind. A good grammarian, skilled in figures, knows French, Geography and the principles of several sciences. Steady but not severe, perhaps rather upon the reserve, but this is safe. He is a Friend from principle, and uniformly consistent in practice, and very well esteemed by all who know him for uncorrupted integrity.

Education amongst us as a Society is at so low an ebb that I part with a person of such accomplishments with a good deal of pain, for though it may be doubted whether the most culpable neglect of parents in providing the proper means of education, or the smallness of those who are qualified to teach exceeds, yet I think it less difficult to engage a few at least to be in earnest for their offsprings' instruction than to raise up persons with suitable qualifications.

I doubt not but there may divers employments offer that would turn out more advantageous in time than the profession he, R.P., is bred to, but I think him so fit for the station that I heartily wish he may be encouraged as he deserves.

I know you are supplied, or at least very lately were, with a very valuable person in Philadelphia, I mean, C. Thomson; [4] I would by no means propose that the Bearer should be thought to fill his place till he chooses it no longer. But if a proper school could be opened in some other place, and I imagine there must be many such in your Province, it would probably turn to the account both of Masters and Scholars. — Would Burlington answer?

How far I may be able to succeed, I know not but I could wish Free Schools erected, for Friends' children only, in different parts of this Nation. Where the Quarterly Meetings are small, I would have two or more join to raise from 30 to 50 pounds *per annum* to give to some Friend schoolmaster who should teach all that come *gratis*, but might have the benefit of boarding. I could wish that something of the like kind might be early introduced with you, and if Friends could be prevailed upon to join in purchasing tracts of land and annexing them to that office, the expense would be easily defrayed, and posterity be great gainers. For where there are posts in any degree lucrative and settled, there will be candidates; and one established school would breed many persons expecting and therefore endeavouring to succeed. The other candidates would supply other places — and you would always have choice.

During the present commotions it seems not a proper time to embark on such an affair, but I think it will be in no way improper to be now and then considering, and even more than considering, how they may be most benefited by their predecessors. If they do not set the like example to those who succeed them, the fault will not then be ours.

Our last Yearly Meeting took some steps to get information what provision there was in the several counties for the education of youth; [5]

201

many answers have already come to the Meeting for Sufferings. These will be digested and laid before the next Yearly Meeting; very probably some farther proceedings will be ordered so that, step by step, a foundation may be laid for giving the youth of our Society in this place almost as good an education as many think fit to give their dogs and horses! For at present many have less expense employed on them — and so much for the public.

I must now turn to a little affair of my own. When Brother Samuel in thy company passed through North Carolina, you were so kind together as to purchase a tract of land for me. If the quit-rents are not duly paid, I apprehend advantage may be taken of it to deprive me of my property. I have wrote to Thomas Nicholson,[6] who has the deeds relative to it, to pay what is due, and if he has no other way to reimburse himself, to draw upon thee for the money. If any draughts of this kind come to thy hand, be pleased to pay them, and I'll order the money to be paid here to whom thou pleases, at sight.

Some Friends here, of whom I am one, have been treating with the London Company for their land in your Province. If we agree with the Company, we shall proceed to sell the tracts most wanted, pretty readily; we don't propose any extraordinary advantages to ourselves, interest for the money advanced and a moderate compensation for the labour. The country will reap no inconsiderable advantage by having tracts of land, now uncultivated because there is nobody to buy, made the property of several and occupied accordingly. If any part should devolve upon me, I know of no higher satisfaction than of devoting a competent share to the service of the Society in your Province, particularly in what concerns [illegible] education [illegible].

We have lately been foiled on the coast of France as you have been at Ticonderoga.[7] A Bystander may perhaps see faults that he himself would have committed had he been the actor. We blame one and we blame another, but the great almighty ruler of all things suffers events to take place as may conduce to the good of the whole. War is not our province and the less we interest ourselves in anything that concerns it, the better, yet it is scarce possible to escape the general contagion; and at least not to blame when obvious mistakes are committed, and not to give some degree of approbation when proper conduct produces proper effects. Peace seems yet to be at a distance. We think France is in distress; they may possibly think we are so. The contest does not seem to be now, as contests of this kind used to be formerly, who should commit the greatest excesses of barbarity, kill the most men and spread ruin and desolation the farthest, but which of the two nations shall bear a heavy expense the longest. The national revenues of France are greater than those of England; the natural and artificial revenues of England were equal if not superior to those of France. The French natural revenues are lessened by a most luxurious Court, the rapine of the collectors, the loss of numbers and the poverty of the rest. The artificial revenues arising from commerce are almost totally dried up.

Our natural revenues are very little affected, our artificial are very little less than in time of peace, so that . . . we seem most likely to bear a great expense longer than the French . . . and must therefore be victorious.

But if the French wheedle us into a Treaty, and grievously overreach us in the bargain as hitherto they have done, it makes very little odds whether we have a peace in a year or twenty. — Private men can only communicate their thoughts to each other as private men, but I think that if those in power would shut up the navigation to Quebec, as they may do, and shut up passages to New Orleans by the Mississippi, which with our superior fleet is not impracticable, to me there seems a speedy conclusion to the French Empire in North America, and this without any considerable danger, only patience and resolution. The Indians will follow the strongest, either through fear or affection.

We see that a bill has passed for regulating the Indian trade, so that the scheme which a few of us here had come into for assisting you is unnecessary. As I doubt not but that John Hunt will give thee full information [8] . . . I shall only add that as we had no design to be great gainers so we must trust that Friends on your side will let us lose as little as possible for our generous intention. [*Passage omitted.*]

J.F.,

P.S. As no other way offers at present to send our Yearly Meeting Epistles to Friends of North Carolina I have committed them to thy care. The packet to T. Nicholson thou will very probably send by post, and if no better method offers, send . . . a few of the Epistles by post under cover.

25th at night   [25.9.1758]

It may not be improper to inform thee that endeavours will be used to lay the whole blame of the late Indian ravages in your province upon Friends, as likewise it will be charged to their account entirely, Teedyuscung's complaints against the Proprietary agents on the score of Indian purchases.[9] I have seen a paper today in which are the following expressions; I imagine it is the report of a committee of Council to the Governor:

We cannot but impute the said Teedyuscung's making that base charge [of fraud] against the Proprietor to the malicious suggestions and management of some wicked people, enemies to the Proprietaries, and perhaps it would not be unjust in us if we were to impute it to some of those busy, forward people who in disregard of the express injunctions of his Majesty's ministers against it, and your Honour's repeated notices thereof served on them, would nevertheless appear in such crowds at all the late Indian Treaties, and there show themselves so busy and active in the management and support of the Indians in these affairs against the Proprietaries.[10]

Though it is not unlikely that the whole of this is not unknown to thee, yet lest it might be so, I thought it not improper to give thee this information with the following most earnest request.

Don't grow warm and impatient; sink quietly down and look for better directions than even thy own. Let every prudent measure be taken quietly to procure the necessary materials for your justification. The transactions are recent and facts may easily be ascertained. Therefore provide everything that the nature of the case will admit of, and get every circumstance authenticated. The whole affair will, I believe, be brought before the K's Council.[11] It therefore behooves you greatly to steer clear of any such imputation. I believe this utterly untrue because I think thee and many others utterly incapable of so dishonest a part, but as others may not think as I do, furnish us with incontestable proofs of your innocence, and such I doubt not may be come at.[12] I think Teedyuscung's evidence of great moment,[13] and get his account of your conduct authenticated by the provincial interpreters in form. To support the allegation that Friends are the chief of these savages, they say that the Delawares demanded the Hatchet at the commencement of the war from the Assembly; that the Assembly refused them permission to strike the French; that the Assembly was influenced by the Quakers; the Indians disgusted at this refusal went over to the French, perpetrated all this mischief in revenge;[14] that the Quakers have by every artifice in their power endeavoured to prevent the Delaware chief from acknowledging this truth, and that in short this is the only true reason why those people busy themselves so much with the Indians. A succinct inexpressible confutation of these calumnies, highly authenticated, would be of great service to you, the Assembly, the Province, and perhaps to America.

B. Franklin is a little indisposed from a cold. I think it will become a regular intermittent.[15] It may confine him from business a short time, but his friends, I think, need not be in any [fear] about his recovery. I think he is intently pursuing the business he came about, but the obstacles are inconceivable; prejudices have sunk so deep that they are scarcely to be eradicated.

I must find an end somewhere, though my affection to thee, the province and . . . many I esteem, would suggest a long train of reflections, but I once more say that I am thy affectionate Friend

J. Fothergill

Ms. autograph letter, Pemberton Papers, Etting Collection, II, 33, HSP.

1. Robert Proud (1727/8–1813), devoted his mature years in Philadelphia to shaping the Friends Public School (Penn Charter) by standards of British classical education. After retirement in 1791, he wrote a two-volume history of Pennsylvania, which still furnishes useful material. — Charles West Thomson, "Notices of the Life and Character of Robert Proud," in *Memoirs of the Historical Society of Pennsylvania*, I (Philadelphia, 1836), 419–435.

2. Assistant to the Headmaster.

3. Silvanus Bevan (1691–1765), the apothecary of Plough Lane, though twice married, had no children. Timothy Bevan, his brother and business partner, married in 1735 Elizabeth Barclay, daughter of David Barclay, merchant and banker. They had two sons, Timothy II and Silvanus III, and a daughter, Priscilla. — Raistrick, p. 284.

4. Charles Thomson (1729–1824), who has been mentioned before as secretary to Teedyuscung at the Easton treaty of November 1756, arrived in Philadelphia as an orphan of ten. Befriended by a Presbyterian minister, the Rev. Francis Alison, who conducted an academy in New London, Pennsylvania, the lad received a classical education which fitted him to become Headmaster of Friends Grammar School. During the 1750's Thomson's interest in provincial affairs led him into close association with Quakers and Indians opposing policies of the Proprietary Government of Pennsylvania. In 1760 he definitely left the schoolroom for the world of politics and trade and in 1774–1789 he served as Secretary of the Continental Congress. — Lewis R. Harley, *The Life of Charles Thomson* (Philadelphia: Jacobs, 1900).

5. At Dr. Fothergill's instigation in 1757, the Yearly Meeting had begun to investigate schools maintained by the Society of Friends. Fothergill's summary of 1760 disclosed that the number of schools was insufficient, that teachers were scarce, poorly prepared, and underpaid, and that the curriculum needed improvement. — Elfrida Vipont, *Ackworth School* (London: Lutterworth, 1959), 17–19.

6. Thomas Nicholson was born in 1715 in Pequimas County, North Carolina, where he died in March 1780. A manuscript journal of his life, placed in the care of

the Philadelphia Yearly Meeting, records his three journeys made "in the service of Truth." In England he traveled upwards of 2,500 miles on horseback. Nicholson was consulted by Lord Granville about his own extensive holdings in North Carolina, known as the Granville District. In 1755 Nicholson was appointed by the Society of Friends to a committee which was to take charge of Quaker publication. This committee established what was practically an *Index expurgatorius*, whereby "no Friend or Friends should write, print or publish any Book or Writing whatsoever tending to raise Contention or Breach of Unity among Friends, or that have not first the perusal and approbation of such Friends as shall be appointed." — Stephen B. Weeks, *Southern Quakers* Baltimore: Johns Hopkins University Press, 1896), 140–142.

7. The French stronghold at Ticonderoga, on Lake Champlain — poetically named Fort Carillon from the bell-like sound of its waves in motion — was ably defended in 1758 by Montcalm and his soldiers. British and provincial troops under command of General Abercrombie met with a disastrous defeat (July 8, 1758) in spite of outnumbering the French defenders. The setback on the coast of France was probably that of St. Cas bay in September. — *NCMH*, VII, 538; Freeman, *Washington*, II, 305, 322; Encyc. Brit.

8. John Hunt believed that the Governor's acceptance, 8 April 1758, of the Indian-trade bill passed by the Pennsylvania Assembly had been instigated by Thomas Penn to frustrate Quakers "who might have" a view to engross trade for themselves. — Thayer, *Israel Pemberton*, 160.

9. The Proprietary party in Pennsylvania resented the influence of the Society of Friends upon the Indians as an intrusion upon its right to formulate policies for government under the leadership of William Penn's sons, residing in London.

10. This quotation is an abridgment of a passage in "The Report of the Committee of the Council appointed to enquire into the complaints of the Indians at the Treaty of Easton the Eighth Day of November, 1756." This report to Governer Denny was read in the Provincial Council on 6 January 1758, but was not published in Philadelphia or entered in the Council's minutes until after the Philadelphia Meeting for Sufferings had twice addressed the Governor, asking for a copy. Their second address, 13 January 1759, which like the first was signed by James Pemberton, Clerk, was longer and fuller than the first. They insisted: "We are the more earnestly engaged to urge this request, as we have received undoubted Intelligence from our Friends in London, that though the Name of our Religious Society may not be Expressly mentioned in the said Report of Council, yet it evidently appears to be designed to lay on us the whole Blame of the late Indian Ravages, as a Paragraph of the said Report communicated to us is to the following Effect" — and continued with the passage almost verbatim as given in Dr. Fothergill's letter. — See *Minutes of the Provincial Council of Pennsylvania*, VIII (Harrisburg, 1852), 236–261.

11. The Privy Council.

12. Charles Thomson had already made a compilation of such material, and manuscript copies had been in England for some months, but his *Enquiry into the Causes of the Alienation of the . . . Indians, etc.*, was not published until about 1 March 1759. See letter of 9 April 1759, below.

13. Actually, Teedyuscung's evidence could not be relied upon. His addiction to liquor had increased his emotional instability. Evidence given by him on the same subject on two successive occasions might be quite contradictory. — Boyd, *Indian Treaties*, 192. Richard Peters described him as follows: "He was born among the English, somewhere near Trenton, is near fifty years old — a lusty, raw-boned man,

haughty, and very desirous of respect and command. He can drink three quarts or a gallon of Rum a day without getting drunk. He was the man who persuaded the Delawares to go over to the French, and then to attack the Frontiers." — Wallace, *King of the Delawares*; Richard Peters, Letter Book, 4 August 1756, p. 115, HSP.

14. Although Teedyuscung practically admitted at the treaty of Easton in 1757 that the French had influenced the Susquehanna Indians to attack the English settlement, he protested that old injustices rankling with the Indians made them ready to listen to England's enemy.

15. Franklin had suffered from a similar illness soon after arrival in England, and at that time had first employed Dr. Fothergill as his physician. — Van Doren, *Franklin's Autobiographical Writings*, 107–108.

To Alexander Fothergill, Carr End, Wensleydale, Yorkshire, 30 January 1759

London, 30.1.1759

Dear Brother,

I had not time to acquaint thee I received thy last kind letter, and the bill inclosed for fifty pounds, which was duly paid, and placed to Sister's account. I have laid out £200 for her in a way that will bring in 24 per cent for 20 months with good security, with £200 more of my own. These opportunities happen but seldom, but the India Captains sometimes want money out and this is the common interest on those occasions.[1]

As the weather will soon permit thee to go abroad with less difficulty, I shall be glad if thou would sometime or other make Bellerby in the way, and let me know thy farther sentiments about it, because I should like to have as much time as I can to prepare by calling in if possible some little sums that are owing me.

I shall be glad to hear that you have got pretty well through the winter; thus far it has been much less rigorous here than usual, but I imagine you have had your share of wet, if not of cold. Sister and myself are through mercy pretty well. She is thin and rather puny from anxious solicitude to do well in every respect, and I am kept from gaining much superfluous weight or strength by my way of life, which is more fatiguing than ever. But at present it seems to be my unavoidable lot, and therewith I labour to be content, and fill up my duty as well as I can in hopes that it must not thus continue to the end of my days, the thought of which would almost freeze very power. With respect to my affairs in the North, I know nothing but that it remains under some kind of deliberation but when or how it will terminate I know not, for here I am at present immoveably stationed. C. Payton is at present with us, on a visit to this city, where her labours though often painful to her self, I believe are greatly helpful to many.

Poor Brother Joseph has had a second loss in his youngest daughter,[2] which was the more painful as the stroke was sudden. — Pray is John [3] yet fixed there? — How does your School at Countersett go on? I am ready to assist whenever I am called upon, if it cannot otherwise be supported.

Thou will see by the public papers, that national affairs go on prosperously; I wish we may be sufficiently grateful. One single man sent from Philadelphia [4] engaged most of the Indians to leave the French and come over to the English interest. This induced the French to abandon Fort Duquesne, which then became an easy prey to General Forbes.[5] I have the person's journal in my hands, and intend to get it published in some of the newspapers. — However the French are now driven from those posts, and the back inhabitants may once more rest in security as the Indians are disposed to peace, and the English to use them better and thereby secure their friendship. Goree, the only remaining place of any strength which the French have on the [west] coast of Africa, is now in our possession.[6] Their trade on that coast is consequently almost destroyed (they have yet a few old settlements but of no force) and these Islands must want a supply of Negroes. — But their Islands by this time are most probably under great apprehensions for their own security. The French at home know it, and are trying to play their usual game of a specious peace to gain breath.

How has thy plantation gone on this winter? The season is approaching for some fresh care; and I could wish thou would employ a little in this most beneficial, pleasing and necessary economy. Plant ashes thick on the highway sides.[7] By this means half the drip falls on the road, which likewise supplies half the nourishment. I know of nobody who has thought of this circumstance. Sow ashes and acorns together — the ashes will shelter the oaks, and may be cut down before those can injure these. — But I have almost filled my paper, and can only add our affectionate remembrance to thee and Sister and family, from thy affectionate Brother.

J. Fothergill

Ms. autograph letter, Fothergill Family Papers, Wallis Collection.

1. This was not a strictly speculative venture. Each captain of an East Indiaman was permitted a fair amount of private trade at his many ports of call. Large profits could thus be made, especially on the China run, where merchandise much prized in England could be obtained. For this trade the captains borrowed the necessary capital. Dr. Fothergill was able to venture a sizeable sum which would be commercially useful as well as profitable to himself. — Personal communication, Professor Lucy Sutherland, Lady Margaret Hall, Oxford.

2. Katherine (1744–1759). Joseph's wife had died in 1758. — Fothergill Genealogy, below.

3. Alexander's son, apprenticed to his uncle Joseph.

4. Christian Frederick Post, a Moravian missionary who had lived for years among the Delaware Indians and had married a woman of that tribe. For more about Post's journal, see letter to I. Pemberton, 9 April 1759, below.

5. John Forbes (1710–1759), a veteran of the War of the Austrian Succession and the campaigns of "the 45" against the Young Pretender, was sent to America in 1757 to command the expedition against Fort Duquesne, where General Braddock had been disastrously repulsed in 1755. Planning a deliberate approach, Forbes led his men through the wilderness in 1758, building a chain of blockhouses along the route while a road was being constructed. As winter approached the outlook was discouraging, but when French troops guarding the fort learned that (partly as a result of messages carried by Post) most of the Indians were withdrawing their support, and that the dreaded British attack was imminent, soldiers and ammunition were hastily loaded into boats and sent down the Ohio under cover of darkness. Just before the last boatload left, on the night of 24 November, French soldiers set fire to the fort, which burned to the ground while lighting their escape. On 25 November 1758, General Forbes raised the British flag over the abandoned site. He was obliged to garrison a small force of soldiers there during the winter, "in order to fix this noble, fine country to all perpetuity under the dominion of Great Britain." — Freeman, *Washington*, II, 306–307, 352–353, 365.

6. The British attack upon French colonial possessions in West Africa culminated in Admiral Keppel's capture, 29 December 1758, of Gorée, a small island off the coast of Senegal. British success in West Africa achieved important economic results by crippling the French slave trade, a serious blow to owners of sugar plantations in the French West Indies who were dependent upon slave labor. — J. H. Parry and P. M. Sherlock, *A Short History of the West Indies* (London: Macmillan, 1956), 119.

7. For some years, Alexander Fothergill had been engaged in the construction of a turnpike between Richmond and Lancaster (see Introduction).

To Israel Pemberton, Jr., Philadelphia, 9 April 1759

London, 9.4.1759

Dear Friend,

Thy vigilance and industry demand the grateful acknowledgment of thy Friends. I cannot make equal return, being every day less and less at my own disposal. Now and then to confer with a few Friends who have your concerns at heart is the most I can do, and to wipe off unjust accusations as opportunity offers.

A piece has been lately published here, some copies whereof thou will probably receive, that I hope will tend insensibly to produce a fairer hearing.[1] It is already got into many hands and is well received. — By this time I imagine some overtures have been made to the Assembly by the Proprietors. I wrote to I. Norris [2] upon the subject, but whether he received it I know not. The purport was only to request that if the terms proposed were such as seemed in the least conducive to peace, that they might be cherished; and if there was any appearance of amicably adjusting the dispute that small matters might not easily set them aside. I remarked that though some part of the prejudice against the Assembly might have subsided, yet the times were still unfavourable enough, and that a dispassionate hearing might be difficult to be procured.

I would not however propose that the Assembly's agents should be ordered to desist from prosecuting their proper business in the meanwhile, till it was obvious that the terms proposed were such as might solidly conduce to establish a good understanding between the Proprietor and the people.

B. Franklin has acquired the confidence and esteem of many persons in high station, and by his clear and solid reasoning has in some degree recovered a favourable ear. I don't however apprehend that the Proprietors are solely guided by this circumstance, but I hope from some inclination to be upon better terms with the people than of late they have been. As this disposition would be of the highest advantage to both, I could only wish to do all in my power to induce the Assembly to cherish it, without at the same time relaxing from the measures concerted for their own safety, till they see how far such a disposition may be confided in.

Your old and faithful servant R. Partridge [3] is now no more. He died of a suppression of urine, the consequence of some gravelly complaints. He went off tender, sensible, and full of hope that all is well with him. R. Charles I suppose will now become the sole agent for the Province, and all connection with the Society here, in respect to the public concern of the Province totally cease.[4] Be this as it may, divers here will I believe at all times be willing to assist you in anything they may, whether the agent thinks it worth his while to keep up any sort of intercourse with them or not. There is a Friend in this place whom we should some of us have recommended to the notice of thy Assembly had the place been vacant, who I believe would have served them both ably and zealously. He is about 44 or 5, in the mercantile way, acquainted with the nature of Parliamentary and public business, cool, friendly and judicious. His name is Jacob Hagen,[5] and I believe he will be nominated one of your correspondents. As he is a person of considerable property, he would have some weight in proportion, and not be considered as a mere solicitor. But I think there is so much due to the person who at present occupies the post, that I think it would be imprudent in me to propose that any steps should be taken to set him aside unless his behaviour should give cause for it.

There is a sum of money due to me in Maryland [6] which I believe will be paid without much difficulty. I have sent by Captain Simpson,[7] who brings this, the proper powers to transact the affair, and must request thy assistance in it. I formerly requested thee to lend me a little help in respect to the land bought for me in North Carolina, viz., to get the quit-rent paid, and to procure a survey that I might know somewhat of its site. All the expenses, be pleased to charge to my account, and if the money in Maryland is paid into thy hands, as I expect, deduct what is due from hence.

I am sorry to hear that a general pacification with the Indians advances so slowly, but the English never act from thinking but from feeling. It behooves those who have the affair at heart to be instant now, both in season and out of season, till the business is done. More attention begins to be paid here to Indian affairs than had been, and I imagine orders will be sent from hence to content the Indians. It is very obvious from F. Post's journal why they repose so much confidence in Friends, and why we of all people are the fittest to transact business with them. They have sense enough to see that those people, who will not take up arms to defend their own, will never by force of arms invade the Indian property.

The second part of the journal will be printed in due time,[8] and if any thing comes to hand that seems interesting to the public, it will be added. I am much concerned to hear of some dissension amongst you. It is not now a time to fall out. There is scarcely anything that can now occur which can justify dissension. From what I hear, some amongst you are straining at gnats and swallowing camels. Rigorously insisting upon points which are disputable; and a man may be very good and think either way; whilst rancour, animosity and fiery ignorant zeal is tolerated, nay commended, when in behalf of an ill-grounded opinion. I say not this to condemn anybody. I am ignorant who the leaders are but I know there are divisions, and am sorry for it, because it is hardly possible to be in such a state and yet maintain Christian charity. Those who think themselves most in the right, ought to show their superiority by bearing with the weak. So did our Saviour whilst on earth; so does his spirit now, or else where should the best of us have been?

Your present state demands of you daily considerations what is the cause. And there is no greater danger in giving an untrue answer than by looking at national faults, misconduct or public vice. Our own hearts and houses claim our first regard in the work of reclamation. By the time we have made any considerable progress here, we shall have learned a little more compassion for those who have not all the strength and all the wisdom that we once thought ourselves possessed of. Believe me I aim this at no particular person. This I know full well that my worthy Friend, to whom I write, from constitution, from habit, from the uprightness of his intentions, from his good wishes to the Society is as likely to grow warm in a good cause, exceeding warm as most people; but this warmth can only beget its like. And it is the pure peaceable wisdom from above only that can guide us in the middle paths of judgement to our own safety, the church's good, and the honour of that great name and cause we mean to serve.

I have heard likewise there is some coolness between W.L.[9] and thyself. Which is most to blame I want not to know. I love you both, and you must be friends. I will hear nothing concerning either of you, neither accusation on one side nor vindications on the other side. I condemn you both. A strange way of doing justice; but one ought to have offended less, the other ought to have borne more; had this been done, you had never disagreed.

Call in no arbiters, but as you value your own peace and the good of Society, be at peace, let the sacrifice be never so great. Till this is done, you cannot prosper in religion, pretend to it as much as you please. As I know nothing of the nature of the difference between you, I must insist upon hearing nothing more from either of you than that you are cordially reconciled; and this, if I have any influence with either of you, I entreat may be done as soon as possible, if it is not already. I should

212

not presume to use such language in any other case, but I am of opinion that where there is concord, piety may flourish; but it cannot with dissension.

Remember me to J. Churchman, W. Brown, thy brothers, and our common Friends. Let me entreat you to be extremely sparing in your commendations, I mean publick commendations in your epistles, of any ministry whatever, however worthy you may think them. In a very late instance you have done no extraordinary honour to your discernment. But I attribute all this to the partial regard you ever show to Friends from Europe, but let not your benevolence appear so conspicuous at the expense of your own feeling and capacity. My Sister joins in sincere and affectionate regard to you both. I am thy faithful Friend

J. Fothergill

Ms. autograph letter, Pemberton Papers, Etting Collection, II, 40, HSP.

1. *An Enquiry into the Causes of the Alienation of the Delaware and Shawanese Indians from the British Interest, and into the Measures taken for recovering their Friendship. Extracted from the public treaties, and other authentic papers relating to the transactions of the Government of Pensilvania and the said Indians, for near forty years; and explained by a map of the country. Together with the remarkable journal of Christian Frederic Post, by whose negotiations, among the Indians on the Ohio, they were withdrawn from the interest of the French, who thereupon abandoned the fort and country. With notes by the Editor explaining sundry Indian customs, & c. Written in Pensilvania* (London: Printed for J. Wilkie, 1759). This pamphlet (the "Enquiry" by Charles Thomson) had been published anonymously about March 1 under the direction of Benjamin Franklin. Post's journal, added by Franklin, was that covering his journey of 15 July–20 September 1758, carrying an invitation from the government of Pennsylvania to the Indians at the Forks of the Ohio to attend the conference at Easton in October. — Thayer, *Israel Pemberton*, 157; *Franklin Papers*, ed. Labaree, VIII, 199, 297–298, 322.

2. Isaac Norris was Speaker of the Assembly. A message to the Assembly from Thomas and Richard Penn, bypassing Franklin, had been laid before the Assembly by Governor Denny on 27 Feb. 1759. — *Franklin Papers*, ed. Labaree, VIII, 178–188, 310n.

3. Richard Partridge had been agent for Pennsylvania since 1740. — *Franklin Papers*, ed. Labaree, V, 11n.

4. Robert Charles, who was not a Quaker, had lived in Philadelphia from 1726 to 1739 as a clerk in the proprietary service and had become thoroughly acquainted with conditions in Pennsylvania. In 1751 he had been formally appointed assistant to Partridge, and in 1754, joint agent. — Wolff, *Colonial Agency*, 119–128, 149–150; Nicholas Varga, "Robert Charles, 1748–1770," *William and Mary Quarterly*, 17 (1961): 211–215.

5. Jacob Hagen (1715–1795), a Quaker merchant whose family, of German origin, had established themselves as stave-makers in Mill Street. — Thomas Mortimer, *Universal City Directory* (London, 1760).

6. This sum was probably rental due from a Maryland tenant on property owned by Dr. Fothergill. The locations of his holdings in Maryland and North Carolina cannot now be traced.

7. Captain Simpson has not been identified.

8. *The Second Journal of Christian Frederick Post, on a message from the Governor of Pensilvania to the Indians on the Ohio* (London: Printed for J. Wilkie) was issued later in 1759. It covered Post's mission of 25 October 1758 to 10 January 1759, on which he carried the word that led the French to abandon Fort Duquesne (see letter of 30 January 1759, above). Both journals were reprinted in an appendix to Robert Proud's *History of Pennsylvania* (Philadelphia, 1797–98) and are available in R. G. Thwaites's *Early Western Travels*. See also Wallace, *Teedyuscung*, 41, 48, 181, 190, 191; Crane, *Franklin's Letters to the Press*, xlvi–xlviii.

9. William Logan. The cause of misunderstanding between Logan and Israel Pemberton is unknown. Their mothers were sisters, daughters of Charles Read, a prosperous Quaker merchant who served Philadelphia as alderman and was elected to the provincial Assembly. — *Hannah Logan's Courtship*, 19, 20.

To Israel Pemberton, Jr., Philadelphia, 11 September 1759

London 11.9.1759

Dear Friend,

In hopes of procuring a conveyance for the inclosed to your Meeting for Sufferings by the same vessel that brings over your new Governor,[1] I snatch a few minutes just to send a hasty line together with my affectionate remembrance to thee and thy family. I am apprehensive that the tide of popular dislike is beginning to run high in this place against the Proprietaries, and as things of this nature seldom keep any due bounds, it is possible that the stream may overflow to your mutual disadvantage.

If more harmony does not prevail among you, of one thing I am pretty certain, that the frame of your Government will be changed; but that you will be no losers by the change is not equally clear to me. There have been bickerings I know between the Governor whilst in a private station and several in the Province. I am satisfied he comes over with a disposition to forget everything on his part; and I persuade myself you will find him, as a friend to justice and the true interest of the Province, ever ready to cooperate in anything that may conduce to the good of the whole.

Meet him in the like disposition and think the Province happy in having a Governor who has a large interest at stake in it; who knows your constitution; has felt the inconveniences and dangers it has been exposed to; and who comes over with fewer restraints to you and a stronger inclination to promote its happiness than any stranger would have had.

Don't imagine I am chiming in with a party, and speaking the language of one side which has views of deceiving the other. No such thing. Uninfluenced by any other motives than a wish to promote harmony amongst you and to preserve your constitution inviolable, I want not that you should give up anything. I want only that a proper temper may be preserved, and that it may be thought that the Governor may possibly be at full liberty to put an end to the disputes that have prevailed in the Province, provided the people in general are as willing as he is to put an end to them. I remember that I am writing to an individual who is invested with no power or influence but that of a private man among his friends and his equals. I don't forget that our Friends are no longer a majority in the Assembly. But I reflect at the same time that if my worthy Friend and such as himself treat the Governor with a cordial regard, and consider him as the friend and deliverer of his country, till they have reason from his conduct to think otherwise, their sentiments will influence many; and instead of being looked upon as the head of a party only, and his endeavours for the public good by these means effectually set aside, he will be looked upon as I believe he is, more at liberty to promote the general good of the Province and as much at least disposed to do it than most of his predecessors. I believe he has been the means of bringing the Proprietaries into different considerations about their interest in the Province and as such, I most sincerely esteem him its friend and benefactor, and wish to have him so esteemed by others.

Last week we received the accounts of the reduction of Niagara, the progress of General Amherst at Ticonderoga and Crown Point.[2] These are affairs of importance to you in the first place, and to us likewise. Prince Ferdinand pushes the French very hard in Germany,[3] the army is almost ruined and their supplies procured with difficulty. Prussia had victory in his hands a few times but would not be content with it. He forced the Russians to beat him against their will.[4] He is meditating revenge, but he has great skill, and superior force to encounter. No mention is made of peace, nor do the French seem ready for it. They have yet great resources, and greater hopes. A change of ministers at

215

home would give them all they want. But this is not likely to be soon effected. A little good news will not content us. Today we have possession of Quebec in the papers, and the people last night were beginning to illuminate. But the reduction of this place will not be so easy, though the loss of Niagara and the advance of Amherst must a little dishearten them.[5] We are but too happy, and oh, could we but be sensible of it! All the appearance of peace at home, great plenty, and commerce flourishing. Farewell my dear Friend, and believe me to be thine.

affectionately
John Fothergill

Brought by Gov. Hamilton

Ms. autograph letter, Pemberton Papers, Etting Collection, II, 41, HSP.

1. The new governor, James Hamilton (*ca.* 1710–1783), member of a family prominent in Philadelphia, had served as governor from 1748 to 1754. Although reluctant to accept this responsibility a second time, he considered it a duty and remained in office four years. The son of Andrew Hamilton, an eminent lawyer, James had inherited a splendid estate, Bush Hill, where he installed the first outstanding collection of works of art in Philadelphia. — Carl Bridenbaugh, *Rebels and Gentlemen* (New York: Reynal and Hitchcock, 1942), 180, 213, 214, 218.

2. Fort Niagara was captured by British troops on 25 July, Ticonderoga on 26 July, and Crown Point on 31 July. An all-out assault was planned to gain control of the St. Lawrence Valley, but little progress could yet be made beyond Lake Champlain since these victories required consolidation. — *NCMH*, VII, 539.

3. In 1758 Parliament reorganized the Army of Observation in Germany, originally led by the Duke of Cumberland, by placing it under the command of Prince Ferdinand of Brunswick and staking victory by a fabulous appropriation of £1,200,000. The subsidy made it possible to secure the best service of any army in Europe. Infiltration of French troops through Harburg became impossible.

4. Frederick the Great had been left free, through Prince Ferdinand's activities, to concentrate his efforts against Austria and Russia. In spite of this relief, he had been defeated by the Russian General Saltykov at Zullichau on 23 July 1759 and at Kunersdorff on 13 August. — *NCMH*, VII, 469–475.

5. General James Wolfe and Rear-Admiral Charles Saunders left England with orders to launch an attack upon Quebec. During the summer of 1759, they sailed up the St. Lawrence and deployed their men in various minor engagements in order to grow familiar with the region. Quebec stood seemingly impregnable on rocky cliffs high above the St. Lawrence. Wolfe waited until the days were shorter to make a surprise amphibious attack. On 12 September, in the dead of night, his troops were landed on the north shore and clambered up to the Plains of Abraham beyond the city. Their unexpected ascent found the French forces totally unprepared and outnumbered. Next day the British were victorious in battle, but both gallant commanders, General James Wolfe and the Marquis Louis Joseph de Montcalm, were mortally wounded. Today a single monument in a little park overlooking the St. Lawrence commemorates the heroism of both generals. The city of Quebec capitulated on 18 September 1759.

To Israel Pemberton, Jr., Philadelphia, 30 June 1760

London, 30.6.1760

Dear Friend,

This comes by my dear and worthy Friend G. Mason who is drawn to visit the churches of America; who and what he is will be better known to those who are alive by feeling for themselves than by any description I can give. He is a native of Yorshire brought amongst us by convincement. He makes my house his home when in London, and we can esteem his company as a peculiar advantage.[1] Susannah Hatton from Ireland comes in the same vessel, a valuable Friend and esteemed in her own country as well as here.[2] May they be made the happy instruments of turning more to reflection from the pursuits of this world to seek after a better country.

It is long since I received a line from thee; perhaps thou may say the same of me, but not I think with equal reason. But we are both excusable, if we suffer no proper opportunity to escape of endeavouring to stir up the pure mind in each other, and lessening our attachment to things that are only for a season.

Through mercy my sister and self are well, and not unmindful of our Friend, though often hindered from manifesting it in the manner we could wish nor so often as would be agreeable. We are in a sort of publick station, the objects of numerous applications of very different natures, so that by much the least part of our time is at our own command. I mention this as a reason for the slow returns I make, as well as my Sister to thy Wife's kind notice of us, and indeed it is no light matter to either of us to be thus deprived of a correspondence which is very grateful to us, but so it has happened, and will do so, I am afraid, at least for sometime longer.

I sent to thy care some time ago a power of attorney to recover a debt in Maryland. As I find some remittances are made to England, if nothing be done in the affair I should be glad that any farther proceedings were stopped. I likewise requested thy care in regard to the tract of land in North Carolina. I have heard nothing further from T. Nicholson, and am therefore afraid lest the quit-rent should be so long neglected that my little properties should be vacated.

We are glad to find that the affairs of your Government wear a more favourable aspect, and we hope the Indians will be more quieted when

217

they find how little assistance they are to expect from the French. For I imagine, after their retreat from Quebec and the loss they sustained there, the power of the French position in those parts must be much enfeebled and leave them as easy conquest if no unforeseen disaster befalls us.

I have little expectation of any effectual relief in the Indian affairs from the Proprietors. I think however the application from the Friends on your side [3] was both prudent and proper, and will be seconded by a few with their best endeavours.

Peace is much talked of here and it's possible it may be near at hand, but I do not expect to see it yet. France is heartily tired of the war, but her allies are not. Whilst France can pay they will not make peace. When the Austrians and Russians must fight their own battles and at their own expense, then peace will soon follow. I consider these two last powers as our high allies; they are in reality joining their endeavours to exhaust France and reduce her to reason. The present war is not so much a trial of force as a war of expense, in which that side will be victorious that can longest hold out. The necessary funds for the present year being therefore raised, and the troops in the field, it seems most reasonable to consider that those who think they may be better, but cannot be much worse, will not be hasty in foreclosing any possible advantage that may arise to them in the course of the campaign.

Farewell, my dear Friend, remember me to thy Wife, in which my Sister joins me, to thy Brothers and our common Friends. I need not request thy friendship to my worthy lodger; thou will feel his worth, and be readier to do, than he to receive, every act of kindness. Remember me sometimes with a line, and think of me as I am,

Thy affectionate friend
J. Fothergill

Ms. autograph letter, Pemberton Papers, Etting Collection, II, 42, HSP.

1. George Mason, of Thirsk in Yorkshire. A few years after this visit to America he left England with his wife and five children to settle "either in your province [Pennsylvania] or in West Jersey." — Gwendolyn Beaufoy, *Leaves from a Beech Tree* (Oxford, England: Privately printed by Basil Blackwell, 1930), 106, 107.

2. Susannah Hudson Hatton (1719–1781), a Quaker minister, was the widow of Joseph Hatton of Waterford, Ireland. Her visit to Pennsylvania in 1760, lasting a year, created many friendships and led eventually to her marriage to Thomas Lightfoot of Uwchlan, Chester County, Pennsylvania, where she settled in 1764. She was active as a Quaker minister for almost fifty years. — Woolman, *Journal*, ed. Gummere, 548–549.

3. The Friendly Association, founded by Israel Pemberton in 1756, aimed at im-

proving relations with the Indians through fairly conducted trading posts. The scheme was opposed by the Parliamentary party. In March 1760, the Association had sent a letter to John Hunt and Dr. Fothergill enclosing an address to the Proprietors concerning the Indian problems. — Samuel Parrish, *Some Chapters in the History of the Friendly Association for Regaining and Preserving Peace with the Indians by Pacific Measures* (Philadelphia: Friends' Historical Association, 1877), 114–116.

To Israel Pemberton, Jr., Philadelphia, 8 September 1760

London, 8.9.1760

Dear Friend,

Inclosed is an answer to the address of your Association [1] which was presented to the Proprietaries soon after its arrival. As it was sent to me sealed up, I am a stranger to its contents, and can only wish it may be agreeable to the views and wishes of the Association.

The Proprietors intended to have communicated the contents, I believe, to the Friends that presented the address to them, and were sent to for this purpose; but it happened they were all out of town but myself and I was engaged so as not to be able to attend at the time they appointed. You are wise and able, and I can only wish that you may be governed aright in your undertaking. In my opinion the sooner you can withdraw from any public concern the better. Your country seems devoted to feel the effects of increased power, which nothing but the hand of Providence can avert. The safety of all consists of a careful humble attention to this; and a living desire after it, truly cherished, will step by step bring forwards to such a degree of establishment as to bear patiently what may occur. [*Passage omitted.*]

John Hunt showed me thy account of our money transactions, with accounts of Indian commerce. As I see commission is charged on your side where no risk is run, it is but reasonable to allow J. Hunt the same, who has had the labour and care in shipping and so forth; to this, add £34 sterling which I have paid on an account relative to your Province and if not for its benefit at least in some degree for its credit, and I shall be content that the profits arising from the money advanced should go to the use of the Association.

The money I hint at was paid on the following occasion. Not long after the *Brief Account of Pennsylvania* [2] was published, one Cross, who resided some time in the Province, wrote an answer to it which though unequal to the former yet had some service. [3] The author, however,

219

besides his labour became indebted to the printer, the pamphlet not selling to expectation, for the sum I mentioned. On this account he applied to B. Franklin, in hopes that as Agent to the Assembly he might procure a reimbursement of a sum which Cross could not conveniently lose. B. Franklin was of the opinion that the present Assembly would not readily be brought to allow such an article, and therefore applied to me to know whether the Society could not find means to raise the sum in question for a person who, at least, intended them a service. This I thought would be as difficult to accomplish as the other; and therefore, as the poor man was very pressing with B.F. for the money, I paid him myself, rather determined to lose the money than that any person should say he had been a sufferer by endeavouring to advocate our cause, though he had done it unasked, and at the same time not in the most satisfactory manner. As this is the case, I think I may reasonably expect a reimbursement of this expense, the principal and interest to it being converted to the Society's use, only making satisfaction to J.H. for his care in proportion to what is required on yours, who ought in this case to have been the foremost in setting us a good example. [*Passage omitted.*]

J. Fothergill

Ms. autograph letter, Pemberton Papers, II, 43, HSP.

1. See the preceding letter.
2. Dr. Fothergill continues to refer to William Smith's pamphlet as "Brief Account."
3. *An Answer to an Invidious Pamphlet, intituled, A Brief State of the Province of Pennsylvania; wherein are Exposed the many false Assertions of the Author, or Authors, of the said Pamphlet, with a View to Render the Quakers of Pennsylvania and their Government Obnoxious to the British Parliament and Ministry* (London: Printed for S. Bladon, 1755). William Smith circulated the story that the author of this account was an attorney's clerk guilty of forgery who had been transported to Pennsylvania for a period of exile.

To James Pemberton, Philadelphia, 2 November 1761

London, 2.11.1761

Dear Friend,[1]

If my leisure and inclination were equal, I should write to thee often for thy friendship's sake and the country's. But I can appoint no substitute in my occupation; each day brings with it full employ to be discharged by no hands but my own. The following occasion however prompted me to borrow an hour to write to thee, and through thee to such Friends as thou thinks proper to consult upon the affair.

From the time we were first considered as a distinct religious Society, we have laid hold of proper opportunities to present ourselves before the Throne, and generally I believe with acceptance and to our own satisfaction. The death of the late King [2] and the accession of the present engaged us to follow the example of our predecessors; and a more recent occasion, the marriage [3] of the King, has again incited us to pay a just and necessary mark of our regard.

It is a favourable circumstance that we have a King of whom it may I think with great truth be said that there are few persons of his age [4] in his extensive dominion who are blessed with a better mind or a clearer understanding. Of both these he has given undoubted proofs, and young as he is, has already brought about by his example solely, several necessary and commendable reformations. He speaks what he means, and he means the happiness of his subjects.

Three days ago we presented an address to him, another to the Queen, a virtuous, sensible, engaging Princess, pleasing in her person and of a character unblemished; as also to the Princess of Wales.[5] On this occasion I could not but regret that Friends on your side the water had never thought proper to address, when much less important branches of society do it daily with approbation.

As it was laid upon me to read the address, and to point out to the King the more considerable of those Friends who were present amongst the rest, I took notice of a native of your Province,[6] upon which the King was pleased to say he imagined there was a very large body [of Friends] if not the largest in that Province than any other part of his dominion. This suggested another reason why you ought to embrace the present opportunity; and give me leave to mention another which I think is not less important. From the conversation I have casually had with some persons of eminence here, I am persuaded that when a peace is once settled, the consideration of the several Governments in America will be brought upon the carpet. How far the respective privileges of the several Governments may be altered or abridged is not possible to foresee; but in all probability the privileges of those will be least attended to who are the most unknown or disregarded.

I could therefore wish that the Friends of the Meeting for Sufferings in Philadelphia, or some other Meeting that may soon happen and be most representative of the whole body, would consider the affair, and it no material objection is urged, would speedily proceed to prepare something of this nature to the King only, upon his accession to the throne and his marriage, together. You are wise and prudent and will feel how far your liberty extends. The liberties we enjoyed under the late reign, the happy commencement of the present, his declaration and conduct consistent with them, will furnish you with abundant matter. Those we have presented are not altogether to my wishes, but they were the best the time allowed us would permit. I shall only add one consideration more respecting the necessity of such an application. You would wish to appear not inconsiderable, yet if you are too small to be seen, or too indifferent whether you are seen or not, how can you expect any notice should be taken of you when perhaps you most need it?

Should Friends think proper to fall in with the proposal, a consideration will arise probably by what canal to convey it. Had your Proprietor been his own friend or yours, to him I should have recommended it, but as I am afraid you have not sufficient proofs that he is either one or the other, perhaps it had best be sent to the Meeting for Sufferings, who will, I doubt not, take what care they can concerning it. [*Passage omitted.*]

My Sister joins me in tender salutation to you both, from thy affectionate Friend,

J. Fothergill

Ms. autograph letter (faded), Pemberton Papers, Etting Collection, II, 46; a clerk's copy also exists: Pemberton Papers, XXXIV, 111, HSP.

1. James Pemberton (1723–1809) was a partner in the export–import business which brought the Pembertons wealth. Educated in the Friends Publick School, he worked zealously in maturity for improvement of education throughout the Quaker schools of the colony. In 1756 he was one of the Quakers who voluntarily withdrew from the Assembly when Indian warfare threatened. In the same year he became the first Clerk of the Philadelphia Meeting for Sufferings. In 1765 he was elected to the Assembly again, and held office for four years. He was a member of the Board of Managers of the Pennsylvania Hospital for twenty-two years and its secretary from 1754 to 1772. At Quaker Meeting he sat for a long period at the head of the gallery on First Days. Both he and his brother Israel were elected to the American Philosophical Society in 1768. James has the distinction of being a founder of the Pennsylvania Society for the Abolition of Slavery; he succeeded Benjamin Franklin as president and held this office from 1790 to 1803.

2. George II died 25 October 1760.

3. The marriage of King George III to Princess Charlotte of Mecklenburg-Strelitz took place 2 September 1761.

4. King George III was twenty-three.

5. Augusta, Princess Dowager of Wales, was widowed in 1751. Mark Beaufoy, a prominent London businessman and one of the twenty-four Friends received by the King and Queen at St. James' Palace, described the presentation in a letter to his sister: "This day, at one o'clock, we were received by the King, Queen and Princess Dowager; the first two at St. James's, the latter at Leicester House, with all the marks of Complacency and Favour that I believe was ever shown on like occasion to any body of people. Dr. Fothergill read the address to the King in the Public Levee Room, and afterwards, as we passed by the Royal Presence, gave our names; and the King was pleased to converse very graciously with several of the members, particularly with Peter Collinson and David Barclay . . . Jacob Hagen, on account of being able to speak the German tongue, was appointed to read the address to the Queen, which being done, it was presented to her, in a fair hand in two columns, the one in English, the other in German, after which she very obligingly entered into conversation with him. On the whole we are much pleased . . . and we think ourselves obliged to the Earl of Bute and the Duke of Manchester who introduced us, the first to the King, and the other to the Queen on this occasion. The Queen is not handsome, but very agreeable, in Stature much as my Wife, has a kind of Smartness in her Countenance, but there is in her Eyes something uncommonly lively . . . her Deportment is sedate, with a Kind Obliging Deference towards those she speaks to, as if she renounced Superiority — and rather confessed this due to those with whom she converses, which according to my idea . . . is the very Essence of good breeding. — Beaufoy, *Leaves from a Beech Tree*, 100, 101.

6. His name is not mentioned.

To Zachariah Cockfield, Upton, Essex, 16 March 1762

London, 16.3.1762

Esteemed Friend,

I have often thought it very hard that because I had done a person a kindness once, he seemed to claim a right to demand my assistance whenever he thought it necessary. I little thought that this would have been so much my case as it is like to be. Thou hast served me once very cordially and effectually and, behold, I am going for the same reason to ask thy assistance again.[1]

The house and about 7 acres of ground contiguous to that thou hast already purchased for me, nearer Ham, I am informed is to be sold. I should be glad to have it, at any reasonable rate, for considerations too obvious to mention. I must, therefore, intreat thee to befriend me in this as thou hast done in the former, and whatever thou thinks it worth I will readily pay.

Some afternoon ere long when the weather is somewhat milder, I will endeavour to come down and confer with thee upon it; but this needs not to hinder thee from taking every needful step to effect the purchase, and if thou pleases, as for thyself. The purchase I have already made is magnified to an hundred acres, all walled in; and if it gets abroad that I have bought a single acre more, some people will imagine that I aim at nothing less than the whole country. Thy obliging readiness to serve me perhaps influences me to use greater freedom than I ought; but as there is no person on whose judgement and disinterested friendship I can more rely, do not wonder that I request thy assistance where I cannot help myself. When we are nearer neighbors, I hope not to forget how much I am

Thy obliged Friend
John Fothergill

Ms. autograph letter, Dimsdale Mss., LSFL.

1. Zachariah Cockfield, a wealthy merchant and ship broker who was Dr. Fothergill's patient, was instrumental in Dr. Fothergill's purchase of land at Upton. — Fox, 82n; *Works*, ed. Lettsom, III, 38–39.

To James Pemberton, Philadelphia, 7 April 1762

London, 7.4.1762

Dear Friend,

I am indebted to thee for several acceptable letters, which I have often wanted to acknowledge, but time was not allowed me. I could not however suffer my worthy Friend W. Logan to return without bringing with him some small proof of my respectful remembrance and a disposition to cultivate it with much cheerfulness, if my leisure was equal to my inclination.[1]

But alas, I am every day more than ever plunged into embarrassments I know not how to avoid. An extensive practice has furnished me with some experience; those who early employed me seem to have a right to my riper judgment; others, who have not the same right, think it hard to be refused. Thus I am oppressed between the upper and nether millstones, deprived of ease and necessary respite; deprived of leisure to cultivate the social connection; and almost deprived of the proper time for looking farther than what concerns this life only. — But I cease not to look about me with some care when and how to extricate myself from a part at least of this oppressive labour. — I distributed the books thou was pleased to send me, as desired; but they came perhaps at an unlucky juncture. Money is much wanted here for numerous purposes, and men part with fifty pounds with reluctance when they know that a little more would purchase them an hundred. The Hospital must however subsist itself as well as possible till better times. I propose to send by Dr. Shippen[2] a present to it of some intrinsic value,[3] though not probably of immediate benefit.

I need not tell thee that the knowledge of Anatomy is of exceedingly great use to practitioners in Physick and Surgery, and that the means of procuring subjects with you are not easy. Some pretty accurate anatomical drawings, about half as big as the life, have fallen into my hands, and which I propose to send to your Hospital to be under the care of the Physicians, and to be by some of them explained to the students or pupils who may attend the Hospital. In the want of real subjects these will have their use, and I have recommended it to Dr. Shippen to give a course of Anatomical lectures to such as may attend.[4] He is very qualified for the subject, and will soon be followed by an able assistant, Dr. Morgan;[5] both of whom I apprehend will not only be useful to the Province in their employments, but if suitably countenanced by the legislature, will be able to erect a school of Physick amongst you that may draw many students from various parts of America and the West Indies, and at least furnish them with a better idea of the rudiments of their profession than they have at present the means of acquiring on your side of the water.

Dr. Chancellor,[6] though perhaps not qualified to take any considerable share in an undertaking of this nature, yet has spent his time here to considerable advantage. I esteem him much, and have no doubt but his diligence and care, improved by the opportunities of seeing a great deal of practice, will render him a very useful member of society.

Should the Managers of the Hospital think proper, I could wish that if the drawings and casts I shall send by the next convoy come safe, that they might be lodged in some low apartment of the Hospital, not to be seen by every person but with the permission of a trustee, and for some small gratuity for the benefit of the House. The drawings are in Crayon, and should therefore not be kept in too dry a place, nor shaked [sic] about too much.[7]

I am coming now to a very tender subject, and must beg thy patience, if I judge amiss, and thy prudent aid, if I judge aright. I have seen your address and dislike it.[8] There is just room and just cause to say more; and not to go as far as may be with truth and sincerity is lessening yourselves. I am afraid we should greatly suffer in our Sovereign's opinion and in the judgement of the public should we offer it. Why do you lay such a task on your correspondents? The Meeting for Sufferings have not yet seen it; it is scarce known to any but ourselves that an address is come over. We must suppress it from appearing, unless you will resume the subject and say something more worthy of the Sovereign, more worthy of yourselves, and less exceptionable to us. Twice I had the privilege of a few moments conversation in both of which he was pleased to ask after you, your numbers and conditions particularly. — But I'll say no more on this subject.

I part with my worthy Friend [9] to whose care I consign this with some regret, saving that his family and his friends require his presence. The Province are I think greatly obliged to him, as he has taken care on every occasion that offered to vindicate their conduct, remove aspersions, place them in a just light with our superiors, and has done them some extensive services. By this means I hope the captive inhabitants will be set at liberty and a better understanding open with persons in power here. He has neither courted the Proprietary family nor shunned them. He wished them well but his country better, and thus without any pay or appointment, he has to my knowledge endeavoured to serve effectually. He brings along with him part of a laborious work that is printing here chiefly at my risk, which I hope will prove a not unuseful present to the public. It is a translation of the Old Testament, to be followed by the New, from the original languages by a self-taught philosopher and linguist in this country.[10] I fancy it will make two pretty large volumes in folio and may come to about 7 Guineas price. It contains a vast fund of useful erudition, and I hope will prove instructive if not entertaining.

Pray how are the Pennsylvania Company's lands supposed to have been sold; if well, it will give the Trustees satisfaction. But they must still regret the loss of poor Friend Rawle.[11]

I am indebted to thy worthy Brother Israel, but I fear I shall scarcely be able to pay him debts at present. Be pleased to communicate to him any parts that may be agreeable to him with the remembrance of my dear love to himself and his family.

G. Mason spent some weeks with us this winter to our great satisfaction and I hope lasting benefit. He often spoke of your families with affection and esteem. A severe rheumatic pain in one arm affected him most of the winter and spring, and is not wholly removed. The last autumn, the winter and the spring till this time have been unusually cold. I question whether we have had four days together from the time called Michaelmas to Lady Day on which there has not fallen either rain, snow or hail. The spring was unusually backward, and though we have had a brigher sky for a week past yet the nights are frosty and vegetation advances slowly.

In respect to public affairs I know nothing more than the papers mention, but I should conjecture that peace is yet very distant. That France will attempt to give us an home thrust, and that Spain will not regard any loss in her colony, if they can either reduce Portugal to the Spanish yoke which sccms not improbable or recover Gibraltar, which though deemed impregnable may perhaps not be found so to fraud or force, and of these there will be no want in our adversaries.

I have borrowed the time I have been writing from my rest, and must conclude in order to get some recruitment for the endless labour of tomorrow. When conversing with my Friends, I know not where to stop till necessity claims pen, and bids me, with all my warmth of friendship, pay her the tribute she exacts. Affectionately remember me to thy family, thy Brother and our common Friends and be assured that I am thine

J. Fothergilll

Ms. autograph letter, Pemberton Papers, Etting Collection, II, 47, HSP.

1. At a meeting of the Board of Managers of the Pennsylvania Hospital, 27 July 1762, "William Logan, lately returned from England, presented a copy of *A History of the Materia Medica* by William Lewis, FRS, being a present to this hospital by Dr. John Fothergill . . . an additional mark of the Doctor's benevolent regard for this institution." This was the first volume received for the Hospital's library. — Pennsylvania Hospital Minute Books, II, 312, 314, on microfilm at APS.

2. Dr. William Shippen, Jr. (1736–1808), son of Dr. William Shippen, Sr., of Philadelphia, was graduated from the College of New Jersey (later Princeton) with distinction as valedictorian of his class. After assisting his father in medical practice for a year, he was sent to London to study anatomy with William and John Hunter, and midwifery with Dr. Colin Mackenzie. With this background he entered the medical school of the University of Edinburgh and in 1761 received his M.D. degree. He returned to Philadelphia in 1762. — B. C. Corner, *William Shippen.*

3. Dr. Fothergill's "Donation of Anatomical Drawings and Casts" is entered as part of the capital stock of the Pennsylvania Hospital, and appraised at a valuation of £350 when received. — Pennsylvania Hospital Minute Books, II, 325–327, on microfilm at APS.

4. On 9 November 1762, Dr. Fothergill's gift was unpacked at the Pennsylvania Hospital in the presence of the Board of Managers, several hospital physicians, and Dr. William Shippen, Jr. The boxes contained anatomical casts, a human skeleton, a human fetus preserved by injection, and eighteen crayon drawings in color, showing various "curious parts of the human body." These drawings, carefully "framed and glaized," were the work of Jan van Rymsdyk, a talented Dutch artist employed by Dr. William Hunter for more than thirty years while preparing his medical atlas, *The Human Gravid Uterus*. Permission was granted young Dr. Shippen to use this donation for the instruction of private classes in anatomy, such as he had attended under the Hunters in London. Shippen's classes mark the beginning in the American Colonies of medical education at the university level, although without academic affiliation.

5. John Morgan (1735–1789) was a member of the first class to graduate (1757) from the College of Philadelphia. Having served an apprenticeship with Dr. John Redman, he enlisted in a provincial regiment and served as lieutenant and surgeon during the French and Indian War. On the advice of Dr. Redman, and with an introduction from Benjamin Franklin, he then went abroad, studying for a year in London with Dr. Fothergill, the Hunters, and William Hewson and for two years at the University of Edinburgh, where he received his medical degree in 1763. For Morgan's career, see Whitfield J. Bell, Jr., *John Morgan: Continental Doctor* (Philadelphia: University of Pennsylvania Press, 1965).

6. In May 1753, a Dr. William Chancellor sold medicines at John Jarvis', opposite Black Horse Alley, Philadelphia; in November 1753 he conducted business at the Sign of the Mortar and Pestle, opposite the Presbyterian Meeting House in Market Street. *The Pennsylvania Gazette*, 21 October 1762, carries a notice of Dr. Chancellor's death.

7. The Managers of the Hospital ruled that the entire collection from Dr. Fothergill should be placed in a locked upper room, suitable for protection from "the curious," and also for Dr. Shippen's demonstrations to his students. Each student would be charged one pistole for the privilege of observing the material. Later, when there were requests to view the collection, "reputable citizens" were granted at stated times admission upon payment of one dollar each. Money received went into the Hospital treasury. — Morton and Woodbury, *Pennsylvania Hospital*, 357–358; G. Canby Robinson, M.D., *Adventures in Medical Teaching* (Cambridge, Mass.: Harvard University Press, 1957), 71, 72; *The Diary and Autobiography of John Adams*, ed. L. H. Butterfield (Cambridge, Mass.: Harvard University Press, 1961), II, 116, 117.

8. The address to the King suggested in the letter (above) to James Pemberton, 2 November 1761.

9. William Logan.

10. Anthony Purver.

11. Francis Rawle (1729–1761), a prosperous young Quaker merchant who had been exceptionally useful to the Pennsylvania Hospital Board of Managers as secretary and liaison officer in dealings with the Pennsylvania Land Company, had died in June 1761 as the result of an accidental gunshot wound. His will left provision for his wife and children, together with a small bequest to the Pennsylvania Hospital, to which he had given devoted service. Morton and Woodbury, *Pennsylvania Hospital*, 394; J. Bennet Nolan, *The Schuylkill* (New Brunswick, N.J.: Rutgers University Press, 1951), 180; information from Whitfield J. Bell, Jr., Librarian, APS, Philadelphia.

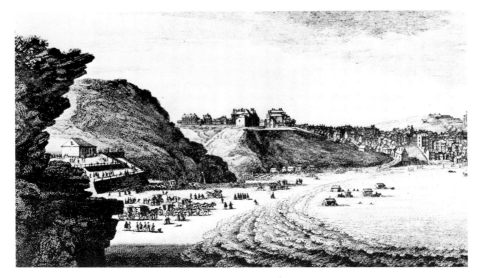

Bathing at Scarborough, 1745

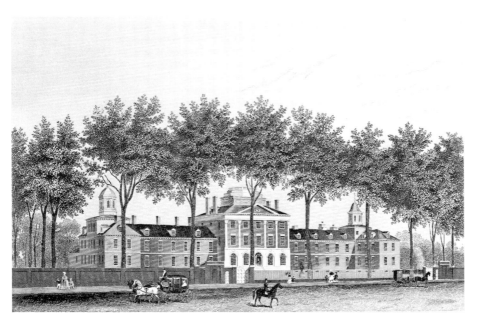

The Pennsylvania Hospital

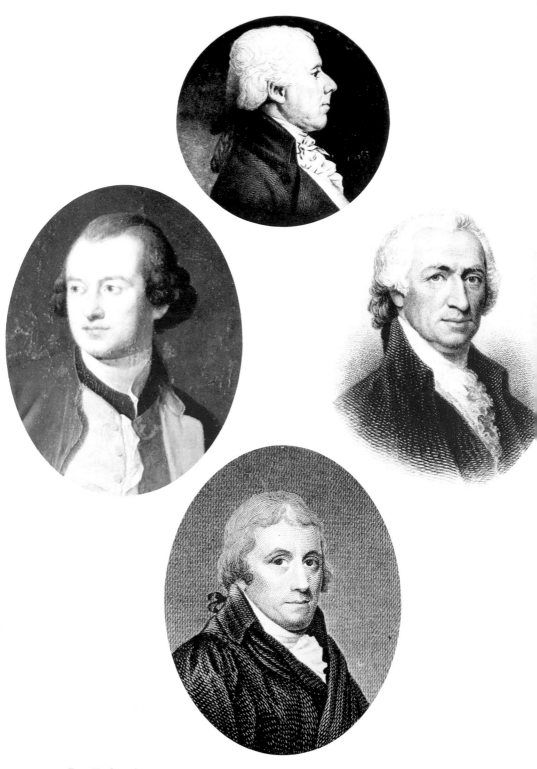

Dr. Fothergill's American friends; top, Dr. Benjamin Rush; center left, Dr. John Morgan; center right, Dr. William Shippen, Jr.; bottom, Dr. Benjamin Waterhouse

To Alexander Fothergill, Carr End, Wensleydale, Yorkshire, 12 August 1763

Scarborough, 12.8.1763

Dear Brother,

This afternoon I received thy very acceptable letter and embrace the first opportunity to answer it and acquaint thee with my intentions.

We propose leaving this place on fifth day and sleep that night at G. Mason's who will conduct us to Thirsk next day to dinner. Here we shall be glad to meet thee to show us the rest of the way to Carr End. We fancy we can get to Bainbridge in our carriage, at least to Askrigg and to leave it, our horses, and servants there; [1] only the saddle horse to carry me, and thou must get one either single or double to carry Sister. [2] We hope to get to Carr End on seventh day evening, and to be at your meeting next day, and set out the following day for Lancaster, to which place we shall be very glad of thy company both as a guide and our Brother.

I should be very glad of thy company here was it not that it would add one more difficulty; I have already more acquaintance than I can satisfy their demands; and a wish to enjoy thy company, too, would rather add to my embarrassment. This prevents me from asking thee to meet me here, especially as I shall have some reliance upon thee to conduct me through a country to me altogether unknown [3] when I leave Carr End.

I intend writing to thee again before we leave this place, but if any accident prevents it reaching thee, I think thou may expect to see us at Thirsk about noon this day two weeks (sixth day), to go that afternoon as far as may be convenient to reach Carr End in the evening of the following day.

Please remember us to Sister and thy family, and accept our affectionate remembrance

from thy Brother
John Fothergill

Ms. autograph letter, Fothergill Family Papers, Wallis Collection.

1. Bainbridge, a pleasant Yorkshire village with an ancient inn, the Rose and Crown, which now welcomes twentieth-century travelers, has been a settlement since the Romans built their fort there on the Brough, a hillside site. Askrigg, a place of greater importance commercially, is proud of a fine market cross and St. Oswald's

Church, dating from the fifteenth century. — Hartley and Ingilby, *Yorkshire Village*, 5, 6, 58–59, 94.

2. James Hack Tuke pictures the cavalcade proceeding from Bainbridge "up the hilly road to Carr End . . . the great London Doctor, with cocked hat and medical wig, sitting upright in his saddle, with Sister Ann, in bonnet and habiliments of the plainest sort, on a pillion, escorted by their brother Alexander, let us hope in dalesman's costume." — Tuke, *A Sketch of the Life of Dr. John Fothergill* (London: Harris, 1879), 39.

3. Alexander Fothergill when surveying the road between Carr End and Lancaster described it as one of the worst in England.

To James Bogle French, Apothecary, 1 Wood Street, Cheapside, London, 19 August 1763

Scarborough, 19.8.1763

My worthy Friend,[1]

It was very obliging to favour me with so agreeable a letter; I felt more anxiety on leaving our Patient in a doubtful situation than on any other; and it gave me vast relief to hear of his recovery.

This place is at present very full, not of invalids, as one would expect, but of the Gay, the young and Expensive.[2] There are indeed more of the former than have been for many years; and a considerable number of my acquaintances from the South especially. Some little business I cannot avoid, but I endeavour to give no cause for uneasiness to my Brethren, and I hope I have succeeded in it.

Dr. Waugh of Malton, Dr. Pettit of London, have attended for some years.[3] Dr. Knox [4] is with the Marquess of Granby. Dr. Mushet is also here, but I have not seen him.[5] Dr. Wood lives upon the spot, and practices among the Lower Inhabitants of the town at a cheap rate.[6] Judge if there be not enough of the faculty to take care of five or six hundred people, nine out of ten of whom are in perfect health. To the Honour of the Faculty [7] be it spoken, we are all on good terms, and live not uncomfortably together.

The balls and assemblies I am told are crowded immoderately; 550 people and upward in a room of not very large dimensions. Here they stew till midnight, come out of a Stove upon a high sea Cliff, with the utmost contempt of cold or Fogs, plunge into the sea next morning, and prepare for another evening's campaign. And all this after they have travelled about 200 miles for the recovery of their health, with many a wise prescription in their pockets. I shall return very knowing in these affairs. I am surprised that my Brethren at Almacks [8] have so little consideration; are they not daily reproaching the English for invidious distinctions, and are they not daily giving the English too obvious instances of their own nationality (excuse a new coined word).[9]

Thus far I have happily kept out of any party disputes, though we have some warm people on both sides amongst us. But the only time I am in public is at the Spaw in the morning. I return before most others get out of their beds; I pay a visit or two, when I have time before dinner; we dine at home, and often drink tea without company (unsociable animals), and when the rest go to the Assembly, a quiet evening's walk, a book or my pen prevent me from thinking time heavy upon my hands. And indeed, I begin to think it high time to retreat from unnecessary dissipation as much as possible, and without being tired of life or out of humour with the world, or disgusted with the pleasurable and the Gay, I think it but wisdom to think in what manner I may best husband what may yet be allotted me of time, thoughts that in my most busy hours seldom forsake me long together, with gratitude I speak it, yet it would do me no harm to be more familiar.

My accounts from Philadelphia are truly deplorable. Have we lost with the ablest pilot this nation perhaps has ever had, all powers of feeling or emotion? [10] Ought not the most general confederacy that was ever formed by savage nations give us a just alarm? Nations that can still drive us into the ocean from which we came, in spite of all our endeavors! [11]

Dreadful indeed must be our case if hostile measures are desired. Common justice and the expense of maintaining a single regiment would make them our friends forever. But he that rules above knows what is best; we are in private stations, and all that is encumbered upon us is to do the duties of them with diligence, integrity and submission to his will. This will make us fearless under every situation. I am glad to find the tumults in Ireland are suppressed. How happy it would be if the Princes of the Blood were to reside there as Viceroys successively! — Adieu, remember me to thy girl, and believe me to be thy assured Friend

J. Fothergill

We shall leave this place next week, but it will be near a month before we reach London.

Ms. autograph letter, Mss. Collection 583, no. 712, National Library of Scotland, Edinburgh.

1. James Bogle added his wife's family name to his own when he married Elizabeth French. In 1757 Dr. Fothergill discussed before the Medical Society the report on a series of experiments "in mixing oils . . . with water, by means of a Vegetable Mucilage," made at his request by Bogle French. The report, with Dr. Fothergill's discussion, was published in the first volume of *Medical Observations and Inquiries*. Some years later, with Dr. Fothergill's encouragement, Bogle French compiled *The London Practice of Physic, for the use of physicians and younger practitioners, etc.* (London: W. Johnston, 1769), "recommended as the first book of its kind." — Fox, 42n; *Works*, ed. Lettsom, II, 25, III, 188.

2. With the rise of the cult of sea-bathing in England about 1760, Scarborough, long frequented for its mineral waters, became even more popular as a fashionable resort. — Hughes, *North Country Life in the Eighteenth Century* (Oxford, 1952), 400, 402.

3. Dr. Waugh is not listed in *Munk's Roll*. Dr. John Lewis Petit, of Huguenot descent, was educated at Queen's College, Cambridge (A.B. 1756, A.M. 1759, M.D. 1763). He was admitted Fellow of the Royal College of Physicians in 1767. Like some other physicians of his time, he probably started practice before writing the dissertation required for a degree. — *Munk's Roll*, II, 280.

4. Dr. Robert Knox (M.D. St. Andrew's, 1750) enrolled in the army in 1765. In 1769 he was appointed physician to Middlesex Hospital; in 1786 he was admitted, "speciali gratia," Fellow of the Royal College of Physicians. — *Munk's Roll*, II, 365.

5. Dr. William Mushet, born in Dublin, probably educated in Trinity College (Ireland), first studied medicine in Leyden and later received an M.D. from King's College, Cambridge, in 1746. He was admitted Fellow of the Royal College of Physicians in 1749. He became an army doctor, rising in rank to the physician-in-chief to the British Army. A baronetcy, offered because of his valor, was declined. Later he became personal physician to the Duke of Rutland, and lived for eleven years in apartments at Belvoir Castle. — *Munk's Roll*, II, 170–171.

6. Dr. Wood is not listed in *Munk's Roll*.

7. "As Physicians are called *the Faculty*, and Counsellors at Law *the Profession*, the Booksellers of London are denominated *the Trade*. Johnson did not approve of these denominations." — James Boswell, *The Life of Samuel Johnson*, ed. Roger Ingpen, II (London, 1907), 787n.

8. Intended as a jocular reference. Almack's was a club where gaming tables were the chief attraction.

9. *Nationality*, to mean the fact of belonging to a particular nation, did not come into general usage until 1828. — *OED*.

10. A tribute to Lord Granville (d. 1 January 1763), whose concern for the welfare of the American colonies had influenced parliamentary policy during his long service as President of the Privy Council.

11. The savage nations mentioned by Dr. Fothergill are the Mohawks, the Oneidas, the Onondagas, the Cayugas, the Senecas, and the Tuscaroras, who formed the confederacy of the Six Nations.

To Samuel Fothergill, Warrington, Lancashire, 15 October 1764

Upton, 15.10.1764

Dear Brother,

Having escaped to this place after a hard day's labour, I sit down to converse with thee a few minutes on the subject of thine which I re-received this afternoon.

But in the first place, I must acknowledge the satisfaction I received from the kind intelligence thou gave us of thy journey.[1] Though I could not always make the returns my affection would have dictated, yet thy care and regard to us should not be nor will be forgot.

When I look toward the Society in Scotland, I easily foresee their extinction without manifest interposition of Divine Providence. But the cause is not solely ours; they are concerned in it, and must bear the chastisement if they wilfully suffer the testimony to drop in their streets.

It gave me some surprise to think that a circumstance that I had not so much as whispered had taken air so publickly but I open my whole thoughts to thee and then thou will be able to judge of the affair. One day it came unsought for into my thoughts to retreat a few months next summer into Cheshire, and it seemed easy to me to do so, and some part of the country not far from Middlewich seemed to be pointed at. I never was in that part, nor know the country, but I should like, if I do make a trial, to be somewhere thereabout.

The views I have in it are by a few months recess from this place to get some time to breathe, and to let the dependence that many have upon me here gradually die away, rather than break it off by violence. Should it in process of time seem more profitable for me to fix there altogether, I should do so. Should it on the other hand look more like my place to be in the neighbourhood of this city, by long and repeated absences I might be wholly forgot.

Thou will see by this sketch how improper it would be for me to think of building or purchasing. I am looking for a quiet place where I have no acquaintance yet not far from those I most love. In the neighbourhood of Warrington, a populous country not very far from Manchester, can I expect to escape a thousand solicitations? My aim is quiet, and if we can procure some decent abode not far from a Meeting, nor far from a market, in a situation not unhealthy, not very populous,

233

where we may have room enough to entertain a friend or two, and live not uncomfortably, be the terms what they may, we shall be satisfied. I want nothing great or elegant or expensive, but if nothing but what is such can be had, I would submit. Should thy affairs lead thee to Middlewich, and thou would call upon Tomlinson, attorney at law there, with my respects, acquaint him with my inclination to pass a few months in that neighbourhood in privacy the next summer, and request him if he hears of any place that may be suitable to accommodate a family like mine — my Sister, myself, four or five servants, with a bed or two for friends, I shall be glad to give any reasonable consideration. I imagine he will endeavour to help me effectually. In this part thou sees there is the forest on one side which is not populous, there is a Meeting; I am not obliged to be every day with one family or another, as I must near Warrington. I can see you occasionally, spend a night or two with my Uncle,[2] and now and then perhaps have him with us. From this thou will see how improper it would be for me to think of building anywhere, and least of all in a place where I should be so totally deprived of the repose I am seeking. Farewell.

J.F.

Ms. autograph letter, Port. 22/106, *LSFL*.

1. Samuel Fothergill had been attending Friends Meetings in Scotland.
2. Probably Uncle Thomas Hough, his mother's brother, at this time an elderly man, who lived in Marsh Gate near Frodsham, Cheshire.

V
1765-1769

By one means or another I have acquaintance
in most of the Colonies of North America,
as well as with the mercantile people in
London who trade thither. It is but too well
known that some acts and regulations have
spread universal discontent, and produced some
very unjustifiable proceedings on the other
side . . . I could not but now and then bestow a
thought upon what might be the most prudent
method of allaying these unhappy discontents . . .

To the Earl of Dartmouth, August 29, 1765

To James Pemberton, Philadelphia, 13 February 1765

Dear Friend James Pemberton,

Had my leisure been proportioned to my inclination, I should long since have answered thy several acceptable and affectionate letters; but I am still in a state of bondage peculiarly difficult to escape from; and to the constant unavoidable engagements I am subjected to, and have been for years past, my silence only must be attributed.

For not to fill up this paper with a detail of myself and occupations, I can only say that I hardly know what it is to be thoroughly unbended, day or night, so many things of various kinds lie upon me to be done.

I have enclosed the copies of some papers that relate to unclaimed shares of the Land Co. in which your Hospital is so happily interested. The money was vested in the funds as early as possible. What claims may arise we cannot foresee, but I hope the interest will be more than sufficient to pay them, in which case the Hospital in the year 1770 will without difficulty be put in possession of 6 to 7,000 £ sterling.[1]

Till that time, you will have no need of an agent as the money is perfectly secure, and should I be then living, or any member of the present trustees, all the care that can be will be taken of your part, and remitted as soon as possible.

I need not point out any manner in which so capital a sum should be employed. But I should think not in building. This money laid out properly would afford a noble addition to your income, and let the present age contribute to the building if it become necessary.

I send this by Dr. Morgan [2] who with Dr. Shippen will I hope do credit to the province. Dr. Shippen has already given proofs of his abilities, and Dr. Morgan has been equally diligent and successful in

237

prosecuting his studies, and comes over with as much reputation as any American that in my time has studied here. I have advised him to set out in practice upon a plan that I think will be more beneficial to the Province, than the present. He will inform thee more particularly of my sentiments. In short I think it would be of great service that a few persons should devote themselves to the instruction of young people in Physick, and if they do this to purpose they must be exempt from the low drudgery of Physick, and act as Physicians only. A few such the Province can support, and they will be more than proportionately useful in consultations.[3]

I hope to send over by the same vessel about a score of Anthony Purver's Translation of the Bible, to the care of Thomas Fisher to dispose of.[4] One copy I would have given to Friends library; another to the Loganian Library;[5] and those who choose it must purchase. I gave the author £1000, have printed it at my own expense; the sale will be slow, and I shall be a good deal out of pocket, so that I cannot be so liberal of an expensive work to my Friends as I could wish. It is spoke well of, by the ablest masters in the Hebrew language, and all allow his Chronology is the best that has been offered. His notes are crabbed (his style being extremely concise) but they contain much useful erudition.

With this I send a tract lately printed here, the work of our valuable Friend J. Griffiths.[6] I was solicitous, as your correspondent to have procured a considerable number for Friends in your province. But I find, he is likely to pay you a visit ere long, and he chose, and I thought the sentiment just, that not many should go over before him. If you think his service beneficial, as the wise in heart will find it is, after his departure you may print an edition for yourselves and the colonies.[7]

Two editions of R. Barclay's *Apology*[8] are now in the press, one in octavo by Clark and Richardson, the other in quarto by Baskerville; when they are printed, you may have some of both.

With respect to public affairs, I have little to say. I think Friends have acted wisely in not interfering with the petition.[9] We will endeavor, if the application for a change of government goes on, to bestir ourselves as well as we can to assist you. A resolution of the House of Commons has within the last few days, given America a dreadful stab and hurt the Mother Country no less; at least in my opinion.[10] But we know not what is best; in things not subject to our decision, it is safest to acquiesce, unless duty calls to more. Whether I shall have leisure to write to thy brother Israel by this opportunity is doubtful. Give my love to him, I received his kind letter sent by Young; but have never seen *him*. He keeps higher company.[11] It is now a time when Friends should endeavor as much as possible to put on the whole armour of light. Nothing less can protect them from the danger at hand. My wishes for thy preservation attend thee. Thy affectionate Friend

J. Fothergill

Ms. autograph letter, Pemberton Papers, Etting Collection, II, 39, HSP.

1. By Act of Parliament in 1760, certain tracts of land in Pennsylvania, New Jersey, and Maryland, held originally by a partnership established by William Penn as the Pennsylvania Land Company, had passed to the control of an English Board of Trustees headed by Dr. Fothergill, henceforth to be known as the Proprietors of the Pennsylvania Land Company in London.

On 26 May, 1766, "sundry papers relating to unclaimed shares of the Pennsylvania Land Company . . . transmitted . . . by our good Friend Dr. Fothergill of London," were produced and read at a meeting of the Board of the Pennsylvania Hospital and were directed to be entered in the Minutes." All shares remaining unclaimed after 24 June 1770 were to "go to the use of the Hospital in Pennsylvania." — Pennsylvania Hospital Minute Book, IV (14 May 1764–1768), 237–246, on microfilm at APS; Morton and Woodbury, *Pennsylvania Hospital*, 240–251.

2. Dr. John Morgan, after taking his medical degree at Edinburgh in 1763, made a prolonged tour on the Continent, seeking interviews with the most distinguished professors and scientists in important medical centers and gleaning their ideas upon the problems of educating would-be doctors. Back in London in the winter of 1764–65, he became a licentiate of the Royal College of Physicians and was elected to fellowship in the Royal Society of London. With foresight he sought acquaintance with Thomas Penn. Early in 1765 he returned to Philadelphia, where, powerfully supported by Thomas Penn's recommendation, he took the lead in starting the first medical school in the American Colonies. Morgan's *Discourse upon the Establishment of Medical Schools in America*, carefully prepared while he was traveling in Europe, was delivered in May 1765 at the commencement exercises of the College of Philadelphia and printed within a short time by William Bradford. (In 1937 the Institute of the History of Medicine at Johns Hopkins University issued a reprint in recognition of the importance of the document to the history of medical education.) The College of Philadelphia gave its first medical professorship to John Morgan. The second went to William Shippen, Jr. Formal instruction in Philadelphia's new medical school started in mid-November 1765 with anatomy classes conducted by Dr. Shippen, and a few days later John Morgan began his lectures on the "Theory and Practice of Physick." — Bell, *John Morgan*; Montgomery, *History of the University of Pennsylvania*, 304–308, 479–483; "An Account of the late John Morgan, M.D.," *American Magazine*, 6 (1789): 353–355.

3. A surprisingly early suggestion of specialization in internal medicine, which Dr. Morgan adopted in his *Discourse*.

4. Thomas Fisher (1741–1810), a successful Quaker merchant of the firm of Joseph

Fisher and Sons, operating packet ships to Europe, retired in middle life to manage his country estate near Logan's Stenton. He was elected to the Board of Managers of the Pennsylvania Hospital, and in 1794 was active in establishing a coeducational Friends boarding school. — Morton and Woodbury, *Pennsylvania Hospital*, 418.

5. The Friends Library was probably kept in the Meeting House at Fourth and Chestnut Streets. — Information from Miss Dorothy Harris of Friends Historical Library, Swarthmore College, Pennsylvania. The Loganian Library was that founded by James Logan, scholar and devoted public servant, who designed and built a small library in Sixth Street to house more than 3,000 scholarly books, a collection unsurpassed in the colonies. By terms of his will he left it with an endowment "to the end that all persons residing in the province educated in reading and writing . . . more especially those who have knowledge of the Latin tongue, or who study the mathematical sciences or medicine . . . may have free admittance . . . with the liberty of borrowing any of the . . . books." — Edwin Wolf, 2nd, "The Romance of James Logan's Books," *William and Mary Quarterly*, 13 (1956): 342–353; Richard M. Gummere, *The American Colonial Mind and the Classical Tradition* (Cambridge, Mass.: Harvard University Press, 1963), 69, 122–125.

6. John Griffiths (b. 1713, Radnorshire, Wales), after living in Pennsylvania in his younger days, returned to Great Britain. His tract is entitled *Some Brief Remarks necessary to be understood . . . by all professing the true Christian Religion, and Principally addressed to the People called Quakers* (London, 1754; 2nd ed. 1765). — Rufus Jones, *The Later Periods of Quakerism*, 2 vols. (New York: Macmillan, 1911), II, 20–22.

7. Griffiths' tract was reprinted in Philadelphia, probably several times. As late as 1781 — after the author's death in 1776 — an edition was issued, "reprinted by Joseph Crukshank."

8. Robert Barclay's work, *An Apology for the True Christian Divinity as the Same is Preached and Held Forth by the People in Scorn called Quakers*, was originally written in Latin and published in 1676 at Amsterdam. An English translation was published there later that year. The quarto edition mentioned here was planned by Dr. Fothergill in cooperation with the famous printer and typefounder John Baskerville (1705–1775). Baskerville insisted on using only the finest paper and best ink for his productions. He admonished Dr. Fothergill, whose hasty letters had a brownish tinge, to supply himself with better paper and a jet-black ink that Baskerville himself used. — Josiah H. Benton, *John Baskerville . . . 1706–1775* (Boston: Privately printed, 1914); William Bennett, *John Baskerville: The Birmingham Printer and His Press, Relations, and Friends*, 2 vols. (Birmingham, England: School of Printing, 1939).

9. In May 1764 the Pennsylvania Assembly had adopted a petition addressed to the King asking him to give Pennsylvania royal instead of proprietary government, and in October it reasserted its will and sent Franklin back to London to pursue the matter. — *Pennsylvania Archives*, 8 ser. VII; 5607–5610, 5688–5690, cited by Knollenberg, pp. 369–370.

10. The House of Commons, by a vote of 245 to 49 had resolved to proceed with the stamp tax proposed in Lord Grenville's budget message of 6 February. The Stamp Act, which was introduced in the Commons on the day Dr. Fothergill wrote this letter, was passed by the Commons on 27 February, and by the Lords on 8 March. — Knollenberg, 224–226.

11. William Young, whose father had a farm and market-garden in Kingsessing, Pennsylvania, not far from John Bartram's plantation, was a self-trained botanical

collector, highly recommended by Dr. Alexander Garden of Charleston, South Carolina, to John Ellis of London. — James Edward Smith, *A Selection of the Correspondence of Linnaeus and Other Naturalists*, 2 vols. (London: Longman, Hurst, 1821), I, 512. Young was invited to England in 1764 to work in the Royal Gardens at Kew. John Bartram protested "Young's sudden preferment" to Peter Collinson, who consequently sought and secured Bartram's appointment in 1765 as King's botanist, "with a salary of fifty pounds a year." — Darlington, *Memorials*, 266–270.

To Samuel Fothergill, Warrington, Lancashire, 28 June 1765

London, 28.6.1765

Dear Brother,

I doubt not but that thou will sometimes be thinking about us, and of our movement to your parts. As soon as we had fixed the time I thought it would be agreeable for thee to be informed of it, and have just devoted the corner of an evening to that purpose.

I think we shall leave this place sometime on the 16th, stay part of the first day following at Coventry, and try to reach our quarters before third day night. Elizabeth Graeme [1] will, I believe, come down with us to Lea Hall, where R. Peters [2] will meet her in a day or two, to go for Scotland.

This week we have put on board the Earl of Chester five cases directed to the care of Hillary and Scott in Liverpool [3] for J.F. When this vessel arrives, thou will please to order all under this direction to be sent as thou advises. We have likewise sent off this week by the carrier, several packages which we hope will be properly taken care of.

As soon as we can be pretty certain of our departure we shall give J. Mollineaux [4] proper notice, and propose to send two maid-servants to be there a few days before us. I am thankful, repeatedly thankful, for the prospect of this recess. It was not of my own contrivance nor willing, but I esteem it as I ought a favourable prospect of escaping by degrees from labours next to oppression.

Much I owe to the public and honestly have I endeavoured to repay the obligation. May they never want persons better qualified than myself to serve them! To me the world has not frowned. I courted not its favours, nor feared the reverse. It is time, however, to think of getting

241

into port, and as the wind serves, I hope to make use of it for this best of purposes, security.

If it will suit thy conveniency to order us a little wine and necessaries of that kind, we shall be pleased. The quantities and kinds will be mentioned below.

As we shall have a stranger with us, and perhaps another to escort her from us, we must not desire thee to meet us at our coming, but as soon as we are fixed and can give thee a morsel in quiet, we shall be truly glad of thy company.

Sometime ago Sister sent down to Henry [5] a box containing among other things the books thou desired me to ask for and the Epistles. There were, likewise, to fill up the box, some clothes belonging to our servants, which Henry will be kind enough to send us with the goods he may have occasion to send to Lea Hall.

He will likewise send us two stoves; one for the large parlour, one for one of the lodging rooms; more we shall order as we may want them. Accept our united tenders of affection to Sister and thyself from thy affectionate

J. Fothergill

Please to procure for us, and send to Lea Hall as convenience may offer

2 gallons of the best French Brandy
3 gallons of good Mountain, and a
gallon or two of any very good white
wine, either Lisbon, Port, or Sherry
that thou thinks is genuine
6 gallons of good Red Port, rather new
than old, as little bordering on the acid
as may be. A rough, good-bodied wine I
like best.

These will be sufficient at present. If more are wanted, we shall order them in time.

Ms. autograph letter Port. 22/107, LSFL.

1. Elizabeth Graeme (1737–1801), a charming blue-stocking daughter of the wealthy Dr. Thomas Graeme of Philadelphia, was described by her friend Dr. Benjamin Rush as "a woman of uncommon virtues and talents, admired and loved by a wide circle of friends and acquaintances." — *The Autobiography of Benjamin Rush*, ed. George W. Corner (Princeton: Princeton University Press, 1948), 320.

2. After many years of governmental service to the province of Pennsylvania, Richard Peters (1704–1776), a talented Englishman who had originally been educated for the ministry, resigned all public office in 1762 in order to accept the pastorate of the united parishes of Christ Church and St. Peter's in Philadelphia. In 1765 he went to England to receive ordination by the Bishop of London, from London to Liverpool where his brother Bartlett lived, and later from there to Lea Hall to consult Dr. Fothergill. Elizabeth Graeme was already the guest of the Fothergills, having come there likewise for consultation with the eminent London clinician before going to Scotland to visit relatives, the Graemes of Edinburgh. — Hubertis Cummings, *Richard Peters* (Philadelphia: University of Pennsylvania Press, 1944).

3. A prosperous Quaker firm in Liverpool, trading principally to the West Indies. The senior partner, Richard Hillary (1703–1789), was the youngest son of Wensleydale parents, Mary Robinson (1661–1733) and John Hillary (1666–1721). The junior partner, John Scott (1725–1791), was Richard Hillary's nephew, the son of his eldest sister Ann (b. 1693) who had married Joseph Scott of Burtersett in 1724. — Yorkshire Births and Burials, LSFL; personal communication from Mrs. Mary Hopkirk of Danbury, West Chelmsford, England.

4. Perhaps an estate agent who would open the house.

5. Probably their nephew Henry Fothergill (1736–1769). — Fothergill Genealogy, below.

To Israel Pemberton, Jr., Philadelphia, 5 July 1765

London, 5.7.1765

Dear Friend,

Inclosed is a copy of the written Epistle from our late Yearly Meeting with some of the acts relating to the Stamp duties lately imposed on North America. If more are wanted, they may be had by applying to us at any time. As a provision is therein made for Friends, it was thought expedient that you should have this act to produce in case of any difficulties arising in this respect.[1]

I received the narrative, and in part approve the charitable design. I say in part, because I think it is necessary first to bring them to be *civil* before they are made *religious*; and I often think it is next to having no religion at all, or worse, to have a bad one. A person of liberal sentiments and education, patient of labour and able to bear much, has found himself engaged as by a sense of duty to attempt the civilizing of some Indians if he can.[2] He is gone to South Carolina and proposes to make a beginning among the Creeks or Cherokees, as he shall find it most proper. He proposes to live among them, teach their children to read, the men argriculture, if they are willing to learn, and cure a few if possible of their wandering life to make them civil, social creatures. He is supported by a few persons here, chiefly Friends, who think him as equal to the task as most, as he engages from principle in the work, and I think much more reasonably than thy Friend. Nevertheless I mean not to discourage his endeavours; I mention these circumstances to show that I am engaged in a like charitable design, and I hope upon a plan not less likely to contribute to their benefit. We may make men Pharisees and formalists; truly religious we cannot make them. God alone can do this; and by his help alone can we benefit our neighbours.

I am much obliged to thy excellent wife for a very kind and acceptable letter. I am just setting out for Cheshire for a couple of months, to recover the power of recollection if possible. Perhaps in a quiet hour I may have an opportunity of acknowledging it to herself. If this occurs, she must be sure I shall not forget her kindness.

Our friend and your Friend, John Griffiths,[3] comes in the ship that brings this. We think he grows in grace and in the knowledge of his Lord and Master. May he reap peace and do you good in the service before him!

We can only pity your distressful situation; torn by divisions within, oppressed by factions without, Government contemned, violence, insecurity, what can be a greater misfortune? But we know not what is best. Let us learn by the things we suffer — patience and experience.

I am, thy affectionate Friend

J. Fothergill

Ms. autograph letter, Pemberton Papers, Etting Collection, II, 50, HSP.

1. Great Britain, having incurred tremendous expense during the Seven Years War, partly in preventing France from acquisition of the American Colonies, felt justified in requiring her colonists to share in the cost of their protection. Taxation seemed the method best suited for gradual fulfillment of this responsibility. The Stamp Act, proposed without previous consultation with those to be affected, passed the House of Commons in February 1765 and the House of Lords in March, to become effective 1 November. After that date, stamps were to be required on newspapers, pamphlets, almanacs, calendars, broadsides, all legal papers, ships' papers, documents, licenses, playing cards, dice, and the tea which Britain, importing and then exporting, sent in quantity to America. Funds collected were to be paid into the Royal Exchequer "towards defraying the expenses of defending, protecting and securing the American Colonies." The "provision . . . made for Friends" refers to the substitution of an affirmation for an oath when legal papers were required. — See Edmund S. Morgan and Helen M. Morgan, *The Stamp Act Crisis* (Chapel Hill: University of North Carolina Press, 1959).

2. The person mentioned has not been identified. His approach to this work resembles that of a modern social worker.

3. John Griffiths is perhaps the Quaker minister mentioned earlier (in letter of 13 February 1765) by Dr. Fothergill, or a younger member of the same family. — James Bowden, *The History of Friends in America*, 2 vols. (London: C. Gilpin, 1850), II, 291.

To the Marquis of Rockingham, 31 July 1765

Lea Hall, Middlewich, Cheshire

31st Inst.

I hope my Noble and Honoured friend[1] will excuse the liberty I take in following him, in his retirement,[2] to express the satisfaction I feel at his being called again into the service of his King and Country.

And indeed the satisfaction is general amongst those with whom I converse; they are pleased with the event, and look up to the throne with gratitude for the choice that has been made of its firm and ancient friends.

Envy and disappointment will without doubt attempt to raise much clamour and discontent. But the Marquis of Rockingham may rest secure of the countenance and support of the truest Friends of their King and Country; and they only wish that no clamour or opposition may discourage a Nobleman in whom they greatly confide, from using his utmost endeavours to restore satisfaction to their Sovereign, Harmony among his subjects, Honour and Security to the whole.

Perhaps in some pensive hour my Noble friend will not be displeased with this assurance from one individual who joins sincerely with many others in wishing him health and success. Having been wearied I have retired for a month or two into an obscure corner of this country, and should have taken the liberty to have waited upon the Marquis of Rockingham before I left London, had my time been my own.

Perhaps I ought to make some apology for this intrusion, but the pleasure I feel at this event, prompts me to express the dictates of my heart, and that I am with gratitude and respect,

The Marquis of Rockingham's

Obliged Friend

John Fothergill

Ms. autograph letter, Wentworth Woodhouse Muniments, R1/487, Central Library,

Sheffield, England, by courtesy of Earl Fitzwilliam and the Trustees of the Wentworth Woodhouse Estates.

1. Charles Watson-Wentworth (1730–1782), second Marquis of Rockingham, had just been appointed Prime Minister. Because he advocated repeal of the Stamp Act, his year as Prime Minister placed him in the ranks of the liberals, closely allied to the merchants who were seeking expansion of trade beneficial alike to Great Britain and the American colonists. — George H. Guttridge, *The Early Career of Lord Rockingham, 1739–1765* (Berkeley: University of California Press, 1952); Lucy S. Sutherland, "Edmund Burke and the First Rockingham Ministry," *English Historical Review*, 47 (1932): 46–72.

2. "Retirement" means simply that Lord Rockingham had left London temporarily to visit his Yorkshire estates.

To the Earl of Dartmouth, 7 August 1765

Lea Hall, near Middlewich, Cheshire

I persuade myself that my Noble and Honoured Friend [1] will excuse the liberty I take of addressing him upon his being called into the service of King and Country.

I congratulate the Public on this event; at the same time I most cordially sympathize in the anxiety which must attend a station from which so much is expected, and wherein so many and unusual difficulties will be found.

One circumstance, however, affords me entire satisfaction, that the same Providence which has led my Noble Friend to this seat of eminence and anxiety, is able to support with strength and wisdom equal to every exigency.

It will perhaps afford some little satisfaction in a pensive hour to know that all those with whom I have conversed, rejoice that the King has been pleased to choose a Nobleman so nearly related to one of the ablest and most upright servants the Crown ever had, and himself distinguished for his virtue and integrity.

People in general seem only to fear lest the clamour which the interested may raise, should drive Lord Dartmouth into his beloved privacy, and deprive the public of his assistance just when he is acquiring the means of serving them efficaciously.

If my opinion may be of any moment, permit me to interest my Honoured Friend wholly to disregard anything of this kind; as ambition has had no share in this call to public service, regard nothing but to fill the post with diligence and integrity; and in this Lord Dartmouth will be supported by the best of all comforts, the satisfaction resulting from an honest discharge of duty; but he will likewise have the collateral aid of the countenance and good wishes of every friend to the present Royal Family, and the public in general.

The fatigue which I have undergone for some time having rendered a few months retreat into the country necessary, I have chosen an obscure part of this county for the purpose, where I am as well accommodated as I can wish, and have leisure to recollect myself and lay in some degree of health for future labour, if Providence sees fit.

There is a person in the city with whom I have been long and intimately acquainted* 2 and whom I can cordially recommend for his probity and general knowledge. His judgment is exceeded by few in commercial affairs, especially those relating to our plantations, in many of which his influence is extensive, as well as among the merchants at home. He was greatly esteemed by the late Lord Granville, and consulted on many occasions. He is a firm Friend to the present family and would serve them from principle and affection. He is under our profession, though perhaps not so strictly educated as some others. As I cannot but esteem his abilities from long acquaintance, and know that he is discreet and sensible, I thought it would not be improper to give Lord Dartmouth this account of him as a person in whom he may thoroughly confide.

I have only to request my Noble Friend will excuse me for thus venturing beyond the limits of my profession. My best wishes, whether in public or in private station, will ever attend him, being with great esteem

his obliged, respectful Friend
John Fothergill

* Capel Hanbury

Ms. autograph letter, Dartmouth Papers, Patshull House Collection, William Salt Library, Stafford, England. This letter carries a contemporary endorsement: "Dr. Fothergill, 7 August 1765." It was originally catalogued: "Autograph letter: 1765 August 7/8," thus giving both the date of its writing and that of its receipt.

1. William Legge (1731–1801), second Earl of Dartmouth and stepbrother of Frederick North (Lord North), son of the Earl of Guilford, had become a dissenter. In 1765, upon the foundation of Lord Rockingham's ministry, Lord Dartmouth, then thirty-four, was persuaded by the Duke of Newcastle to accept the office of President of the Board of Trade and Foreign Plantations. He was also sworn in as one of the Lords of Privy Council. — *The Manuscripts of the Earl of Dartmouth*, vol. II:

American Papers, with an Introduction by B. F. Stevens, being the Fourteenth Report, Appendix 10, of the Historical Manuscripts Commission (London, 1895), intro., iv. v. 17.

2. Dr. Fothergill draws attention to the name of Capel Hanbury, inserted at the end of the letter. Capel Hanbury of Mark Lane, London, a Quaker merchant, had succeeded his cousin John Hanbury of Tower Street (d. 1759) as head of the Virginia Company which imported Virginia tobacco in exchange for British goods.

To the Earl of Dartmouth, 29 August 1765

Lea Hall, August 29, 1765

Lord Dartmouth's most friendly and obliging letter at once relieved me from some anxious fears, lest I had committed an indiscretion in taking the liberty I did, and added if possible to the attachment I felt to my Noble Friend, for his condescension and regard.

I should not so soon have intruded again, had not a circumstance occurred to my thoughts which though out of my sphere, seemed not unworthy of some attention. I shall stand in need of all my Honoured Friend's partiality, I fear, to excuse me from venturing upon subjects so much above my reach.

By one means or another I have acquaintance in most of the Colonies of North America, as well as with the mercantile people in London who trade thither. It is but too well known that some late acts and regulations have spread universal discontent, and produced some very unjustifiable proceedings on the other side. Though it did not immediately concern me, yet I could not but now and then bestow a thought upon what might be the most prudent method of allaying these unhappy discontents, whose effects will be extremely injurious to both countries.

To annul the Acts would perhaps encourage the Americans to oppose in like manner every future regulation, however necessary to the well-being of the whole, if it thwarted the interests of the leading men. To reduce them to reason and subjection to the Acts and regulations by severe and harsh methods would perhaps be alike disagreeable to the Administration at home, and pernicious in their consequence to the Colonies.

What occurred to me to mention was this: that if proper Commissioners could be chosen to go over to America to confer with Comissioners to be chosen by their respective governments upon the subjects of their complaints — if these Commissioners had it in their instructions to assure the Americans that the Government at home intended them effectual relief but that they must first be fully informed of the reality of their grievances — these Commissioners would be able by conversing with different people, seeing the state of the several governments on the spot, to give the Ministry such information as would assist them in settling the affairs of the Colonies in such a manner as might be highly conducive to the interest of the whole.[1]

That the Colonies aspire to Independency has been asserted, but if we treat them with mildness, yet firmly securing the connection by making it their interest cheerfully to obey, this prospect must be at a very great distance. The late attempts to teach them obedience have made them wish for such a situation; and what people wish for they oft accomplish, though under the greatest disadvantages.

It seemed to me that by appointing a proper Commission for these purposes, the Administration might have it in their power to keep between the two extremes of doing everything the Americans wish for and doing nothing. It would please them to see the design of relieving them; they would bear the difficulties till they better felt their real weight, and the Ministry would gain time and proper information to proceed upon with prudence.

I know not what apology to make for these suggestions; if they are weak, they are well intended, and solely in the power of my Noble Friend to deal with them as he thinks fit.

I am glad that Lord Lewisham [2] recovered so happily. Be pleased to present my respects to Lady Dartmouth, and be assured that I am, with great deference and respect,

Thy obliged Friend
John Fothergill

Ms. autograph letter, Dartmouth Papers, Patshull House Collection, now in the care of the William Salt Library, Stafford, England. This letter carries contemporary endorsements: on its wrapper, "August 29 1765"; on its first page, "Lea Hall, 31st Inst." The letter itself is catalogued by B. F. Stevens, editor of the catalogue of Dartmouth Mss., as of 1765, 29 August Lea Hall; the "31st Inst." has been added to indicate the date on which it was received by Lord Dartmouth.

1. This idea of holding an Anglo-American peace conference is surprisingly early.
2. Lord Dartmouth's oldest son.

To Dr. John Morgan, Philadelphia, 7 December 1765

London, 7.XII.1765

Dear Doctor,

This week I received your obliging letter by Capt. Friend, and though I have not yet received thy kind present, I think it not improper to hint my sentiments as concisely as I can respecting the contents of thy last.

It may be necessary to yield to the times and at present to the customs of the place. Get some prudent person to dispense the medicines at home; if fees are offered, refuse occasionally, but not always; if they are not offered, yet visit and prescribe as occasion occurs.

I have no doubt but that when more favourable times return, with such assistants, such countenance and such abilities, a school will be established that will afford many advantages. Pupils soon form very high ideas of their Masters if they are sensible and discreet. These will promote consultations, and call their Masters, or consult them when they can. From these sources advantages will accrue superior to anything speedily to be expected in this place. A single man may risk much, and hope for much. With a family or the prospect of one, a small certainty is better than a great uncertain prospect. For thy own sake, thy family's and thy country's, think only of fixing where thou art, and fear not but in time everything will suceed to thy wishes.[1]

I was pleased to know of thy change of condition. It is at once safe and honorable. I have no reason to doubt of the wisdom of thy choice, and therefore congratulate you both sincerely upon the happy union.[2] It is necessary in every respect that we should meet with difficulties. It is our own fault if they depress our spirits. Difficulties keep our sensibilities alive, and make us alert to our duty. This creates just reputation, and reputation thus obtained is wealth and honour.

As I knew the S. of the Royal Society was oft necessitous, I knew not what degree of credit to give to his request. This made me the more slow in advancing money; otherwise I should have paid his demand, and without the least hesitation.[3]

We have nothing lately published in medicine of much value. Potts' dissertation on the *Fistula in ano* is decisive on the subject and instructive.[4] — Pray, Dr., get us some intelligence of your mineral waters. You must have many towards the mountains, and inquire them out. In Rutty's *Synopsis*, which I know is in some of your libraries, there are

250

ample directions for discovering their properties and affinity to our English waters. Much medicinal help is to be derived from them.[5] The cicuta is not yet discarded. It does not cure cancers but it retards the progress of the most inveterate. It is of use in acrimonious juices. It is mildly anodyne, mitigates pain and increases all the secretions.[6] I hope to send some seeds ere long of the true Vienna kind which seems not to differ from ours. Adieu.

J. Fothergill

Ms. autograph letter, Charles Roberts Autograph Collection, Haverford College, Pennsylvania.

1. Dr. John Morgan, in his *Discourse upon the Institution of Medical Schools in America*, had stressed far ahead of his time the importance of specialization in medical practice. His idea that doctors in the Colonies, as in England, should be released from the task of compounding their own medicines for patients could not easily be realized in the American Colonies: the Pennsylvania Hospital had been obliged to send to London for a properly trained apothecary. Dr. Morgan had become discouraged by professional criticism in Philadelphia and had actually thought of establishing practice elsewhere, perhaps in the West Indies.

2. Dr. Morgan had recently married Mary Hopkinson, the sister of his friend and college classmate, Francis Hopkinson. — Nathaniel Burt, *The Perennial Philadelphians* (Boston: Little, Brown, 1963), 122, 323, 369.

3. The reference is to Dr. Emanuel da Costa, a gifted scientist of Portuguese descent, who held a clerkship at the Royal Society. He was often hard pressed for money, usually in debt, and considered unscrupulous. Dr. Morgan had not yet received notice of his election to the Royal Society of London when he left England; and the arrangements he had made for the payment of his fee were unknown to Da Costa, who apparently sought payment on behalf of Morgan first from Dr. Fothergill and then from Benjamin Franklin. Franklin made the payment for Dr. Morgan in order to acknowledge the honor promptly. — *Franklin Papers*, ed. Labaree, XII, 203, 307.

4. Percival Pott (1713–1788) was a distinguished surgeon of St. Bartholomew's Hospital, London. His book was recently off the press.

5. John Rutty's *Methodical Synopsis of Mineral Waters* (Dublin, 1762) contained a survey of mineral springs in the British Isles. Dr. Fothergill had collected quantities of pamphlets on this subject and gave them to his friend for use in this volume.

6. The reference is probably to *Cicuta*, or water hemlock, a plant containing alkaloids of a strongly sedative nature.

To Lord Dartmouth, St. James's Square, London, 1765

6th Inst., 1765

Dr. Fothergill takes the liberty to present to Lord Dartmouth the papers intended to have been sent to the *Gazeteer* and one of the Magazines. They were wrote with this view, and hopes they would do no injury if they were permitted to be laid before the public, either to the present Administration, the colonies or the Mother Country.

But this he submits entirely to the opinion of his Noble Friend. Dr. Fothergill is now and then putting down some hints relative to public affairs as they occur to him, and shall, as soon as he can, take the liberty of producing them.[1] Dr. Fothergill earnestly entreats Lord Dartmouth to think no more of resigning. He will be pleased to consider that in this respect he is not his own Master. The King, the Public are satisfied of his integrity and good will to his country. That Providence which has so ordered that Lord Dartmouth is called into the service of both will afford abilities adequate to the situation.

An incompletely dated ms. memorandum, Wentworth Woodhouse Muniments, R65/5, Sheffield Central Library, England. It was probably sent by Lord Dartmouth to the Marquis of Rockingham while Prime Minister. By courtesy of Earl Fitzwilliam and the Trustees of the Wentworth-Woodhouse Estates.

1. Dr. Fothergill's hopes were realized. His papers, favoring the American Colonies as an asset of greatest value to Great Britain, were published in a small volume entitled *Considerations Relative to the North American Colonies* (London, 1765).

To James Pemberton, Philadelphia, 25 February 1766

London, 25.2.1766

Dear Friend,

I received thy kind letter (the copy dated 18.12.mo.) and the paper inclosed. H. Brown [1] and myself will by the first opportunity give the satisfaction required.

But at present I must turn to another subject which I hope will afford no little satisfaction. By the clemency of the King, the steadiness, ability and application of the present Ministry, the moderation and humanity of the House of Commons, I hope the Stamp Act is in a fair way to be repealed, your other difficulties removed and your commerce restored to a better footing than ever.

By what means this has been effected, would take up more of my time to mention than I can at present spare. I shall only add that the present Administration have had to contend with greater difficulty than ever any other had upon any occasion. It may justly be thought that the North America merchants here would bestir themselves zealously for their own interests' sake, but they have done more; they have so effectually served the whole British Empire that their diligence, their indefatigable, united, efficacious endeavours to serve the whole community at this juncture ought never to be forgot.[2]

Barlow Trecothick, Esq., Alderman of London, Chairman to the Committee of Merchants, stood a three hours examination at the Bar of the House of Commons; Capel Hanbury near two; D. Mildred a shorter space, but all came off with reputation.[3]

B. Franklin has served you ably and uprightly. He also was examined, and gave the House sufficient proofs of his ability, your distressed condition, and the absolute necessity of relieving the Americans by repealing the Act.[4] The progress of conviction in this affair has not been owing to ministerial interposition. They had many of the King's servants, and I may say a part of the Royal Family against them. But it has been chiefly owing under Providence to the good sense of the ministry, supported in the most consistent manner by a train of evidence, that convinced everybody but those who first framed the shackles, their numerous dependants and the natural enemies to liberty either civil or religious.

In every question concerning the important business a majority of more than 100 in three has appeared so that though the enemies of America, and therein of the public peace, are determined to create all the delay and difficulty they can in passing the bill, yet it is very probable that in the space of a week or ten days the bill for repealing the Stamp Act will be passed in the House of Commons.[5] I make no doubt but this intelligence from all your correspondents will diffuse universal satisfaction through the continent, but I must entreat thee and every person within reach of thy influence to determine with the utmost steadiness to repress every mark of intemperate joy on this occasion.

Nothing has created so great difficulties to your Friends or furnished your opponents with so many arguments against you, as the tumultous behaviour of too many on your side of all ranks. The Parliament saw its authority not only rejected but despised, opposed and insulted. What difficulties has not this madness occasioned to all who endeavoured to serve you! If the people of America give the loose to intemperate joy, the Parliament will doubtless consider it a triumph on your part, and if an ensuing session acts according to such an opinion, and which they most certainly will if your opponents come into power, what then becomes of public safety, mutual security, and the common good?

From the prompt, impetuous temper of the Americans much I am afraid is to be feared, unless those amongst them who are guided by reason and reflection immediately interpose. Demonstrations of joy carried beyond a certain point will be most certainly fatal to both countries; and no person can better serve them than by repressing them.

I could wish, therefore, if the Assembly is sitting when this news arrives, they would immediately take the affair into consideration, and by some public act which the wisdom of the Assembly will better point out than I can suggest, at once decently acknowledge the maternal tenderness appearing in the mother country and prohibit strictly all discrimination of Friends or Enemies on this side the water.

Some weeks ago I wrote to my friend William Logan, though the packet having been detained both your letters will come together. Be pleased, therefore, to communicate the purport of this to him, as I fear I shall scarce have time to write to him by this opportunity, intending to send a few lines to W. Allen [6] to request his influence through the continent to discountenance measures that will unavoidably tend to your undoing. — I hope likewise to get time to write to R. Peters [7] on the same subject, for I am certain that nothing will tend so effectually to establish your friends here, enable and encourage them to serve you so efficaciously, as your prudent, grateful conduct on this occasion. Not publickly to individuals, either as friends or enemies, but privately as may consist with the laws of order and Society.

If P. [8] has pleaded your cause most strenuously don't therefore crown him King of America. If G. G. [9] has opposed you to the utmost stretch of his abilities, don't consign him to be hanged in effigy at every town's end. The greatest may be misled and misinformed. Discourage all this with spirit and intrepidity because it is against the laws of God and man.

Make any use of my letters that discretion points out; I write in great haste and after extreme fatigue; but I thought it would not be doing justice to our friendship if I omitted to give thee some account of your situation.

The Marquis of Rockingham, Secretary Conway, [10] and all the active part of the Administration deserve your grateful acknowledgments, but do this with discretion and not at the expense of your opponents.

I am far from thinking thy acceptance of a seat in the House [11] improper. I wish that every member in it was actuated by the like sentiments, and furnished with equal ability. Nevertheless, we ought always

254

to distrust ourselves and scrutinize severely the motive of our conduct. I feel no uneasiness with thine and wish thee able at all times to act as best wisdom guides, and then thou will help many, as will

Thy affectionate Friend,

J. Fothergill

Ms. autograph letter, Pemberton Papers, Etting Collection, II, 51, HSP. Written before repeal of the Stamp Act.

1. Henton Brown (1698–1775), a member of Gracechurch Sreet Meeting, author of several tracts in defense of the Quaker faith, was a banker who resided in Clapham Common. — Raistrick, 324; J. H. Tritton, *Tritton: The Place and the People* (London: Humphrey, 1907), 152–154. His given name sometimes appears as "Hinton," but his firm is listed as Henton Brown and Son, "opposite the Castle Tavern, Lombard Street," in Thomas Mortimer, *The Universal Director* (London, 1763), pt. III, p. 79. For "the paper enclosed" see the next three letters.

2. A committee of London merchants dealing with North America had brought together a notable group of witnesses to protest against the Stamp Act. For several days early in February 1766 the House of Commons sat as a Committee of the Whole to question these men. Dr. Fothergill goes on to give further details.

3. Barlow Trecothick, born in Boston, Massachusetts, became a successful London merchant and maintained important commercial relations with the American Colonies. — T. D. Jervey, "Barlow Trecothick," *South Carolina Historical and Genealogical Magazine*, 32: 157–169 (July 1931). Capel Hanbury feared that financial failure threatened the Virginia Company, which he headed. He testified that planters in Virginia and Maryland would be unable to meet the demands of the Stamp Act with what "hard money" they kept on hand. Tobacco, in lieu of specie, was customarily exchanged for British goods. Enforcement of the Stamp Act would require military action, and Virginians would then "repell force with force." To ensure continued mercantile prosperity, he considered total repeal essential. — Freeman, *Washington*, II, 156–160, quoting Capel Hanbury's testimony from the Newcastle Papers in the British Museum. Daniel Mildred (1731–1788) was a Quaker merchant familiar with the needs of the American Colonies. — London and Middlesex Births and Burials, LSFL.

4. Franklin was subjected to a grilling examination which it was hoped might confuse him, but he held his ground and came through the ordeal amazingly, to the discomfiture of his questioners. — Van Doren, *Benjamin Franklin*, 336–352.

5. The bill for repeal of the Stamp Act was introduced before the end of February.

6. William Allen (1704–1780), Chief Justice of Pennsylvania, 1750–1774, a man of wealth, culture, and outstanding ability, who had received his legal education in England. — *Franklin Papers*, ed. Labaree, VI, 284.

7. Richard Peters, who earlier as provincial Secretary had upheld the interests of the Proprietors against the Quaker-dominated Assembly, had retired from political life in 1762 to begin another career as rector of the united parishes of Christ Church and St. Peter's. — Hubertis Cummings, *Richard Peters* (Philadelphia: Lippincott, 1941).

8. William Pitt (1708–1778), the Great Commoner, whose oratory in opposition to the Stamp Act helped to change the course of history. — Van Doren, *Benjamin Franklin*, 335.

9. George Grenville (1712–1770), while First Lord of the Treasury and Chancellor of the Exchequer in 1764, had presented a resolution to Parliament in which he expressed the opinion that "it may be proper to charge certain Stamp Duties in the Colonies and Plantations," in order to recoup some of the expenses of the Seven Years War. Nevertheless, he had personal misgivings about the Stamp Act, and four days before the bill was introduced, he met protesting colonial agents to tell them that he regretted causing uneasiness among the American colonists: if a better plan to pay for a British military force to give them protection could be proposed, he would gladly adopt it. — E. S. Morgan, *Prologue to Revolution, Sources and Documents of the Stamp Act Crisis* (Chapel Hill: University of North Carolina Press, 1959); David Lindsay Keir, *The Constitutional History of England, 1485–1951* (London: A. & C. Black, 1953), 258, 259; L. H. Gipson: *The Triumphant Empire: Thunder Clouds Gather in the West, 1763–1766* (New York: Knopf, 1961), 384, 385.

10. Henry Seymour Conway, a man whose distinction is revealed in correspondence with his cousin Horace Walpole, was Secretary of State for the Southern Department during Lord Rockingham's ministry, also leader of the House of Commons. — Knollenberg, 95, 389.

11. James Pemberton, after having resigned from the Assembly in 1756, had accepted re-election in 1765.

To James Pemberton, Philadelphia, 27 February 1766

London, 27.2.1766

Dear Friend James Pemberton,

Having just perused the translation of C. Kreble's letter relating to Benjamin Franklin [1] and communicated it to H. Brown, that no opportunity may be lost in setting him in a just light with these people, be pleased to acquaint them for the present that from my own knowledge I can safely aver that Benjamin Franklin did all in his power to prevent the Stamp Act from passing; that he waited upon the Ministry that then was to have informed them fully of its mischievous tendency, and that he was uniformly opposed to it, to the utmost of his ability; that in a long examination before the House of Commons within these few weeks, he asserted the rights and privileges of America with the utmost firmness, resolution, and capacity.

I can further aver, likewise upon my own knowledge that he had diligently, steadily, and judiciously pursued the business recommended to him when he came over as Agent; and if he does not succeed in it, it will be more owing to the present unfavourable circumstances of the times than to the want of either application or address. He has been an able, useful advocate for America in general, the Province of Pennsylvania in particular during his stay here; and of this they will receive from many persons undoubted information, as well as from

Thy assured Friend
J. Fothergill.

Ms. autograph letter, Pemberton Papers, Etting Collection, II, 32, HSP.

1. A manuscript endorsed "Translation of Caspar Krebles letter to David Dashler and Jno. and Richd. Wister relatg to the reports concerning BF dated Towamencin Octob: 21. 1765" is in the Yale University Library. The text is printed in *Franklin Papers*, ed. Labaree, XII (1968), 329–330. Casper Krible (or Kriebel), a farmer of Towamencin Township, Montgomery County, had emigrated from Saxony in 1734 with nearly two hundred fellow Schwenkfelders seeking religious liberty in Pennsylvania. His letter, written in confidence to friends who knew Franklin personally, pleaded for refutation — for the German community — of malicious insinuations in the German-language press, particularly the charge that Franklin had favored passage of the Stamp Act. David Deshler, one of the men addressed, was a Schwenkfelder merchant, later also a member of the Pennsylvania Committee of Correspondence. John Wister (originally Wüster), an emigrant from Germany, had become a wine merchant in Philadelphia and from 1756 to 1761 had been Franklin's landlord; Richard Wistar, John's nephew, a Philadelphia businessman, was the son of Caspar Wistar (who spelled his name thus), founder, in 1738 at Salem, New Jersey, of the first glassworks in America. — See Samuel Kriebel Brecht, *The Genealogical Record of the Schwenkfelder Families who Fled . . . to Pennsylvania in the Years 1731 to 1737* (New York and Chicago, 1923), 348–49, 1504; *Franklin Papers*, ed. Labaree, *loc. cit.*, and IX (1966), 184n; Burt, *The Perennial Philadelphians*, 109, 110, 239.

To James Pemberton, Philadelphia, 8 April 1766 (I)

London, 8.4.1766

Dear Friend,

Agreeable to thy desire my Friend H. Brown and myself have signed the inclosed which we hope will prove satisfactory.

Before this arrives the repeal of the Stamp Act [1] will be known in America, and I hope we shall receive from your province at least no unfavourable report of your behaviour on this occasion. The Administration who have so steadily countenanced the repeal have had the heaviest opposition in every step that ever an administration had to contend with, the King wavering, the Favorite [2] against you, a great part of the King's servants and even part of the Royal Family your opponents, and what was the heaviest, perhaps, in the scale your own imprudent conduct — I mean the Americans in general.[3]

Against this formidable opposition there was at first only three or four North America merchants amongst whom B. Trecothick, C. Hanbury, D. Barclay and D. Mildred were the foremost and most active; a committee was called, regular meetings established and proper people assigned to wait upon those in town and attend Parliament. Circular letters were sent to the trading towns, to request the concurrence of those who were affected by the Act and Regulations in question and every step taken that the necessity of their affairs or prudence could suggest. It may be sufficient to say that this sub-committee were indefatigable. They gave the ministry such clear and undisguised accounts of the situation of affairs that though they at first seemed at the best inclined to a suspension, yet they came totally into the idea of a repeal.[4]

The Parliament met most strongly prejudiced against America. I need not recount the causes. Pride in the first place, interest in the next, passion resulting from both, worked up by inflammatory writers to an extreme degree. Judge from this portrait what an arduous task the Ministry had to engage in, what a slender support they had reason to expect from a few individuals who were in a good measure unknown to them. But when the evidence they had to produce was laid before the lower House; when the consequence of America to this country began to be explained; the efforts of a misunderstanding ascertained by unquestionable facts; when the chicanery, despotism, obstinacy of those who had promoted the late measures appeared uncontrovertably, numbers daily altered their opinion; and if ever a Parliament was swayed by reason solely, this most certainly has the credit of it, the King, Ministry, the Favourite, part of the Royal Family, the immediate servants of the Crown looking at the Favourite against you. The present Administration is now in power, mostly unknown to the people, treated with contumely by the opposition who valued themselves so much upon their influence and superiority as to have divided all the departments of Government one day amongst themselves. But it seems to me that Divine Providence immediately blasted their pride, devoted them to the humiliating situation they now occupy, and most graciously interposed to save us from the brink of ruin, from intestine quarrels, from the contempt of all Europe, by giving that firmness and unanimity amongst those in power that has once more established harmony amongst us.

In regard to the Act of Right,[5] I hope the Americans will be wiser than ever to take the least notice of it. Suffer it to die away in the obscurity it deserves. I hinted in a former letter the propriety of addressing the King on this occasion, I mean either by the whole legislature of Pennsylvania, or so much of it as can agree upon the subject.

It has been suggested that you ought to address both King and Parliament. But this does not at present appear to me proper. First, I believe it is utterly unprecedented; secondly, it seems utterly improper. The King is the head, and the head only ought to be spoke to. Let him use what language he pleases to the two inferior parts; he may either give the addresses themselves or the substance with his approbation. The lower House is a fluctuating body. If you address them, the whole have the praise, though a formidable minority opposed you to the utmost of their power. Can you thank these for their services?

In the upper House, the case was the same. Divers, and amongst them some of the most considerable personages in the kingdom, have protested against you; their protest is on record. Are they also entitled to your gratitude? They are to your pity and forgiveness.

How then can you with any propriety address the two inferior parts of the legislature? The King solely confirmed what the majority of the others agreed to. — I throw out these hints to thyself just to suggest what occurs to me against this measure, if it should be proposed or urged, as I have heard it hinted; at the same time I allow that reasons may be offered for it which have not occurred to me. This perhaps may come too late to be of any sort of use in this affair, but the incessant calls upon me in the duty of my vocation often render it impracticable to seize the earliest means of intelligence. W. Logan will deliver thee a little pamphlet wrote by a friend of mine on American affairs during the late contest.[6] If it has done no good, it has done very little harm, few having thought it worth reading. I sent to W.L. a pretty full, I can't say complete, collection of pamphlets wrote during this debate. I thought it would be of use to have them in some public library as they may possibly be helpful on some future occasion. I have not had an opportunity of perusing them yet, though I question not but there is much folly and impertinence as well as strong reasoning amongst them.

See R. Peters sometimes, and cultivate a friendly understanding with him. He has known little of us, though he has lived so long amongst you; I believe he wishes sincerely to have an enlarged heart and to meet with such who are honestly travelling to that better country. [*Passage omitted.*]

I know not how many attempts I have made to finish this letter, but it is concluded almost under every disadvantage, fatigue, interruption and some degree of infirmity. Under all these, as thou desires it, I am willing to give thee all the information I can, leaving it to thy own decision to make the use designed of this information.

I think the present Administration are likely to continue much to their own honour and the benefit of this country. They are men of ability, application and integrity; descended from or connected with the ancient firm friends to the present Royal Family, moderate in principle and firm to civil and religious liberty. As such they claim my cordial wishes, and I hope that every Friend to such principles will contribute to support them.[7]

A public demonstration of the allegiance and affection of the Americans to their Sovereign will reflect some little credit to those who have advised him to such prudent measures, and this I think is your reasonable duty.

My Brother Samuel is favoured with tolerable health; we heard from him last week. My sister joins me in kind respects to thyself and family. We are still in the same situation and occupied as usual. [*Passage omitted.*]

From thy affectionate Friend

John Fothergill

Ms. autograph letter, Pemberton Papers, Etting Collection, II, 53, HSP. Written after repeal of the Stamp Act.

1. The bill repealing the Stamp Act, having passed both Houses, received royal assent on 18 March. News of repeal reached New York on 26 April. Nonimportation was at once given up.

2. James Stuart (1713–1792), third Earl of Bute, who had tutored Prince George in boyhood and retained his influence as adviser to the King. — Manfred S. Gutmacher, *America's Last King* (New York: Scribners, 1941), 27, 56, 57.

3. Demonstrations against the Stamp Act had been almost universal in the coastal cities of America. In Boston, effigies of Andrew Oliver, recently appointed Stamp Agent, and Lord Bute were hanged on an elm tree for hours, then taken down and transported on a bier in a mock funeral procession to the State House. That night Oliver's office was torn down and some of the lumber thrown on a bonfire dangerously near his home. In Charleston, South Carolina, St. Michael's bells tolled all day as for a funeral. At night a mob paraded the streets, burned the stamp distributor in effigy, and rushed into private houses to search for stamps, supposedly hidden for future extortion. Upon arrival at Justice Skinner's house, the rioters found he had prepared bowls of strong punch and was waiting to join them in drinking the toast "Damnation to the Stamp Act!" — Esther Forbes, *Paul Revere and the World He Lived In*

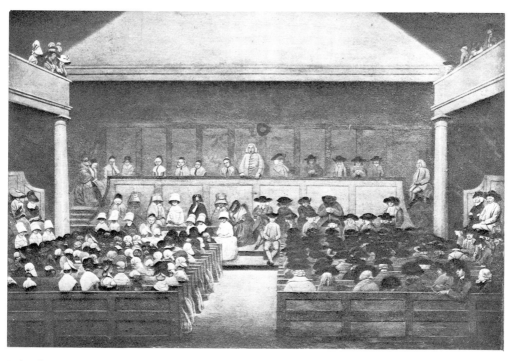

Friends' Meeting, Gracechurch Street, about 1770
The last figure on the platform, at the right of the picture, is said to be
Dr. Fothergill

Respected Friend,   London 29 oct. 1768.

The loss which we have both
sustained by the death of our late very
valuable Friend Peter Collinson, is the
principal occasion of my writing to thee
at this time. I must in the first place
however acknowledge myself indebted
to thee for a box of very curious plants
which I received some time ago, and
which are most of them prosperous, and
all of them would have been so, had my
then Gardiner taken the care of them he
ought: For they came in a very prosperous
condition. The Pittsburgh Iris I lost and
indeed I ought not to think of increasing
my collection; for my leisure to attend to it
seems to lessen every day: For on one
account or another so many people seem
to have claims to my assistance that I

find one for my self.
Accept my kind acknowledgment for thy
kind present, and believe me to be
thy very respectfull Fd

John Fothergill.

From letter to John Bartram of Philadelphia, 1768
(See page 289)

(Boston: Houghton Mifflin, 1942), 96–99; Harriott H. R. Ravenel, *Charleston: The Place and the People* (New York: Macmillan, 1927), 158–159; *The Diary and Autobiography of John Adams*, ed. L. H. Butterfield, I, 259–261.

4. Barlow Trecothick, whose appearance at the Bar of the House of Commons is mentioned in Dr. Fothergill's letter of 25 February, had organized a committee of twenty-eight merchants dealing with North America to protest against the Stamp Act as a threat to commerce. Lord Rockingham helped Trecothick compose a letter which was dispatched to more than thirty manufacturing and shipping centers. As a result, petitions for repeal were sent to the House of Commons from London, Liverpool, Manchester, Halifax, Leeds, Bradford, Birmingham, Witney, Wolverhampton, Coventry, Lancaster, Leicester, Macclesfield, Nottingham, Chippenham, Stourbridge, Dudley, Frome, Minehead, Taunton, Bristol, Newcastle-on-Tyne, and Glasgow. "Utter ruin" of trade was inevitable, they prophesied. — Sutherland, "Edmund Burke, 46–72.

5. The Declaratory Act of 18 March 1766, almost unnoticed because of the excitement over the repeal of the Stamp Act that same day.

6. William Logan carried this letter on his return voyage to Philadelphia, together with Dr. Fothergill's "little pamphlet," published as *Considerations Relative to the North American Colonies* (London, 1765).

7. The Rockingham ministry was short-lived, however. It was succeeded in the summer of 1766 by a new one headed by William Pitt, who very shortly was created Earl of Chatham.

To Israel Pemberton, Jr., Philadelphia, 8 April 1766 (II)

8.4.1766

Esteemed Friend,

We have received thy letter to us dated the 17th of December 1765, and the translation of a letter to David Deshler, John and Richard Wistar, signed by Casper Kreble, dated October 21, 1765, relative to the conduct of Dr. Benjamin Franklin in regard to the Stamp Act and the execution of the trust reposed in him respecting the change of government.[1]

Perhaps there is nothing more agreeable to minds well disposed than to have it in their power to do justice to an injured character, and we have the satisfaction to be able to do this, so far as our testimony may avail, with respect to the person above mentioned.

And we can safely aver, from our own knowledge as well as from the testimony of many persons here of undoubted character and reputation, that Benjamin Franklin was so far from proposing the Stamp Act or joining with it in any manner, that he at all times opposed it, both

261

in word and writing, though in vain, as neither his nor any other endeavour could influence the ministry to relinquish the design.

But if any doubt of his diligence or sincerity in this respect had remained, the evidence he gave before the House of Commons, on the occasion of the bill for repealing this act, was such as to remove every scruple of this kind. For the information he gave the House, the distinct, judicious and convincing proofs he laid before them of the impropriety of the Stamp Act we believe had considerable influence with the Parliament.

In respect to the commission with which he was charged from the Province of Pennsylvania we can assert our own knowledge that he has endeavoured, both by admitting friendly mediation, and by pursuing more vigorous measures when these proved unsuccessful, to discharge his duty most uprightly to his constituents.

And it should rather be attributed to the singularly unfavourable position of affairs both at home and in America, than to the want of industry or address, that he has not hitherto succeeded in his negotiations.

We hope this attestation will fully satisfy Dr. Franklin's friends, and enable them to do his character that justice which we think his steady attachment to the interests of America in general and of his own Province in particular deserves.

We are Thy respectful and assured Friends

Henton Brown
John Fothergill

Ms. autograph letter, Pemberton Papers, XXXIV, 142, HSP.

1. This letter is the formal attestation requested by the Pemberton brothers in order to reassure the German community of Benjamin Franklin's loyalty to the Colonial cause. See the letters of 25 February, 27 February, and 8 April (I), above.

To James Pemberton, Philadelphia, 10 May 1766

Lea Hall, 10.5.1766

Esteemed Friend,

Though J. Reynell[1] will acquaint thee with some circumstances relative to the present situation of your affairs, yet as the packet is about to sail, I knew not how to let it go without a line, as the present conjecture will require thy attentive consideration.

It would require a volume to describe the transactions of the present Parliament with respect to the affairs of America; it may be sufficient to observe that after the most unwearied, obstinate opposition, every circumstance has ended in your favour.[2] Letters in abundance will I doubt not arrive by the packet with the pleasing information, and from persons of much more leisure and much greater ability and acquaintance with the affair. The Quadrumvirate I formerly mentioned, viz., Barlow Trecothick, C. Hanbury, D. Barclay and Daniel Mildred have been incessantly laborious and successful; they have been admitted to the Ministry at all times, have supported them with proper and just evidence, and have acted as became Friends to England, to America, to themselves, to their country and posterity.[3]

The Ministry, the Friends of America, almost totally despaired of affecting any one point beneficial to commerce in general. But on a sudden almost, the opposition seemed to cease, and every necessary regulation was agreed to in the House, and a bill is now framing to enlarge your commerce, to secure you from the tyranny of the West Indians, to open fresh markets, and to render smuggling and other collusive means unnecessary.

A paper, signed by an impartial Bystander, enclosed, wrote by an acquaintance of mine, will give a general idea of the sentiments propagated here, and which I believe are just. Whether it had any weight I know not, nor is it material. This, I know, that your deliverance from the Stamp Act, the present advantages, may be justly ascribed to the secret working of inscrutable wisdom. To the King, to the Ministry, to a few able and willing advocates here under Providence, you owe the most invaluable blessings. In a former, I proposed an early address from your Assembly.[4] It has been queried here, shall it be to the King only or to the King and Parliament, the legislature? I think to the King only. He is head, he is always the King, veritable. The King, your Protector and your Friend. The Parliament, though a majority are your friends, yet what can you say to this majority which the minority could not ascribe to themselves, and by this means cancel the remembrance of their deeds?

Give me thy sentiments when leisure presents on the following question.

By what means can the increase of P.b.t.n. power in America be most effectually checked, consistently with liberty of conscience and the genuis of British freedom? I see that sometime America will be P.b.t.n., a persuasion altogether intolerant, and I could wish to retard it, as long as possible.[5]

I am thy affectionate Friend

J. Fothergill

Ms. autograph letter, Pemberton Papers, Etting Collection, II, 54, HSP.

1. John Reynell (1708–1784) emigrated to Philadelphia from Jamaica before he was twenty. Described as "a valuable member of the Society of Friends," he prospered as a shipping and commission merchant. He was appointed Treasurer of the Board of Managers of the Pennsylvania Hospital at its start, and served as President of the Board, 1757–1764. — Tolles, *Meeting House and Counting House, passim*; Morton and Woodbury, *Pennsylvania Hospital*, 412, 456.

2. Dr. Fothergill was too optimistic. When the duties imposed by the Declaratory Act, passed the day the Stamp Act was repealed, became effective in 1767 opposition and resentment were again aroused in the Colonies.

3. The merchants who had worked for repeal of the Stamp Act were publicly honored in April 1766 at a dinner described by Edmund Burke as "a city feast where the Majority [in favor of Repeal] . . . dined with the North America Merchants. The Company, last Wednesday [April 23] at Drapers Hall, was very numerous and the most brilliant ever seen in London. It is said there were 240 who dined, amongst whom were nine Dukes and a considerable number more of the nobility and members of the House of Commons, who honored the American Merchants with their company." — *The Correspondence of Edmund Burke*, ed. Thomas Copland (Chicago: University of Chicago Press, 1958), I, 251; *Annual Register* (London, 1766), entry for 23 April.

4. See Letter of 25 February 1766; and possibly for the Bystander, p. 261, n. 6.

5. Presbyterians and Quakers were finding themselves rivals commercially and politically in Pennsylvania. Perhaps their distrust of one another had its origin during the seventeenth-century "sufferings" William Penn endured at the instigation of Thomas Vincent, a Presbyterian minister. Penn had openly declared disbelief in the concept of the Trinity. Vincent insisted upon public debate. Penn published a tract, *The Sandy Foundation Shaken* (London, 1668), without getting the necessary license from the Bishop of London. Charged, consequently, with misdemeanor, he was confined in the Tower for nine months. During his imprisonment, he was frequently visited by the Bishop of Worcester, Dr. Edward Stillingfleete, who urged the young man to write another tract explaining his religious convictions. As a result, Penn produced *Innocency and Her Open Face, presented by way of Apology for the Sandy Foundation Shaken* (London, 1669) in which he avoided detailed doctrinal discussion but asserted his firm belief in the divinity of Christ. On 28 July 1669, Charles II, who had promised upon accession to defend the Presbyterian faith, found Penn's expression of belief acceptable and ordered his immediate release from prison in the custody of his father, Admiral Sir William Penn. — Catherine Owens Peare, *William Penn: A Biography* (Philadelphia: Lippincott, 1957), 77–88.

To Dr. Lionel Chalmers, Charles Town, South Carolina, 10 September 1766

Lea Hall, 10.9.1766

Dear Friend,[1]

Yesterday's post brought me thy very acceptable letter. The history of the Bee man confirms the accounts I had received beyond a doubt.[2] That he can collect them together and make them cling about him so safely and so steadily is surprising, but still it is less so than to conceive by what means he can divest himself so soon of his formidable robe, and return his visitants so timely into their hive. I am glad for the sake of these useful creatures, that kind Providence has permitted a method to be discovered by which they may be reserved for fresh labour after they have drudged so hard for the entertainment and advantage of mankind.

I am sorry for our worthy Friend J. Bartram, and could wish most sincerely to suggest anything that may contribute to his health.[3] I suspect, but cannot be certain from the very short account before me, but that it is possible his disease proceeds from small insects burrowing and breeding in the flesh. It [the insect] is extremely small, and is very common in hot sandy countries. There is a very full account of this most mischievous insect in Ulloa's Voyage, Vol. 1, and the method of treating it. They have the book no doubt in Philadelphia; and he will readily discover by the symptoms whether my suggestions are right.[4]

But if the corroding ulcers only proceed from sharp acrimonious juices, I could wish he would make trial of the extract of hemlock internally, and a fomentation made of the Decoction of this plant externally, if the surgeon under whose care he is sees no reason to the contrary. The dose of the extract must be so much twice a day as will *not* create a singular kind of giddiness that always accompanies *too large* a dose of this drug. He may begin with 16 grains twice a day, and increase 4 grains at a time till he finds the quantity that affects him as I have mentioned; the quantity short of this is the right dose, and this may be gradually increased a little farther as he can bear it.

But if before these hints arrive, he finds himself recovering, by all means continue the use of those means reasonably. — He must also determine most resolutely to keep in a lying posture night and day,

265

till his legs are well, or it will be impossible by any means whatever to make him a sound man.

I can give no precise directions with respect to his diet, management, and other medicines. The gentleman who has the care of him will undoubtedly take care to give him now and then a gentle purgative; decoction of sarsparilla, the bark or such other internals as the case in general may seem to require, if the extract does not succeed.

If the case admits of so much delay, or at least is not considerably better when this arrives, I shall be very ready to lend all the assistance in my power, when I have particulars sufficient to enable me to form a clearer notion of the disease than the few hints before me will permit.

The insect I have mentioned is one of the most mischievous kind in being. It is extremely small; it penetrates the skin of the feet and legs without pain, and discovers itself only when it has made provision for many generations of a numerous progeny.

Yes, my Friend, I took notice of the preceding account of rice and so forth, and was pleased to see so many interesting circumstances recorded to posterity. I wish, and at that time particularly I wished, that some person could be found in America capable of describing the present time with the state of agriculture, commerce, and the dawn of arts; and that every 20 years a fresh account of the present state of every colony should be authenticated by their respective assemblies. If the history of the actions of men in civil life are of any use to posterity, what advantages might not be gained by thus taking time by the forelock. — Unfortunately for us, we are introduced at school and in the course of our education, into war, battles, sieges, carnage, and no character is thought equal to that of a hero, a licensed, wholesale *murderer*; we are taught to be in love with Virgil's heroes, Homer's, and in sober prose with the lives of men who made themselves illustrious by slaughter. Multitudes never emancipate themselves from these prepossessions, and it is difficult even for the few who do. How much happier it is for those who have none of these learned prejudices to eradicate, but like a *tabula rasa* are open to the impressions of every useful bias that humanity and philanthropy exult in.

When I look to my Friends in London, the prospect of seeing them well and happy is pleasing. When I reflect that I must exchange quiet for bustle, retirement for dissipation, for ease extreme fatigue, this scale preponderates. But duty calls as well as interest, and where duty leads,

266

pleasure seldom loiters long behind. I have tired thee, filled all my paper, and have only room to add that I am

Thy affectionate Friend
J. Fothergill

Ms. autograph letter, Bartram Papers, IV, 12, IISP.

1. Dr. Lionel Chalmers (1714–1777) of Charleston, South Carolina, was a well-educated Scotsman, highly esteemed by Dr. Fothergill. Chalmers had emigrated to Charleston without a medical degree and entered into partnership in 1738 with Dr. John Lining, to whose practice he later succeeded as the "principal physician" of the city. In 1756, through the efforts of a friend, Dr. Robert Whytt of Edinburgh, Chalmers was awarded an M.D. from St. Andrews *in absentia*. At the time of his death the *South Carolina Gazette* of 12 May 1777 brought to attention his activities as justice of the peace and in the Charles Town Library Society. He left an estate of £24,000, in addition to personal property and nine Negro slaves. He was considered a man "of sound judgment and benevolent heart," who used his knowledge "for the good of mankind, and left behind him the name of an affectionate husband and parent, a skillful humane physician, and a worthy, honest man." — Dr. Joseph I. Waring, "Lionel Chalmers, Medical Author," *Bulletin of the History of Medicine*, 32 (1958): 349–353.

2. Thomas Wildman, "the Bee-master," in the 1760's attracted considerable attention in England by his performances with swarms of honey bees. His *Treatise on the Management of Bees . . . with the various Methods of cultivating them . . .* (London: printed for the author and sold by T. Cadell, 1768) was reviewed in the *Monthly Review* (London), 39:105–110 (August 1768). See also John Nichols, *Illustrations of the Literary History of the Eighteenth Century*, I (1817), 104; V (1828), 787.

3. John Bartram, accompanied by his son William, made a journey of botanical exploration to the southern wilderness of Florida (1765–66), passing en route through Charleston, where they met Dr. Lionel Chalmers. John Bartram was in poor health when he left Pennsylvania. His London correspondent, Peter Collinson, had been much distressed by news from his friend John that he had a troublesome ulcer on his leg. In the spring of 1766, John Bartram concluded his collecting, left William in Florida to raise indigo and rice, and went on to Charlestown. Fevers and jaundice had beset him while traveling, and the ulcer had not healed. — John Bartram, "Diary of a Journey Through the Carolinas, Georgia and Florida from July 1, 1765, to April 10, 1766," *Transactions of the American Philosophical Society*, 33, Pt. I (1942): 1–120.

4. Bartram's letters of 1767 report improved health after exchanging the primitive life of wilderness travel for the comforts and routine of life at home. The infestation suggested by Dr. Fothergill is described in detail by Antonio de Ulloa, *Relacion Historica del Viage a la America* (Madrid, 1748). An English translation, *A Voyage to South America* (2 vols., London, 1758), is listed in a catalogue of Dr. Fothergill's library. The condition observed by Ulloa was caused by a minute insect, the chigoe (English derivative, jigger), but known in Latin America as *nigua* or *pique*. This insect burrows into the skin, necessitating surgical intervention if neglected. — O. S. Ormsby and Hamilton Montgomery, *Diseases of the Skin* (Philadelphia: Lea and Febiger, 1954), 1280–1281; Ulloa, *Voyage*, I, 66–99.

To James Pemberton, Philadelphia, 30 September 1766

London, 30.9.1766

Esteemed Friend,

Be pleased to acquaint the Managers of the Pennsylvania Hospital, that it will not be practicable to receive any part of the interest upon your capital in the bank till the whole becomes due.[1] It was an act of considerable favour, that any interest was allowed. Proper care will be taken by the Trustees, that the Hospital shall receive every advantage that our legislature kindly intended.

I am pleased to find that the Hospital is likely to receive advantage from the Workhouse now establishing in your city,[2] as I am certain from experience of the benefits that may be derived from such institutions both to the public immediately and ultimately by the increase of skill and experience of those who have the charge of the public health. I cannot but wish it success and am glad that it has been in my power in any respect to promote it.

A careful, disinterested inspection into the conduct of your servants of every rank, from the Physician to the lowest menial, will have great effects. So long as a care of this kind to see that everyone discharges his duty with fidelity and skill according to his station, so long will the hospital be prosperous, your credit will increase, subscriptions come in freely, the patients will be satisfied and recover the faster through this satisfaction. But whenever you begin to relax in your care everyone will begin to carve for themselves; one will like ease, and another profit; neglect enters and the fruit of your labours falls off, immature. Your servants will become your masters, and as the corruption of the best things becomes the worst, your ruin will be certain and speedy.

Permit me to request that a particular regard may be had to the conduct of the medical part of your institution, with respect to their cordiality and unanimity. Jealousies and emulations will happen, they are often useful; but if they proceed to enmity, dismiss the person who gives just occasion for it, be his merits what they may. I say, just occasion, because I know that unjust insinuations may be thrown out, but this your sagacity will soon discover.

I am far from suspecting that anything of this kind is in hazard of existing with you. From the little I have seen, I have seen it possible that detriment may arise to the patients from disunion amongst the faculty.

268

By this time I apprehend that by the generous conduct of the late administration and the legislature all your fears are dissipated, and benefits thrown into your lap which you could not hope for. To Providence in the first place, next to our generous Sovereign and the administration then in power, with a few active honest individuals here, you owe your advantages. Remember them with gratitude, and when you see commerce not only reviving but invigorated and extended beyond your utmost expectations, look up to the First Great Cause with reverence.

Dear Friend, When I sat down to write I proposed this as a letter only to the Hospital, but I see that it is improper to be laid before them. Be pleased therefore to acquaint them with the purport of the little that concerns them. Assure them however of my wishes for their prosperity, and that if anything within my reach occurs in which I can be of service, I shall not neglect them. [*Passage omitted.*]

In respect to public affairs the papers will inform you of the alterations and our division of sentiments. My own opinion can avail but little in determining thy judgement, where the facts are so public. I think the Americans have gone unwarrantable and ungrateful lengths in ascribing all their advantages to the late great Commoner.[3] You are less obliged to him than you suspect, but you are Americans, warm, passionate and an Englishman in excess. You are solely obliged to the steadiness of the late administration [4] under Providence and to the few individuals here whom I have formerly mentioned. Lord Chatham coincided in the Stamp Act, I mean in *repealing* it, and by this, gave great weight to the ministry. But he opposed divers of the regulations so beneficial to you, the free ports especially. Abraham Rawlinson of Lancaster [5] was the projector of this scheme; he convinced the North American committee of its utility; they obliged the West Indian committee to be of the same sentiment by clear reasoning; and the chief opposition arose from W. Beckford,[6] and through his friendship with W.P., from the present Lord Chatham. Notwithstanding this duplicity I hope he will serve the Nation both ably and disinterestedly — and I mention these circumstances chiefly to show how much many of the colonies are misled. They overlook those who have actually served them and most essentially; they are erecting statues to a man who however he may deserve it on other occasions, in this has much less merit than you imagine.

I have but little time left by this last ship's departure to pay a transient visit to my friends. My leisure and inclinations don't always keep pace.

Remember me to our mutual Friends, and believe me to be thy affectionate Friend

J. Fothergill

Ms. autograph letter, Pemberton Papers, Etting Collection, II, 55, HSP.

1. Dr. Fothergill is referring to funds accumulated by the Pennsylvania Land Company in London and invested for the benefit of the Pennsylvania Hospital. The capital was kept available for withdrawals upon demand; the interest was banked intact in order to accumulate for future needs.

2. The Almshouse and House of Employment on Spruce Street between 10th and 11th Streets, supplementing the work of the Pennsylvania Hospital, provided care and work for the aged, poor, and needy, and also offered hospital service for unmarried mothers. Certain clinical lectures and demonstrations were later given at the Almhouse to medical students. — G. W. Corner, *Two Centuries of Medicine*, 74.

3. William Pitt's acceptance of a peerage cost him the popularity which his eloquence had won while he was a member of the House of Commons. His sphere of influence henceforth was limited because visitors and newspaper reporters were denied admission to the House of Lords. His health declined during this period, forcing prolonged retirement in 1768. — Knollenberg, 15–17, 240–241.

4. Rockingham's ministry.

5. Abraham Rawlinson, a Quaker M.P., was a member of a family of Furness, Lancashire, with ships, in the lucrative West Indian trade (Raistrick, 302). Rawlinson's liberal principle of free ports did not receive Parliamentary support. Parliament, faced with the necessity of securing revenue "to meet the expense of defending, protecting and securing His Majesty's dominions in North America," passed the American Act of 1764 to levy import duties on sugar, foreign molasses, and European luxury fabrics. — Gipson, *Triumphant Empire: Thunder Clouds Gather in the West*, X, 223–245.

6. William Beckford (1709–1770), considered the wealthiest man in London, was a close friend and political associate of William Pitt. He came from a colonial family whose fortune was made by exporting sugar, molasses, and rum from their extensive West Indian plantations. He sat as M.P. in the House of Commons, 1754–1761; was twice Lord Mayor of London, 1761 and 1768; and in the last year of his life, 1770, presented an address to the King, advocating political liberties for that city. — Lewis Namier, *The Structure of Politics at the Accession of George III* (London: Macmillan, 1953), 55n.

To the Reverend Richard Peters, Philadelphia, 10 October 1766

London, 10.10.1766

Before this comes to hand I hope my much esteemed friend will have received an answer to his case by the conveyance of our mutual friend the Proprietor.[1]

I intend likewise to say something on this subject to Dr. Graeme [2] to whom I shall write by this packet. It is not always right to be talking about Physick to our patients; an expression misunderstood may cause hours of anxiety.

Soon after we got down to Lea Hall, I received a very friendly visit from thy Brother,[3] and if I live to see that country again, I will endeavour to return it. I left nothing undone, that I so much regretted in the country, but I stayed very little from the place of our abode. I had many things to do, much to recollect, and to think of setting my house in order. I consider this favourable retreat from hurry as a time allotted to the most necessary purposes to cultivate and cherish the secret drawings of divine regard, to strive after the one thing needful. — We passed our time in a placid calm; more alone than the last year, but not without the countenances of many we esteem, both of our own and other persuasions.

When I was very young, a story that was told of a person of some distinction in the country where I then lived afforded me at that time and since some instruction. She was so ignorant as to ask of an acquaintance if he thought there were any beggars or poor people went to Heaven, intimating that she should not like to see such mean, low people there. This taught me early to beware of thinking meanly even of those who differed from me with the greatest acrimony, much less to think cooly or in the least disadvantageously of those who stood fair candidates for heaven, be they of what nation, people or tongue whatsoever. There, there is no jar, no confusion, no distance; all is love. Let us then cultivate this universal spirit which is essential to our happiness, both in this life and that which is to be. I have had many advantages, good precepts, good example, circumscribed from many dangers and delivered from many temptations; what, am I not indebted? More than I can ever pay; and may it be my living, dying wish to love him above all who has done so much for me.

My Brother's health is better established; the gravel afflicts him sometimes. I saw him with satisfaction as I think he is gradually refining. We gave comfort to the few of our persuasion, and some little encouragement to live in Love, and fear. Our neighbours in general were not dissatisfied with our being there, and this gives us satisfaction if at least we are no cause of stumbling to any in their pursuit after their duty, whether it be in this or that denomination.

Sometimes when I was in the country I wrote now and then a line or two as my leisure and inclination united, to Betsy.[4] It grew at last into a long letter. I have charged her not to show my letters to anybody, if she chooses to have me as a correspondent. Perhaps, in a fit of pain, some parts may draw off attention a little from it. Give her a dispensation to thyself only, if she thinks it worth while. But excommunicate her wholly, if she trespasses to any other!

This time twelve months, you were tossing in the Downs, and I daily felt for your uncertain situation. But when I considered you [*illegible*], where your station was allotted you by superior direction, I left you, stifled anxiety, pursued my business, and calmly said whatever is, is not only right but best.

We begin to feel the effects of luxury in the want of necessary provisions. The whole compass of our Island will soon be too little to support even the horses we employ. This is the cause of dearness of provisions now felt, at least one principal cause. Mobs and riots now govern us; a prelude to greater misfortunes. We are gone too far in forgetfulness to whom we owe the greatest blessings that mankind can enjoy — life, liberty, property in full security. My best wishes if wishes can avail, attend thee, and that the declining shades of life may be to us both comfortable. My sister joins me in remembrance of sincere friendship and good will.

From thy affectionate Friend

J. Fothergill

Dreer Collection, 150, HSP; a letter without cover or salutation; the context identifies the correspondent.

1. A report from a Philadelphia doctor was sent in the diplomatic pouch, evidently concerning the condition of Dr. Fothergill's "most esteemed" patient, the Rev. Richard Peters.

2. Dr. Thomas Graeme, born about 1688 in Belgowan, Perthshire, Scotland, went to Philadelphia in 1717/18. He served as a member of the Provincial Council, a Judge of the Supreme Court, and after establishment of the Pennsylvania Hospital in 1755, was appointed Consultant in Surgery. He acquired a country estate called Graeme Park where his daughter Elizabeth (see letter of 28 June 1765, above) displayed her talents as a hostess. — Montgomery, *History of the University of Pennsylvania*, 181, 182; *Letters of Benjamin Rush*, ed. Butterfield, 179, nn. 1–4; *Autobiography of Benjamin Rush*, ed. G. W. Corner, 116, 167, 302, 320; Thomas A. Glenn, *Some Colonial Mansions and Those Who Lived in Them* (Philadelphia: Coates, 1899), 367–398; Charles P. Keith, *Provincial Councillors* (Philadelphia: The author, 1883), 161.

3. Bartlett Peters. A letter from Richard Peters to Elizabeth Graeme, 2 July 1765, from Liverpool, tells her of his plans to visit Dr. Fothergill at this time. — Miscellaneous Collections, HSP (unnumbered volume, identified by year of material).

4. Elizabeth Graeme, who had by that time returned to Philadelphia after visits in Great Britain.

To Sarah Titley, Warrington, Lancashire, 6 January 1767

London, 6.1.1767

Dear Sally,[1]

I received thy kind and affectionate letter last night, and communicated the contents to my Brother who was much affected with the account of Sister's misfortune [2] and is now upon the road to Warrington.

He is much recovered and had proposed setting out this morning in a returning post chaise before he received this account. I expect he will reach home by seventh day night and J. Coakley Lettsom comes with him to bear him company.[3] He proposes to be at Hockley this night and will call in his way down at the *Swan*, Coleshill; *ditto*, Litchfield; *Saracen's Head*, Wolseley Bridge; *Dog* at Sandon; *Crown* at Stone; *New Roebuck*, Newcastle; *Swan*, Talke o' the Hill, and C. Vernon's Holmes Chapel.[4] To any of these places an express messenger may be sent and will be sure to meet him, should any appearance of an immediate hazard appear. And I think if appearances grow worse, it would be right to meet my Brother at one of these places with the account, as it may lessen his anxiety as he approaches home. I am much pleased he was with us. He had got some cold in coming up which brought on a fit of the gout. By good nursing and management, it has gone off regularly, and if he does not suffer by an indiscreet endeavour to get home with too much expedition, I hope he will have no cause to repent his journey.

I am much obliged to my kind kinsman, thy husband, for his endeavours to serve me. We have got everything ready to receive any quantity he may provide for us. I would by no means hurt the poor in your part by endeavouring to help those in this; but a small cargo now and then arriving may induce those who have stocks here to part with them at a lower rate, when they know . . . much larger quantities are coming to market.[5]

The fish thy husband was so kind to send us was exceeding fine and claims our grateful acknowledgement. Be kind enough to tell him if I live to get down to Lea Hall and see him not there, we shall begin to think he has some dislike to his wife's relations. For my part I sincerely wish to cultivate a good understanding with him, and hope he will consider me as his Friend and relative . . . Accept our cordial salutations, and be assured that I am thine affectionately.

J. Fothergill

Ms. autograph letter, Port. 22/100, LSFL.

1. Dr. Fothergill's niece, daughter of his deceased brother Joseph. She had married Abraham Titley of Warrington in 1764.

2. The Doctor's sister, Ann, who had fallen from a carriage and broken her leg while on a visit to Warrington, was recuperating in Sally's home.

3 Samuel Fothergill, after his recent illness in London, was accompanied by John Coakley Lettsom on the journey homeward to Warrington by post chaise. Lettsom, "a volatile Creole," born in Little Vandyke, a tiny island close to Tortola in the West Indies, was a protégé of the Fothergill brothers. Samuel Fothergill, one of his legal guardians, had directed his education in England, sending him first to Gilbert Thompson's school in Penketh and later arranging his apprenticeship to Abraham Sutcliffe, a Quaker apothecary in Settle, Yorkshire. Lettsom, in 1767, was a young man of twenty-three spending a year at work in St. Thomas' Hospital in preparation for return to Tortola to practice medicine. He returned to England in 1768, pursued further medical studies in Edinburgh, Paris, and Leyden, in 1769 obtained the degree of M.D. at Leyden, and subsequently attained eminence as a physician in London. — Fox, 99–117.

4. This route was retraced in 1960 by Dr. Booth, who found that many of the inns mentioned were still in operation.

5. Dr. Fothergill and several other prominent Friends were backing schemes to make food cheaper for London's poor. Potatoes, always a staple in the British diet, were being bought at wholesale in Lancashire and sent to London, "where there is more poverty (as well as more wealth) than in any part of the Kingdom." Dr. Fothergill, David Barclay, Thomas Corbyn, and others raised a fund for wholesale purchase of fish for shipment to certain London warehouses where it was sold below cost for the benefit of low-income groups. To lower the price of bread, a recipe for making it with one part potatoes to three of ordinary flour was being sent in circulars to bakers and householders. Bread made by this rule, as well as fish and potatoes, was sold at the warehouses mentioned. Dr. Fothergill and his sister made it their custom to serve these foods once a week as the main course dinner. — Fox, 229–231.

To Humphry Marshall, West Bradford, Chester Co., Pennsylvania, 2 March 1767

London, 2.3.1767

Respected Friend,[1]

I received thy kind letter as well as the box of seeds and the duplicates it contained. I think myself much indebted to thee, and shall endeavour as occasions may offer to show that I am not insensible of thy kindness nor ungrateful.

I knew not whether anything would be more acceptable to a botanist than Miller's *Gardener's Dictionary*,[2] which I hope thou will receive with this, and if thou art possessed of one before, dispose of it and accept the produce as an acknowledgement of thy kindness.

274

As it may suit thy other concerns, I shall be glad if thou would proceed to collect the seeds of other American shrubs and plants as they fall in thy way, and if thou meets with any curious plant or shrub transplant it at a proper time into thy garden; let it grow there a year or two; it may then be taken up in autumn, its roots wrapped in a little moss, and laid in a common box just made close enough to keep out mice, but not to exclude the air.

If thou knows of any plant possessed of particular virtue and that is known by experience to be useful in the cure of disease, this I should be glad to have in particular, both the parts used, and seeds of the same. I accept thy offer to collect for me the curious animals of your country, very readily; and as I may shall readily make such acknowledgements as may be agreeable. And in doing this I shall take it kind, if thou will just point out in what manner I can render the most service.

Except the Rattlesnake I have scarce any of your reptiles, and but few insects. Whatever of this kind occurs may therefore be laid aside for me; the reptiles may be put together in a little common spirit, and the insects stuck through with a pin and fixed on the inside of a box made of soft wood. — Small birds may be gutted and dried, filling them with moss and tobacco dust. Larger birds may be opened and gutted, then filled with salt and pepper.

Whilst however I am putting thee upon these services I must desire thee not to give into their searches so much as either to lessen thy attention to the duties of thy station here, or thy regard to the more essential ones of another life. I endeavour to keep all these things in their proper place; and by no means permit them to interfere with more important considerations. They are lawful but may not be to all expedient, and whilst I am gratifying an inclination the most innocent, I would take care not to hurt another. I shall be pleased with thy correspondence, and if occasion offers, I shall gladly promote thy interest here, as well as contribute to it myself; but still remember these pursuits are not the main business of life, but may be allowable relaxations. My Brother Samuel remembers thy family and speaks of them with esteem. Follow the example of wise men, seek their company, and then thou will become such thyself and an example to others. Farewell

John Fothergill

Ms. autograph letter, Miscellaneous Collections, HSP; printed in Darlington, *Memorials*, 495, 496.

1. Humphry Marshall (1722–1801), son of a Quaker landowner of Chester County, Pennsylvania, was apprenticed to a stone mason at the age of twelve and became adept at his trade, but relinquished it in 1758, when he was married and assumed the management of his father's extensive farm. Like his cousin John Bartram, he was intensely interested in all aspects of natural history, educated himself by reading widely, and became a correspondent of Peter Collinson. In 1764, enlarging his father's house, he added a small conservatory. He became an authority on trees and shrubs, and in 1785 published *Arbustum Americanum, or, an Alphabetical Catalogue of the Forest Trees and Shrubs, Natives of the American United States.* This book, dedicated to the officers and members of the American Philosophical Society, was widely praised as "the first truly indigenous Botanical Essay published in this Western Hemisphere." — Darlington, p. 489.

2. Philip Miller (1694–1771), whose *Gardener's Dictionary*, justly popular, had many editions, had been Curator of the Chelsea Physic Garden since 1722. The Apothecaries' Society had first established this garden in 1675, but found its upkeep expensive. When Sir Hans Sloane bought Chelsea Manor in 1722, he became thereby the Society's landlord, and conveyed the Garden to the Apothecaries for a token payment of £5 annually and an agreement to supply the Royal Society each year with fifty specimens of different useful plants, "well dried and preserved," until 2000 had been accumulated — a promise faithfully kept. — Gavin R. de Beer, *Sir Hans Sloane and the British Museum* (London: Oxford University Press, 1953), 16, 24, 28, 60–62, 111.

To Samuel Fothergill, Warrington, Lancashire, 10 December 1767

London, 10.12.1767

Dear Brother,

I have not been inattentive to thy several very kind letters but was prevented from acknowledging them in the manner I could have wished for want of time. Last week we put on board the *Barnevelt*, George Evans, Master, for Liverpool, a case directed for thee, containing the bookcase I mentioned.[1] Its back may be fitted to any mouldings of the wainscot and is left rough for that purpose. I had it made deeper for my own use, as thou will perceive, but it will not be less convenient to thee, and I am glad of placing it under thy roof.

The carpet was sent down by the wagon yesterday. We thought it rather too valuable to go by water and though it will cost thee something considerable for carriage, yet I hope it will not come too dear, nor prove improper for thy use. It is still plainer than ours at Lea Hall and was it to make over again, it should have been more so, but it will neither, I hope, hurt thee nor anybody else. Its price is about 8 pounds, which I mention only for thy information, that if anybody wants such another, they may know how and upon what terms to come at it. The breadth of each piece is easily distinguished, and these breadths are six shillings per yard.

We hear nothing yet of our potatoes, and yet the wind has blown from every quarter of the compass. Pray let us have them by the cheese ships though the freight is more. They must sail, but the others will not, so long as they can add the least fragment to their loading. Our fish is arrived from Ireland, and we hope to have them here in a few days. We should be glad to have our potatoes also, but they may be detained a month yet. For the future, would it not be best . . . to oblige the Master to stand to all loss, the consequence of delay? I wish it could be done. I see we shall suffer by the triviality of these ignorants.

Through mercy we are pretty well and have suffered nothing from our new abode. Indeed the weather has been with us most uncommonly favourable. When it is a little on the sharp side we find least difference between this situation and the city. We have almost an hour's daylight more. I keep at home to see patients only on the 3rd and 5th day afternoons, by which means I have the 2nd, 4th and 6th day afternoons more at liberty. And I hope gradually to lessen both my business and all other encumbrances. I have been preserved through many dangers, and my life mercifully prolonged to this time, and it is not the least of the favours which I have to acknowledge that I am kept in a degree alive to gratitude.

C. Payton was expected in town about this time. The precarious health of her family keeps her at home where I wish she may be safely and usefully employed till it is a ripe season for her coming. Our niece, Nanny Freeman,[2] has been long indisposed but in a manner I could not understand; within a few weeks, however, she has had a fever and not without some symptoms *mali moris*, which in medicine means not without danger . . . She is now getting better, and I most sincerely wish that with a sound body she may recover a sound mind . . .

By a note I have just received from one of J. Hunt's daughters, we are informed that their Father is expected in London early next Spring. W. Logan's son [3] is returned, had a 14 weeks passage over, and the crew must have perished by famine if they had not met with five successive recruits from vessels met at sea. His return was through a continued storm, and the ship was almost wrecked on the coast of Wales. They

277

lost everything, and were glad of compounding for life itself. At present he is here, more grave, more considerate, more solid than might have been expected. He makes one wish that he might be something more than a wild, unsubdued, unstable American. Samuel Emlen is here, a reputation to his country, a help to society, the pattern of innocence, wisdom and simplicity.[4] J. Roper has been in town on business but our visitors are few, very few. I think it is right. Our religion entering little farther than the ear, it had better die outright than be merely superficial.

I had twenty things to say to thee upon one occasion or another but they have escaped me at present. Thou complains of thy house being damp. Treat with thy tenant of his two years lease and give him a generous conpensation to resign it, if he can do it without injury to his family. If he consents, cut down here and there one of the trees, leave the best bearers of the best fruit. They will be useful and ornamental. At our time of life two years of exemption from great inconveniencies are not to be valued at a low rate. Had we children dependent upon us, other considerations might justly take place. In the course of Providence it is so ordered that we have none to look up to us and call us Father. An exemption from millions of anxieties! It is then but justice that we use the favour of Providence granted us, whether the fruits of our industry or by a more special favour of easy inheritance, to the proper purposes; our own accommodation according to the station in which we are placed; the benefit of the community in general, and our Brethren in particular.

I pity our distressed kinsman, G. Thompson; yet I know not that it is right.[5] Is it uncharitable in me to say that never any man hid his talents more under a bushel than himself? Is nothing wanting to move such a timid, such a bashful, such a cautious, such a selfish soul, gifted with such power, to a proper consideration before it quits this lower stage, and purify it for a happier existence. If I am right, let him suffer here, and may I also rather than — but enough!

My sister is knitting by me, knows I have not been idle today, is ignorant to whom I am writing; I see she wishes me to have done, even if she knew that our affectionate Brother was the present principal object of hers and mine and Sister's and our relations' [regard].

J. Fothergill

Ms. autograph letter, Port. 22/109, LSFL.

1. Dr. Fothergill and his sister Ann were moving to a more desirable location, in

Harpur Street, Bloomsbury, just off Red Lion Square. Theirs was the first house to be occupied in a street taking its name from a fourteenth-century Lord Mayor, Sir William Harpur. They apparently had furnishings to dispose of and were glad the bookcase and carpet would be useful to Susanna and Samuel. — Fox, 268.

2. Alexander Fothergill's daughter Ann (1742–1781) was now the wife of James Freeman of Gracechurch Street, a silk-mercer. — Fothergill Genealogy, below.

3. Billy Logan of Philadelphia, returning from a visit to his father, William Logan of Stenton, was on his way to Edinburgh to resume his medical studies.

4. Samuel Emlen, a Philadelphia Quaker minister beloved by the Fothergills, was "a little man, in person homely to the extreme, of great vivacity and pleasing manner." — Ms. recollections of James Jenkins, LSFL.

5. Gilbert Thompson III (1728–1803) had served as an usher in the family school at Penketh before studying medicine in Edinburgh. Attempting to enter practice in London after receiving his degree, he was too diffident to win the confidence of patients and suddenly surprised all who knew him by taking a position as writing master at a boarding school in Tottenham. He later worked as a "dispensing assistant" in the Bevans' apothecary establishment, until a bequest from his uncle, Gilbert II, of Penketh, encouraged him to try to re-enter practice about 1768. — Nicholas Hans, *New Trends in Education of the Eighteenth Century* (London: Routledge and Kegan Paul, 1951), 116; *Munk's Roll*, II, 290; Fox, 127–128.

To Thomas Penn (?) , 4 February 1768

[Harpur Street,] 4 February [1768]

My worthy Friend,

I have repeatedly perused and considered Dr. Morgan's letter with all possible attention.[1] I have always wished that Philadelphians might take the lead in the profession of Physick, and that it might become the first School in America. It enjoys some natural advantages; its climate is less intemperate, either in respect to heats and colds, than its neighbours. A very hot or very cold country are alike unfavorable to study. It enjoys some artificial advantages. Great freedom and unshackled by narrow prejudices, sentiments of benevolence to all mankind and there is greater perfection than (in most) other Countries. And this is the Air which Science breathes to most advantage. The Hospital, the Academy, the diligence of the Professors of Medicine in that city are daily gaining reputation. Every reasonable encouragement ought certainly to be given them, consistent with the state of the Colony.

I think, however, that application for a Charter is rather too early. I know not that it would be useful for the promotion of Medicine. The skillful physicians will always be found out. And the unskillful deserted, however he may be enveloped with external dignities. Besides it does not appear that they are unanimous with this request. There are many able practitioners in Philadelphia whose names are not on the list. Unanimity is necessary for such an institution. There is a College of Physicians at Edinburgh, at Paris, in London and other places. Experience does not prove they have been of much utility. The pretence of founding these Societies was to countenance and support the regular physician; to suppress quackery. But the effect has generally ended in a sort of monopoly. A few have got into the management of these Societies who have generally found means in order to raise themselves and lay others, not less knowing, able or honest, under great difficulties. All the advantages of a Medical Society may be obtained without a Charter. There has been one in London several years, unconnected with the College,[2] that has communicated more useful knowledge to the world than the College have done in their corporate capacity since the time of their first foundation.

I should, therefore, think it more prudent to delay the grant for a Charter for a College of Physicians in Philadelphia till some stronger reasons occur to make it necessary.[3] They have full scope to render themselves the first School of Physic on the continent, if they continue their diligence and make proper use of the opportunities afforded them; and more I think is not necessary. If we reflect but a moment on the jealous temper that has been raised in this country against America, and is now most unhappily propagated with success, we cannot suppose that a transaction of this kond will pass unnoticed.

I seized the first piece of paper that fell in my way, and find I have made a very bad choice — it is sullied and torn, but I have not time to transcribe it. Excuse it therefore, as well as the liberty I have taken in giving my opinion against my friend's proposal. I endeavour to judge from experience, and my friend from hope. At the same time I wish most sincerely the advancement of physical knowledge on which physical dignity depends. I have very little affection for its happenings, as I think they are made use of more to the benefits of individuals than of mankind in general.

As these are my present sentiments, grounded so far as I know on impartial considerations, I have no objections to their being communicated to those who are engaged in this affair, should it be conducive to obtaining farther lights than theirs. If I know anything, it is I shall

wish well to my profession in general and to Philadelphia in particular.
I am, with much respect,

Thy assured Friend

This letter is published here for the first time by courtesy of Walton B. McDaniel,
2d, Curator of Historical Documents, College of Physicians, Philadelphia. It is a copy
in an eighteenth century hand, unaddressed, insufficiently dated, and without signature. The original letter, now lost, was evidently written by a physician in London
to another Londoner, not a doctor, but a person well informed about Philadelphia.
From its content and phraseology, the letter may safely be attributed to Dr. Fothergill.
It may be assumed that he is writing to Thomas Penn, eldest son of William Penn
and head of the proprietary family.

1. Dr. Morgan's letter to which this letter refers cannot now be found.
2. "About the year 1752, several physicians in London," among whom Dr. Fothergill was a leader, "formed a Medical Society for collecting and publishing . . .
observations and enquiries that . . . deserve the public notice." — *Works*, ed. Lettsom, II, 376. This was the society that issued *Medical Observations and Inquiries*.
3. Philadelphia physicians had to wait almost twenty years for the establishment
of a College of Physicians. On 1 February 1787, *The Pennsylvania Packet* announced
the founding of Philadelphia's College of Physicians by twenty-nine prominent doctors. Among these charter members, Dr. William Shippen, Jr., Dr. John Morgan, and
Dr. Benjamin Rush, whom Dr. Fothergill had encouraged and counseled in their
youth, received special mention as professors in the medical department of the College
of Philadelphia.

To Dr. William Hunter, London, 11 May 1768

Harpur Street, 11th Inst.

Dear Doctor. — [1]

I am greatly obliged by thy kind, discreet and effectual application to
Lord H———.[2] I am not less so to that worthy Nobleman for the part he
takes in this affair. It may perhaps never be in my power to make proper
acknowledgments to either of you for even the inclination of serving me.

I have directed the proper inquiries to be made respecting Dr. Saunders' connections,[3] and will send them the moment they come to hand.
Be kind enough to favor me with a list of the Governors, and if there
are any amongst them to whom I can apply, I will do it with pleasure.
It is my duty, and I am sure it is my wish to deserve Dr. Hunter's
friendship.

It may perhaps be proper to acquaint Dr. Demainbray [4] that the corals
are just as they came out of the sea. They may be easily cleaned by

281

putting them in warm water just acidulated with spirit of sea salt,[5] and then again washing them in fresh warm water. When dry they may be fixed on small suitable pedestals, and either put up in a glass case to secure them from dust, or placed up and down the museum, covered with glass bells. Some are reserved for Dr. Hunter's Museum [6] when it is ready to receive them. At present they may lie where they are as safely as amidst a thousand Hobgoblins, nightly searching for their scattered remains.

Pray, dear Doctor, will it be practicable for Lord H——— to dismiss me with any decency from the Stage? [7] I am brought there to say nothing but what is proper, but to say it and appear in a ridiculous manner. Is not this as great an insult upon me, and even upon any character that is opposite to vice and folly, as can be offered? Buffoonery should only be let loose to prey on these, not to render their opposites in any degree contemptible. If through weakness or indiscretion I slide into mistakes, I bear most patiently the just chastisement, whether public or private. But in this instance I am doubly hurt. I am held up to the whole town to laugh at, and the people with whom I am connected, likewise. Nor does the Faculty [8] in general derive much benefit from the contempt thrown on an individual — though individuals of the Faculty may rejoice at it.

I am Dr. Hunter's obliged respectful Friend,

J. Fothergill

Ms. autograph letter, Hunter-Baillie Mss., I (2), 33, Royal College of Surgeons, London. Dated through internal evidence.

1. William Hunter (1718–1783), M.D., F.R.S., anatomist and obstetrician, had been appointed Physician Extraordinary to Queen Charlotte in 1764. — See *Munk's Roll*, II, 205–207.

2. The Earl of Hertford. In his capacity as Lord Chamberlain, Hertford controlled the licensing of London's dramatic performances. Evidently Dr. Fothergill had been soliciting Dr. Hunter's help to influence Lord Hertford to suppress a certain play appearing at this time on the London stage. (See note 6, below.)

3. William Saunders (1743–1817), who had received his medical degree at Edinburgh in 1765, like Hunter had been a pupil of Dr. William Cullen. He set up practice in London. Joining Sir George Baker in studies of Devonshire colic, he distinguished himself by proficiency in chemistry. In 1769 he was admitted licentiate of the Royal College of Physicians, and in 1770 received appointment to the staff of Guy's Hospital. Twenty years later, during Sir George Baker's presidency of the Royal College of Physicians, Saunders was admitted Fellow, *specialia gratia*, and thereafter served the Royal College frequently as Censor. In 1792 he was the Gulstonian lecturer, and in 1796, Harveian orator. In 1807 he was appointed physician-extraordinarius to the Prince Regent. — *Munk's Roll*, II, 399–401.

4. Dr. Stephen Charles Triboudet Demainbray, F.R.S. (1701–1782), in 1754 had been appointed tutor to the Prince of Wales and after his pupil's accession to the throne continued in service as tutor to Queen Charlotte. In 1768, when an astronomical observatory was erected at Kew, the royal couple's favorite resort, Demainbray was appointed astronomer in charge, and remained at Kew the rest of his life. — Hans, *Trends in Education*, 145.

5. Hydrochloric acid; variously called earlier "muriatic acid," "spirit of sea water," and "chlorohydric acid."

5. These corals, some shells, coins, and curios, and no doubt botanical books were purchased by Dr. Hunter after Dr. Fothergill's death and form a part of Dr. Hunter's bequest to the University of Glasgow, where they may still be seen in the Hunterian Museum. — S. Peter Dance, *Shell Collecting: An Illustrated History* (London: Faber and Faber, 1966), 38, 110–111, 139.

6. Samuel Foote's play, *The Devil upon Two Sticks*, set London laughing in the spring of 1768. In the autumn of 1767, disgruntled licentiates assisted by hired ruffians had broken through the gates into the forecourt of the Royal College of Physicians in Warwick Lane and plunged into the building where the Comitia majora was holding session, demanding redress from restrictions they considered unjust. In the play, burlesquing the episode, scenes of violence were depicted uproariously. Dr. Melchisedech Broadbrim, in Quaker garb of gray and wearing his broadbrimmed hat, made sanctimonious, long-winded pleas for peace in affected, inflated language. Sir William Brown, President at this time of the Royal College, was pictured to the life as a little, round, well-fed gentleman, an open volume of Horace in one hand, a "spying glass" dangling on its ribbon from his buttonhole, trying vainly to retain his dignity. Two little apothecaries dancing about and claiming recognition provided additional comedy. The curtain went down with problems still unsolved. Reviews of this play recorded a full house every evening for many weeks. The performance was considered by critics a triumph of humor. Foote himself took three minor roles in the production, perhaps caricaturing himself in the title of the play: he had hobbled about with sticks ever since he had lost a leg in an accident.

Dr. Fothergill felt that in ridiculing him Foote had ridiculed the customs of the entire Quaker sect. — William Cook, *Memoirs of Samuel Foote, Esq.*, 3 vols. (London: R. Phillips, 1805), I, 139–144; John Genest, *History of the English Stage*, 10 vols. (Bath, Eng.: H. E. Carrington, 1832), V, 212, 213; Lloyd G. Stevenson, "The Siege of Warwick Lane," *Journal of the History of Medicine and Allied Sciences*, 8 (1952): 105–122; B. C. Corner, "Dr. Melchisedech Broadbrim and the Playwright," *ibid.*, 122–135.

8. The medical profession.

To James Pemberton, Philadelphia, 16 September 1768

Lea Hall, near Middlewich, Cheshire 16.9.1768

Esteemed Friend,

If my leisure was equal to my inclination I should more frequently pay thee and my friends in America more frequent literary visits. But my employment being of such a nature that I must do everything myself, I am often obliged to put those things last which I would willingly execute in the first place.

As soon as I received the request of the Managers of your Hospital, I immediately set to work in conjunction with Timothy Bevan [1] to inquire for a proper person to serve them as an apothecary. But we were soon informed that a person had shipped himself from Bristol for your Province on that account,[2] so that we desisted from any farther inquiries, and expect you are served to your satisfaction.

I write this from an obscure place in Cheshire, above 150 miles from London, to which place my sister and myself have retired for a few summers past for about a couple of months, in order to get some little strength both of body and mind to enable us the better to discharge our duties. Hither I bring down a great cargo of letters; but by the time I am a little recruited, letters follow me from home so fast as to leave me but little time to pay any debts to my absent Friends.

Just before we set out, our Friend John Hunt arrived in London. We saw him once or twice; he gave us to understand that he was not determined to return to America, but I hear he is now making preparations for a speedy departure; perhaps we may see him no more, though we hope to be in London in a little more than a week. I have loved and esteemed him much; and it costs me great pain to lose a Friend, and more so when I am in doubt whether or not he is pursuing his own real interest.[3] I dare not sit in judgement or decide upon this occasion. I know, however, it would afflict me much to hear anything but well of him in one respect as well as another. There are wise and weighty counsellors among you, and if ever he should undertake anything that might to them seem hazardous, I most fervently wish he may have an ear to hear, as I do for myself, should any bewildering prospects ever present themselves in an unguarded hour.

Though I am not able to furnish thee with a hint that can avail to the service of America, yet I cannot forbear devoting a part of the paper to that subject; to complain allows some ease to a mind not at ease; and less I cannot do, as I think both you and we are in a situation so critical, that I see nothing but the interposition of divine Providence that can prevent us both from suffering deeply. I speak of Great Britain and America, but write as an Englishman who knows no difference between their mutual interests. What one loses both lose; and what they lose, their enemies gain. What then must we think of those writers and those people in high situations, who are endeavouring both by word and conduct, are sowing the seeds of distrust between them, and precipitately hurrying the weak and inconsiderate of both sides the water into open violence and hostilities never to be forgotten. In my opinion the Americans have right sentiments, but act wrong in the present crisis. The zeal of the Boston men has outrun their discretion.[4] They are not to be vindicated, and if they should push matters to extremities, they must be chargeable with the fatal consequences. The taxes you complain of are unjustly laid upon you. But is open force the way, the proper way to redress? By no means. I believe I am not mistaken when I say that not one half of this nation knew what country their American brethren sprung from, what language they spoke, whether they were black or white, till the affair of the Stamp Act. I don't speak of the lower orders; I question if numbers in the legislature had much clearer ideas. They knew not your relation to us. They judged of you as conquered enemies, or as people revolted from legal Government. The majority of the nation are not perhaps yet much better enlightened, and it will require a long time to erase ill-grounded opinions, and plant better in their place. Those who took your part could not then be heard or scarcely can be at this time, but when the Americans talk of resistance, the whole spirit of John Bull is raised; and if it was his only brother, and by whose benevolence he subsisted, pride and passion would carry him headlong into battle and to violence. This is the temper not only of the mob but their superiors, and we have so many ignorant, inflammatory writers as to keep up this spirit to its full extent in the proportion as fools and knaves exceed wise men in point of numbers. What part your Province will have taken in this coalition I know not. But I do know what I wish; — that you may have stood singly on your own foundation. I would by no means wish that you should silently submit to the impositions in question. Submit, but remonstrate with decency and firmness. Have no glance to the conduct of other colonies. And be not hasty in remonstrating. The conduct of Boston by soliciting the aid of other Provinces has given great disgust, without necessity. They might have obtained their rights by prudent application. They have raised prejudices everywhere against them, and as they have intimated resistance, I should not wonder if they are put to a bitter trial — and all America suffer for their intemperate zeal.

Don't apprehend I am condemning their cause. I have often placed myself in your condition and sincerely wish our legislature had done so likewise. The legislative power in each province, in conjunction with the King's representative only, have the right of raising money. Great Britain has authority to say you shall not hurt us absolutely; you shall help us when we need it, but the measure of this help shall be in just proportion to your abilities, and of this we leave the Colonies and the King's representative to judge. — I have gone thus far only to show that I am with you from principle, but disclaim all violent conduct or opposition to the Mother Country till — oppression without prospect of redress — but this is not your case yet. Soft language, conduct not servile, patience repeated, prudent applications will make those your friends who now through pride and ignorance are your enemies, and will enable such who would serve you from just principles to do it efficaciously. I can scarce acquit myslf of vanity in presuming to throw out hints of this nature to a person who must be more enlightened on these subjects than I am; but by dividing one's grief it seems to be lessened.

I took the liberty to urge your agent B. Franklin to stay here another winter. Much time will be spent on affairs of election this session; but America will nevertheless engross the attention of the public. I already perceive a spirit of bitterness against you prevails through most ranks except the Merchants and the wiser mechanics. Country Gentlemen are almost totally against you, full, as I said before, of the spirit of John Bull. It has fallen in my way to see more of this than I can easily describe in a short compass. I, therefore, thought it was right, necessary that a person so able and so willing to serve you should be upon the spot to render America and its friends all possible assistance, and all, I fear, will be too little.

Should the present Ministry[5] continue in power, there seems little reason to doubt but they will go on enforcing; that a better will succeed is not likely; for as the more able are apprised that they probably may be obliged to pursue measures not quite to their own satisfaction, they generally decline the service of Government. Nor can I blame them. Time may however come when the assistance of such will be necessary and admitted. I am sure that no man can wish more ardently for the happiness of his friend than our Sovereign does for satisfaction of all his subjects. But be these things to ourselves. It fell in my way to have it hinted above, that the Province of Pennsylvania has declined engaging in the Boston resolves, that though you thought your liberties were attacked, yet you chose not violence, or cabal, or resentment to be your advocate; that you would think it expedient as well as other colonies to apply for redress, yet you did not mean to do this in a manner that should embarrass Government, or show resentment to your Mother Country. I hope I was not too officious.

Our summer has been unusually wet and tempestuous. We have had more thunder and lightning, more men and beasts destroyed by it, more destructive floods in almost every corner of Great Britain at different times than has ever been recorded. Much corn, hay, and cattle have been swept off in many places. The harvest very precarious, and the quantity of grain rather moderate than plentiful. I believe we must always for the future be your customers for grain. I scarce expect that this country will be able to spare much to its neighbors, perhaps not have always sufficient for itself. The vast number of horses bred here and kept for use and show eat up the whole country. The winter before this last I was informed that not less than seven thousand quarts of oats per week were consumed in the whole nation! We are going fast with inland navigation. This in time will force out incredible numbers of draught horses, but others will be multiplied in proportion. I expect everybody will ride.

I return my grateful acknowledgement to the Managers of the Pennsylvania Hospital for admitting me amongst them.[6] Perhaps it may not be so much in my power as I wish to serve them, but they will always have my good wishes.

Remember me kindly to thy Brother Israel and his wife, to J. Churchman and William Brown. I could fill up my paper with the names of Friends whom I love and esteem. My Brother Samuel was with us a few days ago, likewise thy valuable countryman Samuel Emlen who was well and is daily growing in wisdom and simplicity. We are not far from my Brother's neighborhood. He now and then sees us and helps to sharpen our faces, as a man does his friends. Thou will see that I write to thyself in general. There are passages that should not go farther, and I trust thy discretion. My sister is well, and joins me in kind respects to thy whole family.

I am, thy affectionate Friend,

John Fothergill

Ms. autograph letter, Pemberton Papers, Etting Collection, II, 58, HSP.

1. "Timothy Bevan and Sons, Druggists and Chymists" succeeded to the manage-

ment of the Bevan firm in 1766. The Pennsylvania Hospital received most of its drugs from this source. — Raistrick, 283, 284; frequent entries in the Pennsylvania Hospital Minute Books.

2. The Managers of the Pennsylvania Hospital paid the passage of Robert Slade of Bristol, England, who came to assume the duties of steward and apothecary, beginning work 30 May 1768. He died unexpectedly on 14 June 1769 and was buried in St. Peter's churchyard. — Morton and Woodbury, *Pennsylvania Hospital*, 528, 529.

3. John Hunt frequently took risks that were unwarranted. He suffered a succession of reverses in the tobacco trade just at the time when he was recalled to London by the death of his wife.

4. On 28 October 1767, protesting the Townshend duties of that year, the Boston Town Meeting had passed a resolution against the importation and use of British goods. Early in 1768, the Massachusetts Assembly had sent a petition to the King urging repeal of the obnoxious acts, and in a circular letter to the Assemblies of the other colonies suggested that they do likewise. In June, the seizure of John Hancock's sloop *Liberty* for illegal entry provoked a riot, and later that month, after Lord Hillsborough, the new Secretary for the Colonies, had ordered that the Massachusetts Assembly rescind its circular letter or be dissolved, that body by a vote of 92 to 17 refused to rescind. Meanwhile, in March the Philadelphia merchants, sympathizing with their fellows in Massachusetts, had resolved that the taxes imposed by Parliament constituted an invasion of American rights; but they did not subscribe to the nonimportation agreement, and in May the Pennsylvania Assembly, when the Massachusetts circular letter was laid before it, took no action upon it. — Justin Winsor, *Memorial History of Boston* (Boston, 1881), III, 22–23; *The Barrington-Bernard Correspondence*, edited by Edward Channing and A. C. Coolidge (Cambridge, Mass., 1912), 162–163; Theodore Thayer, *Pennsylvania Politics and the Growth of Democracy, 1740–1776* (Harrisburg, 1953), 142, 143.

5. The Duke of Grafton's (1767–1770).

6. Appointment of Dr. John Fothergill to the Board of Managers of the Pennsylvania Hospital was seemly recognition of his many valuable services to this institution. In 1771 he was also appointed to "the Corporate Body of the New York Hospital" when a large association was formed to raise funds "to erect an Hospital for the relief of sick and distressed persons . . . which shall forever after be called The New York Hospital." Correspondence between the Governors of the Hospital cannot now be found, but Dr. David Hosack of New York states in a lecture of 1811 that "through the influence of Dr. John Fothergill and Sir William Duncan, contributions were made by many of the inhabitants of London and other parts of Great Britain." — Information by courtesy of Dr. Stanhope Bayne-Jones of Washington, D.C., formerly President of the New York Hospital–Cornell Medical Center; David Hosack, M.D., "A Sketch of the Origin and Progress of the Medical Schools of New York and Philadelphia," *American and Philosophical Register* (New York) 2 (1812): 225–236.

To John Bartram, Philadelphia, 29 October 1768

London, 29.10.1768

Respected Friend,

The loss which we have both sustained by the death of our late very valuable Friend Peter Collinson [1] is the principal occasion of my writing to thee at this time. I must in the first place however acknowledge myself indebted to thee for a box of very curious plants which I received some time ago, and which are most of them prosperous, and all of them would have been so had my gardener taken the care of them he ought for they came in a very prosperous condition. The Pittsburgh Iris [2] I lost, and indeed I ought not to think of increasing my collection for my leisure to attend to it seems to lessen every day — for on one account or another so many people seem to have claims to my assistance that I have less leisure than ever. However I keep a garden still and have an able young natural gardener to take care of it, and though I see it not once a week now, yet when I do see it, it is always with so much satisfaction that I cannot relinquish it but live in hopes of enjoying it one time or another.

I could have wished to offer thee my services in lieu of our deceased Friend, but foresee that I cannot be half so punctual or useful a correspondent. But if in anything I can assist, for his sake as well as thy own, let me know and I will do everything I can.

I called upon my Friend one morning this summer, when he showed me some exquisite drawings of thy son's. [3] He proposed that I should engage thy son to make drawings of all your land tortoises. I wish he would be kind enough to undertake this for me, and at the same time to make some short notes, with respect to their natural history, way of life, places of abode, generation and whatever occurs to him. Twenty guineas was mentioned but I will not restrict him to this sum. Let him take his own time. Send me a drawing or two as time and opportunities offer. If he has been able to divide them into classes or fit proper names, he will be kind enough to mark them, and I'll either pay what he requires, as he may have occasion for it here, or remit it together as he chooses.

I shall be glad likewise to make thee any acknowledgement thou pleases, for any curious plants that may occur to thee. I think it would be a great advantage if thou was to sow a considerable part of most of the seeds thou collects, I mean the new discovered plants, in a little

289

garden at home, and to send over young plants of two years old in boxes, several sorts of plants in one box. Many seeds wholly miscarry with us. The young plants would always find a good market. Seeds might be sent likewise, but young plants I think would be better. I should be glad of a collection of your American Martagons.[4] It has happened that I have seen but a few. Would it not be practicable to send over a root or two of the Colocasia [5] in autumn in a tub of mud or in wet moss? The seeds mostly germinate but the plant perishes, at least all that I have made trial of. I shall be glad to hear from thee when convenient. Direct to me in Harpur Street, near Red Lion Square, London. Anything sent to me to the care of Daniel Mildred, Merchant, will come safe. Let me know what kind of return and how I shall repay thee for thy trouble, and I shall gladly repay. I propose if time permits to give some little account of our deceased Friend in some of our public prints;[6] if I do I shall send one for thyself.

Accept my kind acknowledgement for thy kind present, and believe me to be

Thy very respectful Friend,
John Fothergill

Ms. autograph letter, Gratz Collection (European Physicians), Case 12, Box 20, HSP.

1. On 11 August 1768, at the age of seventy-four.

2. A species found near Pittsburgh, Pennsylvania.

3. On 18 July 1768. Collinson had written to John Bartram from Mill Hill, 28 May 1766: "Billy's elegant drawings are admired by all that see them . . . Mr. Ehret, our famous flower painter, was with me, and I showed him Billy's paintings. He admired, as we all do, his fine Red Centaury; a most elegant plant, if we can but get it in our gardens. His butterflies are Nature itself. His yellow fly is admirable." — Darlington, *Memorials*, 280, 296, 300–301.

4. The Turk's-cap lily — *Lilium martagon* — so-called because of fancied resemblance to the turban worn by Sultan Mohammed I. Another variety is the Scarlet Turk's-cap, *Lilium chalcedonium*; both are known in England today.

5. *Nelumbo lutea* (Willd.) Pers. "Among the earlier drawings [by William Bartram] shown to Fothergill and acquired by him was that of the water chinquapin or American Lotus, *Nelumbo lutea*, miscalled *Colocasia* from its resemblance to an Asiatic plant." — Joseph Ewan in *William Bartram: Botanical and Zoological Drawings, 1756–1788* (Philadelphia: American Philosophical Society, 1968), 60. Peter Collinson had repeatedly asked John Bartram to send him this plant, but as early as 1760 Bartram wrote: "It will be very difficult to send the roots; they are as brittle as glass, and run two or three feet deep in the mud." In February 1768, when William Bartram's drawing reached Collinson, he was delighted with the "inimitable picture" and wrote to John Bartram: "So great was the deception, it being candle-light, that we disputed for some time whether it was a drawing or an engraving. It is really a

noble piece of pencil-work . . . My ingenious friend . . . has amply gratified my wishes to see the *Colocasia*, and I desire no more." — Darlington, *Memorials*, 227, 296, 297.

6. Dr. Fothergill's final tribute to this friend was *Some Account of the Late Peter Collinson, Fellow of the Royal Society* . . . (London, 1770), a biographical memoir, handsomely published in a slim octavo edition, embellished with a full-page engraving.

To Samuel Fothergill, Warrington, Lancashire, 6 December 1768

London, 6.12.1768

Dear Brother,

We can only acknowledge thy kind attention to us in giving us such frequent intimations of thy health; to help it at present seems scarcely in my power. It was prudent to leave Buxton.[1] A longer stay there would have been of no advantage but much discomfort to thyself. Nor can I advise thee at any time to go thither under doubtful circumstances of health. These kind of remedies are more fit to establish good health than to recover it. I could wish thou would not be too solicitous about exercise. When the gouty pains are in any degree present, riding rather aggravates them, and it is difficult to avoid taking some cold. I think it is always best to let the gouty matter spend itself, taking care to avoid such things, both in quantity and kind, experience has taught us to be injurious.

Perhaps it may be worth a trial to take constantly every morning one or two tablespoonfuls of the Baume de Vie,[2] just enough to give a motion the day following. Take the whey and hartshorn as constantly, at bedtime, and be uniformly consistent in diet and liquors. When well, make it a rule to drink no wine before dinner, nor between meals, nor any other fermented liquors, I know the pernicious custom of the country in many places is to bring out these things and urge their acceptance as a test of friendship, but it is a bad one. I don't say this as in any way doubting thy care in this respect, but to strengthen thy hands against imprudent importunity.

Write to S. Emlen, and acquaint him that I received his kind letter from Buxton, and wish he could give the waters so far a trial as they agree with him. His prudent, circumspect feeling will soon give him notice what he may expect from them. I would not wish him to stay there longer than just to be acquainted with their effects, and if these are favorable, leave the place as soon as he will, and return to them at some other opportunity, if such should offer.

I have been twice today at Clapham, twice in the city from end to end, and had not a moment's respite from intense thought the whole day but when I got a little obstructed in passing through a crowd from place to place. Make, therefore, every allowance for me that thou canst. I do this because it seems unavoidable. I have no reason to doubt but that what is best will follow, if I am happy enough to look for it.

Dr. Russell is no more.[3] And on 7th day last, I was sent for in a great hurry to Clapham to see our Friend Capel Hanbury who, from being quite well, was suddenly seized with a stroke of the palsy on his expressive faculty. He knows everybody, has the power of sense and motion, but expresses himself very imperfectly. This is the effect of a most uniform intense application of a capacity inferior to few. I think there seems no immediate danger in respect to his life, but I much doubt his recovery to that clearness he has hitherto possessed.[4]

I accept this as another hint to necessary care respecting myself, and labor to abandon any pursuit that is not conducive to the purpose for which we ought to live. One friend, another companion, a third acquaintance — able, sensible, affectionate — all gliding from my sight! What have I lost within this year! — Through favor, we are well. — Don't let this make thee melancholy. Let it cheer thee that the Brother whom thou loves, hates not instruction.

Farewell, and tell us thou art better when thou canst.

J. Fothergill.

Ms. autograph letter, Crosfield Mss. 73, LSFL

1. Muirhead's *England* still cautions visitors that Buxton's powerful waters should be used only upon the advice of a physician.

2. Literally "balsam of life," compound tincture of aloes.

3. Alexander Russel(l), with his fellow students William Cuming and George Cleghorn, had been a founder of a students' medical society at the University of Edinburgh. John Fothergill was invited to join this society soon after entering the University, and maintained friendship with each of these men throughout life. In 1740 Russell became medical officer to an English "factory" of merchants in Turkey and for fifteen years he served "Franks, Greeks, Armenians, Jews and Turks." He took advantage of his opportunities to study regional diseases, climate, and natural history, and Dr. Fothergill, his constant correspondent, urged him to put the results into a book. Russell's *Natural History of Aleppo* was published in London in 1756,

the year after his return to England. The book won instant success and a Dutch edition appeared in 1762. Dr. Russell settled in London after obtaining an M.D. degree from Glasgow in 1760. He died suddenly of "a putrid fever" in November 1768. A memoir by Dr. Fothergill, read at a meeting of the Society of Physicians in October 1769, appears in *Works*, ed. Lettsom, II, 361–379.

4. Capel Hanbury of Mark Lane died on 9 June 1769. — *Gentleman's Magazine*, 39:319 (1769).

To Susanna Fothergill, Warrington, Lancashire, 26 January 1769

London, 26.1.1769

Dear Sister,

Just to save my Brother the labour of writing, I take pen in hand to acquaint thee that he is well. He has entered the service he came up for, and I trust with satisfaction to himself and to the objects of his mission. He finds nothing to induce him to think that Friends in general do not both open their doors and their hearts to the visit, and a more acceptable companion could not perhaps have been found than Samuel Emlen.[1]

We have both been labouring pretty hard in our different vocations, but as I think his of much greater moment than my own, I should readily bring his Cloak from Troas.[2]

Do not think because I write he is not able or not willing to do it — he is both one and the other; but I thought it an agreeable employment just to let thee see thou art not forgotten by us, nor that my Brother and ourselves are forgetful of thee, though under a multiplicity of engagements.

My chief solicitude is that my Brother may not be more in haste than he ought. I love diligence, but there is such a thing as being too eager and earnest. My Brother is smoking his pipe[3] and little suspects to whom I am writing, but I know when I give it to him to read, he will not be dissatisfied, but will join with Sister, Nanny[4] and myself in cordial salutations from

Thy affectionate Brother
John Fothergill

Crosfield Mss. 74, LSFL.

1. At this time Samuel Emlen and Samuel Fothergill were holding a series of meetings in the homes of well-to-do London Friends, hoping to reawaken them to

active religious concern and to gain the interest of younger people. Some other highly placed dissenters occasionally attended these meetings, among them Selina, Countess of Huntingdon, and Lord Dartmouth. — Woolman, *Journal*, ed. Gummere, 321; records of 1769, Society of Friends, LSFL.

    2. A Biblical reference: "The cloak that I left at Troas with Carpus, when thou comest bring with thee and the books, but especially the parchments" (II Timothy 4: 11).

    3. Indulgence unusual in the eighteenth century for a Quaker minister.

    4. Ann Fothergill, daughter of their brother Joseph. — Fothergill Genealogy, below.

To William Huddesford, the University of Oxford, 5 April 1769

Harpur Street, London
5th Inst.

Respected Friend — [1]

If I had not been interrupted by many unexpected engagements, I should certainly have assured thee by letter of the papers being sent.

All Dr. Lister's papers [2] I bought at an auction about seven years ago. They had been thrown aside in the dust as wastepaper; and very likely if I had not purchased them, they would long since have been annihilated in the pastry-cook's oven.

Dr. Lhuyd's letters [3] I purchased from Dr. Costa; [4] at least I accepted them as payment for a large debt. My views in securing both these parcels of papers were some amusement and enjoyment for myself; some benefit for the publick.

The very active scene I am engaged in, and perhaps may continue in, if health prevails for some time longer, gives me no prospect of the first; and it would be injustice to the publick I wish to serve to detain a treasure in my hands that I cannot enjoy, merely on speculation that I may enjoy it in some future period. — Should I ever have leisure, and wish to peruse any of these papers, I would only desire that upon giving proper assurances that they shall be returned to the College, I may have a sight of them. Whatever use may be made besides, I am sure there is one important lesson that this frivolous Age might learn from them (if the time of learning is not already passed): that the greatest men of the past Century derive their credit from that firmest of all foundations — Virtue. In this term I include Piety, Benevolence and Industry.

What do we not owe, in respect to Natural History to the great Persons whose names appear in this collection.

By making this little present to the University, I seem to have raised myself into some little consequence in my own opinion, and permit me to make use of it in recommending an Edition of Lister worthy of the Author. Let the plates be retouched from as many originals as can be secured. You have some shells, no doubt, in the Museum at Oxford. Procure an able engraver to compare the plates with the originals, and amend them when necessary. When your own treasure is exhausted, come up to this place and get all the aids you can. You will find some if not all you hope for. I would bespeak a copy for myself; and if it is to be published by subscription, put me down for a copy — or more than one, if the subscriptions fall short.

I have kept back one of Lister's pieces. It is a collection of many (not all) of the drawings of the Land Snails; they are coarsely done but expressive. This shall also be sent, if wanted.

I could wish to enlist myself in the number of thy correspondents, was my time my own; I should receive much information from it. I owe much to the publick favour; and though I would not be their slave, yet I would rather wish when I die, they were in my debt rather than I in theirs.

Excuse the manner of my address; I can offer one reason that may plead for me. The sons of Jonadab [5] were recommended for adhering to their father's injunction to abstain from wine and other things seemingly of an indifferent nature. I mean no affront, but to keep myself blameless to myself.

Farewell, and believe me to be thy friend and well wisher

J. Fothergill

Ms. autograph letter, Ashmole Mss., no. 1822, ff. 225–226, Bodleian Library, Oxford. Month and year added in another hand.

1. William Huddesford (1732–1772), Oxford B.A. 1753, M.A. 1756; B.D. 1757, had been Keeper of the Ashmolean Museum at Oxford since 1765. Although he had a living at Bishop's Tachbrooke, Warwickshire, he probably resided in Oxford, where his father, Sir George Huddesford, was President of Trinity College. — University Records, Oxford.

2. Martin Lister (ca. 1638–1712), physician, scientist, and writer, Fellow of St. John's College, Cambridge, had studied also at Montpellier where acquaintance with the Cambridge University naturalist John Ray had greatly stimulated his career. He was elected a Fellow of the Royal Society in 1671. His important tract on spiders, considered by many his most important contribution, together with one on mollusks

and another on shells, was published in *Historiae Animalium Angliae Tres Tractatus* in 1678. In 1683 he received the M.D. degree from Oxford; he had set up practice in York at an earlier date. His *Historiae Conchyliorum* of 1685–92 was a compendium of knowledge, splendidly illustrated with 1,000 drawings reputed to be the work of his gifted wife and their daughter. About the time of its publication, he had moved to London, where he soon attracted a fashionable practice. In 1687 he was elected Fellow of the Royal College of Physicians, and in 1709 he was appointed household physician to Queen Anne. — Raven, 138–140; *Munk's Roll*, I, 442–445.

3. Edward Lhuyd (1660–1709) — the name is variously spelled — a Welshman enrolled in Jesus College, Oxford, left his studies to become under-keeper of the Ashmolean Museum. He succeeded Dr. Robert Plot as Keeper in 1691, and served in that position until his death. When a translation of William Camden's *Britannia* was planned by Bishop Gibson in 1688, Lhuyd undertook to collect materials for it in Wales; after its publication, in 1695, he projected a monumental work of his own, never fully completed, on the geography and natural history of Wales. Sir Hans Sloane, Sir Isaac Newton, and others raised funds for the publication in 1699 of 120 copies of Lhuyd's *Lithophylacii Britannici ichnographia*, a catalogue of the figured fossils in the Ashmolean Museum. Lhuyd's scholarship was recognized by an honorary M.A. from Oxford in 1701; in 1707 the first volume of his projected *Archaeologia Britannica* was published, and in 1708 he was elected Fellow of the Royal Society. After his death, his valuable papers and documents were widely scattered until Emanuel de Costa rescued them. Huddesford brought out a revised edition of Lhuyd's *Lithophylacii Britannici ichnographia* in 1760. — Raven, 435; R. T. Gunther, *Life and Letters of Edward Lhwyd*, vol. XIV of *Early Science in Oxford* (Oxford: printed for the subscribers, 1945).

4. Emanuel Mendes da Costa, F.R.S., was both a scholar and a spendthrift. He could not resist buying valuable books which he wanted to own. Dr. Fothergill had helped him to get a position at the Royal Society, where he worked in the library and rendered some secretarial assistance. Nevertheless, Da Costa was at least once sent to prison because of complaints by creditors. He was the author of two books, *Elements of Conchology* (London, 1776) and *Historia naturalis Testaceorum Britanniae, or the British Conchology* (1778) both largely derivative, both published through Dr. Fothergill's generosity. A number of letters between Da Costa and Huddesford appear in John Nichols, *Illustrations of the Literary History of the Eighteenth Century*, IV (1882), 456–478 *passim*. See also Fox, 210.

5. A Biblical reference: Jeremiah 35:5–10, 18, 19. The reason for introducing this reference is puzzling since Dr. Fothergill had ordered a stock of good red mountain wine and a quantity of brandy to be conveyed to Lea Hall. Among William Huddesford's personal papers in Oxford, some amusing verses have been found entitled "A Parody on Plato's Soliloquys, occasioned by being sick with drinking Punch overnight at Oxford . . . and reading Dr. Cheyne's Essay on Melancholy in the morning." It seems unlikely, however, that Dr. Fothergill had ever seen or heard of Huddesford's verses though he might well have recognized the allusion to Dr. George Cheyne (1671–1743), who, according to the *Concise Dictionary of National Biography*, "published treatises on diet and natural theology."

To Samuel Fothergill, Warrington, Lancashire, 6 April 1769

London, 6.4.1769

Dear Brother,

It is very seldom that I have a letter before me when I return an answer to it. When I read one, I commonly engraft in my thoughts the answer that occurs to me, and this is sometimes so fixed in my imagination that I think I have answered letters in reality when they have only been returned in ideas. For once, however, I will leave my common idle [role] and endeavor to take notice of the several parts of thine which require it, seriatim.

Thy health is the most material article. Be content with thy slow recovery. Whilst thou art acting the part thy best discretion directs, think it is for the best, and not an argument that nature is unhinged or inactive. Perhaps the Bark would come in aid very usefully. Boil an ounce of the Bark, in powder, in a quart of water to a pint. Let it be strained off when warm, and bottled. Put to this decoction half an ounce of the spirit of Lavender. Take three tablespoonfuls twice a day with 30 to 40 drops of the volatile Tincture of Guaiacum [1] mixed with it — so much as shall be rendered rather laxative than binding.

The weather is rather against thee at present, but we may hope to see better days ere long. I have no fault to find with thy present regime. Steady, steady is a good sea phrase.

[*Passage omitted.*]

Last night I wrote to Dr. Pemberton on Isaac Pickering's account.[2] If he receives it before this comes to hand, I know he will soon communicate the contents. A little spite may now and then have good effects. Dr. Ratcliffe [3] once was informed that the place of a poor sick exciseman was greedily being sought after by a worthless fellow. His aid was most humbly solicited, and the moment Ratcliffe was acquainted with the circumstance, from this principle only, he attended with diligence and success.

I would take much pains that a worthless hussy should not riot in the spoils of a whole family who all of them had more merit than herself.

Dr. Thompson is not at ease in London. He will never be able to rise even to mediocrity in his profession.[4] I think he would be a proper companion, as a friend, as a physician under Dr. Pemberton, and a tutor

297

to Isaac. Make it worth his while to accept the charge, and I will endeavour both to accept of it and direct the plan. In this I am acting a just part to all parties whose reciprocal advantage I have at heart. If a word of objection arises I will stop.

The space to be allowed in the Scotch Dictionary [5] is 6 or 7 pages if we please. I am pleased it engages thy attention, and shall do more at Lea Hall when thou hast sketched the plan. I would not advise thee to go to Kirby Lonsdale unless thou cannot help it. I know the consequence if otherwise.[6]

Thy remarks on addressing have had their share of my attention. Previous to thy mentioning it, I had thought of a less exceptionable, more necessary and more consistent measure. Let a strong paragraph be inserted in the printed epistle, advising Friends to beware of entering into that warm party spirit that hath sprung up in this country and elsewhere; charging all to remember the obligations we are under to honour and obey the King, and especially the present Royal Family, from whose progenitors we have received so many favours. To address would expose us to the scorn of all but the present, and the chastisement of a future administration. I leave the attempt to thy leisure, and think it both proper and expedient, I mean a paragraph in the epistle.

Let me hear from thee respecting my proposal of Dr. Thompson as soon as may be, that I may speak to the Dr. about it. £100 per Annum salary; expenses defrayed, is the least that can be offered. Accept our united and affectionate remembrance.

J.F.

Ms. autograph letter, Port. 22/111, LSFL.

1. *Guiacum*, a genus of trees found in the West Indies, also in tropical American localities. From the wood of this genus, especially *Guiacum officinale* and *Guiacum sanctum*, a medicine useful in rheumatism and gout was prepared.

2. Dr. Thomas Pemberton, a prominent physician of Warrington, is evidently the adviser of Isaac Pickering, a young Quaker from Yorkshire.

3. *Munk's Roll* gives no information about a Dr. Ratcliffe. The reference may be to Dr. John Radcliffe (1650–1714), benefactor of the Radcliffe Infirmary and Observatory at Oxford, who "annoyed many great people by his extraordinary candour," or to Dr. John Radcliffe (1690–1724), physician at St. Bartholomew's Hospital, London, "a gentleman of excellent parts and sound learning, whose only crime was his singular modesty." — *DNB*; *British Medical Journal*, 23 October 1875, p. 529.

4. On Gilbert Thompson's diffidence see J. to S. Fothergill, 10 December 1767, above.

5. "A Society of Gentlemen" in Edinburgh was sponsoring an ambitious work of reference under the editorship of William Smellie (1740–1795), an enterprising young Quaker. It was to be published in a series of parts as soon as each was satisfactorily

completed; the first had appeared in 1768. By request, Dr. Fothergill, with help from his brother Samuel, was preparing to contribute an article on the Society of Friends, which appeared in the first complete edition of the *Encyclopedia Britannica; or, a Dictionary of Arts and Sciences Compiled upon a New Plan, By a Society of Gentlemen in Scotland* (3 volumes, Edinburgh: A. Bell and C. McFarquhar, 1771). The article was so popular among members of the Society of Friends that a separate issue, *A Brief Account of the People called Quakers; their Doctrines and their Disciplines*, was arranged in 1773. — Herman Kogan, *The Great E.B.* (Chicago: University of Chicago Press, 1958); John Minto, *A Classified and Annotated Guide to the Principal Works of Reference* (London: Library Associates of the United Kingdom, 1929; supplement, 1931).

6. Kirby Lonsdale in Westmoreland had been selected for a regional Circular Meeting of Friends. To attend the gathering seemed to Dr. Fothergill too great an effort for Samuel, whose health was too precarious to justify the effort and excitement of being with a large group of people.

To William Huddesford, 10 April 1769

Harpur Street, London
10th Inst.

Respected Friend

This day's post brought me thy very obliging letter. I have perused the ms., and wish I may be fortunate enough to be at home when Sir J. Pachel [1] is pleased to call for it.

I think it is a laudable attempt to rescue the name of that great man [2] from oblivion and executed with great candour and precision, so far as there were any materials to proceed upon. Now I hope there are some more to enlarge this work; it will again be revised and in due time published.

I cannot say that I like that method of Biography begun I think by Bayle,[3] and followed by some other writers, of throwing some of the most material parts of their history into the form of notes. Was I to attempt anything of this kind I would leave nothing as a note but dates, and references to dates; and even not these if possible to be avoided. Was I to sit down to write an author's life in a manner that would please myself, I would make myself master of as many facts as I could. I would next endeavour to arrange these facts in the most natural and entertaining manner I could, digesting the whole into a uniform narrative as much as possible. But if it was necessary to introduce letters, they should make a part of the book not of the notes. — And so much for this subject.

Permit me to suggest the following thought, respecting the use that

299

may perhaps some time or other be made of these papers. Would not they afford some help towards forming a *Review of the rise and progress of Natural History in Great Britain from the revival of letters to the middle of the present Century, with some account of lives and characters of the principal promoters of Natural Knowledge,* be a work of vast utility, and reflect honour on the British Nation? To execute this extensive undertaking would no doubt require some labour, some expense, much time and leisure. Many hands make light work. One would take the Botanical, another the Fossils, another the Animal Kingdom; or perhaps these might be subdivided amongst others. The result would be an authentick account of the lives, labours, of all the great Natural Historians this Country has produced; and a concise account of the many discoveries that have been made in this Country exhibited to the World in a manner that may claim the publick esteem.[4] Reserve the account of Dr. Lhuyd for that work, and look out as soon as may be for the proper associates. Proceed with Lister [5] in the manner intended by the University; but at the same time look forward to a more extensive and honourable undertaking, in which I am ready to lend any aid that may be in my power, which I own will be very inconsiderable both for want of time and want of ability.

I don't think the papers I have sent to Trinity college deserve any more notice on my account than that which I have already received from my Friend Huddesford in his letter of this day, full of gratitude, and of more esteem than I am entitled to.

A Friend of mine tells me I have a tolerable good Knack of finding work for my Friends. He judges so because I often propose to him business more proportional to his abilitys than to his inclination! I own it hurts me to see men possessed of Talents above the level of mankind in general, burying them in a napkin. I do not know of anything which would give me more pain than to reside a few months in Oxford. I should discover men of the first rank of understanding, partly for want of experience, partly for want of opportunity, but more from indolence, absorbed in an insignificant round of doing that which the lowest of mankind enjoy as much as themselves: eating, drinking and sleeping.

Adieu, my friend, and think of me as

thy sincere Friend
J. Fothergill

Ms. autograph letter, Ashmole Mss. no. 1822, ff. 227, Bodleian Library, Oxford. Month and year added in another hand.

1. Sir John Peshall or Pechell, Bart. (d. 1778) was a local antiquarian. In 1772 he published *The History of the University of Oxford to the Death of William the Conqueror*, and the following year brought out *The Ancient and Present State of the City of Oxford Containing an Account of its Foundation, Antiquities, . . . Monumental Inscriptions, Mayors, Members of Parliament, &c. The whole chiefly collected by Mr. Anthony à Wood; with additions by the Rev. Sir J. Peshall, Bart.* (London: J. & E. Rivington, 1773). He collected materials for other histories which were never finished. — John Nichols, *Illustrations of the Literary History of the Eighteenth Century* (London, 1817–1858), V, 522.

2. Undoubtedly Edward Lhuyd. Huddesford, at the time of his death, was working on biographical material on Lhuyd and others.

3. Probably Pierre Bayle (1647–1706), whose *Dictionnaire historique et critique* (1697) had gone through eleven editions by 1740 and had been available in English since 1710. Bayle's great work "took the form of, mainly, biographical articles . . . accompanied by voluminous footnotes." — *The Oxford Companion to French Literature*, compiled and edited by Sir Paul Harvey and J. E. Heseltine (Oxford: Clarendon Press, 1959).

4. Richard Pulteney (1710–1801), in his *Historical and Biographical Sketches of the Progress of Botany in England, from its Origin to the Introduction of the Linnaean System* . . . (London: 1790), I, 155–163, succeeded to some extent in accomplishing what for botanical science the purpose Dr. Fothergill outlines.

5. In 1770 Huddesford produced a careful edition of List's *Historiae Conchyliorum*, providing a useful index. A contemporary, the Rev. Michael Tyson, writing 5 November 1772, praised his scholarship while lamenting his recent demise: "Poor Huddesford, he is a loss indeed! with what accuracy he made indexes to those four volumes of original Correspondence of Lister, given to the Ashmolean Library in 1769 by Dr. Fothergill!" — Nichols, *Literary Anecdotes*, VIII (1814), 600.

To William Huddesford, Oxford, 25 April 1769

Harpur Street 25th Inst.

Accept my grateful acknowledgements for the favour of inspecting the digested letters. I could have wished to have perused them; but had I kept them a much longer time it would still have been impracticable.

The genteel manner in which they were offered to the University does the composer of that oration credit. Accept my thanks for this favour likewise; and at some opportunity be pleased to express the satisfaction I feel in having done an act that has received so ample a mark of approbation from the University of Oxford.[1]

I have only time to say at present that I am Friend Huddesford's

obliged and respectful Friend
J. Fothergill

Ms. autograph letter, lacking cover and address, Ashmole Mss. no. 1822, ff. 329, Bodleian Library, Oxford. Month and year added in another hand.

1. The gift of the Lister-Lhuyd papers was formally recorded 14 April 1769, together with a brief description of the contents. A decision to render thanks to the donor reads: *Proponente Domino Vice-Cancellario placuit Venerabili Domui ut gratias Domino Doctore Fothergilli agerentur.* — Information by courtesy of I. G. Philip, former Secretary to the Bodleian Library and since 1966 Keeper of Printed Books, University of Oxford.

To John Bartram, Philadelphia, 1 May 1769

Harpur Street, London
1.5.1769

Esteemed Friend

I received thy acceptable letter of the 26th Inst. on the 17th of last month, and in a short time after I also received the box of plants in pretty good condition. Most of them will live and divers of them are new to me. One of the Ginseng plants [1] is coming up vigorously. I am much obliged to thee for this valuable present, and shall be glad to make returns for it as well as I can. If a copy of Purver's translation of the Bible will be acceptable, please call upon Thomas Fisher in Philadelphia and desire him to deliver one bound, and place it to my account. The author of this great undertaking, like thyself, is self-taught and self-instructed. Almost without any assistance but from books, he has acquired the knowledge of many languages; and the best judges allow that the translation is the most faithful one of the original Scripture that was ever made in the English tongue. Let me know if there is anything here by which I can make thee proper satisfaction, and I will do it cheerfully. I don't want my friends should make bricks without straw.

There will be a considerable demand for American seeds to various parts of Germany, and were there any in town, I know they might be disposed of. I have a nephew by marriage,[2] who lives in our deceased Friend P. Collinson's house and carries on the business of a mercer. If Michael Collinson [3] does not choose to engage in the business of disposing of the seeds, I know I can readily prevail upon him to undertake it. He has no skill in these matters, but he would take care to render a careful account of the sales, and make due remittances. I am afraid of entrusting these things to the care of seedsmen. James Gordon, is, I believe, one of the best, yet one cannot be sure they will always continue faithful and honest. If Michael Collinson will be kind enough to undertake the affair, no person is more proper. I will see him as soon as I can, and endeavour to prevail upon him. Should he decline it . . . send thy boxes to James Freeman, Mercer in Gracious Street; and any instructions thou thinks proper to me, and I will take care they shall be duly executed.

I am pleased that thy son William is engaged in describing the tortoises of your country. America seems to abound in this species of animal more than any other country. As the inhabitants increase, these, as well as the native plants, will be thinned; and it is therefore of some consequence to begin their history as soon as possible. I would not limit him either in respect to time or expense. He may send me his drawings and accounts of their history as soon as he finishes them and I will pay his demands to his order.

It gives me satisfaction to find that our opinions are alike in respect to the propagation of plants by seeds on your side. I think there is a shorter method and less expensive of making a natural soil for all your wild plants than is generally known. In the autumn collect a large quantity of new fallen leaves of all sorts of trees. Dig a large hole in any vacant spot, and fill it with layers of leaves and layers of the earth dug out of the hole. Do this every fall of the leaves, and a good compost will be formed in which all sorts of seeds and plants will flourish. If the earth dug out of the hole is not sandy, this had better be thrown away, and the hole filled with leaves and sand. It will be proper that this should lie to rot two years before it is used, but by making such a preparation annually, enough will be at hand for every purpose. I judge that most of the plant country from Canada to Florida has been the last of all redeemed from the ocean. The soil of these flat countries consists of decayed vegetables and sea sand. In some parts the sand prevails, and with it barrenness; in other places corrupted vegetables, and with them fertility. The soil is good or bad or indifferent as it partakes of the riches of corrupted vegetables or the poverty of mere sea sand. This I only hint as my opinion, and on this opinion I found my theory of this species of fertility. Put me to rights if I am wrong. My gardener has directions every fall to collect a quantity of leaves and treat them in this manner. We reserve this for the use of our wild American seeds, and succeed with them. Be kind enough to get us some plants of those curious oaks and chestnuts. Take them up with large balls of earth; tie moss about them, plant them in similar earth at home till they begin to prosper. The branches of the old plants may be laid down and a numerous progeny may soon be raised to oblige and benefit our country. If all the more curious plants and shrubs were to be taken up while very young and planted in boxes and kept in them, often watered during the summer, for one year, they would succeed with us much better and deserve a better price than from any other management.

I shall expect the *Colocasia* when convenient to send it, and I shall do my best to preserve it. I doubt not that my friend B. Franklin has executed my commission. However I hope to see him shortly, and shall endeavour to inform myself what is done, and acquaint thee with it. The present gardener at Kew is from general account a very ingenious, sensible, honest man. It will be much in his power to determine the royal personages, and I think it would not be improper to write to him, if any plants are sent. His name is Aiton [5] and if a line or two are sent to him, I will take care to convey it safely.

As I wish to make thee adequate satisfaction for the trouble thou has taken, and may take on my account, I should be glad to know in what way I can most satisfactorily make thee compensation. Through the favour of Providence, and much careful labour, I want for nothing, and therefore would desire that all due satisfaction may be given to those who are kind enough to do anything for me.

This perhaps will be delivered by Dr. Rush,[6] a young man who has employed his time with great diligence and success in prosecuting his studies here, who has lead a blameless life so far as I know, and it seems but just that those who have endeavoured to deserve a good character should have it when it may be of use to them.

My engagements and the duties of my station may perhaps render me a very irregular correspondent, but my inclination to show regard to every person who was a friend to my deceased Friend Peter Collinson will always lead me to be as diligent as I can.

I am thy obliged, respectful Friend

J. Fothergill

Ms. autograph letter, Bartram Papers, IV, 21, HSP; printed in part in Darlington, *Memorials*, 339–341.

1. The North American species, *Panax quinquefolium*.
2. James Freeman of Gracechurch Street, husband of Alexander Fothergill's daughter Ann.
2. Son of Peter.

4. One of London's well-known nursery gardeners, who specialized in the sale of North American plants.

5. William Aiton (1731–1793), a Scottish gardener from Lanarkshire, received his first appointment in London in the apothecaries' garden in Chelsea then in charge of Philip Miller. In 1759 his skill was recognized by appointment to the Royal Gardens at Kew, where he greatly increased the collections. With assistance from Dr. Daniel Charles Solander of the British Museum, he later spent years preparing a definitive catalogue of all plants cultivated in Kew Gardens. The first edition of *Hortus Kewensis* appeared in 1789.

6. Dr. Benjamin Rush, at this time twenty-four, had spent three years in Great Britain in medical study. After receiving his M.D. at Edinburgh in 1768, he had gone to London "to attend the lectures and dissections of Dr. William Hunter and Mr. Hewson." He had walked the wards of Middlesex Hospital with "Dr. Mark Akenside, the poet . . . cold and formal in his behaviour to students," and "followed Dr. Huck . . . communicative and friendly" at St. Thomas'. Dr. Fothergill hospitably invited the young Philadelphian to breakfast, and thereafter Dr. Rush returned to Harpur Street once a week to this "early levee." — *Autobiography of Benjamin Rush*, ed. G. W. Corner, 52–56.

To William Logan, Philadelphia, 8 May 1769

London, 8.5.1769

Dear Friend,

I received thine of 2nd and 6th with great satisfaction. I must answer it briefly, as I can, with a little respite from increased occupation.

I had a letter from J. C. Lettsom at Edinburgh, and a postscript in it from Billy the other day. They are both pursuing their studies with great application and great success. Billy's health has suffered, but by a little relaxation this is recovered. He is happy in finding me disposed to give in to his views, and is determined to do all in his power to merit so much condescension. If he proceeds as he now promises (I do not mean in words but in conduct), I hope he will make a useful member of society; and if so, he cannot be very unhappy. — I have been repeatedly thinking that Bristol would be a very proper place for him to set down in. It is amongst his acquaintance, his friends' acquaintance, and the late Dr. Logan's Friends will not forget thy son.[1] I had not mentioned this to him, nor shall I do it unless it falls in with thy own opinion. I think he will be less liable to fall into hurtful extreme while he is under the notice of his Friends here than he probably would be under the warm spirits of America.

The present companion of his studies will I believe fix in London,

305

where he lives.[2] He may make a considerable figure, and as their first introduction would be among the same general acquaintance, an emulation not to their advantage might take place; I will rather call it jealousy. Thy sentiments will induce me to enact the part thou would choose. I am the friend, but thou are the father, and as such have the right to prescribe. I think however that Billy will be rather safer here than in Pennsylvania, and perhaps not less likely to get a decent support.

This comes by Dr. Rush, a young man from your Province, who has behaved himself in such a manner as to gain the esteem of those who know him. He is sensible, diligent, well acquainted with his business, and will be of use in the place of his activity, provided he behaves with the same prudence which he has manifested amongst us, so far as I know, on all occasions. — He has corresponded with Billy; has a great regard for him, and will acquaint thee fully with his present situation and pursuits. I think this young man is very well qualified to give lectures on a material part on medical education, viz., Chemistry, and should be glad to hear that he is promoted to that professorship, in which I think he will appear to considerable advantage to himself and to the Colony, as well as in the practice of physic in general.

I think Thomas Lees may safely adventure to collect a few boxes of seeds, of about 5 or 6 guineas value each, and if they are consigned to my nephew James Freeman in Gracious Street, I will take care that he will use his best endeavours in disposing of them and rendering him a faithful account of the proceeds. I think it will be better to trust them in his hands than in a seedsman's as they will sometimes not scruple to take what they like best for their own use. My nephew is no botanist, but an honest tradesman; and I'll endeavour to point out to him who to apply to for their distribution. Let half a dozen boxes be sent next winter for a trial.

I am much obliged to thee for thy sentiments on public affairs; I wish I could send thee anything consolatory in return. America has no good to expect from the present administration, and how long this may last nobody knows. Great is the power of those who have anything to give. Reason, utility, justice, propriety are all out of the question; that a good and virtuous King should confide in a servant more than in anybody else is a mystery to most folks inexplicable; however it is a proof of some kind of talent in a servant to be able under such circumstances to maintain his ground almost against the united voice of the public.

When our domestic feuds will end is difficult to foresee. — Your treatment of the North American merchants, having made them cool in your service, has given the Ministry the opportunity of representing all America as perfectly satisfied with the administration, a few fractious spirits excepted. I was in hopes that your Agents would have joined together as one man to have undeceived them.[3] If the colonies do not send a few sensible disinterested men to join together and advocate their cause properly here next winter, you will probably repent of your neglect when it is too late.

The Agents are unknown, unconnected, no witnesses of their behavior. For the most part they are pensionaries, or wish to be so, and are either inactive or false to your interests. I except Dr. Franklin, but it is even possible that desperation of succeeding may lessen his assiduity. I see a thousand things said against America in our newspapers which pass for current, and yet I could readily contradict, had I leisure — but we must look higher; we have had a long time of peace and ease in this country; we are grown fat and full, and have forgot the Author of our happiness. It is but rightful you and we should be put in mind of our situation, and may it please the great Author of all good that it may be by lenient means.

I have seen T. Wharton;[4] what progress he is making I know not, but I apprehend that neither he nor anybody else will at present succeed in any application respecting America.

I am glad to hear G. Mason is well, and not dissatisfied that he is leaving a country where it is hard to live and live in innocency and peace. I have received several letters from him, and retain an affection for him and his family whose preservation and increase in everything that may contribute to their happiness I fervently desire. Should I say that I have reason to apprehend some of my letters have not been made use of for the purposes I intended, it may be no improper motive to more care on my part for the future. And as I am open and undesigning myself, I know not how to correspond where I have reason to doubt from experience of the like disposition. I want not to make in thy mind any unnecessary scruples; but caution can do no harm. If I have been misinformed, sooner or later I shall know it, and will then do all the justice the case requires.

I rather think thy two younger sons will reap no great benefit where they are; [5] James Fell lost the great support of his family, his wife. I wish

307

I knew to whom I could properly recommend them for tuition, but the little encouragement given here amongst us for education makes proper masters very scarce. There is a little honest Scotchman in the neighborhood of this city who has not many scholars, who nevertheless, I hope, would do his duty to them. His name is Obed Cook; he lives in the house which was styled the grade school on the Southwark side and was under the care of Jacob Hagen [6] etc. He is valuable, and I think a competent master. His terms are not high, and I think he might be induced to take some pains with them. I don't want to injure J.F., but the loss of a few years in the early part of life is so great, so irreparable, that I think it next to criminal not to give some intimations respecting thy sons' present situation.

We rejoice to hear of J. Hunt and family's safe arrival; [7] remember us affectionately to them as opportunity offers.

I am afraid we are likely to be relieved of a very valuable relation of ours, Henry Fothergill of Warrington, who I fear from the accounts I have received, is in a dangerous situation, consumptive kidney.[8] — We expect my Brother here in a few days, as our Yearly Meeting is at hand. Catherine Payton writes doubtfully of his coming. Ever since I returned from Cheshire I have been upon a stretch without interruption. My business has laid very wide and it has been with unwearied labor that I have been able to accomplish it. We shall go down [9] I hope about the usual time and get a little fresh ability of both body and mind to go on in the track that seems open before me till some favourable opportunity of retreating still more may offer. I borrow the time from rest, much wanted, to write even this abrupt epistle, but I could not permit so favourable an opportunity escape me.

Please to tell T. Lees that I should be glad of some martagon, either roots or seeds, and that he would send some of them and all the herbaceous plants that are curious, annually.[10] Shrubs we seldom lose, annuals and perennials often. We both salute thee and thine very affectionately. Farewell —

From thy assured friend
John Fothergill

Ms. autograph letter, Gilbert Collection, II, 141–143, College of Physicians, Philadelphia.

1. People in Bristol, where James Logan's brother, Dr. William Logan, had long been regarded as the city's leading practitioner, might well have favored a young

Edinburgh graduate of the same name and lineage had Billy been content to stay in England.

2. Dr. John Coakley Lettsom had already acquired an enviable reputation in London for ability and devotion to the practice of medicine, and he continued to advance professionally.

3. Each colony appointed its own agent or agents and while, as in the cases of Richard Partridge and Robert Charles, one man might represent several colonies, there was at this time no formal cooperation.

4. Thomas Wharton and Joseph Galloway, prominent citizens of Philadelphia, in association with the printer William Goddard, in 1767 started an anti-proprietary newspaper, the *Pennsylvania Chronicle*, which, though it had a short existence, aimed to awaken its readers to a sense of public responsibility and the need for their participation in the government of their Colony. — Crane, *Franklin's Letters to the Press*, 38.

5. Billy Logan's younger brothers, George and Charles, had been sent to England to attend a small Quaker school in Gloucestershire kept by James Fell, who proved to be a poor teacher and a strict disciplinarian. — Frederick B. Tolles, *George Logan* (New York: Oxford University Press, 1953), 12, 13.

6. The well-educated Quaker of German descent mentioned in the letter to Israel Pemberton, 9 April 1759, above.

7. John Hunt of London, after the unexpected death of his wife Dorothy, took his two daughters to Philadelphia and established a home in what is now Darby, near the city.

8. Henry Fothergill, Dr. Fothergill's nephew, died as a result of renal tuberculosis not long after this letter was written. Having inherited his father's business, he had for eight years maintained the family home in Warrington for his unmarried sisters. — Fothergill Family Records contributed by the late Miss Mabyn Fothergill of Edinburgh.

9. To Lea Hall, in Cheshire. Dr. Fothergill did much of his writing there while freed from the daily routine of practice. Once a week, however, he went to the White Bear Tavern a mile or two away in the village of Middlewich to see patients, refusing to take fees for this service. — Fox, 23, 24.

10. "Thomas Lees' collections (1767–1771) proved of little value." — Fox, 191n. See letter to William Logan 22 April 1771 below.

To James Pemberton, Philadelphia, 16 May 1769

London, 16.5.1769

Esteemed Friend,

When I perused the affecting account of thy son's indisposition I could not forebear feeling for thy distress, yet was sensible it was not in my power to suggest any means of help.[1] Otherwise I should have replied much sooner. Next to having those with us whom we most esteem is a reasonable hope that they are much happier than we could make them, and such is the consolation of the present very affecting event.

309

Though this is wrote during the time of our Yearly Meeting and many Friends are about us, yet I could not omit furnishing Dr. Rush with this introduction to thee. He has behaved himself in such a manner here, and pursued his studies with so much diligence and success as entitles him to the approbation of his acquaintances here and claims this testimonial of his worth from me. If he is not spoiled by too early an introduction to public favour, I hope he will long continue to deserve it. Difficulties at first setting out are often more instructive than a smoother progress. Not that I want to have difficulties thrown in his way, but let him acquire reputation by his own conduct rather than by the too hasty suffrage of his friends.

He has applied himself to chemistry in particular, as well as to the practice of physic in general. He brings with him a very good apparatus, a present from the Proprietor,[2] and I should be glad to hear that this young man, at some proper time, was prefixed to the Chemical Chair,[3] as I hope he would fill it with reputation to himself and advantage to the Colony.

With respect to the public affairs between Great Britain and her Colonies, little can be said. We have people at the helm who seem to like violence more than peace and would rather command obedience than gain affection. They are deaf to any other arguments than those of necessity, and where the contention will end nobody knows. As I am sure I can do no good, I endeavour to avoid suffering harm by not giving way to unavailing anxiety. Whatever may be for the best I hope will happen, though it may be through much pinching distress to many individuals. Study to be quiet — and do my own business, I wish to make my motto.[4] I think, however, the Colonies will be remiss, if they do not depute some cool sensible men from each colony to come over to join their Agents here and the few North America merchants who may be in business (by that time) and are your friends, in soliciting Parliament another winter, unless you decide to try to have another year on the goods already in America without admitting any more from hence.[5] Either do not resolve, or go through stretch and adhere to your resolutions. Those who are adverse to the Colonies say that you are weary of them already, that the merchants here are indifferent about your resolutions, and that the Ministry know you too well to be in pain about any of your resolutions. But I cannot say more on this subject at present.

I shall rejoice to hear of thy family's welfare, and am thy affectionate Friend

J. Fothergill

Ms. autograph letter, Pemberton Papers, Etting Collection, II, 58, HSP.

1. James Pemberton's son Charles had been obliged to give up his work in the family counting house because of a persistent cough and increasing weakness. He was unable to participate in social life with his young friends. His physicians advised a change of climate. Since he was unable to travel alone, his uncle, Israel Pemberton, Jr., head of the Pemberton shipping firm, provided passage to Barbados in one of the Company's ships for both Charles and a close friend, James Hutchinson (later a medical graduate of the College of Philadelphia). Charles was undoubtedly suffering from tuberculosis. — Personal communication from Whitfield J. Bell, Jr., Librarian, APS.

2. Thomas Penn described his gift as "a Chymical Apparatus . . . a Thing that will be of great Use in the Tryal of Ores . . . such as Dr. Fothergill thought necessary." — Thomas Penn to the Hospital Trustees, 9 May 1769, recommending Dr. Rush, in Thomas H. Montgomery, *History of the University of Pennsylvania*, 487.

3. By unanimous vote of the Trustees of the College of Philadelphia, 23 July 1769, Dr. Benjamin Rush "in consideration of his character as an able chymist," was appointed Professor of Chemistry in the first medical school in the American Colonies. — Montgomery, 488.

4. A Biblical quotation, I Thessalonians, 4:11, frequently used by Dr. Fothergill:
> And that you study to be quiet, and to do your own business,
> and to work with your own hands, as we commanded you.

5. In the spring of 1768 neither the Philadelphia merchants nor the Pennsylvania Assembly took action in response to the appeals of Massachusetts for cooperation in attempting to secure repeal of the Townshend Acts. In the summer of that year, however, a mass meeting in Philadelphia resolved that the Assembly should petition the King, Lords, and Council for repeal. When the Assembly met in September the petitions were sent. The Philadelphia merchants still held back for some months, but in February 1769 some sixty of the most radical signed the Non-Importation Agreement, and before long nearly all the rest had joined them. — Thayer, *Pennsylvania Politics*, 143–144.

To John Gurney, Norwich, Norfolk, 2 November 1769

London, 2.11.1769

Dear Friend,[1]

It gave me not a little concern that I was so engaged in business of such a nature as I could not easily quit, that I could not see thee at Norwich. It was much in my inclination.

I have still less prospect of doing it now, and yet I fear it is as needful as it has been, if I could be of any particular service. For though the

311

accounts I receive are such as encourage me to think that thou art rather growing better and though in no respect worse, yet the disease still remains in some degree, and prevents the full recovery of thy health.

It is not from an opinion that I can be of more use to thee than another, that I wish to encourage thee to attempt a journey to this place, but I think a journey would be of use, and might perhaps be more advantageous than any other remedy. As the conveniencies at Hackney are such as few surpass them, and no care can exceed thy sister's, I press it the more strongly. Stay there as long or as short a time as thou pleases, yet I wish thou would attempt the journey. Make the stages as easy to thyself as may be, and consider that the very change of air and place is a remedy. If I can suggest anything when we meet that may be of use, I shall rejoice most sincerely as having contributed to the happiness of so many people as are interested in thy perfect recovery.

I am not put upon making this request by the anxiety of thy Friends here, though that would weigh with me much, but by the uninterrupted friendship that has subsisted from our first acquaintance; a wish to be as useful as I can to a Friend. My esteem for an invaluable member of Society both general and particular, prompts me to urge it with as much earnestness as is fitting. From the time Dr. Manning[2] first wrote to me I have had not the least syllable from him. I could have wished to cooperate with him to the utmost of my power for thy full recovery. Accept the kind remembrance and cordial wishes for better health

from thy assured Friend
John Fothergill

Ms. autograph letter, Barclay Papers, printed by courtesy of Quintin Gurney, Esq., of Bawdeswell Hall near Norwich, Norfolk, England.

1. John Gurney of Norwich (d. 1779) belonged to a Norfolk family noted in the woolen trade for its exceptionally fine woolen cloth. To keep funds fluid for business use, the Gurneys established a bank in Norwich and allowed their employees to make regular deposits from their wages in savings accounts, an innovation at this time, which taught thrift and encouraged loyalty to the firm.

2. Dr. John Manning (1758–1806) received his M.D. in 1753 at Leyden, was admitted extra-licentiate of the Royal College of Physicians in 1757, and settled in Norwich, where his practice in both city and country was regarded as "highly honourable to himself and beneficial to the public." Indeed, "the excellencies and virtues of his private character no less endeared him to all who knew him; and who did not know him in this wide circle?" — *Munk's Roll*, II, 213; quotations copied from a monument erected in his honor, St. Gregory's Church, Norwich, England.

To Granville Sharp, London, 1769

Harpur Street, London
15th Inst. 1769

Dr. Fothergill presents his respects to G. Sharp [1] and returns the Ms. which his brother [2] was so obliging as to put into the Dr.'s hands. He has perused it with attention, and with much satisfaction. For the honor of his species, he wishes most sincerely that such pungent applications to the hearts of men grown callous were unnecessary.

Could not another argument be drawn in favour of the Negroes from this circumstance that though in the Islands, a man who kills a Black may compound for the crime, yet in England, I believe no such precedent exists. A Master who stabbed his black servant, or any other Black would probably hang for it.

Dr. F. requests G. Sharp's acceptance of a book which at least has the merit of being printed by Baskerville. [3] The sentiments in it are *humane,* and will in so far be agreeable.

Ms. letter, copied in a contemporary hand, from the Letter Book of Granville Sharp, Library Company of Philadelphia (now in custody of HSP).

1. Because this letter is insufficiently dated it is placed last among Dr. Fothergill's letters of 1769. Granville Sharp (1735–1813), the distinguished humanitarian and philanthropist, was the active leader of a movement to abolish Negro slavery in Great Britain's West Indian Islands. The manuscript to which Dr. Fothergill refers was probably that of *A Representation of the Injustice and Dangerous Tendency of Admitting the Least Claim of Private Property in the Persons of Men* (London, 1769).

2. Granville Sharp's older brother, William Sharp (1728/9–1810), was a London surgeon in practice from 1750 to 1787. Possessed of "a handsome fortune," he retired to his estate in Fullham where he died in 1810. — Prince Hoare, *Memoirs of Granville Sharp from his own Manuscripts and Other Authentic Documents in possession of His Family and of the African Institution* (London: Henry Colburn and Co., 1820), introduction, 19–23.

3. Probably Robert Barclay's *Apology*, issued in a sumptuous edition under Dr. Fothergill's auspices in 1765.

VI
1770-1773

My garden is pretty large, well sheltered,
and a good soil. The North American plants
flourish with me exceedingly. I have most of
the plants usually sent over . . . Plants that
are remarkable for their figure, their fragrance,
or their use are exceedingly acceptable . . .
An amusement of this kind will have its use
to lessen the tediousness of old age, and call me
out to a little exercise, when subsiding vigor
prompts to too much indulgence.

To John Ellis, Autumn, 1772

To John Bartram, Philadelphia, 13 January 1770

London, 13.1.1770

Dear Friend,

I have now before me thy two kind letters of the 26th and 29th November last. I have received as well the box of plants, the cask of *Colocasia*,[1] and the Bull Frogs alive. I likewise received a roll of drawings directed to me, all safe and very acceptable.

The plants came in good condition. The roots of the *Colocasia* seemed but in a doubtful situation. However they are planted, part at Kew and part in a little piece of water at Upton, my little residence, and exactly agreeable to thy instructions. We first fixed a basket with a light loamy earth; we then separated the roots, and just covered them with the earth. We then let the basket gently down to the bottom of the water, where they will always be at any time covered with about two feet and a half of water.

A place is not yet fixed upon for the Bull Frogs to be put in. In the meantime however they are kept in a shallow vessel of water, the bottom covered with moss, where they may either put their heads above or under water as they like. We have now a severe frost, but when all this goes off they will be set at large somewhere and in safety. We have none of the kind in England. The King is acquainted with their arrival; also the *Colocasia*, and from whom they come.

My nephew [2] will endeavour to serve thee to the utmost of his power — and on the same terms that our deceased Friend Peter Collinson did. As he is a stranger to the value of the things sent him, please to mention at what price they should be disposed of. I will assist him to the utmost of my power for thy sake as well as my deceased Friend. [*Several lines illegible.*]

317

To John Bartram, January 13, 1770

Mention is made in thy letter about some drawings designed for the Duchess of Portland.[3] I received only one roll, and those directed to me consisting of drawings of the *Colocasia*, a new series of *Momordica*,[4] shells etc., 6 in number. If any are for me, which I hope, be kind enough to give me some intimation of their value, which I will pay to my kinsman. If any of them are designed for the Duchess, be pleased to inform me.

I must still desire that thy son will favour me with drawings of the rest of your American tortoises, with such remarks on them as occur to him. As the inhabitants increase, the species of this and some other animals, as well as vegetables, will perhaps be extinguished, or exist only in some still more distant parts. It would therefore be of great advantage to natural history to have everything of a fugitive nature consigned to paper with as much accuracy as possible; and in inquiring into the value of these drawings, I do not so much want to know at how low a price he can afford them, as what in his own opinion will be a proper compensation for his labour and his time. And whatever be attempted of this kind, let it be well finished; and I hope he will not find me niggardly . . .

I wish it was in my power to assist thee to thy sight; but in part it is the effect of your age,[5] which effect I must likewise feel if I live to your age. Are no glasses of use? Pray, was thee shortsighted when young? If this was the case, glasses rather injure than help the sight. If thou canst find out any way for me to inquire after better glasses, I will do it with satisfaction.

I hope to send thee in the spring some little account of our late Friend Peter Collinson's life and services in respect to Botany. For several years past I have left London about ten weeks in the summer and got about 160 miles from it in order to recruit my strength against winter for the duties of my station. It was in one of these intervals that our Friend was carried off by a suppression of urine. Had I been present I know not that anything more could have been done to have saved him. When I was informed of his decease, partly to indulge my sorrows and partly to pay some tribute to his memory, I employed myself in drawing up a short account of his character. A few copies will I believe be printed this spring for the satisfaction of his Friends, and I will take care that a few be sent to thee.

I have not leisure to become a perfect botanist. I love the vegetable creation, I love its varieties and cultivate it as an amusement. Every new plant is an addition to my pleasure. I have most of the common produce of America, and they flourish with me more than anywhere else. I have my garden in a low sheltered situation where they prosper. My *Kalmias* [6] make shoots of 5 or 6 inches in a summer.

Thy assured Friend
J. Fothergill

Ms. autograph letter, Miscellaneous Collections, HSP; printed in part in Darlington, *Memorials*, 341–343.

1. "Colocasia" or "Nymphaea nelumbo" (now identified as *Nelumbo lutea*) was found by William Bartram in its native habitat in Florida — "its large sweet-scented yellow blossoms lifted up . . . above the surface of the water, each upon a green standard, representing the cap of Liberty." — *The Travels of William Bartram*, ed. Francis Harper (New Haven: Yale University Press, 1958), 69.

2. James Freeman.

3. Margaret Cavendish Holles Harley, heiress of the second Earl of Oxford, married William Bentinck, second Duke of Portland, in 1734. The Duchess maintained her own botanical garden and a private menagerie at Bulstrode Park near Beaconsfield where she also arranged the rarities of her varied collections in a museum which Horace Walpole called "truly magnificent, chiefly composed of the spoils of her father's and the Arundel collections." — Horace Walpole, *Catalogue of the Duchess of Portland's Museum*, ed. W. S. Lewis (New York: The Grolier Club, 1936); Walpole, *Correspondence*, ed. Lewis, I, 114.

4. The wild balsam, belonging to the Cucurbitaceae or gourd family.

5. John Bartram was seventy-one.

6. Kalmias belong to a small genus of North American evergreen shrubs of the heath family, the Ericaceae, which includes the mountain laurel, the calico bush, and lambkill.

To Humphry Marshall, West Bradford, Chester County, Pennsylvania, 15 March 1770

London 15.3.1770

Esteemed Friend,[1]

Though I intended thee a long letter, yet I am through unavoidable engagements obliged to send thee only two or three lines.

I received the seeds, plants and cask with the *Colocasia* in very good order. Nothing ever I believe came over in better condition than the plants. I hope some of the roots of the *Colocasia* will live; but they were some of them quite rotten by the moisture. It will be a better way, I see,

319

to send them over in moss, than in mud and please plan to send me a root or two in this manner next autumn.[2]

Dr. Franklin will send all the instruments thou requests, for which I shall pay him cheerfully. Some of the books thou desires are at present out of print, but I shall get and send the rest of the volumes as soon as I can.

I have sent under Capt. Falconer's care an empty box locked, and the key secured to one of the handles. It is designed to secure any insects that may fall in thy way. The drawers are lined with cork, and it will be easy to fix either moths, flies or beetles upon them so as to come with safety. A great variety of beetles must be found under the best of all your old decayed trees.

Continue to send me such new seeds or plants as occur to thee. Ferns and *Polypodia*[3] of many kinds are yet to be found among you; many water plants likewise, which wrapped in wet moss would come to us safe. A Friend of mine has lately published a tract describing in what manner plants may be best conveyed to us, together with a description of your *Dionaea*.[4] Perhaps it may afford thee some little assistance in sending thy plants over.

I doubt not but you have many curious herbaceous plants yet unnoticed; struck with the green objects of shrubs and trees, these humbler ones have been overlooked. Get a complete collection of these into some corner of thy garden, and send us a few roots as thou art able to propagate them. There are few trees in your parts, and not many shrubs, which we have not in our gardens. We have many herbaceous plants likewise, but I dare say a very small number of those that are natives of your parts of America. Look carefully after some ferns for me; as also bulbous plants, as they flower early for the most part; and all sweet scented or showy flowers, or such as are of known efficacy in the cure of some diseases.

Thy account of the long-lived Tortoise is very agreeable; and I am much obliged to thy correspondent Bartram for some curious drawings. He has a very good hand; and I shall be glad to receive from him all his works, and satisfy him for his trouble when he informs me how much I am indebted.

Perhaps thou will be surprised when I tell thee one of my principal inducements to make . . . collections. It is that when I grow old and am unfit for the duties of a more active life, I may have some little amusement in store to fill up those hours when bodily infirmity may require some external consolations . . .

Farewell, I hope thou will hear from me again, in summer.

J. Fothergill

Ms. autograph letter, Miscellaneous Collections (Scientists), HSP; printed in Darlington, *Memorials*, 501–502.

1. Humphry Marshall had been sending specimens to Dr. Fothergill for several years.

2. This much admired member of the water lily family was never successfully naturalized in Dr. Fothergill's garden.

3. A varied and widely distributed family of ferns, known today as Polypodiaeceae.

4. John Ellis, *Directions for bringing over Seeds and Plants from the East-Indies, and other distant Countries in a State of Vegetation . . . together with a catalogue of . . . foreign plans . . . worthy of being encouraged in our American Colonies . . . to which are added the figure and description of a new sensitive Plant, called Dionaea Muscipula*, etc. (London: Davis, 1770). The plant described is popularly known as Venus' flytrap.

To John Bartram, Philadelphia, 19 March 1770

Harpur Street, 19.3.1770

Esteemed Friend,

Having an opportunity of sending thee the inclosed performance of my Friend John Ellis [1] by a young man who comes over as an apothecary to your Hospital,[2] I could not well avoid just sending thee two or three lines though much straitened for time.

In a letter I wrote to thee some time since I informed thee that my nephew James Freeman had undertaken to transact thy money affairs here, and to assist thee as far as he is capable, that I had passed into his hands ten guineas on my own account, and six more that I had received from John Lawin [3] of which I believe he will inform thee himself.

The Frogs are alive and well but not delivered. The King has been acquainted that they are here, and from whom they come; but the present state of the public affairs leaves him not a moment's time to think of anything else.[4] I will endeavour to provide a place for them in my own garden.

I have no express request to make for any plants in particular; but if anything new occurs, either plants or seeds, I should be very glad to be a sharer.

321

Thy son will be kind enough to continue his drawings of any non-descripts he may meet with, either plant or animals, and I shall endeavour to make him proper satisfaction. I hope soon to send thee a short account of the life of our late worthy Friend Peter Collinson; at least an essay towards his character. A few copies will be printed to give amongst his Friends, and no one is more entitled to this epithet than thyself.

I am, with much esteem,

Thy assured Friend,
John Fothergill

Ms. autograph letter, Bartram Papers, 22, HSP.

1. "The inclosed performance" was the pamphlet mentioned in the preceding letter. John Ellis, F.R.S. (*c.* 1710–1776), had established his reputation by *An Essay towards the Natural History of the Corallines, and other Marine Productions* . . . (London, Printed for the Author and Sold by A. Millar, 1755). He proved the animal nature of corals, tubular hydroids, and polyzoa, illustrating many of them for the first time. This book of only 104 pages was illustrated with forty plates and, in addition, contained a drawing of Cuff's marine microscope. Ellis was appointed agent for West Florida in 1764 and for Dominica in 1770, and improved his opportunities to import plans and seeds from the New World. He corresponded faithfully with Linnaeus, who called him "the main support of natural history in England," adding in a letter of 20 January 1772, "Without your aid, the rest of the world would know little of the acquisitions made by your intelligent countrymen in all parts of the world. You are the portal through which the lovers of Nature are conducted to these discoveries." — James Edward Smith, *A Selection of the Correspondence of Linnaeus* (London: Longman, 1821), I, 279–280.

2. In May 1770 William Smith, M.D., arrived in Philadelphia to become apothecary to the Pennsylvania Hospital. He brought credentials from Silvanus and Timothy Bevan, leading apothecaries of London. Articles of agreement drawn between the Hospitals' Board of Managers and Dr. Smith provided him with employment for three years at an annual salary of £100 Pennsylvania currency, good and sufficient food and drink, his lodging within the Hospital, and laundry as needed. — Pennsylvania Hospital Minute Book, IV.

3. Presumably a botanist; otherwise unidentified.

4. John Bartram was eager to have some American bullfrogs placed in the Royal Gardens. Acknowledgment of such a shipment in care of Dr. Fothergill was of course not to be expected from His Majesty.

To William Huddesford, University of Oxford, 21 April 1770

Harpur Street, 21st Inst.

Dr. Fothergill presents his respects to his Friend Huddesford, and takes the liberty to recommend the bearer, J. Miller, an ingenious painter and engraver and a good Botanist, to his protection and assistance.[1]

He is embarked in a design which will much contribute to facilitate the study of Botany, and comes down to solicit the patronage of your University.

He brings with him a small tribute from Dr. F. to the memory of the late Peter Collinson,[2] for his Friend Huddesford.

Ms. autograph letter, Ashmole Mss., no. 1822, ff. 395, Bodleian Library, Oxford. Date, April 1770, supplied in a modern hand.

1. Johann Sebastian Müller (d. 1790), born in Nuremberg, Bavaria, established himself in England about 1744. His early botanical works were signed "J. S. Müller," but after 1760 he used the signature "John Miller." His work for Philip Miller, curator of the Physick Garden, and for Dr. Fothergill won high praise. In 1770 he published the first number of an elaborate series of botanical plates with descriptive texts, to be issued in fifteen installments. John Ellis informed Linnaeus of the project: "This will make your System of Botany familiar to the Ladies, being in English as well as in Latin." The series was completed in 1776 and published as a whole in 1777: three folio volumes, with the English subtitle, *An Illustration of the Sexual System of the Genera Plantarum of Linnaeus.*
2. John Fothergill, M.D., *Some Account of the Late Peter Collinson* . . .

To Dr. John Coakley Lettsom, London, 11 August 1770

Lea Hall, 11th Inst. [8th mo.] 1770

Dear Doctor,

It was very kind to remember an absent Friend and under such circumstances.[1] I wish thee and thy agreeable consort all the happiness that will do you good. I know she will endeavour to deserve all thy regard and I think thou will not be wanting in affectionate esteem. Set out prudently, husband your mutual regard to the utmost advantage; be moderate in your hopes and expectations, so will you be less exposed to disappointments. It adds to my own satisfaction when I see my Friends

323

acting to the utmost of their abilities with discretion, for then I am sure let what will befall them; they cannot be unhappy. Thy partner will be what thou would wish to the utmost of her power. Be then, thyself, the prudent, sensible, affectionate husband and a consistent character, and she follows then throughout. But I have no right to send such prescriptions — I own it. A wish to see you possessed of all which in this life constitutes happiness prompted the expressions.

I was pleased to hear by my kinsman's J. Truman's wife [2] that everything at your marriage was conducted with much propriety. It is a favour when nothing on these occasions is permitted to happen that gives pain. I had heard by the papers of J.——'s death and could not but be satisfied with his removal. I am sorry that J. Cockfield's wife still continues indisposed. Perhaps it will be necessary to take away 3 or 4 ounces of blood, and if any degree of fever remains to enjoin a total abstinence from flesh meat, to live upon fresh vegetables and tarts and the like, to use no fermented liquors, to drink Salter's or Bristol Waters and milk for her common drink, and to use as little exercise as possible. Step down some afternoon and see her — perhaps a decoction of the Bark joined with Sal. Absin. (?) Lini might be of use.[3] Treat J. Cockfield and thyself with a sight of the Garden, for which I have included a passport [4] which will afford thee a subject for a letter. If Jemmy [5] can bear you company, take him. In viewing the Garden forget the indiscretion of the owner for making a Paradise he never must enjoy, but be pleased with its beauties, and be thankful to the Author of Nature for decorating this globe with numberless beauties. Tell Nancy [6] I believe I shall love her. I am sure I shall if she contributes to make thee wiser and better than thou art. We both salute you kindly.

From thy affectionate Friend
J.F.

Contemporary copy, Dimsdale Mss., LSFL.

1. On 16 July 1770, Dr. John Coakley Lettsom married Ann Miers, a young Quakeress of London, daughter of a wealthy tin-plate merchant. — Fox, 101, 102.

2. No Truman is recorded in the Fothergill Genealogy; the transcriber of the letter may have misread a reference to James Freeman's wife, Ann, daughter of the Doctor's brother Alexander.

3. Various concoctions of "the Bark" — cinchona bark — were popular remedies.

4. Joseph Cockfield, son of Zachariah Cockfield, the shipping merchant who had first recommended purchase of the Upton property to Dr. Fothergill, anticipating a later visit to the Upton garden in Lettsom's company, wrote to a friend in March 1771: "We are to have a passport signed by Dr. Fothergill, or most probably should

be refused admittance. His plants are now become so numerous, that to prevent intruders he is obliged to have recourse to this method." — Nichols, *Illustrations*, V (1828), 804.

5. Probably Joseph Cockfield's young son.
6. Ann, Dr. Lettsom's bride.

To Thomas Fisher, Philadelphia, 20 September 1770

Lea Hall, near Middlewich, Cheshire,

20.9.1770

Esteemed Friend,

I think myself much obliged to thee for thy care and diligence in disposing of A. Purver's Translation. The bill came safe and the account entirely to my satisfaction. Twenty sets more I expect will be come to hand before this time. They were shipped on board the Philadelphia packet, Captain Falconer.[1]

I have allowed William Young, the son of a person in your Province who is now in America searching for plants, to draw upon thee for twenty pounds sterling, should he have occasion.[2] If the books have not put thee in cash for so much when he draws, please to advance it, and charge the commission and so forth and deduct from the balance.

I write this from Cheshire whither I have been obliged to retire a few months in the summer these four or five years past. I am therefore a stranger to the news of the town, and can convey no interesting intelligence. The conduct of New York will embarrass the rest of the Colonies much.[3] I often remember the motto of a noble English family, *Aut nunquam tentes, aut perspici*: Either never begin, or go through stretch. Had I been an American, I think I should have submitted at once to the Stamp Act. But at the same time I would have petitioned, then remonstrated, then resolved to take as little from Great Britain as possible, if no other means could have obtained relief. You began at the wrong end. New York has undone you.

At present the commerce of Great Britain is so flourishing that the non-importation scheme has not been much felt. The Russians being at War cannot manufacture the things they used to do and yet must have. A new door of commerce has been opened likewise through Italy to some remote places behind them. Through Germany likewise our trade flourishes. I know not how our demands could otherwise have been

325

supplied. The merchants trading to America are doubtless great sufferers as well as you by the present mode. What you will determine upon is as uncertain as the relief you may expect from Parliament. I wish prudence, not passion, may dictate on both sides. If you are uneasy we cannot be happy. No more than the body when only a tooth aches.

I am thy obliged friend

John Fothergill

Manuscript autograph letter, William Logan Fox Collection (photostat, HSP).

1. Purver's translation of the Bible, published in 1764, had poor sales in England. When Dr. Fothergill's library was sold in 1781, some twenty copies came on the market.

2. William Young, dismissed from the gardening staff at Kew Gardens when he was threatened with imprisonment for debt, had returned to Pennsylvania. Dr. Fothergill, hopeful for the young man's future, had seen that he received commissions to collect plants for British gardeners and also for the Upton garden, a service for which he was well paid. — John W. Harshberger, "William Young, Jr., of Philadelphia," *Torreya*, 17:92–99 (June 1917).

3. The Townshend duties, except the tax on tea, had been repealed on 5 March 1770. New York merchants, after receiving news of the repeal, had voted to resume importation of untaxed British goods. — Thayer, *Pennsylvania Politics*, 146–147.

To Humphry Marshall, West Bradford, Chester County, Pennsylvania, 11 February 1771

London, 11.2.1771

Esteemed Friend,

I have now before me thy two kind letters, one of the 25th. 5 mo., the other the 19th. 11 mo. 1770. The former contains some pertinent accounts of the medicinal effects of some of your native simples, for which I am obliged to thee. It is quite proper to record all the useful observations relative to your indigenous simples. It requires a long time and much experience to know the use of any one medicine. We are apt sometimes to ascribe effects to the wrong causes; and if a disorder wears off after the use of any medicine, it is usual to place the recovery to the account of the medicine.

The Sassafras Bark,[1] I think, is a good medicine in various complaints; and especially in all such as seem to arise from a thin, sharp scorbutic humour, especially in cold constitutions, or aged people. From its sensible qualities it seems likely to expel wind, correct sharpness of the blood, and if given properly, to increase urine and sweat. Attend to its effects, and give a strong effusion of it in such complaints as may seem to proceed from these causes.

We are so well pleased with our Ipecacuanha; [2] it operates so certainly, so gently, that we shall scarcely be soon prevailed upon to admit of any substitute. I wish, however, your Ipecac may be attended to. Gather it when the leaves are decaying; wash it clean, dry it in the shade, and powder it fine. In case of sickness, where a vomit is required, give ten grains; wait half an hour, give a second dose, and try by such means, how small a quantity will answer the purpose.

I should be exceedingly glad to hear that you had any indigenous medicine or simple that would operate freely and certainly by urine. We want such a remedy much. We can promote all the natural discharges with some degree of certainty, but this. We can vomit, purge, sweat, to what degree we please, but we have no certain diuretic. This is much wanted in the cure of dropsies and other complaints. Listen carefully after such a remedy.[3] And now to thy second letter.

Captain Osborne has been arrived for some time, but has been hindered from delivering his goods by a severe frost, and the want of hands, from pressing. The plants and seeds are, however, at length delivered and sent down to my garden, but I have not yet seen in what condition. We have still a hard frost and much snow so that I must keep them as they are until the weather breaks. In the catalogue I see a great number of curious things, and we shall take all the care we can to raise them, and revive the plants.

The box with Insects, by Captain Sparks, came very safe, and the insects in very tolerable condition for the most part. Some of them had suffered by being put in the box before they were quite dry. I have returned the box for another cargo, if any variety occur, and likewise for any duplicates of as many of those that were first sent to me as may be easily procured, for most of them were damaged. Your cedar is too hard and gummy. It exudes a kind of liquor that spoils insects. Your softest fir would do much better. But my box is preferable to anything. Let the boxes be taken out and well dried before any insects are put in. Let the insects likewise be well dried, and a bit of camphire and powdered pepper be tied in a rag and fixed in each partition.

As I have now most of the common American plants in plenty, I would not give thee the trouble of sending more seeds or plants of this

327

kind I have received from thee, except such as I may hereafter require to make up for defects. Any new kinds, either plants or seeds, will be very acceptable.

William Young sends his plants over very safely, by wrapping them up in moss, and packing them pretty close in a box. They come very safe, and we lose very few of them. He ties the moss in a ball about the roots with a piece of packthread or matting, or hemp strings, and puts them so close as to prevent them from shaking about in the box. It is surprising how well they keep in this manner.

I have recommended the following method to my friends, likewise, of sending over seeds in a vegetating condition. Make a box of any width and length, but not very deep; six or seven inches may be sufficient. Cover the bottom with moss (Sphagnum), not quite dry. On this lay acorns or any large kinds of seeds in patches; that is half a dozen, or half a score together, according to their plenty. Cover these with moss, and strew on the top, in patches likewise, any small scarce seeds. These, sent off in autumn, will be committed to proper earth early in the spring here, and will probably supply us with many plants that we should otherwise procure with difficulty.

I wish we may be successful with the *Colocasia*. We will do all we can, and I shall acquaint thee with the success.

The *Alder* [4] is a fine one; the seeds are taken care of, but try to propagate it both by seeds, layers and cuttings; and let us have a few plants.

I hope to write to thee again by Captain Osborne. In the meantime accept my grateful compliments, and think me to be

Thy obliged Friend,
J. Fothergill

The Mocking-Bird unfortunately perished in the passage. The box for Insects will come by Captain Osborne.

Ms. autograph letter, Miscellaneous Collections (Scientists), HSP; printed in Darlington, *Memorials*, 502–505.

1. The root bark of the American sassafras (family Lauraceae), used as a diaphoretic, a flavoring agent, an aromatic stimulant, also for perfumes, supplying an aromatic volatile oil.

2. A tropical South American plant, *Cephalis ipecacuanhana*, popularly called Brazilian ipecac, the dried rhizome and roots of which were formerly used for medicine and are now valued as the source of emetine. *Euphorbia ipecacuanhae* of the eastern United States, the American white ipecac, has a root with emetic and purgative properties.

3. It was not necessary for American botanists to provide the desired medicament. Not many years after this letter was written a Shropshire doctor learned from an old country-woman that the dried and powdered leaf of the common English wildflower, foxglove (*Digitalis purpurea*), was good for dropsy. See William Withering, *An Account of the Foxglove* (London, 1785).

4. The white alder of North America, *Clethra alnifolia*.

To James Pemberton, Philadelphia, 12 February 1771

London, 12.2.1771

Esteemed Friend —

After many repeated applications to the Solicitor whom the Trustees have employed in the Pennsylvania business, I have this evening obtained the draught of a power of Attorney to enable me, or any other person whom the Managers of your Hospital may think fit to appoint, to apply to Chancery and receive the money due to your Hospital.[1]

It has given me much concern that it has not been in my power to communicate this sooner. But as our Solicitor was best acquainted with the transaction, I thought him the most suitable person to enable me to give the Managers such a draught, as when properly executed, would admit of the fewest possible objections on this side the water.

I could wish to have the name of David Barclay inserted instead of mine. He is more at leisure, and more in the way of transacting such affairs than I am. The Solicitor objected to it, that as I was a person pretty generally known that fewer exceptions would be made, but I think this objection altogether groundless.

I believe the sum now amounts to upwards of seven thousand pounds sterling and I shall be exceedingly pleased to have it speedily remitted to you. I hope indeed the Hospital will not have suffered by the delay, for the declining state of the publick stocks for many months during the late apprehension of war with Spain would have made a very considerable difference in this capital.

Should your lawyers be of opinion that this power is improper in any respect, let it be altered. I am not a judge of these affairs, but I think at least it is long enough and recites so many particulars that it cannot fail of succeeding.

I hope the Managers will attribute this delay to its proper and only cause, the delay of our Solicitor. The day after I received the request to

329

look after this business, I sent him the letter, and desired he would furnish me with an answer speedily. Scarce a ship has sailed or a packet left us but I have reminded him in time. A menace to employ another at length procured this.

I must embrace another opportunity to write to thee further on several particulars. At present I am more indisposed with a cold than I could wish, and obliged at the same time to do very hard duty.

Give my kind respects to thy Brother, to Abel James,[2] J. Hunt and our common acquaintance, and be assured that I am

Thy assured Friend
J. Fothergill

Ms. autograph letter, Pemberton Papers, Etting Collection, II, 64, HSP.

1. It will be recalled that Trustees of the joint-stock partnership known as the Pennsylvania Land Company in London had been empowered to sell certain estates of that company in Pennnsylvania, New Jersey, and Maryland, and distribute the proceeds to claimants. All unclaimed assets remaining in the hands of the Trustees on 24 June 1770 were to be assigned to the Pennsylvania Hospital. Money acquired by sale of property was to be deposited in the Bank of England, from which sums might be withdrawn after proper application, and then placed out at interest in some of the public funds of the Kingdom. Purchase of "3 per cent reduced Bank Annuities" had been a safe and profitable investment. — Morton and Woodbury, *Pennsylvania Hospital*, 250–294.

2. Abel James (1726–1790) and his partner, Henry Drinker, ran an export-import business in their own ships, having a wharf on the Delaware at the foot of Arch Street. Both were members of the American Philosophical Society. — Cecil K. Drinker, *Not So Long Ago* (New York: Oxford University Press, 1937), 5.

To James Pemberton, Philadelphia, 13 February 1771

London, 13.2.1771

Dear Friend,

I have just got the enclosed in time to send by our valuable acquaintance Nancy Pearson,[1] who has been so obliging as to see us as often as her business would permit. We were pleased with it as she acts the part of a mutual Friend; brings us an account of our esteemed Friends with you, and carries back all the intelligence she can get that may be acceptable to you. In the parcel is a letter directed to William Young, Jr. Be pleased to give it to my Friend Israel Pemberton, and request his care in forwarding it, with my kind respects.

In one of your epistles from the Meeting for Sufferings, mention I think is made of remitting one hundred pounds for the service of the Meeting for Sufferings here. I do not recollect it has been received.

The *Select Works of William Penn* [2] will come by Capt. Osborn. It is finished.

You have lost one of your Proprietaries, Richard Penn. He died in a very short time but of an illness that had at times affected him many years, a spasmodic affection of the whole breast with intense pain.[3] His brother bears it as well as can reasonably be expected. My Brother Samuel in company with John Eliot [4] has paid a visit lately to the families of Friends within the compass of Westminster monthly meeting (within which we reside much), I hope to his own satisfaction. We are but few, are scattered thinly, through a large space, and the few zealous ancients that formerly lived in this quarter being removed by death, their successors have been much discouraged and almost lost hope of comfort. Yet there are some valuable young men in the quarter and I hope things will revive.

In respect to publick affairs I know but little. I think we shall have no war; and I believe little will be done in respect to America; if anything, it will be undoubtedly to yours and consequently to our disadvantage. Abel James knows the sentiments of those who have it chiefly in their power to do what is right. But they continue inflexible.

I wish your Province would establish a general Register of births, burials, and marriages — to have an officer, some person who can write and read in every township, to register these circumstances within a few days after the fact, and to transmit the account to Philadelphia annually. Much useful information would accrue from it. If you once think of it seriously, I will send a copy of a bill brought into Parliament here some years ago, and the reason of its miscarriage.

But I am called away, and can only add that I am thy affectionate Friend

J. Fothergill

Ms. autograph letter, Pemberton Papers, Etting Collection, II, 65, HSP.

1. A Quakeress, well esteemed in her ministry; she is not identified in the records consulted.

2. An edition (London, 1771) supervised by Dr. Fothergill; it contains an unsigned preface which he probably wrote.

3. Richard Penn had died on 4 February 1771. His "spasmodic affection" indi-

cates angina pectoris, a disease first described in 1769 by Dr. William Heberden. Dr. Fothergill subsequently wrote two important papers on the subject which demonstrated that the pain was due to disease of the coronary arteries. — C. C. Booth, "Dr. John Fothergill and the Angina Pectoris," *Medical History*, 1 (1957): 115–122.

4. John Eliot of Bartholomew Close, London, whose hospitable home was always open to Friends from the American Colonies.

To Samuel Fothergill, Warrington, Lancashire, 22 February 1771

Harpur Street, London
11 at night, 22nd Inst.

Dear Brother,

It is now just half past ten o'clock at night, the post will call in half an hour, and yet I cannot let him pass without scribbling a line or two. It will give thee satisfaction to hear from us; it will take a little weight from my own mind to write to thee though I have nothing more to say than that we are as well as may reasonably be expected in such a season and such a manner of life as we are cast into.

We have received thy own and our relations' accounts of thy return with great satisfaction;[1] remember the motto I have so often given thee *Nequid nimis!*[2] Write it in capitals everywhere. I endeavour to attend to it, in the midst of seeming hurry. With grateful reverence I acknowledge it; not from myself but, I trust, from the secret motions of better help. I receive the intimations of it with thankfulness and daily wish to follow on, to know.

W. Penn's Select Works will now soon be published.[3] Another edition of R. Davies is likewise ordered, a very valuable piece.[4] B. Richman's crash has hurt abundance, ruined some, and spread general reproach.[5] I wish he may feel as he ought to do, but I doubt it. The wound however deep to many will be alleviated as far as may be. He would make an excellent whitewasher; if the colour would but last.

May a person who needs advice as much as most, and at the same time does not profit by it so much as he ought, presume to give it? Thy affection for me will throw a mantle of oblivion over me if I say anything that does not correspond with thy own reflections. Be short in supplication; use no words not of common use, and the same as seldom as possible. The ineflable majesty of heaven is enough to dazzle all human concepts, yet the "Our Father who art in heaven" is indeed a complete model. Stray from its simplicity as seldom as possible. But I speak with unhallowed lips and therefore forgive me. My wish is as strong that the Father of Mercies may long preserve thee a choice instrument, a silver trumpet that gives a celestial sound, as thine is, that I may be conducted wisely through a thorny, slippery, arduous track to safety and happiness at last. So let it be for us both, saith all within me.

Our mutual acquaintance I think are well. The Friends of this quarter I hope [retain] a grateful savour of thy labours amongst them. I know not what S.L.[6] intends to do, but if he does not appeal against our next Monthly Meeting, I know not what step he should take properly. He has never yet given me his charges in writing. He read them and they are silly enough indeed. But he is perfectly intractable. One of those happy people who never are in the wrong but find all others so. The bell now rings, I mean the postman's, and I have only time to say that so far as we know our affection is undiminished to our Friends, relations, and particularly our Brother. Farewell.

J. Fothergill

Ms. autograph letter, Port. 22/138, LSFL. Month and year supplied from internal evidence.

1. In December, 1770, Samuel Fothergill had been very busy in the work of the ministry, with John Eliot visiting "upwards of fifty" Quaker families belonging to Westminster Meeting. After his return to Warrington, on 2 February he wrote to his brother and sister that he had "silently fed on the pleasure of our late interview." He also reported, "My return home was in much quiet." — Crosfield, *Memoirs*, 499–500.

2. The Latin quotation from Terence, *Andria*, lines 60–61, reads in full: *Id arbitror / Adprime in vita esse utile ne quid nemis* (My view is that the most important thing in life is never to have too much of anything).

3. This edition had been prepared for the press by Dr. Fothergill.

4. Richard Davies (1635–1705) was the author of *An Account of the Convincement, Exercises, Services and Travels of that Ancient Servant of the Lord, Richard Davies, with some Relation of Ancient Friends, and the Spreading of Truth in North-Wales* . . . This Welsh Quaker classic was first published in 1710; a second edition had appeared in 1765, and in 1770 a third edition was produced in Philadelphia by Cruickshank and Collins. The edition mentioned here by Dr. Fothergill was the third English edition (London: Mary Hinde, 1771).

5. Probably Benjamin Richman (or Rickman), "for some years a minister of eminence among Friends in London and Southwark . . . who experienced great vicissitudes in life . . . and whose business . . . was . . . unsuccessful until at last he failed and lost his membership with Friends." Richman's bankruptcy evidently caused heavy losses to Friends who had made investments in his business. He died in Dublin in August 1785. — Quotation from the manuscript Recollections of James Jenkins (LSFL).

6. The initials S.L. refer to Dr. Samuel Leeds, a Quaker who had studied medicine in Edinburgh. After receiving his degree in 1766, he went to London and in 1768 was given a staff position at London Hospital. He made an unfavorable impression. Dr. Fothergill, convinced of Leeds's incompetence, told a senior member of the hospital staff that he feared for the safety of patients entrusted to Dr. Leeds. There were other complaints, and the Board of Governors of London Hospital met the situation by a new ruling whereby all staff members were required to be licentiates of the Royal College of Physicians. — Fox, 74, 75. Since Leeds had never received licensure, he was obliged to present himself at the College for examination by the Board of Censors. Sir Kenneth Robson, C.B.E., F.R.C.P., the present Registrar of the Royal College of Physicians, has kindly supplied from the Annals of the Royal College of Physicians the following abstract: "Dr. Samuel Leeds attended 6 April 1770, and being asked whether it was not his request that the Board would examine him in order to know whether he was qualified to be a Licentiate, replied that it was. He produced a Diploma from Edinburgh, dated 25 August 1766, by which he was created Doctor in Physick. He was examined *in parte Physiologica*, and was desired to return to his studies."

Leeds, completely discredited and profoundly depressed by his failure, sent a letter of complaint against Dr. Fothergill to Westminster Monthly Meeting in November 1770. Upon receiving this communication, the Meeting gave the matter profound attention, since Dr. Fothergill was one of the most highly esteemed members of the Society of Friends. A committee of four members was finally appointed to meet both accuser and accused at a special session. Leeds refused to take part in such a meeting, and wrote another letter repeating his grievances. This letter was returned to him with advice to drop the matter entirely. Weeks passed without definite results until late April 1771, when Leeds appealed the matter to the Quarterly Meeting. — Information from Minute Books of the Society of Friends, supplied by courtesy of Edward H. Milligan, Librarian, LSFL.

To Thomas Bentley, Burslem, Staffordshire, 9 April 1771

Harpur Street, April 9. 1771

Respected Friend,[1]

Two sober young women at Middlewich, possessed of a little property,[2] at my request chiefly propose to employ a little of their property in the pottery business.

The little town is so bare in this respect that if we wanted the most common article in the glass or pottery way it was seldom to be met with; others complained as well as ourselves. Who is there at Burslem, that one could recommend them to, that would not impose upon young, unexperienced girls, but who would be likely to give them proper instructions and furnish them with a suitable assortment of goods in this way for young beginners?

I shall endeavour to take care that their payments shall be punctually made. They may go so far as about 40 pounds at their first beginning, and may advance as they meet with success. Be kind enough to give me a line as soon as convenient, and believe me to be

Thy respectfull servant
J. Fothergill

Ms. autograph letter (30669–55), Wedgwood Museum, Barlaston, Staffordshire.

1. Thomas Bentley (1731–1803), born at Scropton, Derbyshire, settled in Liverpool after his marriage in 1754, and became manager of a warehouse for a Manchester firm. A dissenter with liberal interests, he had assisted in establishing the dissenters' Academy in Warrington (*ca.* 1760), and in building the Octagon Chapel, Temple Court, Liverpool, for a short-lived religious sect known as "the Octagonians," to which he belonged. In 1769 he moved to Burslem to assist Josiah Wedgwood, and in 1771 settled in London to take charge of Wedgwood's warehouse and retail trade. Wedgwood's dinner sets were becoming the fashion in London, especially after purchase of a cream-ware dinner service by Queen Charlotte. Wedgwood, in correspondence with Bentley, urged him to "have the dinner service for David Barclay as fine and neat as possible; the Quakers . . . have been trying my wares, and verily, they find it much to their wishes in every respect. As my future orders from the Brethren much depend upon this set, a word to the wise is sufficient." According to Wedgwood's biographer, Dr. Fothergill and his sister recommended these exquisite productions everywhere. — Eliza Meteyard, *The Life and Works of Josiah Wedgwood*, 2 vols. (London: Hurst and Blackett, 1865–66), II, 1–6.

2. The two young women were named Merrick and lived in the village of Middlewich, Cheshire, near Dr. Fothergill's country house, Lea Hall. — Unpublished note, Dr. Fothergill to Thomas Bentley (30670–55), Wedgwood Museum, Barlaston.

To Samuel Fothergill, Warrington, Lancashire, 11 April 1771

London, 11.4.1771

Dear Brother,

Though I take up a sheet of paper, I recollect the busy time in which it arrives and hope therefore not to fill up more than a page of it.

I should indeed be glad that the short visit of the gout which thou hast had lately may suffice for the season. I am pretty confident that a reasonable attention to the hints I gave will be of great consequence.

We had at Bradford an inscription of a sign which may perhaps have been in every town in England: *Good ale tomorrow for nothing.* I have seen many people trespass my rules *today* and have promised to themselves to perform them better *tomorrow.* I do not think this is thy case.

335

I know thy sentiments better, but one can never be too cautious in trusting to that *tomorrow*. Thy letters to us read affection for us in every instance, and manifest a mind intent on its own improvement and advancement of congenial warmth in others. We accept them as such, and I hope they have the effect thou wishes upon us.

In this packet comes a letter to R. Watson [1] enclosing one hundred pounds; the same I have added to all our Nieces' portions. I have made Nanny [2] a little present also that she may be as little burdensome as possible. We rejoice with you on the occasion as far as we may; but we must have time to reconcile ourselves thoroughly to an affair which was not to us the most desirable thing that could happen. Excuse me for taking this over to another page. I quit the subject wholly when I have said bestow thy approbation slowly, as thou would do thy money, till thou art sure the objects are not unworthy. If they are worthy, they will stay for it till they have deserved it.

Our Friend, shall I say our esteemed Friend, Thomas Whitehead,[3] is no more. He left London some time since and went to Reading. Many illnesses befell him; at last he paid the debt of Nature. Where we have a strong hope that all is well, we mention these things with satisfaction; the same must soon be said of us, and we are happy whatever our situation may be, if the genuinely sensible among us have hope concerning us. Our own approbation or the giddy multitudes, have nothing to do with us. My Sister received thine by the last post, and by her report of the letter she wrote to thee [4] is apprehensive she may soon receive another. I have nothing to do in your quarrel, but when she interferes to save my pocket, surely I ought to take her part. Indeed my Niece's migration is not so pleasing to us as to induce me to pay her passage, though she and her husband and thyself had petitioned for it, unless you had sued in *forma pauperis*. Her happiness is the first object; ours a secondary. When both unite, it's better than when neither.

I dare go no further lest I should begin another page and trespass against my introduction. To say that I wish everything prosperous in thy undertaking in the present scene is saying little. Oh, that wisdom and strength to go in and out before the people may be granted; Farewell. Affectionately,

J. Fothergill

Ms. autograph letter, Port. 22/114, LSFL.

1. Robert Watson of Waterford, Ireland, a Quaker businessman of excellent repu-

tation, was soon to marry Molly Fothergill (1750–1834) in Warrington Meeting House.

2. Molly's unmarried older sister, Ann (1745–1807), one of six daughters of the Doctor's brother Joseph. Four of the sisters were already married.

3. Thomas Whitehead of Peel Meeting, an elderly Quaker minister, who had made a religious visit to America early in life. — Testimonies Concerning Ministers, II, 337, LSFL.

4. In a letter to her brother Samuel, Ann explained one cause of Dr. John's annoyance over the approach of Molly's wedding. Evidently Samuel had hinted to Ann that Dr. John might be willing to pay Molly's traveling expenses to Ireland. This Dr. Fothergill refused to do; he had given £100 to each of his married nieces, paid their wedding expenses, and provided their household linen. He was unwilling to make larger expenditures at this time. Ann thought Dr. John was right. In her opinion "M. and R." seemed to have enough money for every purpose, "and I think I might say to superfluity, at least what our Dear Father would have thought reprehensible." — Fothergill Family Letters, LSFL.

To Robert Watson, Warrington, Lancashire, 11 April 1771

London, 11.4.1771

Esteemed Friend and now our Kinsman,

I have presented my Nieces, when they were married, a small addition to their Fortune.

Molly's husband has the like claim, and though, shall I say in some respects reluctantly, Justice obliges me to comply.[1]

I wish you may be helpmeets to each other. The only alleviation to the concern I feel on this occasion will be to hear that you act as becomes persons descended as you are from the noblest ancestry because they were pious and adorned their stations by their virtues.

Time, and your good conduct, and the reputation thence arising, will make me forget the distance from a relation we have valued, and also from one we wish to esteem affectionately. Farewell —

J. Fothergill

Ms. autograph letter, enclosed in a packet addressed to Samuel Fothergill, Warrington, with the preceding letter of the same date, Port. 22/85, LSFL.

1. Molly's fiancé seems to have had an irreproachable character; Uncle John was reluctant to have Molly marry him probably because she would then live in Ireland, and he would seldom see her. The courtship of the young people had been described to Samuel by Ann in June 1770:

"A young man from Ireland (with a favourable character in his own country) has visited Molly pretty frequently since he came to town. His approbation by her much confirmed, he could not leave the Nation without making his inclination known. — He told his case to Joshua Wilson who encouraged him, and 2 or 3 days ago he came to ask my Brother's (J.F.'s) consent . . . My brother told him he was not left so he could give permission to any application . . . further than that he might interest himself in her welfare as a near relation, that thou was her guardian to be applied to . . . He then earnestly intreated him to impart his Mind to Molly . . . He has spoke to Molly . . . she does not at once dismiss the affair. My Brother advises her to consider it well, and act at least a candid generous part to him, not to let him lose time and labour if she cannot accept." — Letter dated "6th mo. 30, 1770," Port. 22/71, LSFL.

To William Logan, Philadelphia, 22 April 1771

Harpur Street, London
22.4.1771

Dear Friend,

This evening I received thy acceptable letters of 3rd and 6th by the New York packet. This comes by thy Son, who I hope will arrive safe and live to afford thee comfort.[1] When a little more experience, some difficulty and a few years have passed, perhaps the Doctor will begin to think it worth his while to apply his heart to wisdom.

I have entreated him earnestly to shun as much as possible administering any cause of offence to his brothers of the Faculty.[2] As surgery may be his line; if he acts properly, all the practitioners may be his friends or his enemies, just as he behaves. Excuse me for telling the Father that his Son requires the utmost of his prudence to guard him against a multitude of inconveniences. With much sensibility and without experience, he is presumptuous. If he carries this disposition too far into his business, he will be undone. Let him creep gradually into credit. Credit arising from desert, not recommendation solely. — If I regarded him less, I should say none of these things which a father's affection can hardly bear. I am more impartial. I view him in a less prejudiced situation. Keep an equal, steady, affectionate authority over him. Bear now and then with his eccentricities, but don't let them blind thee. May the great father of the family of which we are a part endow thee with wisdom understanding and fortitude to guide this young man safely in the middle path of judgement. If I say he is vain, conceited of his abilities, thinks he is equal to all emergencies, superior to every difficulty that can occur, I should not say too much. Therefore take care of him and lead him to think more humbly of himself, before others tell him so in less affectionate language. Show him this and welcome. I have not a wish in my heart concerning him, but for his good, his interest and reputation. I only fear he will not pursue the proper road to any of them, but will strew his road with thorns and afflict the tenderest of his connections. Let his conduct convince me my apprehensions are wrong, and I will promise him I am strongly disposed to receive conviction.

Thy son and the public papers will inform thee in general of our present situation. I do not however think that we are at the eve of any great calamity, though most undoubtedly, we are verging fast to correction. To describe our present situation, the causes that evidently operate to make us from the most envied of all people, the most contemptible, would require a volume. But the ways of providence are unsearchable and I dare not enter upon the subject. The rumors of war are blown over — that is, between us and Spain. France is too feeble to lend the Spaniard any effectual aid. Russia and the Turk are mutually disposed to a conference. Poland will be divided amongst the neighboring powers,[3] and not improbably to its advantage. For nothing can be more miserable than its present state.

There is one thing which will keep the powers in Europe quiet for another year — a scarcity of provisions. Mutton is here at sixpence a pound; in France still dearer; in Switzerland still more so; and we know not of any magazines of corn of consequence enough to supply us. Our winter has been singularly severe. We have not had the sudden extreme rigour of 1739 and '40, but we have had a uniform continuance of a four months' frost. We are at least six weeks later in all the vegetable products than I ever remember. At the date of this, our gooseberry bushes are not covered with leaves quite expanded, and we used to have the fruit by this time carried about in wheelbarrows. [*Short passage omitted.*]

I cannot give up R. Willan's affairs as lost.[4] He had a grant for five thousand acres in Florida; if any adventurer with you would offer me anything considerable for it, I would put him in possession of the grant which is assigned to me for security of the money I paid him to promote his emigration. The land will be valuable to somebody, at some time. It must surely be worth 150 £–sterling to somebody now. It is not located, nor any cultivation of consequence begun.

Richard Penn is no more. Your Governor will return to Europe, and his younger brother succeed to the government.[5] Whether things will

339

change for the better I know not; I am not acquainted with either. — But the hands he falls into on coming over to you, must determine his future complexion.

I am dishonest sometimes through neglect, never I hope through design. Tell me in thy next how much I am in arrears to poor Thomas Lees,[6] and I will pay it instantly to D. Barclay.

I received the box of insects, but sadly spoiled. The wood was too hard to fix them into, and the seams of the box too wide to keep out the moisture. The seeds he sent were in bad condition, and I wish some other means could be hit upon for his support than making such collections. If he has more time on his hands than he can otherwise employ to advantage, and will collect for me any scarce or new plants and will send them late in autumn, well packed in moss, I will give him as much for a few scarce plants as he may probably receive for a larger parcel and less curious. All early spring flowers of the herbaceous tribe would be acceptable; ferns of every kind, flowering shrubs or forest trees; insects well preserved, land and river shells, great or small. Such things he may be able to collect in his walks through the woods, without great expense or trouble, and I shall endeavour to make him proper satisfaction.

The last two weeks have been filled up with much business among our Friends at Warrington. My niece Molly has thought proper to accept of R. Watson, a young Friend from Ireland. The Monthly Meeting, the marriage, the Quarterly Meeting for the county held at Warrington, the Yearly Meeting at Chester were all held in less than ten days. What a Tempest! I expect they are embarked at Park Gate [7] today for Ireland, my Brother accompanying them, and to be present at the Half-year's meeting at Dublin, from thence to Waterford, the residence of the young couple; from thence home, and to the Yearly Meeting in London to be held this day month. Is this to be called diligence — or something more?

I scribble this at a very late hour and after a very laborious day — all mine are such. This must be my apology for faults almost without number. Now thy son's returned, don't forget me. I will write when I can, and if I do not pay punctually, don't be hasty to declare me a bankrupt. My Sister is gone to bed or I am sure she would join me in affectionate remembrance,

from thy Friend
J. Fothergill

Ms. autograph letter, probably from the William Logan Fox Collection, Philadelphia, and presented to Dr. R. Hingston Fox of London. The letter is now found in two parts, Port. 38/95 and 95a, LSFL.

1. Young William Logan was on his way back to America with his wife. He had received his medical degree from the University of Edinburgh after presenting his dissertation, *De regimine phthisicorum*, 12 June 1770. A printed copy of this dissertation has been contributed to the Library of the American Philosophical Society, Philadelphia.

2. Popular designation of the medical profession.

3. The so-called first partition of Poland — parts being taken by Russia, Prussia, and Austria — occurred in 1772, with Poland agreeing to it in 1773.

4. The same Robert Willan of Yorkshire, temporarily a schoolmaster at Penn Charter School, who had made "a precipitate return" to London years earlier. See letter to John Smith, 20 August 1753, note 2.

5. Richard Penn's son John (1729–1795) had been Deputy Governor of Pennsylvania since 1763. His father's death recalled him to England to help in settling the family estate. During his absence of two years, his brother Richard Penn II (1735–1811) officiated as deputy Governor. Upon John Penn's return to Philadelphia, he once again became Governor, holding office from 1773 to 1776. The Proprietary era then came to a close as the War for Independence progressed. — William R. Shepherd, *The Proprietary Government of Pennsylvania: Studies in History, Economics, and Public Law* (New York: Columbia University Press, 1896), 493, 494n, 571–575.

6. See letter of 8 May 1769.

7. Robert Watson and Molly sailed from Park Gate on the River Dee, near the city of Chester, accompanied by Molly's Uncle Samuel and her sister Ann. Samuel Fothergill, after a short stop in Waterford to see Molly's new home, had a full schedule of Quaker meetings to attend in Dublin and vicinity. Ann remained in Waterford for a short time to help Molly get settled.

To Samuel Fothergill, Waterford, Ireland, 2 May 1771

Harpur Street, London, 2.5.1771

Dear Brother,

We received thy affectionate letter from Warrington and one from Dublin, much to our satisfaction. Some of our Friends from this place have acquainted us in general how you all were, and how you had fared. We rejoice that all was well.

This will meet thee perhaps in thy return at Dublin; [1] it may inform thee that we are well and hope nothing will prevent our seeing thee amongst us at our approaching Solemnity.[2] If thou has leisure at Dublin I have a commission or two which I would wish thee to execute for me. One is to remember me affectionately to Dr. Rutty,[3] and tell him he is in my debt. Another is to see George Cleghorn,[4] if thou has time to spare. Send for him to thy lodgings, tell him thou art my Brother, and

341

that I desired thee to see him as a means to brighten the chain of Friendship between us. We have long been acquainted, long had a mutual esteem, and if he is as good as he knows he ought to be, I shall esteem him more than I can describe. Tell him that I think he exceeds most of his countrymen in respect to sincerity, and for this I love him, and that he is inferior to none of them in regard to the business of his profession, and for this I honour him.

Thou has left our Nieces in a place I am fully a stranger to.[5] But wherever they are I doubt not but they will have as much partiality showed them as will do them good, for the name's sake; our Father and thyself will be long remembered in that kingdom. I cannot soon reconcile myself to some things which do not strike me at first with propriety. All that has passed may be right, and I ought to believe it so, but still I must beg time to be quite pleased with this migration. — I have had an exceedingly labourious winter and spring. I already count how many weeks there are to our retreat into Cheshire.

A daughter-in-law of Cuthbert Higham, and a Friend of the name of Watson from the same part, are in town at present on a visit to Friends. I believe they are well received, and I hope meet with an open door everywhere.

If Dr. Rutty thinks that Purver's translation of the Bible would be acceptable to Friends or others in Ireland and would undertake to mention it to any bookseller there, some copies would be sent over so as to be sold at an acceptable rate, and with the usual proportion to the bookseller. Perhaps 20 or 30 copies might be properly disposed of.

Thou hast heard no doubt of T. Whitehead's decease. Daniel Woodward of our Quarter is also removed; in other respects I know not of much alteration among our Friends.

Dr. Thompson [6] has passed the Meetings, but when or where or how the marriage is to be accomplished, we know not. — Will Logan and Sally are suited.[7] Dr. Lettsom has had a tedious confinement from an inflammation of the eye which is still painful. Nothing decisive is done in Leeds's affair. He appealed against our Monthly Meeting. The committee appointed prevailed on me to consent to an arbitration. I did so for peace sake, and he withdrew his appeal.[8] He can get nobody to act as Arbitrators. Here the thing lies at present. I shall not be in any hurry, but if he does not proceed, I think I shall, and press a complaint against him to his own Monthly Meeting for better reasons than he has to allege against me, but I hope to do nothing rashly or from resentment.

Farewell, dear Brother, farewell. We salute thee affectionately, and without deductions. —

J. and A. Fothergill

Ms. autograph letter, Port. 22/115, LSFL.

1. Samuel Fothergill had been called to attend Quaker meetings outside Dublin and was returning to the city to keep engagements arranged before his departure from home.

2. London Yearly Meeting.

3. Dr. John Rutty (1698–1775), a friend of John Fothergill senior, was an eccentric Quaker physician born in Wiltshire who received his M.D. in 1723 at Leyden. In 1724 he settled in Dublin, where he had a lifetime of practice among the underprivileged of the city, dying "unmarried in rented rooms at the corner of Boot Lane and St. Mary's Lane" in 1775. His numerous writings included *A History of the Rise and Progress of the People called Quakers in Ireland from 1653 to 1700, compiled by T[homas] W[ight] . . . to which is added . . . a Continuation . . . to 1750. With an Introduction . . . and a Treatise of Christian Discipline exercised among the Said People* by J. Rutty (Dublin, 1751); *A Methodical Synopsis of Mineral Waters* (1757), an account of medicinal springs in Great Britain and on the Continent; and *An Essay towards a Natural History of the County of Dublin*, 2 volumes (1772). From 1753 to December 1774, he kept a journal entitled *A Spiritual Diary, with Soliloquies* (London, 1775), published after his death. Dr. Johnson and James Boswell were much diverted by this "minute and honest register" kept by the author. Boswell made a list of the faults Rutty enumerated in these "self-condemning minutes," which included: "indulgence in bed an hour too long . . . snappish on fasting; doggish on provocation . . . too great love for studies of materia medica and meteorology." — Boswell, *Samuel Johnson*, ed. Ingpen, II, 715, 716.

4. George Cleghorn, Dr. Fothergill's close friend and fellow student in Edinburgh, was at this time a lecturer in anatomy in Trinity College, Dublin.

5. Waterford, Ireland, where Ann was helping Molly get settled in her new home.

6. Gilbert Thompson had become a licentiate of the Royal College of Physicians on 25 June 1770. In 1771 he married his former cook, Mary, daughter of William and Ann Edmondson of Wray, Lancashire. If she was not a member of the Society of Friends, the couple would have had to attend special meetings, where she would profess conviction before their intentions received approval. — *Munk's Roll*; information from letters seen at LSFL; Fox, 128n.

7. While still a student, "Billy" Logan had eloped with Sarah Portsmouth, a Bristol belle and daughter of a prominent physician in that city. They were married "by a priest" probably at Gretna Green, Scotland. On 13 April 1770 they confessed that fact to Edinburgh Monthly Meeting, and their repentance was accepted. Billy was readmitted to membership and Sally admitted by conviction. — Records, Society of Friends, Edinburgh. The young doctor died 7 January 1772, only a few months after his return to America, leaving his wife and an infant son. — See appendix to John Woolman's *Journal*, ed. Gummere, 560–561.

8. In April, Leeds had complained against Westminster Monthly Meeting to Westminster Quarterly Meeting. After much delay, a statement was prepared and signed by a committee of fourteen prominent members to the effect that whereas

Westminster Monthly Meeting might have acted upon Leeds's complaints, "nevertheless when the said complaint was united with a cause which the Appellant had refused to submit to the Judgement of the Society, it doth appear to us that their Conduct is excusable. And we do further report that we have heard, conformable to your desire, S. Leeds and John Fothergill until they declined saying any more or producing further evidence on the subject of the charge made by the former upon the latter, and are unanimous in opinion that the said charge is groundless and unsupported by the evidence which hath been produced." As a result, Leeds withdrew his appeal and agreed to settle the trouble by arbitration within the Society. Dr. Fothergill submitted to this plan, but arrangements could not be made until Arbitrators had been chosen by ballot. — Minute Books of Westminster Monthly Meeting and Westminster Quarterly Meeting, 1770–1772, LSFL.

To Samuel Fothergill, Warrington, 7 June 1771

London, 7.6.1771

Dear Brother,

We received the account of thy safe arrival [1] with cordial satisfaction, and review the time of our past meeting with not less. We are now stripped of our Friends and left in this respect to ourselves; but the great father is ever near and his mercy cannot be acknowledged to the full.

C. Payton is at Brighthelmstone,[2] and not quite well. She intimates her intention, if able, to be with us sometime next week, and then go directly home.

A Public Friend from North Carolina is just arrived in Capt. Sparke's vessel by the way of Philadelphia; his name, William Hunt.[3] A young man is also with him as companion who sometimes appears in the ministry. Of the former I have an acceptable account from Thomas Nicholson and James Pemberton; he intends to visit the Nation, and has got a safe retreat at John Elliot's.

Our Nephew from Leeds is in town on his former errand. I doubt not but he will suceed, and I wish the affair, if it must be, might be accomplished in our absence.[4] I have a strong dislike to a Mob. I should study hard to avoid it, if I were under the like circumstances.

B. Bartlett called upon us last night; and wishes to know thy intentions regarding I. Pickering.[5] We told him that thou intended his living under T. Stackhouse's tuition, with C. Rhodes and under the like restrictions. "But was it intended that I.P. should keep a horse?" We told him thou had advised the contrary. Of this he much approved, and will prevail upon his Kinsman to have "no such appendage." I mention this circumstance just to assure thee that I hope your sentiments in divers respects will coincide, if not in all. I have wished that they might be situated not far from us that we may have the better chance of seeing them sometimes.

I had distantly looked at the 22nd of next month as the day of our departure from hence. I will gain a week if I can; I mean to set out a a week sooner; my sister wishes it for my sake, and I do for hers!

Our valuable Friend, E. Beaufoy, has undergone an operation,[6] and is in a hopeful way. I could not refuse being present, and to afford her all the comfort I could. She bore it with the patience I expected, which was as much as human patience could sustain, without even the most silent complaint. — She asked after thee today; and I thought that this account was due to your mutual regard.

If no particular service seems to be before thee at present, let it be thy particular care to regard thy health; and consider how to repair the strength that has been so unremittingly expended, and lay up a little stock for the future. Let us waste as little as we can unnecessarily. I curb myself often, however seemingly I am always engaged. Let us hear from thee frequently. It does us good, and draws us nearer together and to the Spring of all good.

S. Clark sent his letter and the books, and we all thought his proposal just and reasonable. Should any Friend among you decline accepting them on these terms, would it be advisable to offer them the alternative, viz: to return the books unopened and receive the subscription money?

If thou should have occasion to write soon to W. Miller of Edinburgh, I wish thou would enquire of him whether the account of Friends sent down to him was acceptable.[7] If not, I wish it returned as I think it, with a very small alteration, might be made an acceptable present to many, if printed. Please to enquire after it.

Accept our united and affectionate remembrance to thyself, Sister, our near relations. We are favoured with health and a degree of contentment — feeling desires of a relief from bondage and a fuller enjoyment of true spiritual liberty which exceeds the temporal, as Heaven is brighter than the earth, or as Eternity surpasses the limits of time.

Farewell, dear Brother,

J. Fothergill

Ms. autograph letter, Port. 22/116, LSFL.

345

1. From Ireland.

2. Early name for Brighton.

3. William Hunt of Spring Gardens, North Carolina, a young American Quaker related to John Woolman of New Jersey, made a successful religious visit in the British Isles and Holland. While returning from Holland to England, his ship was driven off course to seek shelter finally at Shields on the Northumberland coast. Hunt had fallen seriously ill and had to be carried ashore, where it was discovered he had smallpox. He lived only a few days, and was interred in the Friends burial ground, Newcastle-upon-Tyne. — *Piety Improved* (Philadelphia, 1843), III, 17–20.

4. John Fothergill — Alexander's son — and Mary Ann Forbes of London were soon to be married, and Dr. Fothergill dreaded the celebrations.

5. Benjamin Bartlett's young relative Isaac Pickering, a country boy from Yorkshire, had arrived in London with his friend C. Rhodes to seek proper schooling. Samuel Fothergill was to supervise their education. He selected as tutor Thomas Stackhouse, also of Yorkshire origin, who hoped to attract other Quaker lads and start a private school of his own, perhaps in Knightsbridge — Information secured from other letters, LSFL.

6. Elizabeth Beaufoy, wife of Mark Beaufoy, a prominent London businessman, and sister of Capel Hanbury, head of London's Virginia Company, made an excellent recovery from an operation which required great fortitude in pre-anaesthesia days.

7. Very probably the article on the Quakers written for the "Scottish Dictionary" — the first edition of the *Encyclopaedia Britannica*.

To Alexander Fothergill, Carr End, Wensleydale, Yorkshire, 30 July 1771

Lea Hall, 30.7.1771

Dear Brother,

We are arrived once more at this quiet retreat, and with our usual satisfaction. We came hither last 5th day, found all things well, and have since seen our Brother Samuel, who came over to see us. He is finally recovering from a tedious fit of gout, which however has not affected the principal parts so much as heretofore.

I should willingly hope it may be in thy power to see us this summer; it is long since we had either interview or correspondence. Perhaps Thomas [1] may be spared so long as to accompany thee and it may now be time to have some consideration respecting his future progress.

An unpleasant circumstance of my own,[2] likewise, would make me wish for a little conversation with thee, if it could be done without much inconvenience.

This, however, may be communicated by letter should a visit to us be attended by many difficulties. Thy son, John,[3] is in the way to alter his condition, and I think not unsuitably on the whole. In general young women from the country fill up their stations in town with more satisfaction to themselves and propriety, likewise, as being diffident and attentive to learn, than those who go from London into the country. But there is no rule without exceptions, and I hope the young person whom John is in pursuit of will do credit to his choice.

I think we shall not be absent from this place for a month at least, if at all, nor under any particular engagements. In this time, I hope it will not be inconvenient for thee to see us. Should this, however, be the case, please to inform me by a line at thy leisure, and I shall acquaint thee with the circumstances about which I should be glad to have thy opinion.

Remember us affectionately to our Sister and Nephew William.[4] As he has been so long absent from home, we do not ask him to see us this year; but if we live to come down another summer, we hope he will hold himself in readiness to see us at Lea Hall. Remember us likewise to our friends the Robinsons, Hillarys and other Friends. Sister joins me in affectionate remembrance to thyself.

J. Fothergill

Ms. autograph letter, Fothergill Family Papers, Wallis Collection. Dates of several subsequent letters during this critical period of the Leeds affair are apparently missing, but the sequence of the letters and the months in which they were written are fairly well established by internal evidence.

1. Alexander's son Thomas (1751–1822) had no wish to study medicine but became a lawyer, establishing himself in London. He never married. — Fothergill Genealogy, below.

2. The Leeds case, in which Alexander's legal knowledge was to prove of value to Dr. Fothergill.

3. Although Dr. Fothergill was not enthusiastic about the marriage of his nephew John to Mary Ann Forbes, she proved to be an excellent wife and mother. Four of their five sons grew to manhood. Three of their four daughters lived well into the nineteenth century. Their son Samuel (1780–1822) studied medicine. Receiving an M.D. from Glasgow in 1802, he was admitted licentiate of the Royal College of Physicians in 1805 and was appointed physician to the Western Dispensary, London. In 1810 he was elected to the editorial board of the *Medical and Physical Journal*, retaining this connection until 1822. He should be especially remembered for having extended the study of *tic douloureux* (trigeminal neuralgia) by correctly locating the seat of the disturbance in the fifth cranial nerve, which has three branches supplying sensation to the face. This disease, known today in Germany as *dolor faciei Fothergilli*, is called Fothergill's disease in England.

4. William (1746–1837) in 1782 married his Semerdale sweetheart, Hannah Robinson of Counterset, and in 1788, upon the death of his father, inherited Carr End. In 1837 the estate passed to his eldest son, another Alexander (1788–1843). The late Dr. William Edward Fothergill, an eminent gynecologist of Manchester, and Dr. W. Crichton Fothergill (d. 1968), a well-known radiologist of Darlington, County Durham, were among Alexander's descendants.

To Samuel Fothergill, Warrington, August 1771

Lea Hall, 6th Day even:

Dear Brother,

In answer to thine, yesterday, respecting T. Stackhouse,[1] I think I can inform thee that he has taken a house at Knightsbridge with a view to C. Rhodes and I. Pickering's accommodation. This account I had from B. Bartlett, who has been with him several times on the occasion, and acquainted me with the circumstances I have related.

And I think there will be little room to doubt that T.S. if he gives satisfaction, as I trust he will, may have a succession. J. Revoult is decamped. He had contracted many debts, and his creditors grew importunate. He slipped away to France, and left his wife in deep distress, and his school to his Usher. This has happened since we left London.[2]

I had a letter today from C. Payton; she is much complaining. H. Bradford is removed and has left his affairs properly.[3] She has heard of thy indisposition, and I find her sorrow on the occasion is sincere and tripartite. She feels for thee, for herself doubly, lest thou should be unable to attend at Evesham. She is beating up for volunteers already. I wish thee better success in thy lawsuit [4] than I in mine with S.L. I am cast in 500 pounds damage. Enough I think to pay for nothing. But so 3 out of 5 Arbitrators have decreed.[5] Therefore, do not be too sanguine. Innocence is not always a sufficient protection without a little of the serpent's aid, at least in some cases. Though, I think thou stands a better chance, as the cause if brought into a public court, will be decided by indifferent persons who, strangers to both parties, will determine according to equity.

My sister wrote yesterday to Peggy. We may probably see her tomorrow. If not, we shall judge our proposal was in some respect inconvenient.

We have been here about half our allotted time,[6] and must now have many unavoidable engagements. Many causes have contributed to render this in some respects the least pleasing of our journeys. Yet I am not discouraged by it. Nothing happens but for our good, and I will endeavour to profit by it.

Do not attempt to see us till thou can bear the journey without risking a relapse. I have sent for thy amusement S.L.'s charges [7] and my reply. From these thou will see the general state of the affair. It only remains that I humble myself sufficiently, discharge the sum, sign releases, and forget the injustice done me, leaving the event, and profiting if I can by the mortification.

We are moderately well, not much to complain of, yet below our usual state. Accept our united remembrance of affection from thy

A. and J. Fothergill

I would not have the affair made much of.

Ms. autograph letter, Port. 22/117, LSFL. Dated by internal evidence.

1. Benjamin Bartlett II felt responsibility for the education of his young kinsman Isaac Pickering and Isaac's friend, C. Rhodes. Thomas Stackhouse (from Giggleswick, Yorkshire), ambitious to become a schoolmaster, was willing to make a start with only these two boarding pupils.
2. No further information can be found about this French schoolteacher.
3. A Quaker preacher; date of death unknown.
4. George Crosfield's *Memoirs of the Life and Gospel Labours of Samuel Fothergill* makes no mention of Samuel Fothergill's lawsuit.
5. The Arbitrators, whose decision had been announced on 19 July were Daniel Mildred, merchant; Leonard Ellington, merchant; William Smith, hatter; Lewis Weston, cooper; and John Sherwin, baker. The last three had voted in favor of Leeds. – Fox, 75.
6. Dr. Fothergill and his sister usually stayed in their country house, Lea Hall, for ten or twelve weeks.
7. See the next letter.

To Samuel Fothergill, Warrington, Lancashire, August 1771

Lea Hall [August 1771]

Dear Brother,

It was with regret that I sent thee a packet that I knew would give thee pain, looking at the contents in any manner one can.[1] If I have justly incurred such a penalty, I have acted dishonourably not to say worse. If I have not deserved such a sentence, in what light must we review the conduct of justice amongst us? The whole, however, are not to be blamed. The single difficulty with me is, shall I submit to the Award quietly, innocently condemned, and suffer the affair to slide into oblivion? Or shall I embrace the opportunity which the 3 Arbitrators have afforded me to set aside the Award, and bring the affair to a more equitable hearing?[2]

My antagonist is so thoroughly known by all the Physical people of my acquaintance to deserve the harshest censures that can be given, that they stand amazed at the iniquity of the sentence.[3] The very people to whom I have occasionally mentioned the general equity of our procedure and the pains that were taken to see Justice impartially executed amongst us, stand amazed at the decision, and upbraid me with partiality. Must I clear the Society by showing that it was only a few individuals that connived in the affair, and then perhaps from motives in their opinion extremely charitable? L. wanted money; F. had some.[4] Let us therefore give to him that wants. To enter into a detail of every circumstance, every consideration I have had on this disagreeable affair, which has broken in upon me oftener and more forcibly than I could wish, would be adding to my distress.

I am pretty well informed that the Award may easily be set aside. The enclosed is from a sensible, experienced and I think an honest Attorney, whom I have frequently employed; he has served me diligently, and I believe wishes me well.

Thou will see that L. had aimed at the Arbitrators, and will see his reasons which are conclusive against us. Thou will see, likewise, his answer to some objections that occurred to me against attempting to set aside an agreement in which I had become, and voluntarily, a party. Also some traces that I had endeavoured to make him acquainted with the difficulties I was under on account of the Society. That I had more evidence to produce is most certain, material evidence. The other two Arbitrators will likewise give evidence that I requested the Bonds be lengthened for this purpose. These two allegations are capable of the strongest proof. Shall I, or shall I not, refuse complying with the Award? Do not be hasty in concluding.

I have now travelled through an exposed life many years, and with much more reputation than I have deserved. Shall I be the instrument of creating disputes and animosities in any part of the family? Bringing even the justice of its decision into doubt in the face of the public, and exhibiting an instance of the grossest partiality and injustice, capable of afflicting even the character of this whole community?

As I have passed through good report, shall I not submit to the severe, especially when a conscious innocence assures me I have done no wrong? How much easier it is under such circumstances to stand before the public or the most penetrating tribunal, than when covered guilt seeks a refuge in chicanery.

Let passion subside, and think equitably; if it should be permitted by the great Disposer of all things that I should be trampled upon by one of the most unworthy, so let it be. I would quietly submit, and without envy to injustice still more humiliating. What am I, what is an individual, even of much more consequence, to the peace and quiet of a family that ought to live in love and harmony together? Think not of this affair on a contracted scale. I am undetermined. I am in no haste. Nothing decisive will be done till the first of the tenth month next when the three Arbitrators have awarded me to pay 500 pounds, to sign general releases, and to pay half the expenses of the Arbitration. — I hope to give thee no farther trouble on this occasion. Think of it as little as possible; but if in any clear and favoured moment, best wisdom should open instruction, I hope to receive it as a child and pursue it with just submission.

I believe the retreat of J. Revoult will make no alteration in T. Stackhouse's plan. I should by no means propose him as a master for such a place. His abilities would be more useful in another station. As the private tutor of a few, I think he may render important service to some young people.[5]

We have had an exceedingly fine day after a very rainy one and an oppressive one to me. Dr. Percival[6] and Dr. Haygarth[7] spent part of yesterday and the night with us and exhausted me not a little. Indeed I grow old and weak, I am glad to perceive the effect of advancing old age. In respect to thy own health I know not what to say, any further than that I think no extremity of regimen will be of use. On the contrary, to live under a degree of constant, uniform restraint of appetite is the most likely means of arresting those distresses which are the companions, the followers rather, of the Gout. Yet even in this respect extreme mortification is injurious. The stomach if attended to impartially, feelingly will, like conscience, tell us where should be our *ne plus ultra*.

I hear nothing but our common acquaintance in London are well. Our Nephew has made some progress in his affair; I own I should have liked it better, if I could have been sure it was not of his Sister's manufacture.[8] But what must be, must be. We affectionately salute thee and Sister.[9]

J. & A. Fothergill

Ms. autograph letter, Port. 22/119, LSFL.

1. Papers concerning the Leeds case. Leeds's charges were, in effect, the following: (1) Dr. Fothergill had said that Leeds obtained his Edinburgh diploma "surreptitiously"; (2) Dr. Fothergill in conversation with Dr. Dawson, a colleague of Leeds in London Hospital, had slandered Leeds by describing him as incompetent to care for patients; (3) Dr. Dawson had told Dr. John Coakley Lettsom what Dr. Fothergill had said and Dr. Lettsom had reported this to young William Logan, then enrolled as a medical student in Edinburgh, who had repeated this insult to others — and the gossip ensuing had spread throughout both medical and Quaker circles, entirely discrediting Leeds among acquaintances. (The charges are now on file at LSFL with this letter.)

The Award, served 19 July 1771, at an open Meeting by the three Arbitrators who had voted in favor of Leeds, made public the following demands: "John Fothergill, his Heirs, Executors, or Administrators on Monday 21st October now next ensuing shall between 12 and 1 of the clock on the same day at the bar of the George and Vulture Tavern situate in or near Michael's Alley, Cornhill, pay or cause to be paid to said S.L., his Executors, or Administrators, the sum of £500 of the lawful money of Great Britain. Upon payment thereof, we order, judge and award that the said S.L. shall execute and give to the said J.F., and the said J.F. shall execute and give to the said S.L., mutual and general releases of all Controversies, Actions, Suits and Demands whatsoever from the Beginning of the World to the Day of the Date of the said Obligations, and lastly we order and direct that the Cost of Charges accrued by Reason or Means of this Award shall be borne, or paid equally, by and between John Fothergill and Samuel Leeds . . ." — Minute Books of the Society of Friends, LSFL.

2. Appeal might still be made to London Yearly Meeting. — Fox, 76.

3. Fellow members of the medical profession, particularly members of the Royal College of Physicians, were distressed by these proceedings.

4. The poverty-stricken practitioner versus the opulent physician.

5. Acute observation of the situation of private Quaker boarding schools and their schoolmasters in Knightsbridge — a topic raised in previous letters.

6. Dr. Thomas Percival (1740–1804), born in Warrington, studied medicine in Edinburgh, took his M.D. at Leyden, and in 1767 settled in Manchester. He later had a notable career, not only in private practice and at the Manchester Infirmary, but in backing sanitary reforms effected in Manchester's cotton mills, starting "fever hospitals," systematizing mortality statistics, and fostering cultural enterprises. Dr. Percival published two volumes of *Essays, Medical and Experimental* (1767, 1776), also *A Treatise on Medical Ethics* (1803) which formulated the ethical standards soon adopted by the medical profession in English-speaking countries throughout the world. He was foremost among founders of the Manchester Library and Philosophical Society (1781), serving as its president for twenty years. As a Unitarian, his liberal religious principles made him akin in thought to the Quakers. — E. M. Brockbank, *The Medical Staff of the Manchester Infirmary* (London, 1904); Chauncey D. Leake, "Percival's Code: A Chapter in the Historical Development of Medical Ethics," *Journal of the American Medical Association*, 81: 366–381 (August 1923); *Percival's Medical Ethics*, ed. C. D. Leake (Baltimore: Williams and Wilkins, 1927).

7. Dr. John Haygarth (1740–1827), then Physician to the Chester Infirmary, was another doctor from the Yorkshire Dales. A frequent visitor to Dr. Fothergill during his annual retreat to Lea Hall, only twenty miles from Chester, he first submitted to him his plan to exterminate smallpox from Great Britain by introducing general

inoculation. He pioneered isolation techniques in the prevention of infectious fevers, the first separate fever wards being opened at the Chester Infirmary in 1783. It was owing to his insistence that his friend Dr. Percival founded the "Fever Hospital" in Manchester. Dr. Haygarth moved to Bath in 1798 where he died in 1827. — John Haygarth, *A Sketch of a Plan to Exterminate the Casual Small-Pox from Great Britain; and to introduce General Inoculation (London, 1793), 1, 265, 320; A Letter to Dr. Percival on the Prevention of Infectious Fevers and an Address to the College of Physicians at Philadelphia on the Prevention of the American Pestilence* (Bath and London, 1801); George H. Weaver, "John Haygarth, Clinician, Investigator, Apostle of Sanitation, 1740–1827," *Bulletin of the Society of Medical History of Chicago*, IV (1928–1935), 156–200.

8. Dr. Fothergill believed that his niece Alice, who had married John Chorley of London, a linen draper, had furthered the romance between her brother John and Mary Ann Forbes of London.

9. Samuel's wife Susannah.

To Samuel Fothergill, Warrington, Lancashire, September 1771

Lea Hall, 3rd Inst. 12 o'clock

Dear Brother, —

I have received thy kind note this morning, and as my friend Aiken [1] of Chester is coming to Warrington, I have desired him to be the bearer of this.

I need not say that I am sorry for thy confinement. We must bear it. I wish Dr. Pemberton [2] and Peggy could see us tomorrow. On fifth day I wish to go to Tabley.[3] Some time on seventh day Brother Alex and his son Thomas I expect will be here. Thy company and theirs would be quite compatible. Our Quarterly Meeting is next week; [4] and the next we must prepare for our journey.

I received the enclosed from my Attorney this morning.[5] He proposes a journey to Edinburgh. I cannot undertake it. If it should be necessary I would make it worth Brother Alexander's time and he would do all that's necessary; I think both may be dispensed with.

As the bearer waits, I can only add that we are well, though not a little uneasy at times in being deprived of thy company. Farewell,

From thy affectionate
J.F.

Ms. autograph letter, Port. 22/136, LSFL. Dated from internal evidence.

1. In 1771 young John Aikin (1747–1822) had a surgical practice in Chester. The son of a nonconformist minister, he had attended Warrington Academy and been

apprenticed to a doctor, then studied medicine in Edinburgh. He left without a degree, and after a lean time in Chester gladly accepted an invitation to teach physiology and chemistry in his old school at Warrington. Much later he received his M.D. at Leyden (1784) and practiced medicine, but in his last years he devoted himself largely to writing and editing. *Evenings at Home* (1792–1795), six volumes of "miscellaneous pieces for the instruction and amusement of young persons," which he published in collaboration with his sister, Anna Letitia Barbauld, went through many editions. Other works of his included *General Biography*, 10 volumes (1799–1815), and *Select Works of the British Poets, with Biographical and Critical Notes* (1820). — Lucy Aikin, *Memoir of John Aikin, M.D.*, 2 vols. (London, 1823); *Munk's Roll*, II, 421–423.

2. Dr. Thomas Pemberton of Warrington, Samuel's attending physician.

3. The Vicar of Middlewich has kindly informed Dr. Booth that Tabley, not mentioned in Muirhead's *Blue Guide* nor shown on available maps, is a small village not far from Lea Hall.

4. Quarterly Meeting of Cheshire and Staffordshire combined.

5. Charlton Palmer, a London attorney of excellent reputation. The enclosure is missing.

To Samuel Fothergill, 18 September 1771

Lea Hall, 18th Inst.

Dear Brother,

We arrived safe at our habitation,[1] to which Dr. Pemberton accompanied us. I met with a letter from my attorney recommending my Brother's going over to Edinburgh. I found myself disengaged from a burthen that has oppressed me much for several days, and wrote to my Brother Alexander by the post this morning requesting his speedy compliance.

We intend to stay here a week longer than we at first proposed, partly with a view, if possible, to acquire a little more fitness for my usual engagements, and partly to wait the event of my Brother's journey.[2] Because if he finds that my presence is of any importance I would endeavour to go thither. This I hope will meet thee safe returned from thy laborious exercises and endeavouring at a little rest. Some is yet necessary, at least incessant labour will much retard thy recovery.

The enclosed is to inform Nancy Lee [3] that our journey is postponed a week longer, and if it would not fall out very inconveniently for thyself, I was proposing that A. Chorley, thyself and [Nancy Lee] might come in a Chaise next seventh day week, either to dine, or after, as it might best suit you, to stay with us all night, and return in the Chaise after dinner on first day, leaving her with us. But all this is left; there are other means of getting her to this place, if it suits thy conveniency and inclination better to be with us at any other time.

I met with a very friendly letter from Mark Beaufoy [4] relative to my affair, and strongly pressing me to seek a remedy. I shall say little of my intentions to anybody till the time of determination draws near, and I have gotten such intelligence as may assist me in determinancy. In the meantime it does me no hurt. It is a good medicine, and I take it with satisfaction. I mentioned my situation to Dr. Pemberton, requesting him at the same time to keep the affair for the present to himself as much as possible, only, if he could, to acquaint thee that for the present I had laid my journey aside.

Our Nephew's marriage will I find be put off some time longer, a few days only, on what account I don't know. James Freeman tells me it will be solemnized the 26th, and requesting us to come a day sooner if we could, as it would give them all satisfaction.[5] But as we propose to stay another week here, this will not be expected.

I have no accounts from our Friends in London but such as are favourable. Many are gone to Evesham[;][6] Isaac Sharpless is particularly mentioned.[7]

We silently rejoice in this late renewal of our tender friendship. I took part in it strongly, though I could not give much token of it. Let nothing I have said, respecting thy coming over, influence thee in any regard. Come when thou canst, it will always afford comfort to

thy
J. & A. Fothergill

Manuscript autograph letter, Port. 22/134, LSFL.

1. Presumably after attending Quarterly Meeting.
2. Alexander was going to Edinburgh to interview members of the faculty of the medical school where for two years Samuel Leeds had been a student.
3. Daughter of Alice and John Chorley. — Fothergill Genealogy.
4. Mark Beaufoy (1718–1782), a man of high principles and a loyal Friend, was prominent in London business circles. Although apprenticed to a distiller in Bristol for seven years, he is said to have been so affected by viewing Hogarth's depiction of the horrors of intoxication that he went to Holland to learn "the art of vinegar making," which he practiced the rest of his life as head of a vinegar factory in South Lambeth. — Beaufoy, *Leaves from a Beech Tree*, 62–64, 116, 117.
5. Young John Fothergill was James Freeman's brother-in-law. — Fothergill Genealogy.
6. A "Circular Meeting" was bringing Quakers from nearby counties to Evesham, a town charmingly situated on the river Avon, in a vale noted for its production of fruit.
7. Isaac Sharpless, a Quaker minister born in Prescot, Lancashire, was later iden-

tified with Meetings in Hitchin, Hertfordshire, where he spent most of his life. "A circle of admiring Friends" found an autobiographical tract after his death in 1784 and published it as a memorial: *A Short Narrative of our dear and worthy Friend, written by himself shortly before his decease* (Privately Printed, 1785).

To Alexander Fothergill, Edinburgh, 21 September 1771 [I]

Lea Hall, 21st Inst.

Dear Brother,

I received thy very acceptable letter of the 14th on the 19th instant, about the same time I apprehended thou would receive one from me, which perhaps will induce thee to be at Edinburgh as soon as this. I am glad that the time suits so well thy conveniency.

I have received two letters from Professors Monro and Cullen,[1] strongly urging me to let the affair drop, and sit down with loss, etc. This only gives me to understand they are conscious of neglect, and prompts me the more to endeavour to satisfy myself.

When I took my degree at Edinburgh, I went through the following exercises. I was first examined in private by the professors, in Latin and upon various branches of medicine. Two aphorisms of Hippocrates were then given me by the professors, on which I was required to write commentaries in Latin. These being done to satisfaction, two cases or histories were then given to me which I was to explain — to describe the disease, its course, probability of its event, and method of cure — in Latin likewise. They are now extant in a book that used to be kept at the College, and the Professor was pleased to say that in the last part, [mine] would not have disgraced the first physician.[2]

Now if the mode is the same at present as it was in 1736, Leeds must have produced such exercises to the professors, and as he could not perform them himself — for he could not write a sentence in Latin — endeavours must be used to find-out the persons who did them for him. His last exercise, viz.: his thesis, was wrote in Latin, if not wholly made, by one Brown,[3] a person well-known amongst such kind of students, and whose testimony, if he will give it, would be decisive. — Not, however, forgetting to inquire after the rest.

I have inclosed Leeds own charges [4] that if it is necessary to apply to the University, they may be satisfied that I shall be sufficiently able to defend myself, whether they will do themselves the justice they ought to do or not.

I have wrote to Dr. Falconer [5] at Bath, who took his degree at the same time Leeds did, to request his assistance in tracing out the people who made Leeds's exercises for him; if he gives me any light, I will inform thee as speedily as possible.

To have sent the several letters I received from Professors Cullen, Monro and Hope would have perhaps been of no consequence. Two, however I will inclose. They will show what I have to expect from them. H. Beaufoy [6] may probably be easily found out by applying to William Miller at the Abbey, or near it, a Friend of much reputation, and to whom I shall inclose a few lines. I shall send all the letters open for thy inspection — and seal and deliver them as thou thinks fit.

Please to preserve Leeds's charges; it is the original, and I have no copy. — My answers are unnecessary. Thou will deliver the inclosed or not as thou sees occasion. If delivered, please to put a wafer in them. I shall trouble thee with another, and a larger one too in a little time; not relative to this subject, to Dr. Boswell, President of the College.

Having received from Henry Gurney of Norwich a short sketch of Leeds's way of life, I thought it might not be improper to inclose it.[7] I have requested to have a more circumstantial account, and the dates as far as may be collected.

Thou will probably not think it improper to deliver the inclosed to W. Miller. He was much taken with Leeds, supported him, and wrote to me to lend him £50. (I think it was W.M. or Friend King of Newcastle, who is oft at Edinburgh.) But this I refused.

I mention these particulars to enable thee to judge how far it may be expedient to say anything to him of thy business at Edinburgh. Writing the inclosed have kept me busy together with much other of the same kind.

I received thy letter of the 14th, and was much pleased to find thee so much at liberty. Lest, however, mine of the 15th should have miscarried, I write a second time to Carr End by this post, to forward thee if gone. — We are well, and I find myself much at ease since I have resolved to lay this burthen upon thee. Brother Samuel is bravely. Charles Routh of Manchester was buried last 2nd day.

From thy affectionate Brother,

J. Fothergill

Ms. autograph letter, Fothergill Family Papers, Wallis Collection. The date of this letter like that of the next one is derived from Dr. Fothergill's letter to William

Cullen, 21 September 1771, below. The letter to Alexander mentioned in the first paragraph has not been found.

1. During the thirty-five years since Dr. Fothergill had received his medical degree at Edinburgh, Alexander Munro, Secundus, had succeeded his father as Professor of Anatomy, Dr. William Cullen had left Glasgow to become Professor of the Institutes of Medicine, and Dr. John Hope (1725–1786) had succeeded Dr. Charles Alston as Professor of Botany and Materia Medica.

2. This paragraph is actually a carefully veiled criticism of laxity in Edinburgh's current requirements for granting a medical degree.

3. John Brown (1735–1788), a successful teacher of Latin in a grammar school near Edinburgh, was brought to Dr. William Cullen's attention when the latter was seeking a private tutor for his sons. Brown gladly accepted this position, and subsequently became Dr. Cullen's secretary. He was permitted to attend medical lectures at the University, where his proficiency in Latin led students to seek his assistance in preparing the Latin theses still required for the medical degree. Theses of this period, many of which are rumored to be wholly the work of John Brown, may be seen today in a four-volume set entitled *Thesaurus Medicus* (Edinburgh, 1785). — *Autobiography of Benjamin Rush*, ed. G. W. Corner, appendix I, 362–368.

4. The charges are no longer found with this manuscript letter.

5. Dr. William Falconer (1744–1824), M.D. Edinburgh 1766, continued his studies in Leyden and upon return to England set up practice in Chester, his birthplace. Because of special interest in water-cures, he moved to Bath, which had been famous for its mineral springs since the Roman occupation. Dr. Falconer's skill brought him an extensive practice from patients who frequented this city, which had much of the charm of later German spas. He made many contributions to medical literature of the period. A list of his papers covers more than a page of his biographical memoir. — *Munk's Roll*, II, 278–280.

6. Henry Beaufoy (1750–1795), son of Mark Beaufoy, was probably in Edinburgh at this time on business for his father's firm, in which he was a junior partner. He was later elected to Parliament, and subsequently appointed Secretary to the Board of Control of the East Indian Company. — Beaufoy, *Leaves from a Beech Tree*, 138–154; "Obituary of Remarkable Personages," *Gentleman's Magazine*, 9 (1795): 45, 46.

7. The enclosure from Henry Gurney of Norwich (husband of Betty Bartlett) contains the following information: "S. Leeds is descended from an obscure family not famous for the most delicate conduct, and when first known to me was by profession a Barber. This, I think, must be about fifteen or sixteen years ago when he began to attend our meetings, and, by the indulgence of some, became a member amongst us. His custom in trade in about two years after began to decline, and he attempted, or pretended to attempt, weaving for [his] bread, but was afterwards employed to make an implement used in one of our manufactories which we call Hancks and Slays, which not succeeding, he was assisted to undertake making brushes. All of which filled up his time until he came to London. A little before this time, I heard he entered upon the study of Botany, wherein I believe he did not shine, as he was always short in his stability and attention. I think he must have been about 30 years of age when he first aspired to his Physickal character."

To Alexander Fothergill, Carr End, Wensleydale, Yorkshire, 21 September 1771

Lea Hall, 21st Inst. [II]

Dear Brother,

If my last of the 15th should have miscarried, I must desire thee to set out for Edinburgh, as soon after this arrives, as may be convenient.

I sent it directed by Roachdale, and inclosed in it a Bank note for £20 towards thy expenses, and a letter from C. Palmer.[1]

By this post I have sent a larger packet of letters and papers directed to thee at the post office in Edinburgh. I mention the Bank note, that enquiry may be made at the post offices, if the letter should have miscarried.

As I have wrote to thee pretty fully to Edinburgh; and send this only lest my last should have miscarried, I conclude with our affectionate remembrance to thee, Sister and William.

from thy loving Brother
J. Fothergill

Ms. autograph letter, Fothergill Family Papers, Wallis Collection.

1. Charlton Palmer, the London attorney, had written to Dr. Fothergill: "I cannot but approve of your Brother's journey . . . as it will convince your friends that you are in earnest to defend yourself. The notes on this case seem to have been drawn by an able lawyer, and if they are your Brother's, I should not have been afraid of trusting him with the Edinboro' business without any other agent whatsoever." — The manuscript note from Palmer is in the Fothergill family papers formerly in the possession of the late Miss Mabyn Fothergill and now of her brother, Mr. Edward Rimington Fothergill, Edinburgh.

To Dr. William Cullen, Edinburgh, 21 September 1771

Near Middlewich, Cheshire
21st September 1771

My honoured Friend,

This, I expect, will be delivered by my brother Alexander Fothergill, who has undertaken this journey to Edinburgh at my request. My friends in London, not only of our own persuasion but others, are highly dissatisfied with the award against me, and insist upon my endeavouring to vindicate myself from the stain of defamation, and to such an amount as to require so large a restitution as £500.

I have yielded to their importunities; and, conscious of my innocence, both in act and intention, I am in hopes of giving ample proofs of it.

I ask nothing from the Faculty. My proofs will be of another kind; my opponent did not, he could not, perform any of the usual exercises expected from the Candidates for Degrees. Should proofs of this kind be laid before you, your own honour is engaged to disavow the impostor, not for my sake, I ask it not, but for your own. To be mistaken or deceived is not a crime. It happens to individuals, it happens to bodies, and is excusable. But to persevere in a mistake, and countenance imposture, makes those who do so partners in the guilt. A man who is capable of sitting for months together attending lectures in a language of which he knew not a sentence, and make notes of it at the same time, is surely a first-rate genius. The Professors could not suspect that such a case could possibly happen; but if it is proved to have happened will it turn most to the credit of those who have been imposed upon to conceal or to disclaim the imposition?

I have wrote to Dr. Monro on the same subject, and likewise to Dr. Hope. You will please to confer together, and consult the credit of our Alma Mater. I have wrote to a gentleman of Cambridge to procure me, if he can, the usual form of their suspensions, and on what occasions they are principally issued.

I have enclosed a letter from Dr. Watson [1] in London, which I received yesterday, together with a very polite letter from the man in the world, except Leeds, from whom I should least of all have expected it, Sir William Browne,[2] mentioning the motives that induced him to propose me to the College as a Fellow, which were much in my favour, so that his motion, I believe, was honourably intended, though it miscarried. I am very glad it did so; for if they would not have given me my proper rank and standing I would not have entered the College. I am much better pleased to remain where I am; and I will endeavour to act in such a manner as to afford no disgrace to the corps I am in, nor the corps itself to the profession.

At leisure moments, and they have been extremely scarce with me, I have looked over your Pharmacopoeia, and taken more liberties in retrenching than perhaps I ought. I could wish to have had more time, and been at home, but these are impracticable. I have wrote three or four hours almost every day since I came down, for other people not myself. MSS. on one subject or other were put into my hands, by my friends when I left London, and some I have been obliged to rebuild from the foundations.

As I received the request to look over the Pharmacopoeia from Dr. Boswell, I could not refuse sending him the short notes I had made, which I have sent in a packet addressed to him, to my brother's care.

Be kind enough to make my acknowledgments to the gentlemen of the Medical Society for their very polite letter. I hope to acknowledge it myself when I return to London. I am, with great respect, Dr. Cullen's assured friend,

John Fothergill

Published letter: John Thomson, *An Account of the Life, Lectures and Writings of William Cullen, M.D.*, 2 vols. (Edinburgh: Blackwood, 1859), I, appendix, 654–656.

1. William Watson (1715–1787), apprenticed to a London apothecary in 1730, began the practice of medicine in 1738. He was elected Fellow of the Royal Society in 1741 and received its Copley Medal in 1745 for his "surprising experiments in electricity." He received medical diplomas, *honoris causa*, from the universities of Halle and Wittemberg about 1757, and in 1759, after taking the usual examinations, was admitted licentiate of the Royal College of Physicians. In 1762 he was elected physician to London's Foundling Hospital, an office held during the rest of his life. While Sir John Pringle was President of the Royal Society (1772–1778), Dr. Watson was elected vice-president. In 1784 he was admitted Fellow of the Royal College of Physicians, and served as Censor in 1785–86. He was knighted in 1786, but "did not long survive that honour," dying in May 1787. — *Munk's Roll*, II, 348–350.

2. Sir William Browne (1692–1774), an able physician known for many personal eccentricities, took his medical degree in Cambridge in 1721. He was admitted Fellow of the Royal College of Physicians in 1726 and elected Fellow of the Royal Society in 1738/9. In 1748 he was knighted by George II. In 1749 he settled permanently in London and became extremely active in the Royal College of Physicians, holding many offices, including the presidency in 1765–66. Sir William and Dr. William Heberden had actively supported Dr. Fothergill's candidacy for fellowship in the Royal College of Physicians in 1771, but had been unsuccessful. The *Comitia* vote was thirteen to nine against giving this honor to the Quaker physician, because of the publicity which had arisen from the Leeds case. — *Munk's Roll*, II, 95–105.

To Alexander Fothergill, Carr End, Wensleydale, Yorkshire, 10 October 1771

London, 10.10.1771

Dear Brother:

By yesterday's post, I received thy last kind letter and the inclosed papers, very safe.[1] I was with C. Palmer this evening, who is quite satisfied with the affidavits, and we are both satisfied likewise that no such thing would have been obtained without thy assistance. It is full and decisive with respect to the first charge, which was the most important, and this being proved, the rest are necessary consequences.

I shall procure from C.P., in a few days, proper evidence that Leeds's rejection from the Hospital was in consequence of his own ignorance and misconduct, as also from the College, that he was inadmissible to practice from obvious inability. C.P. tells me that if L. proceeds to Law, he must apply to the [Court of] King's Bench for a rule to show cause why I do not submit to the Award. I allege the matters contained in the affidavits. If the Court approves, the Award is set aside. If it disapproves, an attachment is issued. He says that I need not attend at the time and place appointed to pay the money. L. will probably empower an attorney to attend and receive it, who will wait the hour and then make affidavit of my non-appearance. He (C.P.) advises me to take no kind of notice of the appointment, keep on the defensive, and avail ourselves of their accusations as far as we can. How will it suit thy convenience to be in London about two, three, or four weeks hence, or sooner? I think it will be a most material point to have the case settled before it goes to counsel, and I think thy presence would be of considerable service both in presenting the evidence and instructing counsel. C.P. has the matter at heart and I am sure would be pleased with so able an associate.

Thou will see that more depends in this case in collecting and arranging our forces than merely in giving battle in court. Consult thy own convenience in the first place. I do not find that much has been said about the affair in my absence. The 3 [2] are, however, pretty loudly condemned when it is mentioned, and a wish is uppermost that I might be justified some way, though by what means, as the case is quite new, many are at a loss to determine. Don't give yourself the trouble of a further diary. I am quite satisfied that thy expedition was as painful as the event favorable.

I am sorry that I cannot recollect Dr. Grant.[3] Is he of this place or of Edinburgh? I ask because there is a Dr. Grant here from Scotland with whom I am well acquainted. Is the Dr. G. of Edinburgh a relation of the Dr. G. of London? I wish to know because I would acknowledge his civilities.

I really pity the Professors. They wish to serve me, but dare not for false shame. Brown's deposition will ruin his interest with them. I should be sorry that he should suffer for his honesty. I must not forget him when the affair is at an end.[4] Sooner it would be improper.

If it suits thee to come up at all, do what seems most easy, and come up in the most convenient manner to thyself. I am sorry that I have cost thee already so much fatigue. I am got into Harness already and begin to feel the difference between the ease of Lea Hall and the bustle of this place. I must, however, go through with it a year or two longer, if I live, but shall be looking out carefully when and how and where I may bid adieu to a laborious practice. I am not sorry for Leeds' impertinence on one account. It has been the means of a more frequent and necessary communication between us. This, I hope, will not be forgot when this occasion has ceased, but that we shall continue the same brotherly intercourse when such causes are no more. I shall secure for William, *Miller's Abridgement*,[5] as soon as I can. Remember me to him, to sister, and be assured that I am

Thy obliged and affectionate Brother,
J. Fothergill

Ms. autograph letter, Fothergill Family Papers, Wallis Collection.

1. Alexander had procured affidavits in Edinburgh supporting his brother's stand in the Leeds case.

2. The Arbitrators who made the award to Leeds. The case aroused widespread disapproval. The accusations against Dr. Fothergill seemed preposterous to his colleagues. Prominent Friends were greatly distressed by the turn of events which had revealed weakness and dissension within their ranks. Londoners in general thought the affair had been completely mismanaged. It was unfortunate that of the five Quakers chosen to be arbitrators, the three in agreement were respectively a hatter, a cooper, and a baker, men totally unacquainted with the medical problems underlying the Leeds case. They mistakenly believed that Samuel Leeds was the victim of undeserved oppression.

3. The name Grant appears frequently in Edinburgh Directories of this period. The Dr. Grant of London favorably known to Dr. Fothergill was undoubtedly William Grant who received his M.D. from Marischal College, Aberdeen, in 1755. He set up practice in London and was admitted licentiate of the Royal College of Physicians in 1763. Between 1771 and 1782 he published seven octavo volumes principally dealing with his study of fevers. He acquired a "well-deserved reputation" in the metropolis, and was on the staff of the Misericordia Hospital, Goodman's Fields. — *Munk's Roll*, II, 256, 257.

4. No personal communications between Dr. Fothergill and John Brown have been found. The Leeds case did not affect Brown adversely. He continued his medical career in Edinburgh, and in 1778 was awarded an M.D., *honoris causa*, by St. Andrews. Meanwhile he had started an independent course of medical lectures advocating ideas about the cause and treatment of disease quite at variance with Dr. Cullen's.

A bitter quarrel ensued, but the Brunonian System as set forth in *Elementa Medicinae Brunonis* (Edinburgh, 1780) won acceptance by numerous physicians in Europe, and to some extent impressed Benjamin Rush, whose own personal philosophy of disease and its treatment aroused unfavorable comment from his Pennsylvania colleagues. — Thomas J. Pettigrew, *Medical Portrait Gallery*, IV (London: Whittaker, 1840), 1–12; *Autobiography of Benjamin Rush*, ed. G. W. Corner, appendix I, 365, 366.

5. *The Gardener's Dictionary*, compiled by Philip Miller of the Apothecaries Garden in Chelsea, went through many editions. The *Abridgement* was a boon to amateurs.

To Dr. William Cullen, Edinburgh, 15 October 1771

London, 15th October 1771

[*Short passage omitted.*]

My brother succeeded so well as to get an ample affidavit from J. Brown, which, with the evidence I have obtained from other quarters, will, I hope, enable me to justify myself, whether my opponent thinks fit to lead me into Westminster Hall or to bring the matter again before our own people, from whom I have every thing just and reasonable to expect. And it is not more to be wondered at that he prepossessed three weak, though honest, men in his favour so strongly as to render them deaf to all reason or force of evidence, than that he should have had art enough to obtain a degree from gentlemen so eminent for their knowledge and abilities.

It hurts me not a little that the affair has already been so widely published. But the circumstances unfortunately rendered it impossible to conceal it. The gross ignorance of Leeds, the injustice done me on his account, the partial decision in his favour, all contributed to interest a multitude of persons in the event. The University will be the greatest sufferer. Should a professor of any eminence appear at Leyden, the Americans would flock thither, and others would follow them. This may be thought to be the language of resentment: it is not. Experience will demonstrate the reality of this suggestion.

As I have not time to write at present to Drs. Hope or Monro, or any other professor, be pleased to acquaint them, as occasion may offer, with the account I have given of the two young men who are the bearers of this, and introduce them as they may appear worthy.

The College here, I find, have enacted some new by-laws, not upon the whole more liberal than the former. A person who has studied at *any* University two years, may, if found properly qualified, be admitted a licentiate. After standing on this list seven years, he may offer himself as a candidate to become a Fellow of the College. He must then be examined in Greek, *ad aperturam libri*, in Hippocrates, Galen, and Aretaeus, besides his other exercises; and, after all, be ballotted for. No person practising midwifery is to be admitted, be his qualifications what they may.

We shall take no steps at present, but endeavour to keep ourselves together, and watch opportunity.

Perhaps it may not be improper just to mention, that I procured inquiry to be made in the University of Cambridge, whether they ever degraded any graduate, on what account, and in what manner. I find they have degraded several, but chiefly on account of immorality, or flagrant misbehaviour, or infidelity: none on the account of fraudulently obtaining a degree. It may, however, be worth while to consider if a degradation may not be justly founded on the legal proof being adduced that Leeds' exercises were not performed by himself, which he had produced to you as his own; for he did not perform any one of those exercises which he exhibited. But I shall say no more on this subject than that the University is more concerned in it than they are aware of. Whether he is degraded or not, my defence is the same. Believe me to be, with great respect, Dr. Cullen's, and all the Professors', assured friend,

J. Fothergill.

Copy of letter published in Thomson, *An Account . . . of William Cullen*, I, appendix I, 656, 657. The passage at the beginning of the letter was omitted by Thomson.

To Samuel Fothergill, Warrington, Lancashire, 31 October 1771

London, 31.10.1771

Dear Brother, —

This I hope will meet with some favourable symptoms of amendment. I am an invalid myself and this is the sixth day inclusive since I have been out of doors. The effect of a cold seemed to be at first some gouty symptoms accompanied with a fever. I am still lame of one knee, with an uneasy pain in my opposite side. But upon the whole I am better,

I do some business at home unavoidably, which retards me in my recovery. I have allowed myself the remains of this week to rest, and hope to get out a little at the beginning of next week.

I am much at a loss what method to propose for thy more perfect recovery. A change of air I think would be of use, but this is impracticable. An equal attention to diet and a total abstinence from spirits I think would do a great deal. Wine but sparingly and frequent attention to have loose stool. — The artificial Baume de Vie I once prescribed would I think be singularly useful. A small dose taken almost daily, and for a considerable time. Whatever is to be done, must be done by gentle methods, and a diet regulated with much attention.

Sister would inform thee that I had taken no notice of the Award. Two days ago L. called upon me to know if I intended to comply with the Award or not. I told him that I did not intend to comply.

Yesterday he brought with him 3 Friends of our Monthly Meeting,[1] a little irregularity in the point of number for the first visit, this. James Marston, S. Parkinson,[2] and another whose name I cannot recollect nor where he lives, — but a little bulky, self-sufficient looking man. I explained to the Friends in Leeds's presence the reasons that induced me not to comply, particularly the gross partiality manifested by the Arbitrators in refusing to grant me what is allowed of the greatest of all criminals, time to produce evidence. I entered little into the affair in general as I told them that would require proof on one side as well as the other, but in respect to this circumstance of refusing to hear evidence though long within the limited time, and refusing likewise to strengthen the Bonds both which facts my opponent knew to be true. I did not hesitate to think they were sufficiently strong to build my defense upon them, had I no other argument to adduce, as they were a direct attack upon the fundamental maxims of Arbitration. Let both sides be fully heard. My opponent did not offer the least contradiction to this. Save that I had limited the time myself. For this I told him the reason, a consciousness of innocence and the proofs of it were sufficiently strong to have operated on impartial men; but when I saw that these were not sufficiently favourable, and knew that I have much effectual evidence, though not within call, I told him that as he had himself proposed a longer time, no inconvenience could have arisen to his cause by allowing the time I had first thought unnecessary. It seemed as if the Arbitrators were pleased with the opportunity of deciding speedily; and that more obvious, more irrefrangible proof would have given them more perplexity, as they seemed rather to wish to find me guilty than innocent.

After a solid pause, S. Parkinson declared that he had not freedom to advise me to comply with the Award, nor the contrary. The other two Friends declared their opinion, full as strongly against my complying.

I told him before we parted, and before the Friends, that if he felt in doubt how far the Friends belonging to the same Monthly Meeting [as I] might be swayed in their judgement, I would give him free leave to bring with him any others whom he might apprehend were less inclined to think as I did, and the more so, as I was so much strengthened by their judgement. Adding that I should readily follow him through whatever road he should go that was just and honourable to a full and public inquiry into this transaction. And so here I stand.

J. Townsend wrote to me in his manner very passionately to comply. Jacob Hagen [3] came up on this same account today. J. H. had heard no particulars. I believe he was less satisfied with his own opinion before we parted. However, I am easy in proceeding as I do, and hope it will terminate properly. As I expect it will come before the Yearly Meeting, I would endeavour, at least I could wish it was effected, to have such a number of serious, judicious Friends sent up as representatives that a proper choice might be made for the Committee. This must be a matter of some consequence. — Farewell.

J.F.

P.S. I. Pickering saw us in morning; I introduced him to Thomas Stackhouse whom I had sent to, and it was agreed that he should go to Knightsbridge beginning of the week.

Ms. autograph letter, Port. 22/121, LSFL.

1. Samuel Leeds had taken upon himself the duties of an investigator, bringing with him three tradesmen, members of the same Meeting, to interview Dr. Fothergill. The surname of the third, which escaped Dr. Fothergill's memory, was Marshman.

2. Stanfield Parkinson, "an unlettered man," was evidently spokesman of the group. He was a Scot, the son of a Quaker brewer of Edinburgh, Joel Parkinson, known slightly to John Fothergill, Jr., while a medical student in Edinburgh. Joel Parkinson, after the death of his wife, moved to London with his two sons, Stanfield and Sydney, and renewed acquaintance with Dr. Fothergill at Quaker meetings. Stanfield was an upholsterer by trade, and ran a small business of his own without financial success. — Information from Fothergill's preface to Sydney Parkinson, *Journal of a Voyage to the South Seas*, ed. J. C. Lettsom (London: Charles Dilly, 1784), 2.

3. Jacob Hagen, a man of reputed good sense, was distressed by the trouble and wanted it ended magnanimously by Fothergill to rid him of current accusations of persecuting another member of the Society of Friends.

To Samuel Fothergill, Warrington, Lancashire, 20 November 1771

London, 20th Inst

Dear Brother,

The sight of thy handwriting rejoiced us greatly. It was kind to take so much pains to abate our anxiety, and we hope that another post will bring us still more favourable accounts.

Desire thy assistants, when they observe thee begin to breathe with difficulty when thou drops asleep, to awake thee gently and bring thee some sustenance immediately. That terrible distress upon waking is the effect of weakness, and may be lessened much by awaking thee gently when that strength begins which will at length awake thee, and in a hurry not to be described.

My opinion of the opiate remains altered. It saves some present disquietude, but renders it more permanent, and is undoubtedly mischievous. I wish a part of the blister upon the thigh may be made perpetual; that is that it may be kept running a considerable time. I shall write to Dr. Pemberton by this post, and we shall hope to hear from one or other of our relations as frequently as possible. — I may inform thee that Leeds made complaint to our last Monthly Meeting against me, and a few days after made his Bond a rule of Court in the King's Bench.[1] Thither I am following him, pretty well prepared I think; it cannot be decided this term nor extend beyond the next. I would much rather have received justice from the hand of the Society than from a Court of Law, but as he had led me thither, I must unavoidably follow.

To hear of thy recovery would, however, be of much more consequence to me than the issue of this affair can be, go which way it will. We salute thee affectionately and [so do] all our Friends,

J. and A. Fothergill

Ms. autograph letter, Port. 22/122, LSFL. The date 20.11.1771 is added in another hand.

1. Leeds appealed to the Monthly Meeting to make Dr. Fothergill pay the award, and then took his case to the Court of King's Bench.

To Samuel Fothergill, Warrington, Lancashire, 7 December 1771

Harpur Street, London
7.12.1771

Dear Brother,

We received thy lively and affectionate remembrance of us with much thankfulness. I trust thy health will gradually become established. The most formidable symptoms are at least at a stand. Dr. Pemberton acts judiciously in every respect but when he relies more upon my opinion than his own. I wrote to him on receipt of thine and one from him. He will inform thee of the results.

There are many Friends here very anxious for thy recovery, and often enquire after thee with, I believe, a godly solicitude. Mark Beaufoy's family have sent early and late. T. Bevan and wife likewise, and many more.

Through favour I am much recovered and nearly in my usual state of health. I was struck considerably by an anomalous disease much akin to the gout but not fully so. I was the longer in recovery as I had many demands upon me and of serious kinds. My business as usual claims much of my attention. My dispute with Leeds does not affect me any otherwise than as it involves too large a part of our Society here in division, and will entail upon many no small disgrace. I have found out however what I never once suspected. Knowing that I envied no man, I did not think of any envying me, but it is far otherwise. I suspect that many in secret wish that I was guilty; and what they wish, they readily believe. But I will leave such to their own punishers, and study to be quiet and mind my own business.[1] The sensible and judicious amongst us are, I believe, not dissatisfied with my refusal; and such as are at present doubtful, will I hope see cause to be of the same opinion. When thou art well enough to think of these things, I have more to say. At present mind only the recovery of thy health and looking often — as I know thou dost — to the arm that secretly sustains . . .

Whilst things were rather in a doubtful way, Sister and I had been consulting how to render thee any further service. Had not the accounts been favourable, she would have come down to have assisted in anything she could. If her presence, even now, will add to thy comfort, we are both willing it should still be [arranged]. But we would not add to thy encumbrances in any way.

369

Though we rejoice to see thy handwriting, we are sensible how much this indulgence costs thee — therefore don't let us have satisfactions that are too expensive [of thy strength].

We join in affectionate remembrance and in humble thankfulness for thy continuance with us. May it remain with us as a bond of affection beyond the ties of nature merely. Farewell. Salute our Friends, our relations, from thy affectionate

J. and A. Fothergill

Ms. autograph letter, Port. 22/123, LSFL.

1. The oft-repeated Bible text from I Thessalonians 4:11 is again stated.

To Alexander Fothergill, Carr End, Wensleydale, Yorkshire, 18 January 1772

Harpur Street, 18.1.1772

Dear Brother,

I did not expect when I received thy very acceptable and affectionate letter to have been so long without acknowledging the satisfaction it gave me. Thy candour and openness are worthy of thyself; adhere to thy resolution and it will make us all happy, and may the God of our Fathers look down and strengthen thy resolves. Acknowledge thy mistakes [1] to thy Friends. The wise in heart will pity, help, and cover; others will be convinced by such conduct of their imprudence and uncharitableness. It is a sure mark of a good disposition to own where we have done amiss. I shall rejoice to hear that a just concern to shun all occasions of improper conduct replaces thee in the full confidence and esteem of thy best Friends. My heart is full of affection, and I embrace thee with kindness and brotherly regard.

My account from our Sister at Warrington by this day's post continues favourable. Brother cannot yet stir or stand, his breath is so much affected by the least motion; yet he can bear to lie down, takes nourishment sufficient, and recovers a little strength. Sister and the rest are well.

Thou wishes to know something of my affair.[2] It is put off to Easter Term, by the request of Friends, that endeavours may be used to terminate the matter amongst ourselves.

It is scarce credible that a person who has spent upwards of thirty years in this city, in an uniform endeavor to discharge his duty with integrity, to help every body, to hurt none, and was glad when he could reflect any credit upon his profession and do them no dishonour, should now find the generality of that body warmly interesting themselves against him, condemning, without hearing him, and apparently desirous of finding him guilty. But this seems at present too much the case with many, and they seem eager to condemn me because I will not demonstrate my guilt by conforming to the Award. Some that I had esteemed sensible, judicious, and my intimates ever since I came to this place, are inclined to this side. A few, however, and those of the most reputable and judicious amongst us are differently persuaded, and stand by me firmly. The affair was obliquely brought into the Quarterly Meeting about two weeks ago. Much was said to dissuade us from going to Law.[3] Leeds at length offered to defer the trial, if I would consent. I did consent, and proposed that from signing this agreement no evidence on either side should be produced. — I find he had no affirmation or affidavit made, and of course could have produced no evidence this term, but must have moved for time. The court would not have granted it, and of course the business would have been decided next week.

I wished, however, that it might be terminated amongst ourselves, and I hope it will. The Quarterly Meeting appointed a numerous and judicious committee. If the matter is brought before them, I am not in much doubt of the event. — L. had complained to my Monthly Meeting that I had not complied with the Award. Before they had determined or could determine, he complained that I had gone to law with him. He appealed against them for a delay of justice, and the committee is appointed on this appeal, not the merit of the case. Their report will be made next second day,[4] and the same committee will probably be appointed on the case itself. — I am thus far easy in the affair, and whether I am condemned or not, I know my innocence both as to act and intention; no small comfort this. Thou will hear further from me as occasion requires. I was satisfied and so were many others with thy opinion respecting the aggressor in this case. With love to Sister and William,

I am affectionately thine

J. Fothergill

Ms. autograph letter, Fothergill Family Papers, Wallis Collection.

1. Alexander's errors at this time are nowhere described in detail.

2. Leeds's case, taken to the Court of King's Bench in November 1771, would normally have come before the court in January 1772.

3. Samuel Leeds had stubbornly refused advice given by Westminster Monthly Meeting to withdraw complaints against Dr. Fothergill. Westminster Quarterly Meeting had repeatedly urged this solution, holding adjourned sessions twice, but Leeds continued to hold his fixed idea, in opposition to members distressed by the development of factions within the Society. — Information by courtesy of Edward H. Milligan, Librarian, LSFL.

4. Monday, 20 January.

To Samuel Fothergill, Warrington, 25 January 1772

London, 25.1.1772

Dear Brother,

Not knowing but our Sister may perhaps be set out before this arrives, I address it to thee. Though the roads and weather considered, I could almost wish she might remain till there is some little alteration in her favour where she is.[1]

Her journey gave me great ease. I have no doubt of its being both useful and satisfactory. She has seen thee I hope in a fair way to get better, though by slow gradations. For thy own sake and thy Friends', I wish it would be rendered more speedy, but I see not by what means certainly to effect it. Better weather will do much, and I shall not fail to suggest such hints as may occur to me to Dr. Pemberton or Dr. Turner.[2]

This morning at breakfast I was a little surprised by a visit from our Brother Alexander. — He came last night to Gracious Street and left his family well. He proposes to stay here two or three weeks, in which time I hope he will write to thee. I know not at present that he has any other errand to this place than to see if he can render me any service in this troublesome business.

The Committee appointed by the Quarterly Meeting have met many times, and have spent much pains on the subject. They are not yet agreed upon a report, and when they will is uncertain. It is in agitation to advise us both to stop all law proceedings. To this I shall not consent but upon terms:

1. that the Award is quashed.
2. that if any point of Law arises it shall be refered to Council.
3. if any Question is started respecting medical abilities, it shall be referred to Physicians.

These are points that will not be granted; and unless they are granted, it is my present opinion that I ought not to comply.

Do not think of writing a line to me. S. Titley[3] will be thy scribe. Dictate to her thy complaints and thy wants, and I will endeavour to relieve and redress.

Through favour I am well, and not discontent. I shall be more happy than I can easily express when I can hear of thy recovery. — My tenderest regards attend you.

From thy affectionate Brother,

J. Fothergill

Ms. autograph letter, Port. 22/133, LSFL.

1. Ann had gone to Warrington in December to help care for Samuel during his serious illness. — Crosfield, *Memoirs*, 574.

2. Probably Dr. Pemberton's associate.

3. Sarah Fothergill Titley, Dr. Fothergill's niece, the wife of Abraham Titley of Warrington.

To Mark Beaufoy, Cupers Bridge, South Lambeth, London, 27 January 1772

Harpur Street, 27.1.1772

Dear Friend M. Beaufoy,

I have perused the enclosed account of J. Higman's indisposition.[1] It is a very uncommon one and will, I am afraid scarcely admit of much help.— There is, however, one cheap and I think not improper remedy that he may try; and if he finds the least benefit, let him continue it steadily for some months.

Let him drink a pint of Tar-water[2] every day, one third at a time; he may take it either warm or cold as he likes. It may be made by letting a quart of Norway Tar fall into ten quarts of clean cold water in as small a stream as may be. It need not be stirred, but after they have stood together about 48 hours, the liquor may be poured through a flannel into bottles for use.

If it is found upon trial to disagree, let it be omitted entirely; and when Spring is so far advanced as that Dandelions[3] may be got, let the tops and the roots of this plant be well washed, bruised and the juice strained off. Six or eight spoonsful of this juice may be taken in the morning and at noon.

373

Bathing in warm sea-water[4] two or three times a week, when the warm weather approaches, may also be worth a trial. A Tub may be filled with sea water if he lives near the sea, and a pailful or two of the same water made boiling hot may be put into it. He may plunge over-head and put on his clothes without much wiping, and then use what motion he can; or if none, he may be put into a warm bed and lie there till he is quite dry. If these directions are of use to the poor man, I shall be pleased. I cannot recollect anything more likely to do him good and with very little expense. He may continue the kind of diet that he finds to agree best. Please give my respects to W. Phillips,[5] and believe me to be

thy affectionate Friend,

J. Fothergill

Ms. autograph letter, Gibson Mss., IV, LSFL.

1. Neither the patient Higman nor his physician, Dr. Phillips, has been identified.
2. George Berkeley, Bishop of Cloyne (1685–1753), extolling the virtues of tar-water, temperance, and early hours of repose, recommended this concoction as "a cordial not only safe and innocent but giving health and spirit as surely as others destroy them. I do verily think there is not any other medicine whatever so effectual to restore a crazy constitution and cheer a dreary mind, or so likely to subvert that gloomy empire of the spleen." — George Berkeley, *Siris: A Chain of Philosophical Reflexions and Inquiries Concerning the Virtues of Tar Water* (Dublin, 1744); ed. A. A. Luce and F. E. Jessop (London: Nelson, 1953), V, sec. 106, 66, 67.
3. Dr. Fothergill suggested use of a plant which twentieth-century nutritionists have found to have an unusually high content of vitamin A.
4. Coastal watering places rose in public favor about 1760 because physicians began to recommend sea-water bathing in addition to taking the waters of various chemical content at the Spas. Spending the holidays at seaside resorts became fashionable, and swimming became a favorite sport for the young and athletic. — Hughes, *North Country Life*, 28, 29.
5. Enclosed with this letter was one from Dr. William Phillips to Mark Beaufoy giving some details of the illness from which his patient Higman was suffering, and adding a report that Samuel Fothergill "whose life was despaired of" earlier was now showing signs of improvement.

To Granville Sharp, London, 2 February 1772

Harpur Street, London

[Feb.] 2nd. Inst. [1772]

I have perused the Arguments of Council on Somerset's affair[1] with satisfaction, and wish the event may be favourable to publish Liberty.

I should have returned the ms. before, but have been prevented from perusing it as soon as I could have wished. As many and great Expenses must have attended this controversy, I shall be very ready to contribute my mite towards them, and when the affair is terminated, go which way it may, I shall be pleased with an opportunity of confirming on this matter and do everything in my power to lessen the Burthens by dividing it.[2]

I am
Thy respectful Friend
J. Fothergill

Ms. letter, copied in a contemporary hand, from the Letter Book of Granville Sharp, Library Company of Philadelphia (now deposited at HSP).

1. Granville Sharp had become actively interested in the plight of a Negro slave, James Somerset, taken by his master, Charles Stewart, from Virginia to the West Indies and thence to London. Somerset took advantage of a chance to disappear in the metropolis, and after a series of misadventures appeared at Granville Sharp's residence with a tale of his misfortunes and pleading fear of revenge by his master. Sharp furnished funds to secure legal help, with the result that Somerset's case was argued in the Court of King's Bench, Lord Mansfield presiding. Appeal was opened in February 1772 by Mr. Sergeant Davy on the principle of the essential and constitutional right of every man in England to the liberty of his person unless forfeited by the laws of England. Argument was prolonged, and further consideration of the case was deferred till May. The second hearing was opened by the query: Whether a slave coming into England becomes free? Lord Mansfield himself consistently maintained that Somerset was as fully entitled to the rights of a human being as any man listening in the courtroom. Stewart's counsel argued that Stewart had a legal right to hold slaves by the laws of Virginia; it was therefore unjust to deprive him of this legal right when he sailed from country to country on his lawful business, taking with him a slave. This argument was met with a statement from Lord Mansfield that Stewart maintained home and business in Jamaica, not in Virginia, and while living in London was financially aided by West Indian merchants. The case was decided in Somerset's favor. — Hoare, *Memoirs of Granville Sharp*, 69–94.

2. Sharp did not find it necessary to accept Dr. Fothergill's offer of financial assistance.

To Samuel Fothergill, Warrington, 13 February 1772

London, 13.2.1772

Dear Brother,

Our Sister is returned to us safe. She has given me an account of thy situation. I had a letter from Dr. Pemberton after her arrival on the same subject. I shall write to him by this post, and shall devote a little time to thyself.

The oedematous swelling will, I hope, gradually subside.[1] But there are two things that will retard it: one is thy not lying down at nights; the other is sitting all day in the same place and almost the same posture. These must be altered.

By sleeping in a posture so erect, the fluids naturally sink down to those lax and unresisting parts; and by sitting they are retained there. As the swellings are not painful, except from weight and a little tension, a little motion can neither give much pain nor do any harm. On the contrary, it will be very beneficial by promoting a motion of the stagnant juices. I must intreat some little exertion. It is of great, great consequence.

It gives me satisfaction to find that the castor oil agrees so well. Whilst it answers the purpose easily, continue it, taking now and then a little more. — Be sparing of liquor of any kind, and in diet reflect that exercise is necessary to convert it into proper aliment. Forbear sometimes, I don't mean to excess, but to save Nature as much unnecessary trouble as possible. — *Sunt certi denique fines, quo ultra citraque nequit consistere rectum.*[2] This is not beyond the bounds of thy scholarship — but it will be easy to get it interpreted, and not beyond thy power to make a practical commentary upon it.

I will recapitulate my directions: Endeavour to lie down by degrees in thy usual position. Endeavour to use some limited motion, and bear a little inconvenience in endeavouring it. Continue the castor oil while it agrees. Be moderate in respect to quantity both of drink and food. And even try to use thy hands in some motion, if thy feet are not willing to obey the dictates of thy wish.

How many neat walking sticks has our Father cut for his acquaintances by the fireside!

Nothing material has happened in my affairs since I wrote last. As much low, dirty cunning, I see, will be practiced as can properly be continued, but I am not discouraged. The most sensible and judicious, I hope, are not against me.

Brother Alex. is still here, and not unusefully employed. He is doing what he can to draw up a short, intelligent narrative of the whole.[3]

No steps are taken yet, farther than I mentioned, in respect to the Tithes affair. We are a little unfortunate in respect to the time, as two other matters have drawn the attention of the Clergy and Parliament. One is the matter of subscription, which is rejected; the other is a national concern: that no tithes shall be demanded where the claim has lain dormant upwards of sixty years. This will probably be rejected this session, but it will be brought up again and again till it is carried. There is scarce a gentleman in the country who is not interested in it.[4] The Princess Dowager's death [5] will likewise retard public business. It will present an unanswerable pretext to the Ministry to be dilatory.

I have spared thee as much time as I can. We unite in affectionate remembrance and in grateful acknowledgments to the author of all good for thy restoration. Farewell.

J. Fothergill

Ms. autograph letter, Port. 22/131, LSFL.

1. Samuel's illness appears to have been progressive cardiac failure causing severe dropsy. He had suffered repeated attacks of rheumatism in early manhood, as recounted in Crosfield's *Memoirs*. Samuel's heart disease may, therefore, have been of rheumatic origin. Modern physicians would advise such a patient to be propped up with pillows at night to a sitting posture, since lying down (as advised by Dr. Fothergill) would no doubt cause difficulty in breathing. Castor oil was advised to promote loss of fluid from the body. What Samuel Fothergill actually needed was a good diuretic, but in 1772 no effective diuretic was known to the medical profession.

2. The quotation, when made in full, begins *"Est modus in rebus"* and may then be translated freely as follows: "There is measure for everything. There are fixed limits beyond which, and short of which the right goal cannot be reached" (Horace *Odes* IV. xii. 126).

3. The long-drawn-out Leeds affair.

4. The Society of Friends were not alone in seeking readjustment of taxes imposed by Parliament and long outmoded.

5. The Princess Augusta, aged fifty-two, died 8 February 1772 from an abscess in the throat which had caused her months of great suffering.

To Samuel Fothergill, Warrington, 17 March 1772

London, 17.3.1772

Dear Brother,

It seems long since I wrote to thee, and long since I heard from thee. The accounts we have received, upon comparing them together, seem more favourable than they have been, and in this we rejoice.

After thou finds some ability to get abroad, I wish thou would engage a Post-chaise to take thee out, two or three times a week, as it suits thy inclination and ability to travel.

I say nothing of medicine, as I find by Dr. Pemberton's letter yesterday the last has not answered my expectation.[1] — Rest a little, except from castor oil, and an infusion of horse-radish root, mustard seed bruised, each an ounce, black cinnamon, quarter of an ounce, in a bottle of raisin wine. A glass of this may be taken twice a day, with 8, 10 or 12 drops of vinegar of squills.[2]

If thou knew how much I felt from the descriptions of thy situation! There is nothing I could have said would have given a moment of easiness. It amounted to a full proof of a confirmed increasing dropsy; than which, under certain circumstances I know of nothing more certainly though slowly fatal. I am glad to find these circumstances are altered, that thy bulk diminishes; I mean the fullness of thy belly and lower parts, that strength is returning, and some other appearances of amendment. — I wish their continuance, and hope to receive an account of it from thyself speedily.

Please to acquaint Dr. Pemberton that I received his acceptable letter, sent the enclosed to his son, and shall write to him when I find a necessary occasion to give him the trouble of a letter. I know his engagements and know it sometimes straitens him to answer me.

Brother Alexander is still here and not unuseful. Had it not been for the idle disputes on as idle a subject, the Marriage Bill,[3] I hope by this time we should have been excused from the ecclesiastical and other courts. The Acts of William and George the First for the necessary recovery of Tithes,[4] and so forth are designed to be extended to any sum whatsoever; at present the mode is limited to ten pounds. A restrictive clause is added limiting the claimants of Tithes to this mode only, except when the title is in question. Administration takes this upon themselves, and though we are consulted how far this method coincides with our opinion, and every intimation for our security properly regarded, yet we are not called upon to solicit. Nor is it proposed that we shall take any public part in carrying the bill through either house. In this affair our Brother is of use; he attends the Solicitor, rectifies his notions, and sees that nothing is admitted contrary to plan.

My own affair is gradually advancing towards a proper decision. With some difficulty, it was brought before the Quarterly Meeting again. The same committee is drawn to prevail upon us to stop all proceedings at law and submit the decision to Friends entirely. To this I can have no objection; it is my wish; and will, I hope, be urged to mutual advantage

378

and the Society's necessary information on many material points of discipline.

We are favoured with health and a temper of mind not unforgetful of the favour. I shall write when I can. I have had a very labourious winter, and already begin to long for a retreat. Remember us affectionately to Sister, to our relations, and be assured that we are as much as ever

thy
J. & A. Fothergill

Ms. autograph letter, Port. 22/130, LSFL.

1. Samuel's illness had become more incapacitating.

2. Squills are the fleshy inner scales of the bulb of a liliaceous plant, *Urginaea maratima*. Vinegar of squills was considered to be useful as a diuretic and was also prescribed for cases of croup, bronchitis, and dropsy.

3. The Royal Marriage Bill had been proposed to put an end to uncertainties about the right of succession to the throne, especially if and when a member of the Royal Family should intend to marry a person not of noble rank.

4. Payment of tithes, a tenth part of annual income, exacted by law for support of the Church of England, naturally irked members of the Society of Friends and other dissenters. Failure to pay tithes had long been severely punished by government fines, distraint of goods, and imprisonment. Quakers had always considered such taxation a Hebraic custom "abrogated by the coming of Christ" since "the Gospels give no sanction to tithes and the disciples were freed from all obligation thereto." A movement was under way toward securing legislation to relieve all dissenters from these taxes. — Joseph Besse, *A Collection of Sufferings of the People called . . . Quakers*, 2 vols. (London, 1753), I, 20–23; Joseph Davis, *A Digest of Legislative Enactments, relating to the Society of Friends, commonly called (Quakers) in England* (Bristol, Eng.: Wansbrough and Saunders, 1820), section on "Tithes and Other Ecclesiastical Demands," 51–65.

To Samuel Fothergill, Warrington, Lancashire, 28 March 1772

Harpur Street [London], 28 inst.

Dear Brother,

Though I know not how to promote thy recovery at present by any prescriptions, yet it is so long since I wrote and I received so much satisfaction from thy last, that I could not contentedly let another post go away without a letter.

The weather has been so favourable that I doubt not that it has invited thee abroad and contributed to thy advance towards better health,

379

at least I hope so, and perhaps chiefly because I ardently wish it. — I leave thee therefore under thy present program, and when any doubt or difficulty arises, thou will please to inform me. Not knowing thy present precise situation prevents me from doing more. We sympathize with thee much; having so many urgent occasions of distress about thee. Our Sister's enfeebled state, our relations approaching dissolution, and they own infirmities — any of them just causes of anxiety.

Brother Alexander, I apprehend, wrote to thee before he left London, and pretty fully on many points. I wished him to have come down by Warrington, but his affairs did not allow it. He has been very diligent in my affairs, and not unusefully. He would acquaint thee with the issue which is that the affair [1] must be terminated in a Court of Law. The Arbitrators, I mean the three, are inveterate. And there is nothing that they can do against me that will be left undone.

The Royal Marriage Bill [2] has much postponed our affair,[3] but it is now again resumed. I expect it will be moved in the House speedily, not as coming from us, but as taken up by the House for the public good. The bill consists of an extension of the Acts made for the recovery of Tithes under 10 pounds to any sum without limitation to be recovered by justice's warrant and a clause restricting the claimants of Tithes to this mode only, except where the title is in question. So that without any bustle, I hope both the Exchequer, Ecclesiastical and all other oppressive courts will be shut up on these accounts; a favourable intervention truly, and gratefully to be acknowledged to providence, as well as to the immediate instrument.

Sister Ann soon got better of her disorder, but much needs rest both for body and mind. Accept our united and most affectionate remembrance.

From thy A. and J. Fothergill

Ms. autograph letter, Port. 22/129, LSFL. Dated in full from internal evidence and a memorandum in the hand of George Crosfield on the letter.

1. The Leeds case.
2. The Royal Marriage Bill, enacted by Parliament later in 1772, clarified existing confusion and settled questions about the right of succession to the throne and about marriages between members of the Royal Family and commoners.
3. A proposal to relieve Quakers and other dissenters from taxation to benefit the Church of England.

To Samuel Fothergill, Warrington, Lancashire, 4 April 1772

London, 4.4.1772

Dear Brother,

Thy acceptable letter by yesterday's post relieved us much. From the circumstances it describes, I hope the disorder is gradually declining. I am sorry that the Castor Oil does not now answer the purpose so easily and effectually as it has done. And this disappointment engages me to write to thee the earlier, though much unfitted for it this evening by extreme fatigue.

On the other side is an Electuary[1] which I think is not difficult to take, and may probably answer the purpose of procuring a motion every day. Show it to Dr. Pemberton or Dr. Turner, and have their opinion.

If the Electuary cannot be taken, or if it does not answer the purpose, perhaps 3, 4 or V grains of fine Socotrine Aloes,[2] the like quantity of unwashed Calx of Antimony made into pills with any Syrup might answer the purpose well.[3]

The draught on Betson etc. will be cheerfully paid, and we shall adjust that readily. If more is wanted, please let me know.

My affair at last must be terminated in Westminster Hall.[4] L. thinks he has a better chance there than in the Society. He refuses to submit to Friends, and will be supported in his refusal. — What will be the consequence, I know not. I own I little suspected that after having endeavoured to serve anybody at the expense of health, strength and pocket, I had so many enemies.

The Bill[5] I mentioned to thee has been read in the House and ordered to be printed. So soon as I can get a printed copy I will send thee one by the Coach. What the result will be, I know not, but thus far we have met with very little opposition.

Let us hear from thee when it meets thy inclination and ability. Get abroad as much as may be. Farewell, dear Brother, and think of us as affectionately thine.

J. Fothergill

Ms. autograph letter, Port. 22/128, LSFL.

1. A medicinal preparation consisting of a powdered drug mixed to a paste with syrup, honey, or a conserve. Information "on the other side" is missing.

2. A nauseous bitter purgative made from a kind of aloe obtained from Socotra, an island in the Indian Ocean.

3. Oxide of antimony was used as an emetic, or for diaphoretic action to produce sweating.

4. The Leeds case was to be heard by the Court of King's Bench in Westminster Hall.

5. For relieving dissenters from taxation to benefit the Church of England.

To Samuel Fothergill, Warrington, Lancashire, 9 May 1772

Harpur Street, London
7th Day, evening

Dear Brother,

I have been uneasy with myself today that I did not send a line or two last night, as I might have informed thee the sooner that I got home safe in good time without any accident or delay, and found my sister and family well and no material want having arisen during my absence. — I am thankful for these favours and likewise for a circumstance which in the midst of all thy distress will afford thee some little satisfaction. The case between me and Leeds was yesterday decided in the Court of the King's Bench, and the Award set aside as partial and therefore corrupt and unjust. The Court did not even permit my counsel to plead — but condemned him on his own evidence.[1] The Society has suffered nothing on this occasion. The affirmations his party brought did not contradict any circumstances we had alleged, nor was there anything passed that could give any handle to traducers. For this I am thankful. Friends in general rejoice much, and I hope all occasions of further dispute will subside. His party indeed threaten fresh prosecutions in other courts, but I trust I have nothing to fear from them. Leeds appealed or rather gave notice of an appeal last 4th day to Westminster Monthly Meeting, but it was literally a day too late, the time limited by the Yearly Meeting for such notices being expired.

The bill of relief in respect to Tithes is withdrawn by the request of Friends. They found the influence of the Church was such that the restrictive clause could not be obtained; and less than that they did not care to ask for. For this, while I live I think not to forget them, but to keep an eye frequently on that paragraph of the Epistles which relates to Faithfulness . . .[2]

The mentioning of these circumstances has detained me longer than I could have wished from [consideration of] thy own health, a circumstance of more importance to me than rest. On my return I had full leisure to think of it fully, to weigh every circumstance, and to ask myself carefully what further steps could be taken for thy assistance. To say that I anxiously wish it, is not enough. Dr. Pemberton will be kind enough in a few days to inform me of what has passed since I left thee. I shall correspond with him as diligently as may be. Please to tell him that I have a little mistaken the Rye Poultice — it is under.

I have wrote too much at once. We will one of us do it frequently, though less at a time. Accept from us both our fervent desires that every blessing, every comfort, may attend in thy truly distressed situation. — Farewell — from thy affectionate

J. and A. Fothergill

Rye Meal   one pound
Salt   two ounces
Baume   four ounces
and as much water as will make
the whole by kneading into a proper consistence.

Ms. autograph letter, Port. 22/127, LSFL. Dated from its reference to the Leeds case.

1. The trial took place on Friday, 8 May 1772. Presiding at this session of the Court of King's Bench, Lord Chief Justice Mansfield (William Murray, 1706–1793), after hearing testimony from Samuel Leeds and witnesses called in his behalf, threw the case out of court. Lord Mansfield's ironical summing up of a situation which seemed to him preposterous produced laughter in the crowded courtroom. Leeds, completely discredited, left London shortly and went to Ipswich to work as an apothecary. It was reported that funds were sent regularly from London, very likely by Dr. Fothergill, for Leeds's relief during the months that elapsed before his death in 1773. — Fox, 74–78; "Records and Recollections of James Jenkins," Ms. Journal, LSFL.

2. "Moreover, it is required of stewards that a man may be found faithful" (I Corinthians 4:2).

To Samuel Fothergill, Warrington, 20 May 1772

London, 20.5.1772

Dear Brother,

Though I have shut up the intercourse on thy part, it ought not to deprive thee of every bit of comfort which our near and affectionate remembrance can afford thee under deep distress — distress in body and often weighed down with affliction and trials within. But be of good comfort, receive that consolation from others which thy feeling, sympathizing heart has been the means of conveying to many. I am with thee often in mind, and if I knew how to add to thy ease and thy health in the least degree, I need not tell thee how much it would add to my own happiness. I wrote pretty freely to Dr. Pemberton; he will acquaint thee with the purport, and you will all act I know for the best.

We were pleased to hear of the safe arrival of our relations, though from Dr. Pemberton's account of poor A. Titley,[1] I much fear that their meeting would be with that alloy which waits upon every stage of mortality. We have passed three days in anxious suspense, hoping we might have heard from some of our relations whether there was any prospect of a change for the better. Many, many friends here are very anxious about thee, and I believe the prayers of many honest hearts are for thy preservation amongst us. But the event must be left where it ought to be in the discretion of Sovereign Wisdom.

In respect to myself and my own affairs I am easy with whatever happens. Thy recovery is more to us than anything besides. I hear not of any new proceedings in respect to the Leeds affair; nor does it appear that the Society has suffered in this determination — the blame being laid where it was only due, on the Arbitrators. They are silent, and I shall endeavour to do nothing to provoke them or promote dissention. I regret most that we are sunk to so low an ebb as to look towards such as chiefs amongst us of so much vileness. But this should teach us humility, and send us to seek for that wisdom which is from above.

Give my love to Nanny.[2] Tell her she must be kind enough to write to her Aunt or me frequently, and give as particular an account of thy situation as she can. Nothing that concerns thee will be indifferent to us. Sally Titley[3] has endeavoured to give us all the comfort she could. I fear she now stands in need of comfort herself. Remember us to Sister,[4] and affectionately, for we know her distress and that she suffers much, I mean for thee whom she sees with the eyes of affection. Express to those about you all you would wish to say to us. Some of them will gather it up and convey it to us.

If I should mention all those who inquire after thee, I must fill a volume. Let it suffice that the living part of God's heritage sympathize with thee. Farewell, our Brother, our Friend, our Joy in that which is only deserving the name.

Farewell, affectionately from thy J. Fothergill.

Ms. autograph letter, Crosfield Mss. no. 80, LSFL.

1. Abraham Titley.
2. Ann, the only one of Joseph Fothergill's daughters still unmarried.
3. Sarah Fothergill Titley, usually called Sally by her Uncle John, whom she called "Uncle Doctor."
4. Susanna, Samuel's wife.

To Samuel Fothergill, Warrington, 9 June 1772

London, 9.6.1772

Oh, dear Brother, what comfort did thy letter give us! We rejoice with thankfulness and trembling! And recover hope which we had almost lost.

Thy vacant seat at our table, and at the Meetings,[1] hourly reminds us of thee and our own distress, but we leave this and submit the whole to Divine disposal.

The affairs of the Meeting go on well. The Americans help us much. John Woolman is solid and weighty in his remarks.[2] I wish he could be cured of some singularities but his real worth outweighs the husk. The few expressions thou gives in trust to our relation, I shall communicate to Jonah Thompson, and propose that he shall mention them near the close of this Meeting.[3] Joshua Strangman is our clerk.[4] He does his business pretty well, and better I think than most of the Midland clerks, of late. — I shall write to thee when I can, as I know thou longs to learn how matters are conducted in the Camp.

Sister and our relations are well. W. Jepson[5] is with us, and is remarkably solid and composed, yet cheerful and easy.

I rejoice much to hear that Brother Alex. has been at Warrington. Oh, how I long for his return to the paths of his ancestors!

Accept the united strong and affectionate remembrance of this family from thy

J. Fothergill

Ms. autograph letter Port. 22/126, LSFL.

1. London Yearly Meeting was in session. It was at this Meeting that the Society of Friends passed its first Minute protesting against Negro slavery. — Fox, 222.
2. John Woolman (1700–1772) of Rancocas, West Jersey, now remembered chiefly for his Journal, became a Quaker minister in 1743 and traveled in the ministry throughout the rest of his life, both in the Colonies and in England. His work for the abolition of the slave trade was constant and notable. After attending London Yearly Meeting in 1772, he traveled northward through Yorkshire on a tour of

religious exhortation, arriving in York in September to attend the county's Quarterly Meeting. It was reported that he appeared "much out of health" at this time. Early in October he fell seriously ill from smallpox and died in York, on 7 October 1772. He was buried near the Church of St. Mary, the Elder, in the Friends' burial grounds. — Janet Whitney, *John Woolman, American Quaker* (Boston: Little, Brown, 1942).

3. Jonah Thompson read these "expressions" as an informal message from Samuel Fothergill to London Yearly Meeting. See Crosfield, *Memoirs*, 521–522.

4. Crosfield (p. 522) prints the first part of this sentence as "Joshua Strangman (of Leek) is the clerk." A firm active in Waterford, Ireland, during an earlier period, Strangman, Courtenay and Ridgway, Exporters of Beef and Rawhides to England, Holland, Spain, and Portugal, is mentioned by James Jenkins in his manuscript "Recollections" (LSFL) because he first secured employment through the senior member of this firm, Joshua Strangman, a Quaker.

5. William Jepson, a Quaker minister, was the husband of Dr. Fothergill's niece Hannah, fourth daughter of Joseph Fothergill. — Fothergill Genealogy, below.

To Sarah Titley, 12 July 1772

London 12th Inst. 1772

My dear Niece,

Though my mind has been agitated of late on various occasions yet I cannot forget to feel a little for others.[1] I could not lessen thy distress, but I sympathize with thee and wish for a proper opportunity to tell thee so. It is some consolation to us under distress that others would lessen our affliction if they could.

Thy kind, affectionate, constant attention to our Brother and to his relations claims my grateful acknowledgement. In the first place it might in part seem to be a duty but affection mingled its kindness and induced thee to leave nothing undone to him, to us, and to everybody that thy own afflicted situation would allow. Accept our united acknowledgements for thy kindness to our beloved Brother. — Thy own sufferings have been great. In part they are at an end, except when recollection calls to thy view that thou had once a companion that loved thee tenderly, whose happiness while he was himself was centered in thee, and who found in thy duty and affection to him all the solace, the reasonable comfort he could feel. Thy unremitting attention to discharge every duty to him, must now be the source of some consolation to thyself. Look steadily at this when distressing apprehensions would arise, and I am sure this reflection must calm every disquieting consideration.

Like thyself I feel a vast void in my enjoyments, and begin to feel the attachments to this life much loosened. It ought to be so; and these afflicting circumstances, whilst a hope that the objects of our affection are bettered by the change, should instead of urging us to give way to ineffectual sorrow, prompt us to persevere with more ardency the path which they trod to a more peaceful habitation. Think of recovering thy health; dismiss all unavailing anxiety as much as possible. Look to our Brother's doctrine and example. We hope to do the like, and to trust in the gracious help that supported him through moments of his conflict.

Remember us affectionately to thy Sister, to thy Brothers, our Sister and our Friends.[2] The post is waiting while I just subscribe myself thy affectionate.

J. Fothergill

11th Inst.

We propose to set out the 20th Inst. and hope to be at Lea Hall the 24th at night.

Ms. autograph letter, Port. 21/138, LSFL.

1. Samuel Fothergill, greatly mourned, had died on 15 June 1772; Sally's husband, Abraham Titley, had died at Buxton on 1 July. — Records of Lancashire Burials, Friends House.

2. The reference to relatives includes Sally's sisters and their husbands and Samuel Fothergill's widow, Susanna Croudson Fothergill.

To James Pemberton, Philadelphia, 29 August 1772

Lea Hall near Middlewich, Cheshire 29.8.1772

Estemed Friend,

A few days ago I executed a power of attorney to enable my brother agents, David Barclay and Dr. Franklin to receive from the Bank of England the money due to your Hospital. The detention of this money so long from the Managers has given us all considerable uneasiness. It chiefly arose from the dilatory conduct of our Solicitor who, however, has not wanted frequent admonitions from us all.

The sum will be between 6 and 7000£ sterling, and will probably be remitted to the Managers this autumn. I know it will not be kept on this side the water an hour longer than can be helped.[1]

I think myself not a little fortunate for having suggested the thought to the agents for this affair, and I feel a sensible satisfaction in thinking

387

that the distress of many may be alleviated and at so little expense to myself. It is indeed entailing an additional care upon the Managers of that useful charity; but as it enables them to fulfill the intentions and wishes of those who first gave the institution existence, it will add proportionately to their satisfaction.

Permit me just to mention what has sometimes occurred to my thoughts respecting its disposition. I would by no means be thought to dictate in the least. I know my own unfitness and the abilities of the Managers too well. — Would it not be proper to invest 6 or 7000£ of the money in proper securities, land or otherwise, towards the constant support of the House, and employ the residue according to the immediate exigencies of the House? I know not whether the Hospital is furnished with iron bedsteads; they are said to answer well in ours, and are much more easily kept free from bugs and other troublesome vermin.

Please to give my respects to the Managers; I am much obliged to them for many instances of their regard. I wish them satisfaction and success in their endeavours and shall at all times be glad to promote them.

I am

thy assured Friend
John Fothergill

Ms. autograph letter, Pemberton Papers, Etting Collection, II, 66, HSP.

1. The Managers of the Pennsylvania Hospital wished to draw £3000 from the trust fund set up in 1766, in care of the Bank of England, from unclaimed assets of the Pennsylvania Land Company. Dr. Fothergill, David Barclay, and Benjamin Franklin were the trustees of the fund. The Managers of the Hospital were concerned lest the growing political tension between Great Britain and the American Colonies might prevent the transfer of the balance of the fund from the Bank, via the trustees, to the Hospital.

To John Bartram, Philadelphia, Autumn 1772

London [Autumn] 1772

Esteemed Friend,

Constant and various engagements have long prevented me from writing to thee. For some years past I have retired from London to a considerable distance for about two months in order to recover strength sufficient to undergo the duties of my profession. Here I used to have

Esteemed Friend

Near Middlewich } 29. 8mo
(Cheshire) 1772.

A few days ago, I executed a power
of attorney, to enable my brother Agents,
David Barclay & Dr. Franklin to recover
from the Bank of England, the money
due to your Hospital. The detention
of this money so long, from the mana
gers, has given us all, considerable
uneasiness. It chiefly arose from the
delatory conduct of our Solicitor; who
however has not wanted frequent ad
monitions from us all. —
The sum will be between 6 & 7000.
Sterling; and will probably be remitted
to the managers this autumn. I know
it will not be kept on this side the
water, an hour longer than can be
help'd

Please to give my respects to the Managers; I am
much obliged to them for many instances of
their regard. I wish them satisfaction and suc
cess in their endeavours; and shall at all
times be glad to promote them.
          I am thy assured Friend
                  John Fothergill. —

From a letter to James Pemberton, 1772

(See page 387)

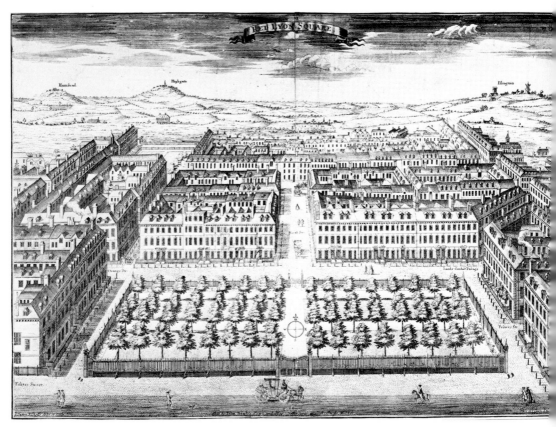

Red Lion Square, looking toward Hampstead, Highgate, and Islington

a little time to correspond with my distant Friends; but last year I was wholly prevented.

I desired my nephew James Freeman to acquaint thee with this, and to desire thy indulgence, hoping to be able at some time or other to acknowledge thy kind remembrance. I hope he acquits himself to my satisfaction. He is a sober, diligent young man and wishes to oblige me and my Friends.

The Frogs came safe and lively. I transcribed thy account of them and had it delivered to the King with an intimation that they were in my hands, and should be sent whenever he would please to order.[1] No order ever came to me. — In a little place where I keep a few gold fish I put the frogs and fenced it in, in such a manner as I thought they would be forthcoming whenever they were called for. A small communication, between the place I had allotted for them and a large canal, underground, and of which I was ignorant, afforded one of them the means of getting more liberty. The other is still a prisoner, is still alive, and my gardener who sees him frequently tells me he is increased in size. I imagine they are quite forgot, and will never be called for, and having once made the offer, through a channel of some consequence, I shall make no further overture. As I have no chance of recovering the animal that has escaped, I think to let the one that is confined have a chance to escape likewise into the same water; perhaps they may find one another.

In a letter to my nephew thou intimates that probably William Young may have endeavoured to raise some prejudice against thee. He has not. He durst not attempt it, as he knew my esteem for thee. He never spoke one word to thy disadvantage. My silence has been solely owing to incessant occupation. I have endeavoured to assist this poor man, and have aided him considerably; but he will not succeed, nor can he be supported.

A few weeks ago I received a letter and some drawings from thy son William in Carolina. For his sake, as well as thine, I should be glad to assist him. He draws neatly, has a strong relish for natural history, and it is a pity that such a genius should sink under distress. Is he sober and diligent? This may be an uncommon question to ask a Father of his son, and yet I know thy integrity will not suffer thee to mislead me. I would not have it understood that I mean to support him. I would lend him however some little assistance if he is worthy. He proposes to go to Florida.[2] It is a country abounding with great variety of plants and many of them unknown. To search for these will be of use to Science in general; but I am a little selfish. I wish to introduce into this country the more hardy American plants, such as will bear our winters without much shelter. However, I shall endeavour to assist his inclination for a tour through Florida; and if he succeeds, shall perhaps wish him to see the back parts of Canada. Many curious flowering plants will doubtless be found about the lakes that will grow anywhere.

We have totally lost in this country the *Tetragonotheca*.[3] Will it be possible to get some seeds, or a few roots of it? I believe nobody in America knows it or where it is to be found but thyself.

My garden is pretty large, well-sheltered, and a good soil. The North American plants flourish with me exceedingly. I have most of the common plants usually sent over; but have room for everything. I am fond of the Ferns. I have several from America, but not all. I do not want to have a specimen of everything that grows in my garden; but plants that are remarkable for their figure, their fragrance, or their use are exceedingly acceptable.

I must own that with this inclination to increase my collection of plants, I have very little time to spend amongst them. I see them now and then, transiently. But I look forwards, and that it is not impossible but I may live long enough to think it proper to decline all business. Then an amusement of this kind will have its use to lessen the tediousness of old age, and call me out to a little exercise when subsiding vigor prompts to too much indulgence. — I hope thou will perceive from this that my regard for thy deserts is undiminished, and that for thy own sake, as well as for my deceased Friend Peter Collinson, I am

Thy assured Friend
John Fothergill

Ms. autograph letter Bartram Papers, IV, 18, HSP; printed in Darlington, *Memorials*, 343–346, omitting paragraph about the frogs in his pond at Upton.

1. Certain letters written by John Bartram to British correspondents and now in the library of the Natural History Museum, South Kensington, London, are also available in photocopy at the Historical Society of Pennsylvania. In one of these letters, unaddressed but undoubtedly written to Dr. Fothergill, John Bartram naïvely describes some bullfrogs he has shipped from Pennsylvania to England: "I have put into a barrel two frogs, and I think they are male and female. There is numbers of them in my fish-pond amongst the Colocasia, on whose broad leaves they love to sit and air themselves on other leaves that riseth two or three feet above the water like a canopy — but here they seldom roar — its on the borders of a pond amongst

grass, or where they can rest their feet, with their heads above water that they may be heard to roar quite half a mile, roaring like a Bull. Our Gentry catches them and esteems them more delicious than any chicken. If put in St. James's Park, they would surprise and delight all adjacent inhabitants. I hoped they would be put in Kew Gardens until they increase in numbers."

2. John Bartram and his son William had visited Florida in 1765–66. See letter to Dr. Chalmers, 10 September 1766, above.

3. *Tetragonotheca helianthoides*, an erect, perennial, composite plant growing in Virginia and southward, one to two feet tall, with pale yellow sunflower-like flowers, is described in *An Encyclopedia of Plants . . . indigenous, cultivated, or introduced to Britain*, ed. J. C. Loudon (London: Longmans, 1841). William Bartram reported finding it about Alachua Savanna, Florida. — "Travels in Georgia and Florida, 1773–1774," annotated by Francis Harper, *Trans. A.P.S.*, 33:149, 224 (1943). Harper gives its common name as pineland ginseng.

To William Bartram, Charles Town, South Carolina, 22 October 1772

London, 22.10.1772

Respected Friend,

I received thy obliging letter, and the drawings that accompanied them. They are very neatly executed, and I should be glad to receive the like of any new plant or animal that occurs to thee. If it was possible to be a little more exact in the parts of fructification and where these parts are very diminutive to have them drawn a litle magnified, I should be pleased and at the same time, if the plants or seeds of such curious plants could be collected and sent hither, it would be very acceptable.

I should have wrote by the person who brought thy letter and the drawings over, but he went away before I was apprized of it. I shall desire Dr. Chalmers of Charles Town to make thee a little present for the drawings, and I should be glad to contribute to thy assistance in collecting the plants of Florida, if thou would suggest what terms might be agreeable. That no time, however, may be lost, should this come to thy hands at Charles Town, I shall desire Dr. Chalmers to confer with thee on this subject, and to render thee such assistance as may be immediately wanted.[1]

The drawings I could wish to have pretty correct, and shall be willing to make due acknowledgment for them. As I imagine thou art well acquainted with the method of packing up plants and seeds, I shall say not much on this head.[2] All bulbous roots are easily managed. Let them be taken up when the flower fades, dry them a little in the shade, put them in a box, either wrapped up in papers or in dry sand, and they will come very safe.

Acorns, nuts, kernels of fruit or stones of fruit and all the larger seeds come very safe in moss. It should be rather dry than moist, as it imbibes a good deal of moisture from the air. When the seeds, acorns and so forth are got together, make a shallow box of any dimensions. Cover the bottom with moss, then lay the seeds and so forth in little distinct patches. Lay a covering of moss, then a layer of seeds, and so fill up the box. A few gimlet holes may be bored in the lid and sides, to let in some air; this may be kept in the cabin and will come safe.

Plants and shrubs of any kind may be taken up in autumn. Wrap the roots with the earth adhering to them in moss. Cut off some of the branches, or long tops, and lay them close in a box, and so close . . . as they shall not be shaked loose by carriage. If the moss is a little wet, it will be no worse. The seams between the boards of the boxes need not be very close, just to keep out mice and other such-like vermin. Carefully packed in this manner, they will preserve their vegetative powers many months, and if they arrive here in any of the spring months, it will be better than in the depth of winter. Dr. Chalmers has some very fine plants of the *Anisum stellatum*.[3] If he will be kind enough to let me have a couple, please to pack them up in the manner I have mentioned. Let a box with wide sections be made, capable of containing them. Cover the roots well with moss, cut off a few straggling branches, lay them in the box and secure them well from shaking. In this manner, if they are kept on the quarter-deck or anywhere in the ship where they will neither be drenched with sea water nor roasted in the ship's hold, they will come safe, requiring no water nor any other care.

In this manner all kinds of plants and shrubs may be conveyed, and if thou undertakes the journey to Florida, endeavour to send a few things by every opportunity. Plants taken up anywhere in winter, or in the spring before their usual time of vegetation, will come best to us and at the most proper season. Thou will please to put down such circumstances relative to the place of growth and appearance as may seem necessary, and a good dried specimen with the flower perfectly formed would be acceptable. And as all the plants from Florida must be inhabitants of the Greenhouse, if not the stove in this country, I should not be solicitous about the tree kind, especially if they exceed in height about 15 feet, because we cannot easily give taller trees the shelter they require. All fragrant shrubs or plants, or such as are remarkable for the beauty or singularity of their flowers and foliage will be most acceptable. I am not so far a systematic Botanist as to wish to have in my garden all the grasses or other less observable humble plants that nature produces. The useful, the beautiful, the singular or the fragrant are to us the most material. Yet despise not the meanest; land, river or sea shells would also be acceptable, or correct drawings of them, where the original cannot easily be produced. — Mind thy studies. In drawing thy hand is a good one, and by attention and care may become excellent.

But in the midst of all this attention, forget not the one thing needful. In studying nature forget not its author. Study to be grateful to that hand which has endowed thee with a capacity to distinguish thyself as an artist. Avoid useless or improper company. Be much alone, and learn to trust in the help and protection of him who has formed us and everything. Fear him, and He will raise thee, Friend, and keep thy foot from sliding. For thy Father's sake I wish thee all good, and for thy own a constant reverent heart and hope in that Power who is ever near to help those who confide in him. — I am, and wish to be thy Friend —

J. Fothergill

Ms. autograph letter, Bartram Papers, IV, 23, HSP; printed in part in Darlington, *Memorials*, 345–346.

1. Dr. Fothergill's interest and financial support enabled William Bartram to pursue his project, which resulted in notable contributions not only to natural history but to the literature of exploration. Dr. Chalmers continued to act as Dr. Fothergill's fiscal agent, supplying funds to William from time to time. — *Travels of William Bartram*, ed. Harper, xix; John Livingston Lowes, *The Road to Xanadu: A Study in the Ways of the Imagination* (Boston and New York: Houghton Mifflin, copr. 1927).

2. "This letter is notable as embodying one of the earliest sets of instructions ever issued for an American biological expedition." — Francis Harper, in *Travels of William Bartram*, xix.

3. *Anisum stellatum*, starry anise, was the name applied to certain aromatic shrubs of oriental origin that had been known in England for many years. Today the Chinese anise — the true star anise — is assigned to the genus *Illicium* as *I. verum*. Specimens of similar shrubs were sent to John Ellis by the Governor of West Florida in 1765 and to Peter Collinson by John Bartram in 1767. William Aiton at Kew raised a few plants from seeds given him by Ellis, who in a paper read to the Royal Society on 30 December 1770 described the purple anise, *Illicium floridanum*, as a distinct species. The yellow anise found blooming at Salt Springs, East Florida, by John and William Bartram in 1765–66 was still mentioned as *Anisum stellatum* in John Bartram's journal published in 1769, but finally recorded as *Illicium parviflorum* Michaux. — *Travels of William Bartram*, ed. Harper, Annotated Index, 532.

To Dr. Lionel Chalmers, Charles Town, South Carolina, 23 October 1772

London, 23 October, 1772

Dear Doctor Chalmers,

I was unfortunate enough not to receive thy letter that mentioned the seeds; how it miscarried or where I know not. Otherwise I should have done my best to have sent everything I could get, and to this day very often regret the loss of that curious cargo of plants I sent from hence a few years ago.

I am sorry that the young man [1] I took the liberty to recommend to my Friend's notice came at so unfavourable a season and so unprepared. He is young; but instructed as well as I could get him, and he must endeavour to shift for himself. I have done as much as I am sure was dependent on me. I thought him too valuable to be wholly lost to the community.

Another person of the like stamp though turned to a different part of natural history claims a little of my assistance; it is the person to whom the enclosed letter is addressed. He is the son of that eminent naturalist John Bartram of Philadelphia; bred to merchandise, but not fitted to it by inclination at least. He is not quite a systematic botanist. He knows plants and draws prettily. I received a letter from him this summer from Charles Town, offering his services to me in a botanical journey to the Floridas. If he is still at Charles Town, be kind enough to enquire for him, deliver the letter that accompanies this, enquire into his situation and his views, and lend him any assistance that may seem expedient, at my expense.

I have told him that I should leave everything of this kind to thyself. I was thinking to give him ten guineas to fit him out with some necessaries immediately, and to allow him any other sum not exceeding 50 £ per annum for certain. In consideration of this sum he should be obliged to collect and send to me all the curious plants and seeds and other natural productions that might occur to him. Any extraordinary expenses in packing or conveying his collection to the necessary post I should not object to paying. Likewise I would make him allowance for his drawings, proportionate to their accuracy. Birds, reptiles, insects, or plants should be drawn on the spot. For any moneys advanced to him,

394

please to draw upon me on sight. I would wish to encourage, not to injure him by proposing a provision that may make him idle.

If I may beg one or two of those fine *Anisum stellatum* I have given here directions how to pack them so as to be no trouble to any captain. Be kind enough to favour me in return with any commissions I can execute and I will do the best I can to observe them. I have three fine plants of the Anisum and hope to increase them. Their fragrance and foliage make them favorites.

I have sent with this an odd production, but I think not a useless one.[2] The author I do not know, nor am acquainted with anybody that does know him. His style is bad; the printer has done him all possible injustice; and yet I think there are some original sentiments that deserve attention. We have passed the age of Theory; we wish to see anything that may assist us in the *cure* of diseases, not to help us to talk about them. Some hints respecting mercurials are valuable.

I do not recollect anything published here of much moment in the practical way lately. Dr. MacBride [3] has published his Institutes of Medicine; Dr. Cullen,[4] a systematic division of disease; and somebody for him, a *Materia Medica*. But these are all in the new style. They do not smell of the lamp, and will not long outlive the day. — I think my Friends at Edinburgh are making, some of them at least, pretty hasty strides to the suppression of medical science — we have believed *too much* and for this reason they believe *nothing*. Baron Dimsdale [5] will ere long publish an addition to his treatise on inoculation. It will contain a short account of his operations in Russia. He has been kind enough to communicate everything to me, and his readers may depend on his narrative.

When a packet sails from Charles Town, give me two lines. I will return four when I can get any leisure. In the meantime be assured that I am

thy much obliged Friend
John Fothergill

Ms. autograph letter, Bartram Papers, IV, 26, HSP.

1. Unidentified.
2. The author and title of this "odd production" are unknown.
3. Dr. David Macbride (1726–1778), born in Ireland, the son of a Scotch Presbyterian minister, studied medicine in Edinburgh and pursued advanced study in anatomy and obstetrics in London with William Hunter and William Smellie. Dr.

Macbride was the author of three highly praised volumes. His *Experimental Essays* (London, 1764) attracted favorable attention and was revised and enlarged in 1767. His second book, *An Historical Account of a New Method of Treating Scurvy at Sea* (1768) prescribed the use of malt as the most effective treatment. A third book, *A Methodical Introduction to the Theory and Practice of Physic*, was published in 1772. His name does not appear in *Munk's Roll*, II, because he was a dissenter without London professional connection.

4. Dr. William Cullen's publications of this period were *Synopsis Nosologiae Methodicae* (Edinburgh, 1768), and *Lectures on the Materia Medica as Delivered by William Cullen, M.D.* (London, 1771).

5. Thomas Dimsdale (1712–1800), of Quaker ancestry and the son and grandson of surgeons, became expert in the process of inoculation to prevent smallpox and the subsequent care of the inoculated, and in 1767 he published an account of his methods. In 1768, through recommendation by Dr. Fothergill (to whom application for advice had been made by the Russian Ambassador), Dr. Dimsdale went secretly to St. Petersburg and inoculated Her Majesty the Empress Catherine and her son Alexander, the Grand Duke, a delicate boy of fourteen. When the news of what had happened was made public, the Russian nobility became "mad for inoculation." In gratitude for Dr. Dimsdale's services, the Empress showered him with gifts — including £10,000 and an annuity of £500 for the rest of his life — and gave him the title of Baron. Returning to England, he was elected Fellow of the Royal Society of London in 1769. His financial status now enabled him to establish a banking house in London under the management of his sons, while he devoted himself to his specialty in a private hospital at Hertford, isolated from the town so that his patients could benefit from country surroundings. In 1784 he retired from practice, except for treating the poor, and began a political career as Tory member for Hertford, a post relinquished in 1790 when his son Nathaniel succeeded him. Although Dr. Dimsdale had forfeited membership in the Society of Friends by "marrying out" in youth, he was buried by his own desire in the Quaker burial ground of Bishop's Stortford. — I. M. Graham, "Two Hertfordshire Doctors," *Transactions of the East Hertfordshire Archaeological Society*, XIII, pt. I (1952): 44–54; Fox, 84–96.

To Humphry Marshall, West Bradford, Pennsylvania, 6 February 1773

London, 6.2.1773

Esteemed Friend,

I received thy box of insects very safe, and in very good order. Many of them are nondescripts, and the rest are in excellent order, a few excepted, which had suffered before they were put into the box. Let it be well dried in the sun or before a fire before any others are put into it, and deliver the key to the Captain, as before, which saves a great deal of trouble.

I wrote a pretty long letter last fall which I hope thou received; it would account for my long silence [1] and inform thee how well satisfied I was with the plants thou had sent, and of their success. I believe we have lost some of them; the alder is alive and prosperous and many other curious plants. All the acorns succeed, as also the other seeds. But there is no necessity for dividing the box into partitions; if the acorns are laid upon a layer of moss, then covered with another layer of moss — upon this any other nuts, fruit or seeds, and so on till the box (which should rather be shallow than deep) is quite full, they will come safe. Small seeds may be put in papers and laid towards the top.

I must desire thee still to proceed in thy vegetable researches, as it falls in thy way. Bulbous roots of all kinds are easily conveyed. The orchis likewise may be easily sent. Let them be taken up when the flower fades, with a large clod of earth about them, pick this off carefully, that none of the roots may be broke and dry them a little in the shade. Wrap them in papers, keep them from vermin, and put them up with the other plants, or in a little dry box by themselves. — I had an orchis sent me from Philadelphia in a letter, which is very prosperous. — Don't forget the fern tribe. This is a very pleasing part of the creation; I have some very rare ones, and one in particular from some part of Philadelphia by William Young.

I have sent the 2nd part of Linnaeus [2] and shall not omit the rest as they are published. I have also sent a few numbers, (all that are yet published) of a very useful work for young Botanists,[3] now carrying on here. There are 3 plates to each plant, and one sheet of description. The coloured plates make the price high, and the whole when finished will come to upwards of 15 guineas. These [parts] will not be half the money; and in respect to use are as valuable as the whole together. I shall continue to send them to thee, as they come out, which is very slowly.

A set of William Penn's *Select Works*,[4] some smaller pieces, and the insect apparatus will make up my present cargo. I consider myself much in thy debt and shall procure thee anything here thou chooses to have to the value of ten guineas, or make thee a remittance of that sum if thou chooses it, which may entitle me to thy future regard in these respects, for the labourer is worthy of his hire.

The insects were divers of them singularly beautiful, the moth tribe especially.

We have not yet succeeded with the Colocasia. I think the water about the city does not suit it, but try to get us some good roots. I think by the help of such a bended fork as is used by farmers to drag the dung out of their carts, tied to the end of a long pole, would fetch up a good root; and I am persuaded it would come as safe in a box of wet moss as by any means whatsoever. The best time would be to take it up late in autumn and send it here by the spring ships. I see by the Chinese drawings [5] that it grows in shallow ponds very freely as well as in their deep waters.

We have got the true Tea Plant at last in England.[6] We are endeavouring to propagate it, and hope we shall succeed, not so as to raise it as a commodity but merely in this country as a curious article. It would thrive in Virginia and Maryland extremely well. I propose to send thee a pretty good account of it, wrote by an acquaintance of mine.[7]

I think the account of the Deluge contains as many things untrue as true. I have it not by me; but if I meet with it, I will endeavour not to forget it.

This little cargo I expect will be delivered by Dr. Parke, whose conduct has gained him esteem, and whose usefulness to the community I trust will gain him deserved reputation.[8]

I am, thy obliged friend
John Fothergill

Ms. autograph letter, Miscellaneous Collections, HSP; printed (with omissions) in Darlington, *Memorials*, 510–512.

1. The letter mentioned, written in September 1772, is printed in Darlington's *Memorials*, 506–510. Since it duplicates the substance of other letters about Samuel's illness and the Leeds case, it is omitted here, but a passage of particular interest is quoted in part IV of the Introduction, above.

2. *Institutes of Botany, containing accurate, compleat, and easy descriptions of all the known Genera of Plants, translated from the Latin of the celebrated Charles von Linné*, by Colin Milne (London: part I, 1771; part II, 1772; no more issued). Dr. Fothergill had sent the first part to Marshall in April 1771. — Darlington, 505.

3. John Miller's *Illustration of the Sexual System of the Genera Plantarum of Linnaeus*, in Latin and English (London: The Author, 1777), first issued in parts, beginning in 1771.

4. Dr. Fothergill's edition, previously mentioned.

5. A set of Chinese drawings is listed in the catalogue of Dr. Fothergill's library sold by Sotheby's in 1781.

6. John Ellis, after many failures, by 1768 had produced a tea plant from seed; this specimen he gave to the Royal Gardens at Kew. Dr. Fothergill, likewise after

many failures, by 1771 had succeeded in establishing an imported plant at Upton; it was visited in March of that year by Joseph Cockfield and John Coakley Lettsom. After Dr. Fothergill's death, Lettsom transplanted from Upton a small tea tree which flourished in his garden. — Fox, 196–197; Nichols, *Illustrations*, V (1825), 804; Fothergill's *Works*, ed. Lettsom, III, xl–xliii (notes).

7. John Coakley Lettsom, *The Natural History of the Tea Tree* (London: Dilly, 1772).

8. Dr. Thomas Parke (1749–1835), a Quaker physician born in Pennsylvania, held a staff position at the College of Philadelphia. Granted a short leave of absence, Dr. Parke sailed for England to visit London hospitals under guidance of a former classmate working with Percival Pott, the surgeon. While making their rounds, the two young men encountered Dr. Fothergill, who was much impressed by Dr. Parke. This favorable opinion was amply justified. Throughout his lifetime, Dr. Parke devoted himself to his patients, especially to those mentally disturbed. He was the favorite pupil of Dr. Benjamin Rush, received promotion rapidly, and succeeded Rush as physician to the Pennsylvania Hospital during a period of momentous change because of war, ravages of yellow fever, and reorganization of the College of Pennsylvania. — *Letters of Benjamin Rush*, ed. Butterfield, II, 653, 654, 658, 677, 687, 708, 1186. Personal communications from Dr. Whitfield J. Bell, Librarian, APS.

To John Ellis, Gray's Inn, London, Summer 1773

Lea Hall, Middlewich, Cheshire
[Summer] 16th Inst. [1773]

Esteemed Friend —

I left London with great regret for not having it in my power to call in Gray's Inn. Every day I proposed it to myself, and was continually disappointed of the time I had allotted.

I received the plate by yesterday's post and think it extremely well done.[1] Be kind enough to give him the money he asks for it and recompense him to his wishes for anything else he may execute. I will acknowledge it at my return.

It has occurred to me within these few days to propose to thy consideration a short excursion to the seaside and even to try sea bathing. I am sure it would contribute to thy health in general and most probably help thy eyes not a little. Choose any place that may be most agreeable, and drink for two or three days, previous to bathing, about half a pint of sea-water or so much as may be sufficient to procure one or two laxative stools. Then try Sea Bathing. Go into the sea two or three morn-

399

ings together just to make it familiar, and then bathe every other morning, and drink the water on the intermediate days.

Take half a drachm or two scruples of the Vegetable Aethiops [2] every night, either mixed with a little simple syrup into the form of an electuary, or taken in a few spoonfuls of water.

I propose this process on many considerations. The air itself will be extremely beneficial, and if neither the water nor bathing should have all the effects one could wish, yet I am sure it must be right to spend a few weeks out of London somewhere, or else another winter's confinement will be distressing indeed. If any doubt arises concerning this process either let me know or ask Dr. Pitcairn's opinion.[3] But I hope what I propose will appear too reasonable to admit of any doubt. I have mentioned no place, as my Friend Ellis is much better acquainted with the several bathing places than I am. Margate has its advantages [4] in respect to use, as one may bathe at all times. — I beg that this proposal may be thoroughly considered as I hope it may be of lasting benefit.

I am, with great esteem
thy assured Friend
John Fothergill

Ms. autograph letter, Ellis Collection, Linnean Society, London.

1. Just which plate had been prepared cannot now be determined; possibly it was the engraving for Ellis' description of the coffee tree, mentioned in the letter to William Logan, 28 June 1774, below.

2. *Vegetable Aethiops* was made by burning to blackness a seaweed, *Quercus marinus*, or sea oak. The dosage would contain iodine as well as the salts of sea water.

3. Dr. William Pitcairn (1711–1791), a Scot from Dysart, Fifeshire, studied with Boerhaave in Leyden and received his medical degree at Rheims. He was private tutor to James Hamilton, the sixth Duke of Hamilton, at Oxford. They traveled together on the Continent. In 1749, when the Radcliffe Library opened in Oxford, Dr. Pitcairn received a medical degree, *honoris causa*, from the University. This made possible his election as Fellow to the Royal College of Physicians, to which he gave loyal service, finally becoming its president in 1775. He held this office until his retirement in 1785. He was physician to St. Bartholomew's Hospital from 1750 to 1780. At Islington he maintained a botanical garden, "second only in size and importance to Dr. Fothergill's at Upton." — *Munk's Roll*, II, 172–174.

4. Margate's advantages were recognized later by Dr. Fothergill's protégé, Dr. Lettsom, who founded there, with other public-spirited citizens, the General Sea-Bathing Infirmary, which later, after enlargement, became the Royal Sea-Bathing Hospital. — Fox, 106–107.

To William Bartram
In Care of Dr. Chalmers, Charles Town, South Carolina,
4 September 1773

London, September 4th, 1773

Respected Friend,

I received thy letter from Charles Town together with the drawings. The bird is extremely well executed; the *Starry Anis* was done in a hurry and too picturesquely. A little practice will soon bring this to rights.[1]

I am pleased that so favourable a passage has been opened into the Cherokee country by the assistance of my worthy Friend Dr. Chalmers and Commissioner Stuart,[2] to whom I am not quite unknown and to whom for this instance of his friendship I think myself under great obligations.

I cannot expect great things from this first summer. I hope, however, to receive both seeds and plants in the autumn. Do not strive to send all at once but take proper opportunities of conveying things to Charles Town at every proper opportunity. I need not give any directions about packing the plants as doubtless thou has frequently seen how this is done by thy Father. Orchids and other bulbous roots may be taken up as soon as the flowers decay; carefully separated from the earth, then dried a little in the shade, to prevent their rotting and then put into a box filled with dry sand, or very dry moss. — Lady slippers, and other vernal bulbs may be collected easily.

In meeting with any new plants in flower, draw the flower and a leaf or two carefully on the spot, and mark the outline of the branch or shrub. The rest may be finished at leisure. The same may be done with any other article of natural history that deserves notice.

There is a young man from England,[3] engaged in the service of a company at Charles Town; he travels into the Cherokee country, and though unacquainted with Botany has sent me many rare seeds, and some plants packed up with much judgement, which are now recovering from that voyage. It may not be improper at some time to go with him, as he will be able to point out things which he has not been able to collect. — Write to me as often as opportunity offers. Boxes or parcels

401

may be directed to me in Harpur Street near Red Lion Square, London. Letters to me in London by the post or packet will be sufficient. Let me know if any particular conveniences are wanted.

It will be right to keep a little journal, marking the soil, situation, plants in general, remarkable animals, where found, and the several particulars relative to them as they cast up. Land and river shells will be acceptable, as also any rare insects.[4]

Take care of thy health, continue thy journey in such a manner as to visit the most likely places for plants at different seasons. Mark the places they grow in, whether in swamps, dry banks, under shade or in the open country. These circumstances will assist us in their culture here.

When any opportunity offers of examining hard wood of any kind, observe if it appears variegated or fit for any cabinet use. This may sometimes turn out to advantage. It will be necessary to send thy journals, when it can be done safely, to Charles Town for safety lest they should be lost or stolen, which would be an irretrievable loss. I would rather wish the remarks made on the drawings for their explanations as the name or description of plants or animals was wrote on a separate paper with numbers or letters of reference, than to mark them on the back. At the foot of the drawing would be better, but a separate paper would be best. I would rather, however, recommend it to thy care to procure the plants or seeds themselves than the drawings only. Drawings of birds, snakes and such subjects as can not easily be sent hither would be acceptable.

I have requested Dr. Chalmers to render thee all proper assistance, and doubt not of his best endeavours.

Let me hear from thee as soon and as fully as is convenient. I shall write as often as I can. I find acorns of all kinds may be safely conveyed in moss, and so may all the larger seeds and berries. Get a shallow box about 6 or 8 inches deep of any length or breadth — suppose 2 feet long by 15 wide. Cover the bottom of this box with moss, not quite dry. Upon this moss lay a layer of acorns, seeds or berries, each little parcel at some distance from each other. Cover these with another layer of moss, and on this put likewise another layer of acorns, seeds and so forth.

The largest may always be left the lowest, and the smaller above. In this manner all the acorns, stone fruit, berries of the [*illegible*] and other seeds of like kind may be sent in the best state I know. The box must finally be filled with moss pressed down so close as to prevent its contents from shaking out of their places. The moss should be barely not quite dry, and if bits of sticks with notches marked for numbers I, II, III and so forth be laid with each parcel, and a list with corresponding numbers be sent with them, we can easily separate them. If such boxes of seeds could be brought over in the Captain's cabin or between decks, they would come much safer than if put into the hold. Though indeed if the seeds should germinate in the moss, we can readily pick them out and plant them. All seeds I should be glad to receive in autumn, as well as the bulbous or tuberous roots, as these for the most part come out early in the spring. Likewise herbaceous plants that die down in winter may come very properly at this season. But shrubs of any kind may be taken up early in the spring and sent by the earliest ships. They then arrive when our extreme rigorous weather is over and they recover themselves fully before the ensuing winter.

I do not want every little diminutive plant that grows. Drawings of such would be sufficient. But plants remarkable for their beauty, fragrance, singularity of appearance or known usefulness, I should be glad to possess. I am, with much respect

Thy Friend
John Fothergill

Ms. autograph letter, Bartram Papers, Autograph Collection, IV, HSP; not included by Darlington in *Memorials*.

1. William Bartram found the purple anise (*Illicium floridanum* Ellis) in 1772 in or near the area of Monroe County, Alabama. His drawing is reproduced on plate 3 of his *Botanical . . . Drawings*, ed. Ewan.

2. John Stuart (*ca.* 1700–1779) was a Scotsman who emigrated to Georgia in 1733. When Georgia was threatened by Spanish invasion in the 1750's, Stuart had a period of adventurous life at sea. Later he volunteered for army service in Tennessee where, it is reported, he was promoted through the ranks to become second in command at Fort Loudon. Returning to South Carolina, he married, set himself up as a storekeeper in Charleston, and became acquainted with the Cherokees and other Indians who frequented this trading post. His friendly relations with these Indians led to his appointment as Superintendent of Indian Affairs for the Southeastern Colonies. Because Stuart had penetrated into remote country with Indian guides and had made rough sketches of difficult routes, his advice was sought when a cartographic survey of the entire region was undertaken. His careful contributions proved invaluable while some of the best maps made during the colonial period were being prepared. Stuart's popularity in Charleston came to an end in 1776 because of his Tory principles; he was forced to leave the city, and returned to Great Britain, where he died.

— William Bartram, "Travels in Georgia and Florida, 1773–1774: A Report to Dr. John Fothergill," annotated by Francis Harper, *Transactions of the American Philosophical Society*, 33, pt. II (1943): 223 ff.

3. Not identified.

4. Instructions begun in an earlier letter are continued at this point. The "little journal" has long since disappeared, but the manuscript report to Dr. Fothergill covering 1773–1774, now in the British Museum (photostats at the American Philosophical Society), was published in 1943, as cited in note 2 above.

VII
1774-1775

Perhaps my penchant for America may sometimes
give a caricature to its enemies; be it so.
But who could quite command himself when he
sees the foundations of a most glorious fabric,
rising fast to meridian splendour, dug up by
piecemeal, through ineffective ignorance and
pride?

To Gilbert Ironside, 22.12.1774

To Dr. Lionel Chalmers, Charles Town, South Carolina, 7 January 1774

Dear Doctor,

I hope before this comes to hand some of my letters will be received. I have delayed writing longer than I could have wished, not from design but perfect inability.

The contents of this box are for William Bartram. It is chiefly paper for putting his specimens in, and a couple of little boxes to carry with him in collecting plants, etc. Be kind enough to send him a little of the paper now and then as opportunity may offer.

The Ms. is not yet gone to the press, and it must be delayed a few months longer.[1] Some late decisions in law have made the Booksellers extremely reserved in respect to purchasing copies. The affair will be brought early into Parliament, and if literary property is secured, they will then be ready to treat for copy. It will make a quarto of moderate size, and I shall endeavor to get at least £50 for the copy, and a few sets for the author and his friends. I shall perhaps shorten it a little by erasing here and there mere speculation. There is a passage likewise respecting the orgasm to which the sex are liable which will either be reserved in Latin or omitted. I shall not neglect the work, the moment the booksellers are disposed to treat on the subject.

I hope to get the time protracted for a premium on Blacklead.[2] Send just enough to ensure this, and then be sparing until the demand increases. I mentioned that it might be converted to great use as a paint in your hot country as in ours. If it finds its way to such a general use, its value will always be considerable.

I have saved the greatest part of the [*illegible*] plants I received last summer. They shot out from the roots and will in another summer be considerable plants. It is a fine addition to our Greenhouses. I have one plant in the natural ground under a glass case. We have now a sharp frost; if it stands this, I hope it will under the cover endure many more and prosper in summer.

I shall be glad to receive some account of our fellow adventurers and their success as soon as convenient. Draw upon me for my deposit as well as on W. Bartram's account as occasion requires. Do not let me run too deep into debt. I rather wish to pay small sums as they become due than run on to large accounts. If the [illegible] I sent out arrive safe and are of the right kind, I shall be pleased; if they do not succeed, let me know. Permit me likewise to propose a proper Garden for Carolina.[3] I would have in it as many of the elegant flowering plants or shrubs as the country produces. — I call myself a sensual botanist. Plants remarkable for their form, foliage, fragrance, elegant flowers, utility, are my objects. Mosses, grasses and the like I leave to others. Ferns indeed and the *Polypodiae*, I love. They are all elegant. From such a collection more pleasure must arise than from anything we can send except our bulbs. Those I sent, I hope came safe. I will send anything that is desired.

Farewell, my Friend, and believe me thine,

J. Fothergill.

P.S. Please to place to my account all expenses of carriage etc., as well as the freight of this box and anything I may send to W. Bartram.

J.F.

Printed by courtesy of Dr. Joseph I. Waring of Charleston, South Carolina, who discovered the original manuscript in the Charleston Library Society.

1. Dr. Chalmers' manuscript to which Dr. Fothergill refers was eventually published as *An Account of the Weather and Diseases of South Carolina*, 2 vols. (London: E. and C. Dilly, 1776). A London reviewer complimented the author as follows: "When Dr. Chalmers transmitted his present laborious and useful work from America to be printed in London, we presume he little expected that all intercourse between this country and that from which it was sent would have been interdicted before publication . . . We hope however that men of science, and especially those in pursuit of medical knowledge, will never be at variance . . . In treating of the diseases of South Carolina, Dr. Chalmers discovers himself to have been a very accurate observer and a judicious practitioner." — *Monthly Review* (London), 54 (1776): 275, 284.

2. Graphite; deposits had been discovered in South Carolina, as Dr. Chalmers' book noted. The review cited quotes Dr. Chalmers discussing minerals: ". . . we have also antimony, alum, talk [talc], blacklead, marle" (*ibid.*, p. 278).

3. One of the oldest landscaped gardens in the United States, started by Henry Middleton in 1741, is on the Ashley River near Charleston, which has many notable gardens of later date.

To Carolus Linnaeus, Uppsala, Sweden, 4 April 1774

4th April 1774 London

[*Translation*]

I am very grateful to thee [1] for the letters which I lately received. I had long been thinking of writing to thee for various reasons, but hesitated for fear of disturbing thy precious and valuable leisure without good cause. Thy very kind letter, however, gave me courage, and therefore accept what I have to offer.

It was our Collinson who taught me to love plants. Stimulated by his companionship, who could fail to be enthusiastic about plants? I need not tell thee who and what he was. He persuaded me to create a garden. Many items he gave me himself; others I collected as opportunity occurred, and so there was born no mean Gaza [2] of plants, under a proprietor but little trained in botany, but burning with a love of plant life.

Clinical practice occupies practically the whole of my time and perhaps will continue to do so as long as my strength is not entirely broken by age. I confess I cannot willingly refuse help to those who fostered my interests and kindly supported me when I was younger. Perhaps some day it will be given to me, worn out with work and cares, that I may endure the tedium of life and old age amongst Flora's lovely treasures.

Berlinus,[3] soon after he reached Africa, went to join the great majority. It was that fatal fever which in hot damp regions so surely slays a man before his time. When first stricken by the disease, trusting his own opinion too much, he refused medical treatment long established by experience. Confused and disturbed, he soon died — a great and wellnigh irreparable loss to Botany.

Smeathman is, I hope, among the living.[4] He has sent a large number of insects, many of them rare. No plants, no seeds — not a single one. By great misfortune, it happens that no ships have returned [directly] from Africa to our shores. Laden with the wickedest of cargoes [5] — men torn from everything that makes life worth while — they proceed to the West Indian Islands, and after a long delay return thence to England. Because of this long detour, everything dies. We have decided to send out a ship which under Smeathman's direction, if he is still living, will go to Africa and returning to us directly, will bring, we hope, an immense treasure of natural objects. We have written to Smeathman telling

409

him to come home as soon as possible. Rebuilding his strength under a cooler sky, he can return to Africa next autumn. If there is any young man at the celebrated Linnaean School, vigorous and able to withstand hard work and a hot sun, and thoroughly imbued with the love of plants and of natural history, who wishes to offer himself as a companion for the journey at the beginning of the summer, please inform me.

I am indeed surprised that Solander[6] should show so ungrateful a spirit towards his teacher, supporter and greatest helper. This, however, is what should be thought about it: It is not by his own will. What God commands should either be done or not undertaken at all.

I have sent a son of that venerable old man, Bartram, to Florida in the southern part of British America, to collect plants there.[7] If he sends any that are new or rare I shall gladly share them with thee. From these shores we received *Illicium annisatum*[8] which I gave to Miller last summer, to send to thee.

I am grateful to thee for having wished to number me among the lovers of plants, but looking upon myself as merely an inadequate adjunct of science, I blush. Thy kindness will always receive from me the honour it deserves, and grateful recollection of what thou hast done.[9]

I have decided to send thee that plant as soon as possible, if fortune favours my prayers for a vigorous shoot this summer. I fear this letter will be unintelligible, for my long disuse of Latin makes it impromptu. If anything is not clear, pray let me know next time. Would that I had attained a leisure full of strength and knowledge of important subjects, so that I could make one moment of life happier for the great Linnaeus. Farewell, most esteemed Friend, than whom none has been more deservedly praised and who is held in the highest honour by all.

Farewell.

Ms. autograph letter written in Latin, Linnean Society, Burlington House, London; translated by Nathaniel Booth and Dr. George W. Corner, Sr. For original Latin text, see Appendix, below. The customary salutation and complimentary close were omitted by Dr. Fothergill.

1. Carl von Linné (1707–1778), founder of the modern system of botanical nomenclature, described himself in various roles as doctor, professor, Royal physician, knight, and nobleman; he claimed authorship of seventy-two books. — Hagsberg, *Carl Linnaeus*, 206–208.

2. This allusion is obscure.

3. In 1771, Anders Berlin, a pupil of Linnaeus, went by his advice to London to work in the British Museum. Two years later he was sent to Africa to assist Henry Smeathman who was already collecting natural history specimens on the west coast

of Africa. Berlin fell victim to a tropical fever, very likely malaria, and died, an exile from home. — Benjamin Daydon Jackson, *Linnaeus*, adapted from the Swedish of Theodor Magnus Fries (London: H. F. and G. Witherby, 1923), 240.

4. Henry Smeathman's journey to the west coast of Africa was promoted by a number of subscribers, including Dr. John Fothergill, Dr. William Pitcairn, and Joseph (later Sir Joseph) Banks, who contributed a large share of necessary funds. Dr. Fothergill presented the traveler with a small well-stocked medicine chest, together with prescriptions for treatment of tropical diseases and a few medical books. Smeathman sent more than 6,000 species of plants to the British Museum, as well as specimens of insects, minerals, and shells. His notable paper, "Some Account of the Termites of Africa and Other Hot Countries," was published in *Phil. Trans. R. S.*, 71:138–145 (1781). — See letter from Smeathman quoted in *Works*, ed. Lettsom, III, 177–196.

5. Reference to the flourishing slave trade which supplied the sugar plantations in the West Indies with their employees.

6. Daniel Carl Solander (1736–1782), son of a country clergyman in Sweden, was educated in Uppsala and became a favorite pupil of Linnaeus. In 1759 he was sent to London to assist Joseph Banks at the British Museum. He lived in London the rest of his life and became so engrossed with his work that he entirely neglected writing letters to his mother and to Linnaeus, both of whom were greatly grieved. — H. C. Cameron, *Sir Joseph Banks, The Autocrat of the Philosophers* (London: Batchworth Press, 1952), 15; Sir James Edward Smith, *A Selection from the Correspondence of Linnaeus and Other Naturalists*, 2 vols. (London: Longman, Hurst, Rees, Orme, and Brown, 1821), II, 1–4; J. C. Beaglehole, *The Endeavor Journals of Joseph Banks*, 2nd ed., 2 vols. (Sydney: Angus and Robertson, 1963), I, 24–27; Roy A. Rauschenberg, "Daniel Carl Solander, Naturalist on the 'Endeavor,'" *Transactions of the American Philosophical Society*, n.s., vol. 58, part 8 (1968).

7. See letters to William Bartram, above.

8. The plant described by John Ellis in his paper on "A new species of *Illicium Linnaei* or starry Aniseed tree lately discovered in West Florida," read before the Royal Society in December 1770, was *Illicium floridanum*, the purple anise; the plant here mentioned was probably the yellow anise (*Illicium parviflorum*) discovered by the Bartrams in 1766 and found again by William in 1772. — See Francis Harper's comments on John Bartram's diary of 1765–66 and William Bartram's report to Dr. Fothergill, 1773–74, in *Trans. APS*, 33: 45, 74, 191, 208 (1942–43).

9. Linnaeus had given the name *Fothergilla* to a genus of shrubs of the witch-hazel family imported from America by Dr. Fothergill.

To James Pemberton, Philadelphia, 28 June 1774

London, 28.6.1774

Dear Friend,

This comes by my Friend Mary Worley,[1] whom I must recommend to thine and thy family's very friendly notice. Sometime since my Friend William Logan requested me to look out for a proper person to fill up

411

a very necessary station in your city, viz., that of a Midwife — in looking round amongst my acquaintances I could pick upon no one so proper as the person I now recommend to thy notice.

She was not educated amongst us but joined us, I believe, on the clearest conviction; she is of a good family, but they turned their backs on her when she came amongst us. She submitted to labours with great content for a maintenance. From the account I had heard of her (for she lived at Worcester), I thought her very proper for the occupation. She has at my request undertaken and will I doubt not fulfill it to her credit and general benefit. — Watch over her for her good, and guard her against the intoxication of success, for if she has health, I do not much doubt but this will attend the knowledge she has acquired.

There is about the sum of £500 in the hands of the Trustees of the Pennsylvania Company due to the Hospital. I shall see Dr. Franklin soon, and shall confer with him on the subject in order to its being put into your possession.

I say nothing of public affairs. Before we are deprived of our liberties, it may be no unnecessary scrutiny to examine how we have used them? Ere long we may do it, and regret the blessings being no longer ours. Indeed the times are dark — and without pretending to see further than other men, grievous difficulties and sore distress may soon awake us to better considerations, when it is too late. — You know by this time what America has to expect — what measures you are taking we know not. The best would be, if deep considerations of our trespasses, neglect and ingratitude could take place in every mind, and prompt us all in every station, every condition to look to him whom we have offended, and by a more perfect resignation to his will be prepared for what in his providence he may see fit to come upon us. — My sister joins me in remembrance to thyself, family and relations.

I am thy affectionate Friend,

John Fothergill

Ms. autograph letter, Pemberton Papers, Etting Collection, II, 67, HSP.

1. Mary Worley, employed as an actress in a provincial theater at a salary of £300, had evidently become a "convinced" Quaker. A copy of a letter she wrote to the manager of the theater asking for release from her contract states in part: "If you was to forse me on the theatre, instead of playing I would preach to the People. As to the Penalty, I am unable to pay it, having no fortune except what my Brother pleases to give me . . . Whilst the Almighty blesses me with health, I am able to get an honest livelihood and the poorer, the better, for what has a Christian to do

with the pomps and vanities of this World, which he has promised to renounce? . . .
I will intrude on your patience no longer, having said enough to convince you of
the inability of my ever returning to the abominable theatre." — Robson Mss., Society
of Friends, Worcester, England. Mary Worley became for a time "a steady Friend"
at Worcester and, it was reported, "followed Clear Starching for a livelihood."

To William Logan, Philadelphia, 28 June 1774

London, 28.6.1774

Dear Friend,

The bearer, Mary Worley, is the person I have engaged to come as a
Midwife,[1] a station that I think her very well qualified for both by
nature and instruction. She has spared neither application nor expense
to acquire a thorough knowledge of her business, and I think I may
safely say without deprecating anyone that she comes over as well qualified both as to practice and instruction as any of her own sex (and
perhaps most of the other) as ever came to America.

There is only one exception. She is single — and if she should marry
and have children, it might cause a temporary inconvenience to some.
In every other respect so far as I know she is unexceptionable.

I must desire thee to lend her what assistance she may want, till she
gets into business and draw upon me for what thou advances. Help her
to a proper situation, which should be near the center of Friends, in a
respectable part of the city, in a place easy to find and not difficult of
access.

Though the present state of her finances may require economy, yet
I could wish she might be provided with respectable apartments, and
where there is a prospect of her continuance. For it would be very improper that she should frequently change her place of residence. She
has prudence, presence of mind, and principle which I hope will preserve her from giving any cause of uneasiness to those who have occasion
either to employ or recommend her.

We are preparing to set out for Cheshire where I hope to have leisure
to write thee a longer letter. I have sent the books I promised thee under
her care, which please to distribute as thou seest occasion. There are
also two copies of a treatise on Coffee;[2] put one into thy own library
and present the other to the Philosophical Society.

413

Enclosed in the same box is a small one for Humphry Marshall — be kind enough to forward it to him by some convenient opportunity.

I can say nothing on public affairs which thou knows not — and feel already. It seems to me that your liberty is near an end, and ours will soon follow after. We deserve no better, but the subject is afflicting.

My sister joins me in remembrance.

John Fothergill

Ms. autograph letter, Pemberton Papers, Etting Collection, II, 65, HSP.

1. See preceding letter.
2. John Ellis, *An Historical Account of Coffee, with an Engraving and Botanical Description of the Tree, to which are added Sundry Papers relative to its Culture and Use as an Article of Diet* (London: Dilly, 1774). The American Philosophical Society still has upon its shelves the copy brought by William Logan as a gift from Dr. Fothergill. The volume contains Dr. Fothergill's own amusing account of how he became a coffee drinker. In the autumn of 1765, George Scott, then Governor of Dominica, had sent the famous London doctor three bags of coffee, samples grown and "cured" in different years on the island, "intended for whatever experiments you may think proper." From this time forward Dr. Fothergill drank coffee regularly, telling his cook to make the drink in the usual manner "only 1/3 stronger," adding "in the French fashion" an equal quantity of boiling milk, and very little sugar, "since on weak stomachs it is apt to become acid, if too sweet." Governor Scott had recommended coffee as "one of the best breakfasts in the world for the honest, brave people of the foggy island of Great Britain, where such a multitude of accidents happen from low spirits." He continued, "But what effects Coffee or Tea have upon the body or mind, you, Sir, must be the best judge, as it is your principal study and profession to know the economy of the human frame; mine, having been that of arms, and at present to preside over this Island; from whence I shall with pleasure send you annually as much coffee of whatever sort you may want for your own use while I remain here, being very much, though unknown, Sir, Your most obedient, humble Servant." — *Works*, ed. Lettsom, II, 329. The review of Ellis' book in the *Monthly Review* (London), 50:397–398 (June 1774) concludes "with a few observations extracted from a letter written by Dr. Fothergill to the author" — on the value of coffee as a beverage and the economic possibilities of coffee as a commodity.

To John Bartram, Philadelphia, 8 July 1774

London, 8.7.1774

Esteemed Friend,

I received thy very acceptable letter of the 14th of April last and am pleased to find thy health so well preserved in the evening of life.

I had a letter the other day from Dr. Chalmers, who mentions that he had a letter lately from William, who was going towards East Florida, and well. I have received from him about one hundred dried specimens of plants, and some of them very curious; a very few drawings, but neither a seed nor a plant.

I am sensible of the difficulty he is at in travelling through those inhospitable countries; but I think he should have sent me some few things as he went along. I have paid the bills he drew upon me; but must be greatly out of pocket if he does not take some opportunity of doing what I expressly directed, which was to send me seeds or roots of such plants as either by their beauty, fragrance or other properties, might claim attention. However, I shall hope he will find means of fulfilling my orders better than he has done hitherto.

If thy son John [1] meets with anything new in his travels about the country, I should be glad if he would send me at least a part of his discoveries; and I hope I may be able to content him for his trouble. I am obliged to him for the seeds of the Orange-coloured Hibiscus.[2] I have a good many plants of the *Illicium*. I have planted these in the natural ground, and shall give them a little shelter in the winter. It has a most grateful fragrance, and will be a pleasing greenhouse plant.

Please let him know that I received the turtle [3] in good health, and shall be much obliged if he will procure me a male and a female Bull-frog. Mine are strayed away notwithstanding my best endeavours. If they are put in a little box of wet moss, they will come safe; at least I received a little American frog, the *Rana ocellata*,[4] in a box of plants, filled with moss. They should be sent in autumn.

I shall be much pleased to see the Tetragonotheca. There is not, I believe, a plant of it now in England.

We have got the true Green Tea Tree. I have a plant in the natural ground near five feet high. Mine has been sheltered in the winter, but old James Gordon left his exposed to all weathers, and yet it thrives very well. We shall propagate it as fast as we can.

Do not imagine that all the people in this country are against America. We sympathize with you very much. It may be our turn to suffer next. We hope, however, that the impending storm may blow over, and that you may be able to act your part properly.

I am thy assured Friend,
John Fothergill

The original manuscript letter cannot be traced at HSP; a printed version is found in Darlington, *Memorials*, 347, 348.

1. John, Jr., was encouraged by his father to become a botanical collector but never attained the distinction his older brother William achieved.

2. Probably *Hibiscus coccineus* but possibly *Pavonia spinifex.* — See William Bartram, *Travels*, ed. Harper, Annotated Index, 526.

3. Dr. Fothergill had much earlier requested William Bartram to send him drawings of turtles seen during travels with his father. The manuscript Minute Book of the Society of Physicians, now at the Royal College of Physicians, crediting Dr. Fothergill with the gift of a turtle upon several occasions, contains an entry which shows that the Doctor's interest in this species was not entirely zoological; members of the Society of Physicians were apparently delighted to feast upon turtle soup at meetings held in the Strand at the Crown and Anchor.

4. *Rana ocellata* is the Linnaean name of a South American frog with eye-like spots. The specimen mentioned here, presumably from the southeastern region of the North American colonies, was no doubt also a spotted variety incorrectly identified. — Information from Dr. R. G. Zweifel, American Museum of Natural History, New York.

To John Ellis, Esq. [without address] 14 July 1774

Lea Hall, Cheshire, 14.7.1774

Esteemed Friend, —

I have perused the Ms. on Breadfruit and Mangostan since I came down hither, and have returned them as soon as I could.[1] For a great part of the time I have been here I was quite unfit for any kind of labour, and since then I have been obliged to do no more than has been consistent either with my inclination or my health — and yet must leave many things untouched.

I think very little alteration or addition is necessary to either of these pieces. In two or three half sheets of paper which accompany them I have proposed some alteration in the method. — The Mangostan has been longer known; I would prefix that, and the extracts concerning it, in the order of time.

What relates to the Breadfruit should then follow, as we have been but lately acquainted with it. The testimonys concerning this likewise should be placed in their proper order. — I have made no attempt at the description of the cases. I could not rightly understand that which I received in thy obliging letter of the 30th Ult. — There is an ingenious Carpenter in Holborn who has made me several of these boxes of the last construction. His name is Bevan; he lives almost opposite to the Upper Turnstyle. Please to order him to make a box with Dr. Badenach's [2] improvements; from this lot a drawing and description [should] be made. The box may be made on my account — I shall send it probably to some [distant] part of the World. — And if a box of this kind was kept ready, made for the inspection of the curious, or sent to the Society of the Arts etc.[3] — it might be the means of obtaining still further improvements.

My references will, I believe, be very readily found out by the Printer, though I could wish it was not put to the Press before I return which will be, I hope, in the first week of October. — I would look over every revised sheet and correct such lettering mistakes as have escaped me.[4] — I have taken no notice yet of the endeavours to be used in order to obtain these two trees in perfection. I think a plan might be formed that would be practicable. — Government will doubtless send back the Native of Otaheite some time.[5] When this is done, let interest be made to bring back the Breadfruit, the Mangostan, and what is of no less consequence to this country, the *Winterania* [6] from the Streights of Magellan.

There is in agitation a subscription for this last purpose, solely. And if the West Indian Gentlemen, who are ten times more interested in the affair, would join properly, it is not impossible but in the course of a year or two, we might be in possession of this and various other valuable articles which will not otherwise find their way to us in a century.

In a scheme of this kind I can only propose and contribute. To solicit others I have neither time nor inclination. — I think I can depend upon four or five hundred pounds and about two thousand, with the aid of a ship from Government, would perhaps perform the whole completely. — At present however reserve these suggestions *in petto* till we meet.

I am, with much respect,

Thy Friend

John Fothergill

Ms. autograph letter, Ellis Collection, Linnean Society, London.

1. Dr. Fothergill and John Ellis were hoping to introduce mangostan and breadfruit into the West Indies to supplement the food supply. The former, an East Indian tree, *Garcinia mangostana*, bears a fruit said to suggest a combination of peach and pineapple; the latter, *Artocarpus incisa*, found by Captain Cook in the South Sea Islands (1768–1771), was an important source of carbohydrates in the native diet. It was ultimately Captain Bligh in the *Bounty* who was sent by the British Government to transport the breadfruit from Tahiti to the West Indies, an attempt initially foiled by the famous mutiny.

2. James Badenach was a ship's surgeon on H.M.S. *Princess Royal* in the summer

of 1771 when with "twelve sail of Indiamen" and the *Endeavor* she was in a convoy being escorted to England by H.M.S. *Portland.* — H. C. Cameron, *Sir Joseph Banks, The Autocrat of the Philosophers* (London: Blatchworth Press, 1952), 38n. It is evident that Dr. Badenach had studied the problems of bringing exotic plants from the Orient.

3. The Society for the Encouragement of Arts, Commerce, and Manufactures, founded in 1754, ancestor of the Royal Society of Arts.

4. John Ellis, *A Description of the Mangostan and the Bread-Fruit . . . To which are added, Directions to Voyagers for bringing over these and other vegetable productions which would be extremely valuable to the Inhabitants of our West India Islands* was published in London by Dilly in 1775. Boxes of three styles were illustrated.

5. Omai of Otaheite (Tahiti), a young man in his early twenties, was brought to London in 1774 by Lieutenant Colonel Furneaux on the *Adventure*. As a protégé of Joseph Banks, he became the sensation of London society. Fanny Burney described him as "extremely graceful, so polite, attentive, so easy that you would have thought he came from some foreign court." In a portrait now on display at Castle Howard, Sir Joshua Reynolds depicted Omai dramatically — standing outdoors, tall and straight, wearing a turban, dressed in flowing robes, against a faintly suggestive landscape, revealing a glimpse of the sea, a shadowy palm tree, and distant tracery of the precipitous mountains of his homeland. In July 1776 Omai was sent home on the *Resolution*, commanded by Captain Cook on his last voyage of exploration. Omai, universally admired in British society, found readjustment difficult after his return to Tahiti. He died before three years had passed. — *The Endeavour Journals of Joseph Banks*, ed. Beaglehole, I, 102–103; Alan Moorhead, *The Fatal Impact: An Account of the Invasion of the South Pacific, 1767–1840* (New York: Harper and Row, 1966).

6. *Drimys winteri* Forst., called *Winterana aromatica* by Lettsom, a tree unknown to Europeans until it was discovered by Dr. John Winter, who sailed with Francis Drake in 1577 to the Straits of Magellan and in 1579 brought back to England from the regions of Tierra del Fuego pieces of its aromatic bark. Named by botanists of the period *Cortex Winteranus*, it is known in modern times as Winter's bark. This bark was beneficial medically as a stimulant, tonic, and antiscorbutic agent. — Dr. Fothergill's paper, "Some Account of the *Cortex Winteranus* or *Magellanicus*, with a botanical description by Dr. Solander, F.R.S.," was presented before the Medical Society in London, 22 November 1773, and published in *Medical Observations and Inquiries*, V (1776), 41–55; see also *Works*, ed. Lettsom, II, 163–177.

To James Pemberton, 23 August 1774

Lea Hall, Near Middlewich, Cheshire
23.8.1774

Dear Friend,

I wrote to thee a few lines not long since by a Friend who went from London to serve your city in a very important business. I hope she

418

arrived safe and may have afforded some satisfactory proofs of her abilities. I mean Mary Worley.

We have been at this place near a month in order to recruit our health and strength to undergo the duties of our station as well as we can, I mean my sister and myself. We are both somewhat better for the recess. I told thee there would be some little assistance more for your hospital which I know would be pleasing news to thee as thou hast its prosperity so much at heart. I sometimes chide myself for being anxious for America, during her present trials, as I know how little my anxiety can avail for her benefit, and what a multitude of able people are engaged in her service both on this side the water and on yours.

I know not well how to be totally silent on the occasion. If my opinions coincide with the judicious on your side the water, every little will add to their strength. If they are foreign to the purpose or unserviceable, thy friendship for me will make the proper use of them; conceal the mistaken but well intended zeal of a Friend.

I shall say nothing of the several acts passed here last sessions relative to America.[1] You all know full well their terms. And we shall on both sides feel their baneful influence, if there be not more wisdom and good sense on your side the water than on ours.

The papers from America tell us that a general congress is to be held in your city; perhaps it is already held and their resolutions taken.[2] If this is so, I trust that the most moderate, as being the wisest plan of procedure is adopted. And I can scarcely admit of a doubt but it is so, when I reflect that a measure of the last consequence to this country, to your own, and your posterity must be agitated by men of whose penetration, good judgement, and stability, I have reason to think most favorably.

I have often asked myself what I [would do] in the like critical situation, called upon one hand by everything that is valuable in this life to take most deliberate council, and urged on the other by the popular warmth of men actuated by more passion perhaps than experience to engage in measures that admitted of no recovery, if these measures were not dictated by the most solid wishes.

I will not presume to enter into a field so replete with difficulties on all hands. I will simply offer what at present seemed most likely to have been my own opinion, supposing I had no better information of affairs than I have at present.

My first wish would be to choose out of so large a congress, a few sensible sedate persons from each colony, to come over to this country immediately, and in the meantime to recommend on your side the most perfect submission to authority. No inflammatory publication, no more non-importation schemes, nothing that your enemies or the ignorant misguided people here could have made use of to your disadvantage. You suffer more by the passionate resolves of some insignificant assemblies, I do not mean provincial ones, than the people of America can easily conceive.

The business of this committee should be to apply to the members of both Houses, individually, at least such as can easily be come at and by a little moderate conversation, give them full information of your situation, apprise them of the state of the dispute between you, and with great moderation yet proper firmness, urge their attention to the mutual reciprocal interests of a great empire. Their application should be indefatigable. They should interest all their Friends here of any weight in the same solicitation. No part of the legislature should be omitted. The Provincial agents here would lend you some assistance in finding out our particular connections. You must even submit to intreat for that which you have a right but no power to demand. Any other mode of application will be fruitless if not injurious. Fruitless because the generality of men, even the highest, do their duty not solely because they ought to do it, but because they are compelled to do it, either by dint of unremitting solicitations, or for fear of losing some advantage. Whatever mode of procedure is adopted, if something of this nature is not attempted, both you and we are, I am afraid on the brink of a fatal precipice. Petitions, memorials, addresses, with whatever cogency of reason they are composed will be totally inadequate. They will be treated as your agents, as ex officio businesses, and will soon have their quietus.

I am much in doubt, I confess, what success even such a personal application might have. It has been, unfortunately, for America, the interest and inclination of too many persons in office on your side the water to represent the people there, just in the light that so many here wish to view them — as hostile in their intentions to their mother country and the objects of correction and restraint. Perhaps a remembrance that the ancestors of most now in power were a century ago sufficiently humbled by the progeny of those whom they now look upon with a vindictive detestation. Their dependents are catching, or affect to have

Carolo Linnaeo   Londini. 4to Ap. 1774.

Johannes Fothergill S.

311

Gratissimae a te litteras nuper accepi. Diu quidem in animo fuerat, varias ob causas Epistolam tibi mittere. Dubius tamen haerebam, ne me, justa ratione, otium teti charum, preciosum adeo, frustra tererem. Animum vero addidit amicissima tua Epistola, & quae impostri vellem sic accepi.

Collinsonius noster, me plantas amare docuit. Ejus consortio potitus, quis plantas colere non potuit? Quae Quales he fuerit Dicere non opus est. — Hortum instruere suasit. Ipse dedit multa, alia congerere occasio stimulavit, & sic nata est Gaza haud mediocris plantarum, Sub domino Scientiae Botanicae leviter imbutae, flagrante tamen vi Botanica Amori.

Bases Chinica inopere totum occupes & dum vires aetati non penitus fracto fuerint, forsan occupabunt. Aque fatror opem iis ferre renuo, qui mihi fautores, qui sese benignos, opitulatores, aetate minorem sese ostenderent. — Foth.

From the Latin letter to Linnaeus, 1774
(See pages 409 and 506)

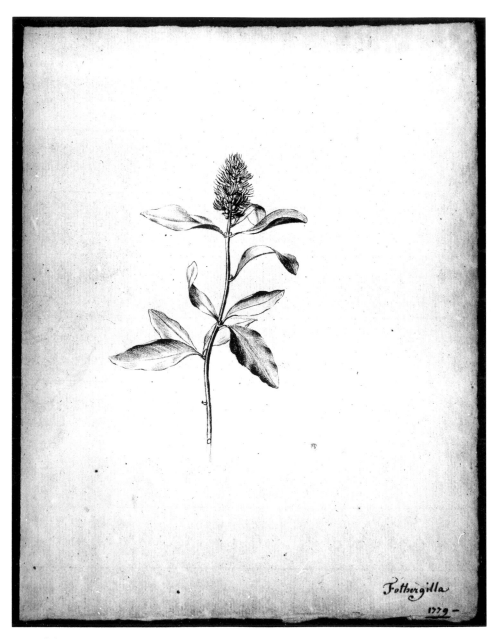

Fothergilla

1779 —

Named by Linnaeus in honor of Dr. Fothergill. From a manuscript at the American Philosophical Society

catched, the like resentment against America, and every little ebullition of Patriotism on your side is worked up into a studied rebellion. I suspect that this is one *secret* unheeded motive to that unparalled act of oppression in respect to Boston.

Should you adopt a measure of this nature and depute a number of judicious, moderate persons, persons who have hitherto kept out of all passionate procedures, I think you would be able to do much for the service of both countries. You would be able at least to give such a color of moderation and justice to your claims, that the ill-informed though well disposed people of this country would concur in your interest and join in your cause. You would be able at least to learn fully what was ultimately designed in our councils in respect to America. And if you found that their resolutions to oppress you were unalterable you would then be at liberty to provide for your own safety, and you would have all the people of sense and moderation here on your side.

I thought I could scarcely dispense with myself from saying this much on the present afflicting subject. But I do not think myself so competent a judge of what you ought to do, as to expect that hints like these can be of moment in your deliberations.

I partly wished that Dr. Franklin would stay here till your determinations are made known to him. Should you think that conciliatory measures ought to be attempted, though he may not perhaps be heard impartially by a few, yet he retains considerable influence with individuals and might render a commission like this proposed very considerable services.

Once more I have only to request that if these suggestions appear altogether unserviceable and improper, the letter that contains them may be immediately destroyed.[3] I shall write to no person else in the province on the subject at this time. Perhaps I may hint something of the kind to Dr. Chalmers at Charles Town to whom I hope to write in a few days. I am thy assured Friend

J. Fothergill

Ms. autograph letter, Pemberton Papers, Etting Collection, II, 69, HSP.

1. The Tea Act of 1773, permitting the East India Company to export cheap tea directly to the Colonies but continuing to tax the Colonies for its importation; the Boston Port Act and the other "Intolerable" Acts of 1774 intended to curb insubordination in Massachusetts; and the Quebec Act of June 1774 extending the jurisdiction of that province to the Ohio. — E. H. Channing, *A History of the United States,* III (1912), 128–142.

2. The Continental Congress met in Philadelphia for the first time on 5 September 1774.

3. Nothing came of Dr. Fothergill's suggestions, but the letter was not destroyed.

To Robert Watson, Waterford, Ireland, 29 August 1774

Lea Hall, 29.8.1774

Dear Kinsman,[1]

Yesterday, and not before, I received thy very acceptable letter, and was pleased to hear you were safely arrived where, I am sure, after so long an absence you were welcome guests to an aged, anxious Parent.

It afforded us satisfaction to hear thy Mother was somewhat better. Thy arrival and Molly's would be a cordial to her, for I have no doubt but Molly has conducted herself in such a manner, as next to her own offspring she is as dear [to your Mother] as can be.

My Sister continued in much suffering after you left us, but within these ten days has continued to recover. She is thin and weak but the pains are abated and she is able to get out in a carriage. But we have given up all thoughts of seeing Warrington this season, as she is far from being as well as she used to be when we left this place, and by one means or another our stay this time will be shorter than usual. Nanny and Betty[2] came to us a few days last week. Peggy and Hannah with little Hannah Jepson[3] came hither last night — are tolerably well themselves and left the families at Warrington very comfortable. Sally is on the eve of being finally engaged. The last visit the Dr. made to her was a fortnight ago. He paid us a How-d'ye-do visit and said not a word of his connection forming at Warrington, no more than if we were totally unacquainted with her and unconcerned for her happiness and further well-being.[4]

I am much obliged to thee for thy kind offers; we make use of them freely, and consider ourselves as your debtors for many marks of your regard. I had a line from my Friend J. Jacobs some time since and requested him to send some of the oranges here, some to London. If no opportunity of shipping them to either place has offered, I think it would be better as the season is advancing to send them all to London: To the care of J. Freeman.

We still propose, if my Sister continues to recover, to return home through Yorkshire by moderate journeys. To be at their Quarterly Meeting is our object where we may see some of the remaining contemporaries of our Father, at least some who knew him in early life. We know there is no sanctity in persons nor in places as such, yet the remembrance of those who have gone before us, if it does not help us to more fervor and excite us to more diligence, it at least creates a wish to do so, in that fight which we must all be engaged in, if we finish our course as they did — and even that will not be overlooked.

When we look towards London it is always with a mixture of diffidence and satisfaction; with diffidence as well knowing the dangers that surround us on all hands, and yet with some degree of satisfaction as we know it must be for the present, as it has long been, our home, and where we have witnessed such gracious preservation.

My Sister and yours and Hannah all join me in affectionate remembrance, and we hope it will not be long before we hear of your welfare. I trust that neither distance nor time will ever lessen our affection for you nor our fervent wishes for your happiness. — You know where to seek it, and may the author of everything that is good, awaken your minds oftener than the morning sun to seek him with full purport of heart. — Farewell, my dear Relations, and believe me to be

Your affectionate Uncle

J. Fothergill

Ms. autograph letter, Port. 22/87, LSFL.

1. With the passage of years, Dr. Fothergill had become quite reconciled to his niece Molly's marriage to Robert Watson of Waterford, Ireland. The Watsons, Robert and Molly, had evidently been visiting in England.

2. Two of Joseph Fothergill's daughters — Ann, still unmarried, and her sister Betty Chorley.

3. Two more of Joseph's daughters — Margaret Kendall and Hannah Jepson, with Hannah's child.

4. Sally Fothergill Titley, widowed in 1772, had indeed become engaged to Dr. William Hird, long esteemed by Dr. Fothergill. It was to be a second marriage for each of them. Dr. Hird had been a prominent physician in Leeds for many years. He was appointed physician to the Leeds Infirmary in 1767, the year of its foundation, and continued to serve in this post by annual election until 1781, with the understanding that "he would give attendance as frequently as his private employments admit of." The *Leeds Mercury* of 25 October 1774 announced: "On Wednesday, William Hird of this town, M.D., was married at the Quaker's Meeting House at Warrington to Mrs. Titley of that place and niece to Dr. Fothergill. They went to live in the fashionable seclusion of Butterworth's Yard." — "Leeds From Past to Present," *The Yorkshire Owl*, VIII, no. 15 (8 July 1896). Information by courtesy of Dr. Stephen Anning, F.R.C.P., Leeds.

To James Pemberton, Philadelphia, 4 November 1774

London, 4.11.1774

Dear Friend,

This comes to convey a few lines from our Meeting for Sufferings to yours; and also a short remembrance to our brethren in New England. We could wish that some solid judicious Friend might convey this to them in a personal visit; if so they find themselves engaged, we should be glad to be informed of their situation through such a channel.

We have taken but little notice in the Epistle of your sentiments in regard to the paragraph in R.B.'s Apology.[1] We wish there never may appear upon record that a diversity of sentiments has ever arisen between you and us on any occasion, however unimportant. Perhaps it may be my fault that you have come to your present conclusion, that the paragraph ought to be retained. I should have suggested some of the reasons that induced Friends here to act as they did. In short, the book from whence this quotation is taken is no other than a mere romance. It is the production of a zealous Mohammedan and ought to be considered . . . just as little as Telemachus[2] and other moral legends of the like origin, written to show the writer's sentiment. It does not appear that R.B. ever saw the book itself, though he saw the quotation, nor that he knew the work was of this stamp. Shall we then persist in supporting an authority so feeble? Our doctrines need no such feeble support; we hope therefore you will withdraw this injunction to perpetuate a mistake, and as softly as you please. We hope never to give you any occasion to think we mean to give up any part of our professed principles, nor any sound reason that may be alleged in defense of them or for their support.

I wrote to thee some time ago by M. Worley who at the request of some friends in your Province I had prevailed on to go through a course of instruction to qualify her for being useful . . . At the time I proposed it to her, I knew not that there was the smallest exception to her character in any respect; but on application made to the Monthly Meeting of Worcester, instead of a certificate I received the enclosed, very much to my concern.[3]

I need not tell thee that the affair is a tender one and requires much prudence. That she is not totally wrong I have not the least apprehension; that she may have been previously is not impossible. I think she

424

cannot now be guilty of any such mistakes. Please see to her, show her this letter and tell her that if she has been unawares overtaken in anything amiss, she will for her own sake acknowledge it to the Friends at Worcester, who I doubt not will cheerfully render her situation as truly satisfactory to herself as possible. But I leave the affair wholly to thy discretion.

Sometime I suggested what appeared to me not an improper step for your Congress to take; [4] whether they have or not, I still think they would be most likely to succeed in this way than in any other. The representations, unless backed by weight of influence here, will signify nothing. We have a new Parliament unexpectedly, but I do not imagine this will at all alter the plan of procedure with respect to America. We shall be glad to hear of your welfare by every convenient opportunity.

What I am now going to mention must be considered simply as my own proposal, and nothing farther built upon it than as a private opinion.

The Pennsylvania Land Company still have some property amongst you which partly from the circumstances of the times, partly from the inactivity of our Agent lies undisposed of, and it may so remain for a considerable time. It occurred to me just to mention to thyself if it might not be advantageous to your Hospital as well as to the Proprietors here, if you were to become the purchasers of the remaining part of our property in your Province. Should this sentiment deserve consideration, I rather think (though I can only mention it as my opinion) that the Trustees would be easily disposed to make the Hospital a better bargain than they would to individuals. Would it then be improper to inquire of our Agents into the value of what remains undisposed of, and to make some proposal to the Trustees? If it is considered, the expense of commission, the loss of time and many other circumstances which I have not leisure to mention — a compromise might turn out greatly to the benefit of both parties.[5]

If this seems not an unreasonable suggestion, please to give it a thought, inform me of thy sentiments and I shall cheerfully contribute all in my power to bring it such an issue as may be just and equitable to the Proprietors, yet generous to you. I am

Thy affectionate Friend
John Fothergill

P.S. I had proposed writing a line by this conveyance to my Friend

425

William Logan, but I find I shall be disappointed. Be kind enough to mention to him M. Worley's affair, and confer with him on the subject. He, as well as myself is interested in it. I cannot learn that there was ever the least suspicion of habitual intemperance — only that an artful bad person has betrayed her into a discoverable weakness. This however is, I hope, entirely rectified in her conduct and must be kept confined to the knowledge of a very few for obvious reasons . . .

J.F.

Ms. autograph letter, Pemberton Papers, Etting Collection, II, 70, HSP.

1. The paragraph mentioned refers to a book "translated from the Arabick" which tells of one Hai Ibn Yokdan, who attained a state of holiness so great that he had "immediate Converse" with God. The paragraph appears near the end of section xxvii of the discussion of Propositions V and VI in editions prior to 1765 of Robert Barclay's Quaker classic. It appears in the Baskerville edition of 1765, in Richardson and Clark's London edition of that year, and in Joseph Crukshank's Philadelphia edition of 1775, but is omitted in some later editions, including three examined by courtesy of Professor Frederick B. Tolles: those of J. Phillips (London, 1780), Joseph James (Philadelphia, 1789), and Kimber, Conrad and Co. (Philadelphia, 1806). Dr. Fothergill's irenic counsel did not obviate dissension. In the nineteenth century the paragraph became "a weapon in theological controversy." — D. E. Trueblood, *Robert Barclay* (New York: Harper and Row, 1968), 158–161.

2. An English translation by John Hawkesworth of Fénelon's popular tale, *Les Aventures de Télémaque fils d'Ulysse*, had been published by W. and W. Strahan in 1768.

3. The enclosure has disappeared.

4. The peace conference proposed in a letter from Dr. Fothergill to James Pemberton, 23 August 1774.

5. This proposition was left hanging for years while relations between the Colonies and the Mother Country became constantly more strained. The Pennsylvania Hospital Minute Books contain various letters from Dr. Fothergill dated 2.11.1778, 31.1.1780, and as late as 8.5.1780, asking repeatedly for an accounting with definite information of the value of the Pennsylvania Land Company's property still undisposed of. The final reply from the Hospital's agents, made on 11 November 1780, reached London after Dr. Fothergill's death. The agents stated that it had not been in their power to comply with his requests since "Samuel Shoemaker, our partner in the Agency, left the city with the British Army, and took the books and other papers belonging to the Company with him, so that we have neither the Cash nor Property in our hands." By that time funds were desperately needed. A draft for £250 was urgently requested "upon the most advantageous terms," since "all prospects of expansion are blasted in this once prosperous land," which required more than ever the services of the Pennsylvania Hospital. — Ms. Minute Books, the Pennsylvania Hospital, now available in microfilm at Library Hall, the American Philosophical Society, Philadelphia.

To William Logan, Philadelphia, 5 November 1774

London, 5.11.1774

Dear Friend,

It is now a long time since I either heard from or wrote to thee. This however has not been owing on my part to design or neglect. I have been very little a master of my time of late. At night when others are at rest I sit down to converse with my absent friends — the only respite I have from incessant and unavoidable labour. I have been returned to this place from our usual Cheshire retreat a few weeks. There I intended to have wrote to many of my American friends, but various interruptions and my necessary employments filled up the whole of my time. We were however much better for our journey — I hope both in body and mind, and once again with our friends here in much peace and satisfaction.

Our Quarterly Meeting in London falling somewhat later than usual, we took that of York on our way home. Sarah Taylor [1] accompanied us from Manchester, and Rachel Wilson likewise attended, and though the meeting was unusually small from a long continued wet season, yet I hope the meetings were endowed with a degree of divine regard. When we left York we went to Knaresborough, where my sister wished to pay a visit to the place where our honourable Father's remains were deposited.[2] I knew she wished to do so, and am glad it was in our power to see that the wild beasts of the field had not trod down the sepulchre of our Father. We were not hurt by our journey; we rejoiced at the remembrance of his care, his kindness, his life and his removal. If we wept, it was not from sorrow.

We got safely to London, and I am just as much engaged as I know how to accomplish, though the town is still empty of a great part of its inhabitants, I mean of those to the Westward. The new Parliament will meet ere long, and I suppose if they do anything in respect to America will pursue the same line as far as they are directed. — What the consequences may be to you, by this time you most probably know much better than we.

In one thing I should have acted, I think, somewhat differently. If I had thought it requisite to shut up the Port of Boston, I would have taken care to prevent any Congress. What yours has determined, or may determine, cannot by us be guessed at — but I would have distrusted them wherever they had met. — Had I thought proper to proceed upon

427

the plan of compulsion, I never would have waited the event of their deliberation. They should have been sent hither, the moment they arrived in Philadelphia! Don't imagine by this that I think the colonies are acting wrong in taking measures for their common safety. I only mean to say that if I had begun to govern arbitrarily I would have gone through stretch. — But I did not intend to say anything on this subject, and therefore think nothing of it. — In respect to your Congress I cannot but wish they may have deputed a few prudent persons from among themselves to come over to this country immediately, to settle with Adminisration and the Parliament a line of future accommodation.[3] Remonstrances, petitions, resolutions and so forth signify nothing; they are not attended to — I wrote sometime since to a Friend in your city upon this subject. Thus it cannot be supposed that any hints on this side can be of much use on yours.

I find I shall be a small sufferer by these disturbances. I must have no plants this season from my Friend Marshall who has supplied me with many rare plants and some curious insects; so my hobby horse must starve!

I shall be pleased to hear in thy next that M. Worley succeeds amongst you, and that she behaves in every respect to Friends' satisfaction. Give my respects to her if she is with you. The time allotted me is so short that it allows me only leisure to say this much, and to assure thee that we often remember thee and thine with satisfaction and are thy affectionate Friends

J. & A. Fothergill

Ms. autograph letter, William Logan Fox Papers, Philadelphia; in photostat copy, HSP.

1. Sarah Taylor of Manchester, a well-known Quaker preacher, was an intimate friend of Ann Fothergill. When they corresponded they addressed each other as "Dear Cousin," although no blood relationship is traced in the Fothergill genealogical records. Perhaps the term "Cousin" was used like "Coz," simply as a term of endearment.

2. It was at this time that Dr. Fothergill and Ann met their brother Alexander in Knaresborough, and with him visited their father's grave (see Introduction).

3. Dr. Fothergill had not relinquished his idea that a peace conference in London might be efficacious. — See his letter of 23 August to James Pemberton.

To Lieutenant-Colonel Gilbert Ironside, Bengal, India, 22 December 1774

London, 22.12.1774

My worthy Friend,[1]

I am so many letters in thy debt — and a variety of other obligations, that it has long been a burthen to me; equally difficult to discharge the obligations as to bear the continual reproaches of a neglect bordering on ingratitude. Suffice it to say, that at the time when the ships sail for India I am incessantly engaged; in the less occupied part of summer I do not write, not knowing but something of consequence may occur to be said — and thus season after season passes, with the same intentions and the same want of execution.

The last communication I received was this season, containing the seeds and letter from James Kerr.[2] I am greatly obliged to you both for the favour, and have endeavoured to serve him as efficaciously as I can. The Directors have recommended him by name to the Governor and Council in India. I shall write to him I hope by this conveyance, and point out to him what to do on the occasion.

In the preceding season I received, along with some instructive papers from the same hand, some very curious accounts and drawings of an ancient city. I have hesitated much whether I ought to lay these before the public in some proper manner, either by the Royal or Antiquarian Society. These papers would have been very acceptable to either and to many curious people — but as I hope they are to make a part of a history of Indostan, I rather chose to keep them back than to diffuse them amongst my acquaintance till I had thy own permission. The account of the funeral tragedy I received long since should have been presented to the public as well as these, if I thought I should not have been acting a part that friendship and delicacy might have condemned me for. Let sometime or other the world be favoured with such an account as my Friend can give — these specimens assure me of it — as much superior to the general histories of travellers as Tacitus and Livy excel our present historians. — Tell me what I am to hope for in this respect; and if nothing but slight sketches, yet massy compared with others, must be given to the public, let me give them as they come to hand.

I take it for granted that all of our political pieces are constantly and

429

regularly sent to India. I have enclosed one,[3] however, because its object is a most important one, and the conduct of Administration relative to the subject, of the highest consequence to the British Empire. I must in the first place inform my Friend, that I have been on the side of America from the time the Stamp Act was first proposed, and have therefore beheld with much anxiety the subsequent measures of Administration, which have brought us to the brink of a gulf, which without the consummate prudence and the interposition of Providence will swallow up the honour, wealth, power, and consequence of the British Empire irrevocably.

Having thus described my complection,[4] it will be easy for a more disengaged spectator to make the proper allowances for a degree of Party zeal which, whilst it is solely disinterestedly pointed to measures not to men, is not altogether culpable.

I do not therefore hesitate to say that these measures have been uniformly oppressive — I do not think they have been so, as the American suppose, systematically — but merely from that kind of disposition which leads John Bull always to think of his own importance in the first place, and to hate most heartily any other person who dares think he may be mistaken; the right and the wrong of the thing never makes a part of his consideration when his supposed consequence is doubted.

Officers were sent from hence in civil departments extremely odious to the people of America. These officers being true John Bulls, as well as those who sent them, soon quarrelled with people who did not wish for their company. They complained of insults which they had drawn upon themselves, and indignities they suffered from want of sense. They soon found by complaining, that they rather afforded satisfaction at home than received the censure due for their officiousness. They provoked still more, and found themselves always great gainers by magnifying those very sufferings which their own imprudence had produced. There was not an office but was filled with such kind or description of American faction: perverseness, misrule, nay disloyalty. Everybody about the Court and the Parliament spoke the same language, and produced a temper most perfectly inimical to the inhabitants of that vast continent.

At the same time the people of every rank, almost, in this country were perfectly strangers to their power, usefulness, loyalty. Everything that could lessen and depreciate was most greedily listened to, and all the branches of Legislature thoroughly imbued with an opinion that they could do what they would, and that a people so contumacious ought to be chastised, restrained, circumscribed within narrower limits. Hence a series of Acts which will everlastingly disgrace the annals of the present time. They begin to find the infant grown too much a man to be whipped like a schoolboy — and see with amazement, what they ought long since to have known, that between two and three millions of people in a country abounding with all the necessaries of life, cannot easily be kept in subjection by 8 millions of people, at the distance of more than three thousand miles. They are stunned with the view of an object as clearly defined. We have 5 or 6 thousand men in a Province where they can muster above 50,000 effective men, well trained, armed, disciplined, and led by officers who fought at Louisburg, Martinique and the Havannah.

Gen. Gage must be very sensible that he owes his existence to the moderation of the Bostonians.[5] With France, Spain, and all the nations of Europe trembling at our rapid progress to a grandeur and force unknown in these parts of the world, jealous to an extreme, how can we spare troops sufficient to subdue such a Country? Yet this is one Province only. I should not doubt but a confederacy would bring into the field near 100,000 men.[6] What force have we to oppose such an array of Englishmen, rendered desperate by the prospect of oppression?

These and many other considerations have thrown Administration into the deepest perplexity. How it will terminate cannot be divined. I hope, however, less impetuous counsels will prevail, and that the Legislature will think it most expedient to endeavour to bind those in a firm connection of mutual interest, which I believe they think, and which I am fully persuaded of, that it never will be in our power to cement to us by any other means.

I do not quite give our Superiors [7] the credit which the Congress does — of endeavouring to enslave them by System. I believe they are very happy if they can find expedients for the present moment — so far, indeed, System may prevail, that if a man is proud, haughty, overbearing, his councils will retain a tincture of his disposition.

Perhaps my penchant for America may sometimes give a caricature to its enemies; be it so. But who could quite command himself when he sees the foundation of a most glorious fabric, rising fast to meridian splendour, dug up by piecemeal, through insufferable ignorance and pride?

Cast an eye upon the Possessions of all our neighbours — are they not so many pledges for their good behaviour, whilst we and the Americans are one? Was another war to break out between Spain and us — not Puerto Rico, nor Cuba, but Spanish America, itself, would be a proper object of our pursuit.

We can send twenty men to all these places while Spain could send one. Shall we dismember such a part of the British Empire for moonshine? But I ought to quit the subject. I should grow too warm. — Should anything in the book way that I can supply be wanting, be kind enough to let me know. I know not how else to be of any use in return for the favours I have repeatedly received.

Pray give my cordial respects to thy very valuable consort [8] and her sister. The unavoidable, incessant engagements of my profession have prevented me from giving those proofs of my esteem, which their own good qualities, as well as their near connection with my Friend, justly claimed from me.

We seem to want for a few years some unfeeling Asiatic despot to seduce us in some order. Perhaps atrocious crimes were never so oft committed in this country from the time of its being first inhabited. The signal clemency of the Prince, our sanguinary laws — [*illegible*] including those we have — the increase of prostitution, all unite in rendering those who have anything to lose extremely insecure. No endeavours seem to be used to effect an alteration. Principle in general is lost, and the appearance of it despised. Our newspapers furnish the neighboring nations with the strongest proof of national barbarity: they reproach us with it continually. How far the riches of the East may have contributed its share towards national corruption, I know not. Those who take up with first appearances, charge a great deal to this account. I think, however, the West Indians have done more to corrupt us — not by means of immoderate wealth, but by example; they are the most strongly disposed to sensuality of most people who have a claim to the title of Britons. Accustomed to libertinism with their slaves from a very early period, they retain this inclination through their lives.

It is some loss likewise to the publick that there is very little religious persecution. For though it might hurt those who had the power to persecute, by cultivating the harsher dispositions, yet it seldom failed of amending the objects of it, rendering them cautious, humane, circumspect and devout — excellent qualities.

The people of our Profession,[9] who are pretty numerous in Pennsylvania, have behaved well in these contests. They did not add to a flame they could not control. They wished to obtain redress by less violent measures — by Petition, by reason, by experience — but the exasperated Bostonians were incapable of listening to such counsels.

Pray tell me what progress my Friend is making in the History of Indostan. Let J. Kerr add his remarks in Natural History — it must be a valuable collection. Let me have the satisfaction of serving the office of a whetstone once more.

Dr. Cleghorn published his account of Minorca; Dr. Russell of Aleppo at my instigation. They have acquired much reputation, and have done their country most signal service. Another Gentleman is doing the same for Carolina; [10] I am not idle in my sphere, though of me it can only be said *Mutas agitat inglorius artes*.[11] May health and happiness — every precious blessing — attend my Friend and his connections, is the wish of

John Fothergill

The seal which was sent to me some time ago by my worthy Friend, writes me William instead of John. It makes no difference in reality, as nobody in this country will ever be able to read it. If it would not, however, be too much trouble to get another engraved, I could wish to have the alteration made.

P.S. 24th. Since I wrote the preceding, I have been favoured with a sight of a part of your new code of laws [12] — I am not a competent judge of its merit — but I think I can perceive in it a tincture of that humanity which does honour to our species, and to our nation in particular. I never have drunk in those absurd notions which are vended here by the ignorant and malicious, of the rapine, cruelty, and despotism said to be exercised by our countrymen in India in a general way. I could not think of them so far lost to the feelings of humanity. We are too generous and brave to be cruel. I am glad that this production gives the lie to this kind of malevolence. — Let us, however, cultivate benignity, both between ourselves, and with those we live amongst, and Heaven will never forsake us.

Adieu

Ms. autograph letter, Charles Roberts Autograph Collection, Haverford College; lacking name and location of addressee; entry, in modern hand: "said to have been addressed to G. Ironside, then in India." This ascription is supported by Dr. Fothergill's preface to James Kerr's paper cited below.

1. Gilbert Ironside (1737–1802) bore the name of his paternal grandfather, Bishop of Bristol and Hereford. Gilbert II was the son of Edward Ironside of Twickenham and London, a banker who was elected Alderman and later Lord Mayor of London. Young Gilbert was educated in Winchester School. He sailed for India in 1757 on the *Prince George* as ensign in an independent company, became lieutenant in 1759, captain in 1763, lieutenant colonel in 1768, and colonel in September 1774. A paper by him, "Of the Culture and Uses of the Son or Sun Plant of Hindostan, with an account of the manner of manufacturing the Hindostan paper," was published in *Phil. Trans. R.S.*, 64:99–104 (1774). In 1786 he retired and returned to London, where in 1802 he died at his home in Upper Brook Street, Grosvenor Square. — Information by courtesy of C. M. H. Burton, India Office Records, Commonwealth Relations Office, London.

2. James Kerr (1738–1782) was "an attentive, able naturalist, assistant-surgeon to the civil hospital at Bengal," according to Dr. Fothergill's prefatory note addressed to the Medical Society in London; his paper, "transmitted by the learned and worthy Lieutenant-colonel Ironside to J. Fothergill," was published under the title "An Account of the Tree producing Terra Japonica" in *Medical Observations and Inquiries*, V (1776), 148–159, and reprinted by Lettsom in Fothergill's *Works*, II, 191–199. Kerr's dates are given in *Roll of the Indian Medical Service 1615–1930*, compiled by D. G. Crawford (London: W. Thacker and Co., 1930).

3. The enclosure has disappeared. It was very probably a copy of Thomas Jefferson's pamphlet, *A Summary View of the Rights of British America*, noticed in the London *Monthly Review* for November 1774 (51:393): "This summary . . . affords a concise and spirited review of the rights and grievances of the Colonies deduced from their first settlement and proposed as the subject of an address to his Majesty from the several '*States of British America.*'" The "humble and dutiful address" that Jefferson outlined contained the forthright statement: "Single acts of tyranny may be ascribed to the accidental opinion of a day; but a series of oppressions . . . pursued unalterably . . . prove a deliberate and systematical plan of reducing us to slavery." The Continental Congress in October adopted a much softened petition to the King, but along with it sent printed copies of a Declaration of Rights voted by the Congress on 14 October 1774 and of the agreement — the "Association" adopted and signed on 20 October — for successive steps toward complete nonimportation of British goods. These documents reached Benjamin Franklin in London on 18 December. — *The Papers of Thomas Jefferson*, ed. Julian Boyd, I (Princeton University Press, 1950), 119–137; *Journals of the American Congress*, I (Washington: Way and Gideon, 1823), 46–49; Van Doren, *Benjamin Franklin*, 502.

4. State of mind; ideas. Meaning and spelling are both obsolete now. When this letter was written, Dr. Fothergill, Benjamin Franklin, and David Barclay had already begun their series of anxious meetings in a fruitless attempt to work out a means of averting war between the Mother Country and the Colonies.

5. On 17 May 1774, General Gage, "an amiable, well-intentioned gentleman who had married an American wife," in addition to his military command had taken over the responsibilities of civil governor of Massachusetts in the place of Governor Hutchinson, who had returned to England. — Channing, *A History of the United States*, III (1912), 139.

6. "The number of personnel in the Revolutionary War is not known; estimates range from 184,000 to 250,000." — *Historical Statistics of the United States: Colonial Times to 1957* (Washington, D.C.: U.S. Dept. of Commerce, Bureau of Census), 131.

7. The abbreviation *Sup.* appears in the manuscript letter.

8. Ironside's marriage to Letitia Roberts, daughter of the Vicar of Aldford, Cheshire, took place in May 1763 in Calcutta. — Information through the courtesy of C. M. H. Burton, India Office Records, London.

9. The Society of Friends, not the medical profession.

10. Dr. Lionel Chalmers of Charleston.

11. Dr. Fothergill quotes part of a passage from Vergil, *Aeneid* XII. 396, 397:

> *Scire potestates herbarum usumque medendi*
> *Maluit et mutas agitare inglorius artes*

(He sought to know the virtues of herbs and their use in healing; and, unknown to fame, to practice the unsung arts).

12. Warren Hastings, designated Governor-General of India by the Regulating Act of 1773, had sent to Lord Chief Justice Mansfield — "21 March 1774 (per *Resolution*); duplicate 25 August 1774 (per *Swallow*)" — two chapters in English translation of a digest of Hindu law being drawn up at the Governor-General's instigation by a group of revered Hindu scholars in an effort to establish a code for the fair and effective administration of justice under the new system. In 1776 this compilation was published in London as *A Code of Gentoo Laws, or Ordinations of the Pundits, from a Persian Translation made from the original written in the Shanscrit Language*, translated and edited by Nathaniel B. Halhed. — See G. R. Gleig, *Memoirs of the Life of the Right Hon. Warren Hastings*, I (London: Bentley, 1841), 398–399.

To The Earl of Dartmouth
at his home, St. James's Square, London, 12 January? 1775

Harpur Street, London
12th Inst.

My noble Friend,

I scarcely know how to attempt to write, nor yet am wholly at ease to be silent on the present interesting situation of this kingdom.[1]

It may seem vain for a private individual to offer his opinion in a case of so great consequence, and especially in an affair so remote from his situation. Permit me to mention a few of the circumstances which have led me to be acquainted with America. If they appear of any moment, I know they will have weight with the Nobleman I am addressing, both from the partial regard he is pleased to pay me as well as from the circumstances themselves.

My Father, a man of the middle rank of life — plain, simple, judicious — visited America three times in the course of his life — all the inhabited parts at very distant periods. A Brother, whom I lost a few years ago, likewise passed through the continent not many years since. Some others

435

of my relations, many of my acquaintances of whose good sense and probity I could not admit of a doubt have likewise at different periods seen the whole country. I have corresponded with some of the most sensible people in most of the Colonies for upwards of thirty years on different subjects with men of different professions, and have been occasionally even visited by them for the like period.

With some little inquisitiveness, some little knowledge of the general history of the globe, some acquaintance with what passes commonly in the world, a very mean capacity must have unavoidably acquired not from system but by accident, perhaps, a general idea of the country, its inhabitants, its connections, its prospects. Such is the little stock upon which I presume to form any ideas of this most important subject.

America is now grown too great to be humbled by this country without such an exertion of force as might, like what happens in the human frame too frequently, bring on such an Hemoptoe [2] as would end in a fatal consumption. We might harrass, vex, destroy a large territory, many people, retard their progress toward greatness, but never, never hope to subject them to Great Britain. This, at least, is my firm belief and founded upon what appears to me indubitable evidence.

What remains to be done? The *Hints* we have offered (D.B. and myself) would secure their Obedience and our Superiority. — Grant them rather more than less. — Make it evidently their interest to be our Friends, to allow us an exclusive trade, to consider us, as they have done and always will do (if we act our part as we ought) as their Parents, Guardians and Friends, and everything will soon return to Peace and Harmony.

It requires a large capacious heart to take in the consequences of a disunion with such a country. This little island will soon become the prey of any bold invader the moment we are separated from our Colonies. — Where are our resources against France, against Spain — much less against both *United?* — View our debts, consider our inability to feed ourselves with bread. See France and her Colonies united — Spain and her distant possessions one Empire. What can Great Britain and Ireland oppose to such powers? Do, my Noble, much-esteemed Friend, forget the little trifling quarrels fomented by mischievous people for the ruin of this great Empire, and give America *all* she asks. [3] Was my life worth pledging, I think I could do it safely, that she will amply repay the condescension. Violent measures will ruin us both — partial con-

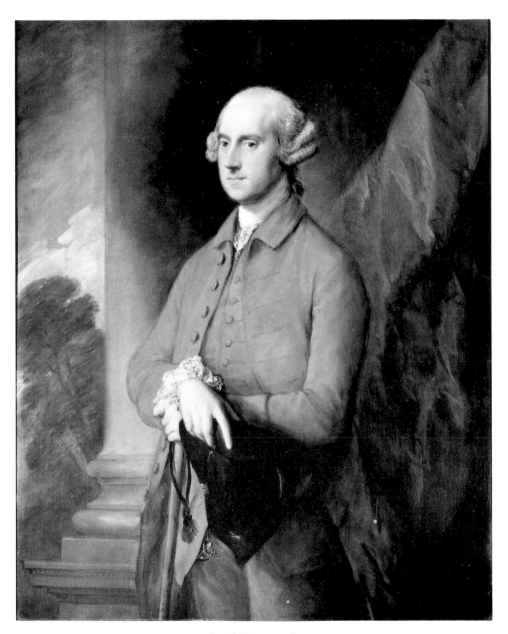

Lord Dartmouth

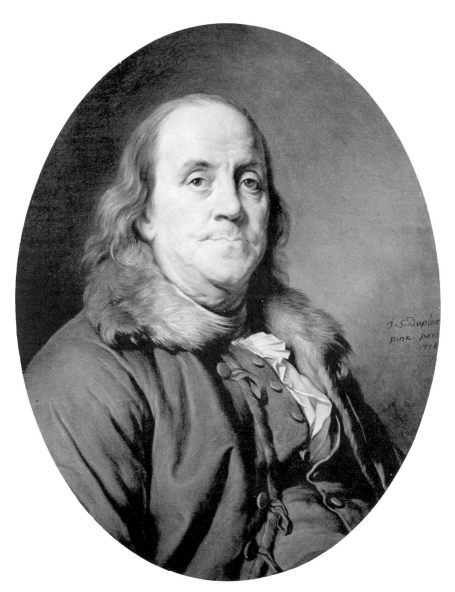

Benjamin Franklin, 1778

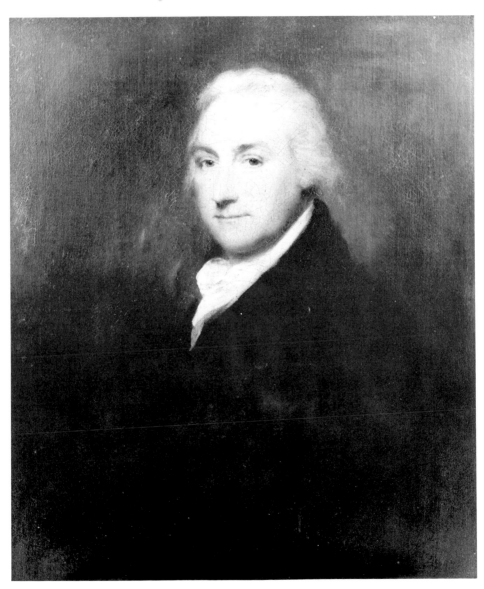

David Barclay

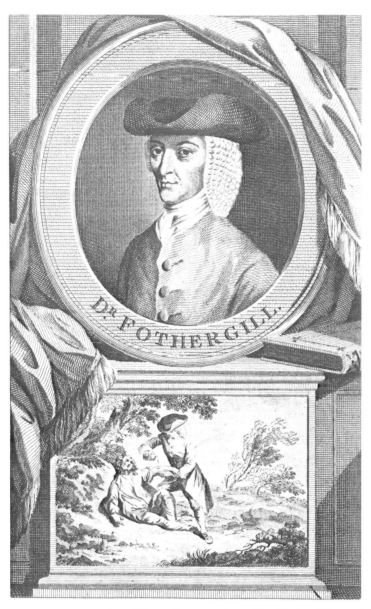

Frontispiece from John Elliot's edition (1781) of Dr. Fothergill's works

descension will pave the way to future and worse misunderstanding. A generous mind will open itself to the liberal plan of human felicity and regulate its actions accordingly.

Excuse this hasty effusion of a mind ardently wishing for the happiness and security of mankind in general, and not less for the honour of Great Britain and those great names who are now permitted to be in such a situation as to decide upon the nation's prosperity and their honour and reputation forever.

I am
Lord Dartmouth's
obliged, respectful Friend,
John Fothergill.

Ms. autograph letter, Dartmouth Family Papers (seventeenth and eighteenth centuries), Patshull House Collection, William Salt Library, Stafford, England.

1. Dated only "12th Inst.," the manuscript letter is endorsed: "Dr. Fothergill 1775 America." It seems probable that it was written in January while, according to Benjamin Franklin's account (*Benjamin Franklin's Autobiographical Writings*, ed. Carl Van Doren, New York: Viking, 1945, pp. 373–374), the "Hints" for reconciliation with the Colonies drawn up in December were still being considered. See Introduction, pages 27–29, above.

2. Haemoptoe: a variant form of *haemoptysis*, expectoration of blood from the lungs or bronchi.

3. Dr. Fothergill undoubtedly here refers to the "humble petition" from the Continental Congress, which had been adopted in October 1774 and reached London 18 December. According to Franklin's account (*Franklin's Autobiographical Writings*, ed. Van Doren, 364), this petition had been favorably received by the Secretary of State for the Colonies (Lord Dartmouth himself), who had subsequently assured Franklin that the King had been pleased to receive it very graciously, and had promised "to lay it, as soon as they met, before his two Houses of Parliament."

To James Pemberton, Philadelphia, 26 January 1775

Harpur Street, London
26.1.1775

Dear Friend,

We received the Epistles of the Yearly Meeting, and Meeting for Sufferings of your Province and have presented them where they will in due time have proper consideration paid to them.[1] It was very kind to convey us likewise a copy of your address, which was seen by none but ourselves. A copy of it got abroad by some means, before the proper time, but not from ourselves. We mention this for thy satisfaction, and that no blame may rest on thee, from any supposed leakiness of thy correspondents here.

We may safely, we think, inform thee that the conduct of Friends in general on your side of the water has been prudent, nay more, praiseworthy; to keep in any degree of order so many young, fiery, unexperienced persons as must be growing up among you is indeed an arduous task, and in which you have been enabled to succeed, we doubt not, beyond your own expectations.

Government is well informed of your sentiments and conduct — they coincide so much with their wishes that you may be assured they are pleased with your conduct. They wish that all America was like-minded. Indeed our principles hold to this patient acquiescence. We have actively no share in legislation. We must therefore submit to the powers that are. On your side you seem thus far to have done everything in your power to promote conciliatory measures; nor have the like been wanting on this side the water by the few who have access to people who have anything to say or to act upon this great and important subject.

If we should here give thee our sentiments on the present state of affairs, we do it as simply private conjecture and wish what we may say to be considered merely as private opinion. Keep this explanation constantly in view, and we may then proceed farther in opening ourselves on the present situation of affairs.

There is a part of Administration which we believe has the King's confidence most, who are utterly averse to temperate measures and who will leave no stone upturned to engage both countries in hostilities. They are the descendants of those people who have in every reign since James I adhered to unlimited monarchical principles, adverse to civil and religious liberty. Too many of these are about the King and have been so from his earliest infancy. People of these principles prevail in the Cabinet.[2]

The other part retain some regard to the principles of the Revolution, but yield, and yield, and yield to the others [3] with the specious hope of moderating the flame of the first, but it is to be feared from a secret love of power and a most certain conviction that it ceases the moment they refuse to comply with every mandate.

We need not suggest to thee what is likely to be the fate of America from such counsel, and from which nothing but supreme interposition seems probable to divert them. To gratify their pride and resentment they would not hesitate, we fear, to sacrifice the happiness of the whole community.

The Landed interest are not your friends, and the commoners of great rank are many of them your enemies — the *dignity* of Parliament sticks so closely to them — the very badge of their preference to a mere fox hunter, will lead them to give and grant — to anybody, all the people in America. Even the mercantile interest is not all on your side. Those trading to North America must be so, if they are true to their own and their country's benefit. The rest see that if goods are not wanted for America, they must be bought cheaper for other markets. Thus from pride, interest and general ignorance of what you are, whence you are sprung, the benefits resulting to us at present, still greater and greater in future, your fast friends on this side the water are reduced to almost an insignificant number. From the temper of the Parliament, from the language of the Ministry, from the disposition of the King, there is too great reason to apprehend that violent measures will be pushed, at least will be attempted. — One may compare wars in general to opening a vein, but intestine quarrels are like cutting arteries. The first soon close, the last are scarcely ever healed but with exceeding difficulty.

There are a number of Americans, and English who have been in America, who are the greatest foes to both countries. Their daily business is to incense, to irritate, and to precipitate the public mind to do mischief. They have lost all love of their country, and would feel no pain in seeing every calamity fall upon both to satiate their revenge. These then finding the completion of the Court inclining to harsh proceedings are goading them on to severities. These are the pests of both countries.

We cannot wonder that many among you, we mean of other professions, should be driven to as great an extreme on one hand as we seem madly to incline to on the other.[4] They remember who they were that drove their ancestors into exile, and whose spirit seems to animate their descendants to render this exile as humiliating as possible.

But we leave these reflections; let us keep to that patient moderation that becomes us. — Though we live in this world and enjoy the position allotted us by Providence and which we ought to do with daily gratitude for the favour, yet when we think aright, we know that our kingdom is not of this world. Let us therefore studiously endeavour to keep out of every consultation on these subjects to the utmost of our power, and by preserving and possessing our minds in quiet and subjection to better rule, we shall be able either to act with propriety or to bear with fortitude whatever may be permitted to befall us. We need not suggest to thee the necessity Friends are under on your side to act with the greatest circumspection — neither to incline so far to the fiery popular side which like many amongst us led by those unfit directors, pride and passion, would sacrifice every substantial benefit in life; nor on the other, leave so much to the inflated vapours of arbitrary dictates as to yield assent to its encroachments on everything that is valuable to mankind.

We doubt not but the same reply which conveys this will bring over with it very interesting particulars of your present situation. There are some in power who give into the measures, with a hope that they may intimidate and induce you to meet them a little more than half way. At the same time we suspect that the greater leaders mean all that they say, and think of nothing less than treating America as a conquered country.

We need not suggest to thee what thy own thorough knowledge of this important concern suggests to promote every reasonable yet firm conciliating measure. Petitions from Assemblies will be treated perhaps with a little more consideration than they have been, at least they will afford a handle to those in Administration here who affect to be your friends — if they are not so in reality — to advocate your cause.

Yet it seems not an easy matter to frame a petition for redress of grievances, whilst all the colonies have resolved as one man to redress their own grievances, by subjecting Great Britain to all the disadvantages they can.[5] This will be a tender point. If you now break through your resolutions, you afford your enemies the triumph they expect, at least which they wish.

We are pleased to hear that the troubles with the Indians are at present pacified.[6] The Government's conduct is by no means relished here. Neither is making war with the Indians nor making peace, as they might have been considered as a thorn in your sides.

Whatever may be the result of these affairs, we have none of us been wanting, as opportunities offered, to render the best services we could to our Friends in America as well as to the inhabitants of that vast region in general, by endeavouring to convince those we had access to that however some warm spirits might have erred both in expression and in act, yet that the generality deserved the generous confidence of the British Nation. When all is said that can be said upon this unpleasant subject — here it must stand — that if we all are happy enough to be preserved, in that calm, quiet, steady refuge which is open to all, we may be instrumental in acting as eyes to the blind, feet to the lame, and supporters to those who need it most. We cannot forget the poor suffering Friends in New England. We hope the Meeting for Sufferings in Philadelphia will get proper information of their state, and communicate to Friends here. We wish likewise that our Friends in Philadelphia would have an eye to Rhode Island and take some little care that the active intemperate zeal of a mixed race may not involve us in some difficulties.[7]

As thou had been kind enough to enter freely into the state of affairs amongst you, so in the same freedom and without reserve, we have treated briefly of the state of things amongst us here, which we leave to thy discretion to make use of as occasion may require. — It may probably be some time before the Meeting for Sufferings may reply to your Epistle; lest it should be so we have been the more explicit in this letter . . . We are thy affectionate friends, John Fothergill

Ms. autograph letter, Pemberton Papers, XXXIV, 171, 172, HSP.

1. The Yearly Meeting for Pennsylvania and New Jersey (24 September to 1 October 1774) had circulated an Epistle signed by James Pemberton as clerk "to our Friends and Brethren in these and the neighboring Provinces," urging obedience to law, discouraging writings and other measures tending to promote disaffection, and affirming loyalty to the King.

2. James VI of Scotland, taking title as King James I of England upon the death of Queen Elizabeth I in 1603, had strengthened the nation, in spite of the opposition of Parliament, by successfully uniting Scotland and England into one realm ruled by a single sovereign. His belief in the divine right of kings was revived by George III and his Tory associates — in the early years of his reign most notably the Earl of Bute, and by 1775 Lord Sandwich and Lord George Germain. Lord North, currently Prime Minister, did not dissent, although his private views were more liberal and pacific. — Trevelyan, *American Revolution*, pt. II, ch. I.

3. The Glorious Revolution of 1688 gave the Crown to William of Orange and his wife Mary (daughter of James II) upon their acceptance of a parliamentary Declaration of Right strictly limiting the power of the monarchy in order to give parliamentary leaders opportunity to voice the rights of the British people. Lord Dartmouth and Lord Hyde were among those liberals in the Administration who very reluctantly yielded to adverse pressure. — *Ibid.*

4. A reference primarily to the Scotch-Irish Presbyterians.

5. A reference to the non-importation, non-exportation, non-consumption Association adopted in October 1774 by the Continental Congress.

6. "Lord Dunmore's War" had concluded in October with the defeat of the Shawnees in the Ohio country.

7. This allusion has not been identified. Dr. Fothergill did not condone slavery

(see his letter to Granville Sharp, above), but he greatly deplored dissension within the Society of Friends. Rhode Island Quakers, led by Moses Brown, had been very active in persuading the New England Yearly Meeting of 1774 to proscribe slaveholding by Friends and in supporting a bill to end the slave trade introduced in the Rhode Island General Assembly in June 1774. Dissatisfied by this bill as amended, Brown and other Quakers were in 1774–75 carrying on an active campaign against the slave trade. — Mack Thompson, *Moses Brown, Reluctant Reformer* (Chapel Hill. University of North Carolina Press, 1962).

To The Earl of Dartmouth
at his home in St. James's Square, London, 6 February? 1775

Harpur Street, London
6th Inst.[1]

I wish it had been in my power to have informed My Noble Friend that our negotiation had been successful. But it is not. And this, not owing to our want of attention or willingness to promote a reconciliation, nor to any opposite or refractory disposition in ———.[2] Our difficulty arose from the American Acts — the Boston Port Bill, the Massachusetts and the Quebec Acts.[3] As a concession to pay a tax was the *sine qua non* on this side, so a rescinding of those Acts, or rather repealing them, is the term of reconciliation on the other.

As we had no permission to give any hopes that these Acts would be repealed, to ask for anything less would not be satisfactory on the other side, and therefore an assembly of delegates, authorized to treat upon the means of establishing a good understanding between the members at variance, would be wholly ineffectual.

We found that the delegates to the late Congress [4] were chosen in the respective provinces by the people who have a right to vote for representatives, and in general by no other, so that whatever may be thrown out to the contrary, we apprehend will be found not to be authentic.

The party we conferred with would have no objection to meeting with the Noble Lords who were pleased to intimate that our endeavours to promote a reconciliation would not be unacceptable, and to consider the whole affair with the utmost candor and privacy, could it in the least contribute to avert the evils, which are inevitably impending without some intervention, upon both parts of our Empire. Was the whole of America as cordially disposed to peace and as sensible of its advantages as Lord Dartmouth, I think there would be no difficulty in accomplishing it, but I see and perceive so strong an assent another way that I despair, without the intervention of Omnipotence, of any reconciliation.

The only thing left for the generality of these devoted Countries is to look for superior protection. The great will always be the great, in every revolution that can happen. The poor will always be the heirs of misery, let who will be their superiors. A numerous, a very numerous part of both Countries, the middling class, who bear all Burthens, who produce all the strength and happiness of states, they must be the sufferers.

Should the King's servants happily coincide in adopting the simple plan of pacification which our Noble Friends so generously concurred in, and include the repeal of the Acts above mentioned, we have not the least doubt but America would immediately return to every just expression of duty, both in language and in conduct. The party we conferred with,[5] should this be tacitly consented to, would have not the least objection to petition for the restoration of Peace, offer on the part of Boston to pay for the tea, though at the risk of his own private fortune, and endeavor *bona fide* to concert every means of a lasting and reciprocally beneficial union.

Should it, however, be determined to proceed with force to reduce the Americans to a different way of thinking, and subject them by hostile means, I most sincerely wish that the Enemies of my Noble Friend, if any such there are, may enjoy the power of issuing such a sanguinary commission.

I am, with the deepest sense of the confidence reposed in me,

Lord Dartmouth's obliged, respectful Friend,

John Fothergill

Ms. autograph letter, Dartmouth Papers, Patshull House Collection, William Salt Library, Stafford, England.

1. The calendar of Lord Dartmouth's papers in the 14th Report of the Historical Manuscripts Commission (Appendix, Part X, vol. II, p. 266) gives the endorsement on this letter as "Dr. Fothergill 6 Febr 1775"; Carl Van Doren (*Benjamin Franklin*, 514–515) is certain that the letter was written on 16 February; while comparison with Franklin's account of the negotiations (*Franklin's Autobiographical Writings*, ed. Van Doren, 381–385) suggests that it may have been written after the meeting of 17 February. Fox, however, prints the letter from a rough draft in the Barclay papers, partly in David Barclay's hand, and gives the endorsement as "Dr. F. to Ld. D. 6th 2/mo. 75. copy." — Fox, 332–333, 398.

The decisive rejection of Lord Chatham's conciliatory resolution offered in the House of Lords on 20 January, and of his detailed plan for conciliation introduced on 1 February, had discouraged the trio of negotiators, but apparently hope had been reawakened, and on 4 February they met in Harpur Street to consider the "Hints" again, with modifications probably suggested to David Barclay by Lord Hyde. Franklin found some of the terms acceptable but others impossible of acceptance. At another meeting on 16 February a further revision of Franklin's list of points, this time called "A plan," was produced by David Barclay. The discussion was inconclusive, but Franklin indicated to the other two that he would undertake, himself, to pay for the tea destroyed at Boston, "if, there were, as they supposed, a clear probability of good to be done by it"; and he agreed to draft a petition to the King urging that a commission with power be sent to meet with assembled delegates of the Provinces to "settle the means of composing all dissensions." The next day, 17 February, there was another meeting of the three at Dr. Fothergill's, to which Franklin, according to his own account, took drafts of a memorial to Lord Dartmouth engaging to pay for the tea on specified conditions, the petition to the King, a letter of similar content to Lord Dartmouth, a list of "Remarks" on the propositions discussed at the previous meeting, and another sheet of notes as a memoranda for the conversation. The others listened sympathetically, but were sure that Franklin's first requirement, the repeal not only of the Boston Port Act but of all the punitive "Massachusetts Acts," would be definitely unacceptable. Accordingly, says Franklin, "I pocketed my drafts." The conversation with his friends continued, however, and he declared his willingness "if this was thought proper . . . to attend them to the ministerial persons they conferred with."

2. Benjamin Franklin.

3. The Boston Port Act had effectively closed that port to commerce as of 1 June 1774. In May, the Massachusetts Government Act had practically taken away the rights and privileges granted by the provincial Charter; the Quebec Act, extending the jurisdiction of the Crown to Ohio, had aroused resentment for several different reasons "from the first and best people in all the colonies," according to Governor John Penn. — Thayer, *Pennsylvania Politics*, 154–161.

4. The First Continental Congress, held at Philadelphia in Carpenter's Hall from 5 September to 26 October 1774. Governor Penn's maneuver in having Pennsylvania's delegates to the First Continental Congress elected by the Assembly gave them legitimacy; the Massachusetts delegates were elected by the House just before Governor Gage dissolved the General Court. Other delegates not chosen by their respective legislatures were chosen by duly elected conventions.

5. Benjamin Franklin.

To James Pemberton, Philadelphia, 17 March 1775

Harpur Street, London
17.3.1775

Dear Friend,

Though I am exceedingly straitened for time by constantly increasing applications in the duty of my profession, I could not let my friend Dr.

Franklin return without some proof of my remembrance of my friends in America, though this is the only letter I have time to write at present.[1]

Perhaps Dr. Franklin will inform thee at some time or other that David Barclay and myself have not neglected taking every step in our power to promote a reconciliation, though ineffectually. The present troubles must continue till both sides are more disposed to a good understanding — and indeed if bloodshed may but be prevented, the continuance of this kind of war — Acts of Parliament on one side, resolutions on the other — may be continued till both sides being tired, they may think it worth while to lay passion and resentment aside, and think of ways and means to cement a better understanding. We have labored so much in the affair as to be thoroughly satisfied that no good can be done at present. We are heady and high minded, and must perhaps by the means of your steady adherence to prudent resolutions be brought to more just sentiment. On this subject I may have occasion, perhaps, to speak more freely hereafter, and indeed I must trust to the leisure of my Friends here to acquaint thee with many things that pass here in which America is much interested. To enter upon the subject is too much for me. I shall only here observe that Friends here have thought it expedient to present a petition to the King, that every means might be tried to effect a reconciliation without bloodshed, and that it has not been unfavourably received. It was delivered this day, and it was proposed to the Meeting for Sufferings to appoint a committee to draw up an answer to the Epistle received from your Meeting for Sufferings,[2] which will probably be done in the course of next week. We have seen the Testimony given out by Friends and the Nation has seen it.[3] We doubt not but it was thought right and proper such advice should be given.

I believe we shall send you a copy of our Petition in which we have endeavoured to be as general as possible.[4] Whether it will be published here by Authority or not, we know not yet. I think it will be your great safety and wisdom to keep close to one another, to yield to the times; neither to relax your care one over another, nor to lean to the violent, nor to join the obsequious. Your all in this life is at stake — life, liberty, and property. — I had wrote the enclosed [5] to thyself sometime ago at the time I was answering a letter which we, your representatives, had received from thy Brother Israel. I did not find time then to transcribe it with the necessary alterations, and I have now much less ability. As it may contain some little information of the present condition of the times, I send it as it is. Make no public use of it. It contains my own opinions solely. A few words more and I must have done, and this to thyself. If America relaxes, both you and we are undone. I wish Friends would studiously avoid everything adverse either to Administration here, on one side — or to the Congress on the other side. Submission to the prevailing power must be your duty. The prevailing power is the general voice of America. You are contending for your privileges by the most innocent yet effectual means of waging war, showing your usefulness. From the little I have had an opportunity of seeing, it seems to me that an oppressive, unjust, tyrannical spirit possesses the chief in power here who are as regardless of the happiness of America as the mandarins of China, provided they should not be losing, themselves, by the contest. — Mind your own business, and neither court unworthily the favors of your superiors on this side, nor oppose with vehemence the party which steps forward for the protection of your liberties, which are all at stake.

J.F.

Ms. autograph letter, Pemberton Papers, XXXIV, 173, HSP.

1. Franklin had learned late in January of his wife's death on 19 December. He had now concluded his arrangements for returning to Philadelphia, and planned to sail on 21 March. With him he carried several of Dr. Fothergill's letters to Pennsylvania Friends.

2. "Held in Philadelphia the 5th day of the First Month 1775." This Epistle, signed by John Pemberton, Clerk, urged that Friends abstain from public office and from all activities tending to "contend for liberty by any methods or agreements contrary to the peaceable temper of the Gospel," and that they remember that "to fear God, honor the King, and do good to all men, is our indispensable duty."

3. The Testimony of the people called Quakers, given forth by a meeting of the representatives of said people, in Pennsylvania and New Jersey, held at Philadelphia the twenty-fourth day of the first month, 1775, signed by James Pemberton, "Clerk at this time," noting that "we have grounds to hope and believe that decent and respectful addresses from those vested with legal authority" would be effective, "publicly declared" against illegal actions and reaffirmed loyalty to the King.

4. A copy of the petition was enclosed with the Epistle from the London Meeting for Sufferings 24.3.1775. The London Epistle is transcribed in the Minutes of the Meeting for Sufferings in Philadelphia, 8.6.1775. The original petition, "asking that the sword may be stayed and other means tried to procure a firm and lasting union with the Americans," carrying sixty-one names including that of John Fothergill, is listed in the Manuscripts of the Earl of Dartmouth, II, 294.

5. "The enclosed" has not been identified.

To William Logan, Philadelphia, 18 March 1775

Harpur Street, London
18.3.1775

Dear Friend,

I have just received thy kind letter by way of Liverpool and doubt not but the packet will be forwarded to me in due time. I have received your Epistle and Testimony — [1] the last has been laid before Parliament by the Ministry as a proof of your approbation of the measure carried on against the liberties of America. I must confess that I know not how to express the concern which so much of thy last and present letter as related to America gave me. I can only say at present that we are quite of opposite opinions on the present subject, a case that has not hitherto happened in the whole course of our correspondence.

I have not time to say what mine are, nor upon what they are founded. This would require more time than the short pittance of an hour which is only left me to say this much and to acquaint thee with a few other circumstances before our mutual acquaintance, Dr. Franklin, leaves us.

Yesterday Thomas Corbyn, Jacob Hagen, D. Barclay and myself,[2] by direction of the Meeting for Sufferings presented a Petition to the King, entreating that every means might be tried to effect a reconciliation with America without bloodshed. We were favourably received, at least in appearance. Friends here are in general as unanimous and anxious for the preservation of the civil and religious liberties of our Friends in America, as on the preservation of theirs perhaps our own may under providence depend. Some of you seem to be very little acquainted with the general state of things here, or are very indifferent about them. But time will manifest all things. Whether our Petition will be published or not I know not, but as we shall soon write to the Meeting for Sufferings in Philadelphia, we shall probably send the purport if not a copy to them. Till we see whether it will be published by Authority, we shall scarce think it prudent to print or publish it ourselves.

We have lost our very valuable Friend Rachel Wilson [3] in this city. She came up under much suffering before the oppressive measures taken against America and wanted admittance to the King. Every avenue was barred against her. She was suffering with an inflammation of the liver, a complaint which she was disposed to, and the consequences removed her from us yesterday. Her valuable husband was in town and had been

447

very instrumental in promoting a petition. She was removed the night after it was presented. — May I speak to thee in confidence? I think ———— wish to reduce all America to the Standard of Quebec and Canada, an abject slavish people to be governed solely by the will of ————.[4]

I am satisfied that those who have stood up in defense of your liberties have carried some things to an extreme. But if the principles on which they act are just, shall we reprobate them because their supporters are not perfect, have committed excesses and often act from prejudice, passion or interest?

I shall request Dr. Franklin to get a few of you together — he knows my sentiments fully and the pains which D. Barclay and myself have taken in these affairs. — Listen to reason; make every allowance for his resentment for unmerited injuries, — for his sentiments bordering on the republican — for his passion for the freedom of America — and yet there will so much sterling reason still be left, as I hope will meet thy doubts on these affairs.

I have only time and space left to say that my Sister joins me in affectionate remembrance, though she never loved thee less than at present.

Farewell

J. Fothergill

Ms. autograph letter, William Logan Fox Collection, Family Papers, now in photocopy, HSP.

1. See the preceding letter, notes 2 and 3.

2. The same group of Friends who had been working on behalf of the American Colonies for at least twenty years.

3. Rachel Wilson, known for her commanding presence and beautiful voice while active in the Quaker ministry for thirty-six years, was the wife of Isaac Wilson of Kendal. She was the mother of three sons and "seven beautiful daughters." Through marriages of the children, she became the ancestress of many able, distinguished Quakers. — *Piety Promoted*, III, 92; Jenkins' manuscript "Recollections," LSFL; Fox, 342n, quoting from the "Pedigree of Wilson of High Wray."

4. "I think the Administration wish . . . all America . . . to be governed solely by the will of the King."

To Benjamin Franklin (Embarking for Philadelphia), 19 March 1775

Harpur Street, London
[March] 19th Inst. [1775]

Dear Doctor,

Be kind enough to take charge of the inclosed and convey them at thy leisure.[1] ———— is a staunch anti-American.[2] I have received a letter from him today by way of Liverpool which hurts me very much. Get him, James Pemberton and two or three more together, and inform them that whatever specious pretenses are offered, they are all hollow, and that to get a larger field on which to batten a herd of worthless parasites is all that is regarded. Perhaps it may be proper to acquaint them with D.B.'s[3] and ours, united endeavors and the effects. They will show at least, if not convince the most courtly that nothing very favorable is intended if more unfavorable articles cannot be obtained.

Pray, is Sir John Pringle[4] a thorough anti-American? Though for answering this idle question I will not put my old friend to the trouble of an answer in his last moments before sailing for America.

Farewell, and befriend this infant growing Empire with the utmost exertion of thy abilities and no less philanthropy, both of which are beyond my powers to assess. A happy, prosperous Voyage! Pray see Betsy Ferguson[5] sometime and tell her she must trust me for a letter till summer.

J. Fothergill

Ms. autograph letter, Papers of Benjamin Franklin, Collection of Henry Stevens of Vermont, Library of Congress, Washington, D.C.

1. Benjamin Franklin left London the next morning. On the voyage to America he was accompanied by his grandson, William Temple Franklin. They reached Philadelphia on 5 May. — *Franklin's Autobiographical Writings*, ed. Van Doren, 399.

2. See the preceding letter. William Logan's name was here discreetly omitted.

3. David Barclay's. In the course of the voyage home, Franklin wrote down a full and colorful account of these negotiations. — *Franklin's Autobiographical Writings*, ed. Van Doren, 347–399.

4. Sir John Pringle (1707–1783), military hygienist and distinguished physician, had a career of varied experience which led to early publication of two important books: *Observations on the Nature and Cure of Hospital and Jayl Fevers* (1750); and *Observations on the Diseases of the Army* (1752). These books effected necessary and lasting reforms in army camps, hospitals, and prisons. Dr. Pringle settled in private practice in London after returning from military service during the War of the

Austrian Succession. His character and skill soon led to appointment as medical adviser at Court, where he became a favorite with the Royal Family. In 1775 he was appointed personal physician to George III. He had been elected Fellow of the Royal Society in 1745 and Fellow of the Royal College of Physicians in 1763, knighted in 1766, and in 1772 elected President of the Royal Society. Dr. Pringle's long association with the King effectually silenced at this time any expression of his personal political views. — *Munk's Roll*, II, 252–256; *DNB*.

5. Betsy Ferguson was known earlier in life to Dr. Fothergill as Elizabeth Graeme, daughter of an eminent Philadelphia physician. She had sought Dr. Fothergill's medical advice during her visits to England and Scotland and had been guest of Dr. Fothergill and his sister at Lea Hall. In 1772 she had married secretly in Philadelphia an enterprising Scotsman, Henry Hugh Ferguson (or Fergusson), to whom she had been introduced by Dr. Benjamin Rush. Later, Ferguson proved to be an adventurer who brought her much trouble. In 1775 he disappeared suddenly, leaving an explanation that he was called to London on business. When next seen in Philadelphia, he entered the city with General William Howe's army of occupation, serving as commissary of prisoners. He succeeded in impressing his wife Betsy with a fantastic scheme he had formed to bring about a quick peace through his acquaintance with General Howe. She responded by advancing funds and signing financial papers to back this scheme, which accomplished nothing. Ferguson soon disappeared, leaving her without the resources of her inherited estate. It was reported that her financial papers had been found and confiscated. After the close of the war, thanks to the efforts of Dr. Benjamin Rush and other friends, some of her property (real estate) was restored to her. Although she was never in want thereafter, she was obliged to live in sadly reduced circumstances. The fact that she never complained about her misfortunes endeared her more than ever to her lifetime associates. — *Letters of Benjamin Rush*, ed. Butterfield, I, 177–179.

To Humphry Marshall, West Bradford, Pennsylvania, 23 August 1775

Lea Hall, Middlewich, Cheshire

23.8.1775

Esteemed Friend,

I am much obliged to thee for several kind letters, and a box of plants, amongst which are some new ferns and a few other rare plants. For these and many others I am still in thy debt, but at present without any opportunity of repaying thee.

I sent the last numbers of the plates that are published and am not quite sure that I did not send one twice over. If I did, only let me know it; it need not be returned. I hope it will be finished next spring; [1] and I shall send it as I may have opportunity.

At present I cannot expect anything, as all intercourse between Britain and America is cut off, and I am afraid for a long time. Be attentive however to increase thy collection at home, by putting every rare plant thou meets in a little garden, and as much like their natural situation — as shade, dryness or moisture — as possible. For instance, most of the ferns like shade; these may be planted in some north border, where the sun shines but little except in the morning, and so of the rest.

A little mattock and a spade are the best instruments for taking up plants. With the first, make a little trench round the plant, at some distance; then raise up a large ball with the spade; the earth may then be gently pared away, so as not to hurt the roots; and in this manner it may be safely conveyed any whither, and in any season.

I write this from Cheshire, 160 miles from London, to which place I retire for a couple of months every year. Nearer London I should have no quiet. My garden is about 5 miles from London, warm and sheltered, rather moist than dry; and I have the satisfaction of seeing all North American plants prosper amazingly. There are few gardens in the neighborhood of London, Kew excepted, that can show so large or so healthy a collection.

I have there likewise a fine young Tea Tree. It is now, my gardener writes me word, 7 feet and 1/2 high, extending its branches in proportion. It flowered last year in autumn, and will do so this. It is in natural ground but sheltered in winter by glass, and covered at night with a mat. It is the finest Tea Tree in Europe. We are endeavouring to increase it both by cuttings and layers.

Many of thy plants are there in good perfection. The poor turtle came to us alive, and continued some months. We suspected he had got hurt on board ship, as he looked uncommonly heavy about the eyes, and did not care for stirring. He had water enough, and land at his choice, and also the shelter of a warm hovel. I am not, however, the less obliged to thee for thy kind attention.

When once communication is opened, let me know how I can most satisfactorily to thyself discharge the debt I have contracted, and I will do it speedily. I have forborne taking any notice till now of the public distress that now afflicts America, and must soon in some shape come home to ourselves. I do not think that our superiors will at all listen to any terms but such as must be disagreeable to America. I therefore expect that much mischief will be done; that a large army will be sent over; and that orders will be given to wage war in every part of America. I have no other foundation for this opinion than from what appears to be the

451

general tendency of the preparations and the infatuation of the time. It seems not unlikely but we may be rendered a severe scourge to each other. It will be happy for those who know where to seek for a quiet habitation both internally and externally.

This I wish most sincerely for all my friends, myself and everybody. What little lay within my reach to do I have endeavoured to do it honestly — but it's all in vain. Providence may see fit by this dreadful work to bring us back to ourselves, and rouse us to better consideration. Many lives will be lost; many fine fabrics demolished; the labor of ages ruined; and all this chiefly at the instigation of some proud discontented people who have been in office in America: and I am sorry to join with them the generality of the Scotch, many of whom being high in authority here, and seeing the ———— rather set against you, urge on these violent councils; in the first place to gain favor with ———,[2] and in the next, to wreak their revenge on the English, by setting them to work to destroy one another.

Whilst the packets continue to sail it will not be very difficult now and then to send little parcels of seeds to thy assured friend.

P.S. I omitted to mention in the inclosed that the two little owls (by Captain Falconer) came very safe and healthy. We put them into an open and proper cage, secure enough from vermin of any large kind, — as rats, weasels and the like; but one morning the larger was found killed, and its brains picked out. We attributed this to its mate; but if so it was not from want, as they always had plenty of victuals.

The instruments are all sent by Dr. Franklin; and I shall call to pay for them in a few days. If a bill is not enclosed with them, I think it is not improper for thy own satisfaction to know that they cost £14.16s.6d. Captain Falconer is very careful of everything sent under his care for me; and as we are at a considerable distance from one another, I do not sometimes see him to make proper acknowledgments. As thou mentions J. Hunt's name, it puts me in mind to ask whether thou received the ten guineas I sent by him. Farewell.

Ms. autograph letter without signature, Miscellaneous Collections (Scientists), HSP; printed in Darlington, *Memorials*, 513–518.

1. "The plates" refers to John Miller's *Illustration of the Sexual System . . . of Linnaeus*, first issued in parts; it was published complete in 1777. See letter to Marshall of 6 February 1773.

2. Darlington (p. 514) adds a footnote: "The *King*, is obviously the word intended

to fill the blanks, prudently left in this letter. The same prudential motive, no doubt, induced Dr. F. to omit putting his name to this, his *last* epistle to our countryman."

To James Pemberton, Philadelphia, 23 August 1775

Lea Hall, Middlewich, Cheshire
23.8.1775

Dear Friend,

[*Passage omitted.*]

I hear by the papers that your Governor is arrived here and is said to have brought a Petition from the Congress.[1] If that is true, I should hope some good may come of it, as I think his Friends would not suffer him to bring a Petition along with him, even officially, that it might enable him to a cold if not contemptuous reception. I will presume this to be the case, I mean that the Petition is likely to be received with favour. In this case, it will be a mutual happiness to both countries. I doubt it, however, — but I will not fill up this letter with dire forebodings to America first and then to the whole Empire of Great Britain. It is more than probable we shall never subdue you. — We, when I say we I mean those above [in power], but we shall struggle hard and run the risk of sending ourselves, if you are first plunged, to the bottom. Fatal, fatal error! The revenge of a few discontented people in office — what dreadful havoc will it make? But it is indeed to you first, and next to us, a time of great sifting, and those who look forwards even amongst us cannot but be alarmed for the public safety. For you, our brethren as a Society, I lament every day. Oh, that the weight of sacred wisdom may press all to that foundation on which alone they may stand securely, and extend a hand of help to those who are in danger of swimming with the tide of confusion till they perish.

What difficulties must attend you at a time of such extensive defection from Principle! But we trust you will be enabled by him whose cause you serve to serve it wisely, efficaciously to the safety of many, and the honour of the profession. Often is my mind with you — and the fervent wish is not long together absent that you and we may be clothed with wisdom and strength equal to the day.

Whatever effects besides this chastisement may produce, if it leads us to a more circumspect humble walking, a more constant feeling after

453

life to animate us, a nearer union with each other and the family of the righteous everywhere, much good will arise from it to ourselves, to our fellow professions; and who knows but through the intercession of many, the impending calamity may be withheld.

Remember me to thy brother, to Samuel Emlen, J. Hunt when thou sees him, and I wish to be remembered by you and every living member in the family.

Our Friend William Delwyn [2] has occasionally visited us. We esteem him much, we believe he has endeavoured to conduct himself blamelessly in all things, and by the general account we hear has acquired much place in the minds of many. It may perhaps be as well to wait for proper opportunities of conveying letters by private hands, as by the Packet, for though we shall neither of us enter deep into the state of the time, yet some caution may be necessary.

We are favoured with a moderate degree of health, and propose returning to our usual abode in London towards the end of next month. I am

Thy affectionate Friend

J. Fothergill

Ms. autograph letter, Pemberton Papers, XXXIV, 175, HSP.

1. Although battles between British troops and colonial forces had already occurred at Lexington and Concord (April), Ticonderoga and Crown Point (May), and Bunker Hill (June), the Second Continental Congress voted in July to petition the King once more, urging him to stop hostilities until a plan could be worked out for peaceful cooperation between the American Colonies and Great Britain. This "Olive Branch" petition, with other documents, was carried to England by Richard Penn, younger brother of Governor John Penn. On 21 August, Penn and Arthur Lee, colonial agent for Massachusetts, requested permission to call upon Lord Dartmouth with the petition to be presented to his Majesty. Lord Dartmouth was at his country estate and the interview did not take place until September 1, when Penn and Lee were told there would be no answer to the petition. Their letter dispatched to Congress on 2 September with the news of this response did not reach Philadelphia until 9 November. — *The Declaration by the Representatives of the United Colonies of North America . . . Their Humble Petition to His Majesty* (London, 1775); Peter Force, *American Archives*, 4th ser. III (1839), 1863–69, 1870–78, IV (1840), 225, 627; E. C. Burnett, *Letters of Members of the Continental Congress* (Washington: Carnegie Institution, 1920), I, 157–162 and notes. The "Olive Branch" petition, carried by Richard Penn to London, may now be seen in the museum of the Record Office, London.

2. A well-known Quaker from Philadelphia who traveled in the ministry of the Society of Friends on both sides of the sea.

To Israel Pemberton, Jr., Philadelphia, 5 September 1775

Lea Hall, Middlewich, Cheshire

5.9.1775

Dear Friend,

I received thine, and my Sister thy wife's affectionate letter at this place, a quiet retreat to which we remove every summer for the sake of a little quiet which we have no other means of enjoying. We have not therefore seen James Hutchinson,[1] who brought thine and many other letters. At our return home, which will be, we hope, at the end of this month, we shall endeavour to render him any assistance in our power. I have wrote to my nephew James Freeman about him.

This comes by our Friend William Delwyn, who during his residence amongst us has gained by his steady, prudent, friendly conduct the regard I believe of all who know him . . . I must refer thee to him for everything concerning us, as it may not be safe to enter much into public concerns. — Be it known, however, that many amongst us deeply sympathize with you under your most afflicting situation. America has nothing to expect from hence but severity. If one might reason upon the righteousness of a cause by the temper of those who are engaged in it, ours cannot be a good one. I believe there is no scheme, however contrary to the principles of religion and humanity, that should be offered as likely to subdue America that would not be adopted. In another light than that in which it was then proposed — "To your tents, oh Israel" — may now be repeated "to those tents let us retire who have the favours of Providence to submissive contrite hearts, showering upon them."

I did not know that I should have time to convey a line to thee by our Friend, and therefore had wrote to him as fully as I could that if through the favour of Providence he arrives safe he may acquaint thee with our sentiments concerning you. I know not that as a body, or as individuals, we have omitted anything that might . . . prevent these vigorous proceedings. But it seems as if through a judicial blindness we were permitted to become each others' scourges.

About ten weeks each summer we escape to this place . . . Here I excuse myself as much as possible from the labours of my profession, both for time to look around me . . . and to acquire strength to discharge the duties of my station; was I nearer London, I should seldom be free from applications.

We received thy kind communication of my Brother's letters, but as yet have made no progress in selecting any passages that may be of general use. I do not forget the business, but I could wish . . . to be better qualified . . . my mind would prompt me to engage in it warmly . . . If I found freedom and leisure . . . I should sit down to the work with pleasure.[2]

My sister joins me in very affectionate remembrance to dear Father's and our Brother's friends. Farewell,

J. Fothergill

Ms. autograph letter, Pemberton Papers, XXXIV, 176, HSP.

1. James Hutchinson (1752–1793), son of Catherine and Randall Hutchinson of Wakefield Township, Bucks County, Pennsylvania, graduated with honors from the College of Philadelphia, was accepted as an apprentice by Dr. Cadwalader Evans, and proceeded to study medicine at the College. His proficiency in chemistry led to his selection as apothecary to the Pennsylvania Hospital, where he took up residence in 1773 while completing his medical course. At commencement exercises in 1774, he received his M.D. and a gold medal in recognition of his attainments, particularly in chemistry. Through the generosity of Israel Pemberton, who had taken particular interest in this young man's progress, he was sent to England for a year of special study under the guidance of Dr. John Fothergill. Because James Hutchinson wished to become a surgeon, he was introduced to London's famous surgeon Percival Pott. The young American soon demonstrated ability which finally won him the special privilege of assisting Pott during operations. He also attended Dr. William Hunter's lectures and John Hunter's classes in their anatomy school. — Whitfield J. Bell, Jr., "James Hutchinson (1752–1793): A physician in politics," in *Medicine, Science, and Culture, Essays in Honor of Owsei Temkin*, edited by L. G. Stevenson (Baltimore: The Johns Hopkins University Press, 1968), 264–283.

2. Dr. Fothergill never found time to prepare an edition of Samuel Fothergill's letters. A privately printed volume entitled *Letters Written by the late Samuel Fothergill*, without editorial ascription, bears the imprint of High Wycombe, 1803. A great many of Samuel's letters are included in *Memoirs of Samuel Fothergill* by George Crosfield, whose wife, Margaret, was the daughter of Betty Fothergill Chorley, daughter of Joseph Fothergill.

To Dr. William Hird, Leeds, 26 September 1775

Lea Hall, Middlewich, Cheshire
26th Inst.

Esteemed Kinsman,

I received both thy very kind letters, and am much concerned for our Niece's suffering and disappointment.[1] I was afraid those dreadful spasms were a prelude to what followed, and as all human precautions were taken, it is our duty to submit. She has met with many difficulties, and being no stranger to affliction, I know her prudence will now be exerted to bear what has happened with due resignation, and to improve, as she has done, every disappointment to her benefit. We affectionately sympathize with her, and gratefully acknowledge thy attention and care for her and for us on this occasion.

My Sister is gradually recovering a tolerable share of health from a long and debilitating pain in her feet and ankles, with an irrefrangible coldness. We have had a good deal of quiet since we came down, which has helped her much.

We were at Warrington last week and passed a few days in that almost desolate place — *desolate* I mean only with respect to those whom we have ever looked up to with affectionate esteem. Alexander and Betsy [2] live happily and deserve by the prudence of their conduct all the countenance we can give them, and they possess our regard. The poor girl has just had a similar, though a less misfortune, than her Sister — a miscarriage. We hope, however, she will not be much a sufferer by it.

We are now in expectation of seeing some of our relations from Leeds in a few days. The next week after is our Quarterly Meeting, and then the time of our leaving the country advances fast upon us. I never thought of business with any degree of anxiety — rather [with] pleasure — before this time. But the remembrance of a most laborious winter is not yet worn off.

I have finished one or two papers for our Medical Society since I came hither. Most part of the Volume is printed, and I expect it will be published early this winter.[3] There are a few interesting papers in it from various hands.

I now wish for a little time to do myself a piece of justice — I mean in respect to Parkinson's accusations in the preface to his Brother's Journal.[4] The poor fellow is now confined in a Mad House, and is likely to remain there while he lives.[5] Everything has been sold, and he left just enough so satisfy his creditors — but nothing for his helpless children. There were 400 copies of his work unsold; I had the offer of them and purchased both them and the plates. I propose to print a short justification on the same paper and with the same types, and add it to the books in my possession, with a table of errors which his Brother has made in his work. This at least will be doing myself some justice. Poverty and pride

457

hurt the poor fellow's intellect. In hopes of gaining wealth and reputation from his Brother's work, he trampled on justice and gratitude.[6]

Remember us to thy Sisters Hustler and Hird if they are still at Leeds, and likewise to our Niece Nancy. We shall be pleased to hear that Sally continues to recover — and are thy very respectful

J. & A. Fothergill

Ms. autograph letter, Port. 21/143, LSFL.

1. Dr. Fothergill's favorite niece Sally — Sarah Fothergill (Titley) Hird — had been delivered of a stillborn infant.

2. Alexander Chorley of Warrington had married Sally's sister Betsy (Betty) in 1770, not long after her return from a visit to Uncle John in London. — Fothergill Genealogy, below.

3. Volume V of *Medical Observations and Inquiries* was published in 1776.

4. *A Journal of a Voyage to the South Seas, in His Majesty's Ship, the Endeavour. Faithfully transcribed from the papers of the late Sydney Parkinson, draughtsman to Joseph Banks, Esq . . . Embellished with views and designs, delineated by the author* (London: Stanfield Parkinson, 1773). Stanfield Parkinson's only pride in life had been his younger brother Sydney's success. Sydney, a botanical artist working in James Lee's nursery garden in Hammersmith, had attracted the attention of Joseph Banks, and in 1769 was chosen to join the natural history expedition sailing on H.M.S. *Endeavour* under the command of Captain James Cook. Sydney produced hundreds of drawings of exceptional merit but died of a tropical fever and was buried at sea in January 1771. Stanfield knew nothing about what had happened until the *Endeavour* reached England in July of that year. Overwhelmed by grief, he demanded everything Sydney had left. The bulk of Sydney's work, belonging by contract to the British Museum, was already in the possession of Joseph Banks, but after some contention, in order to make peace Dr. Fothergill suggested that Banks send Stanfield £500 and also lend him papers found in Sydney's cabin. Dr. Fothergill himself undertook to return the papers describing the voyage as soon as Stanfield had inspected them. Unfortunately, while waiting, Stanfield had engaged an experienced hack writer, William Kenrick, to prepare Sydney's papers for publication. Meanwhile, John Hawkesworth, a well-known man of letters, was already at work on Captain Cook's journals, having been appointed by Lord Sandwich, first Lord of the Admiralty, to publish the official report of the *Endeavour* voyage. An appeal was made to Chancery to stop publication of Parkinson's book, and an injunction was granted but shortly withdrawn. Both books were published in 1773. Hawkesworth's bulky three volumes were an instant success with the public. Parkinson's little book, scarcely noticed, might have been a memorial to Sydney, but had been spoiled by a preface — written by Kenrick but signed by Stanfield Parkinson — denouncing Joseph Banks, John Hawkesworth, and even Dr. Fothergill for injustice. — *The Endeavour Journal of Joseph Banks*, ed. Beaglehole, I, 24, 27, 28, 47, 56–62; II, 190, 323; E. J. Willson, *James Lee and the Nursery Garden, Hammersmith* (London: Hammersmith Local History Group, 1961), 42, 56–60; Joseph Banks and Daniel Solander, *Illustrations of . . . Plants collected in 1770 during Capt. Cook's Voyage Round the World in H.M.S. Endeavour . . . with determinations by James Britten*, 2 vols., printed by order of the Trustees of the British Museum: Volume I (1900), plates 1 to 150, displaying Parkinson's work; Volume II (1905), containing Parkin-

son's unfinished work with notes on habitat, form, and color, completed later in the eighteenth century by accomplished botanical artists at the British Museum.

5. Stanfield Parkinson, hopelessly paranoid, was confined in St. Luke's Hospital, London. He lived only a short time longer. His wife had died shortly before his commitment.

6. The British Museum Catalogue records "a reissue of the Parkinson book with 'Explanatory Remarks on the Preface to Sydney Parkinson's Journal . . . by John Fothergill' inserted . . . London, 1773 (1777?)." In 1784 Dr. Lettsom revived interest in Sydney Parkinson's work by publication of a new edition "to which is now added Remarks on the Preface by the late John Fothergill, M.D., F.R.S., and an Appendix containing an account of the voyages of Commodore Bryan, Monsieur Bougainville, Captain Wallis, Captain Carteret, Captain Clerke; printed for Charles Dilly in the Poultry and James Phillips in the George Yard, London"; priced at £11.11.6.

To William Logan, Philadelphia, 4 October 1775

Harpur Street, London

4.10.1775

Dear Friend,

Before this arrives thou will probably have received several letters from me, with an account of thy Son's arrival and his present situation.[1]

This morning I received the enclosed from Dr. Sims [2] concerning him, which I hope will afford thee satisfaction. — "As to our young friend G. Logan, I have the satisfaction to inform thee that I believe he, myself and family are mutually agreeable to each other; we had today some little conversation about terms. He desired me to mention a sum; I asked if he should think much of seventy pounds, from his first coming to his going to Edinburgh, the autumn of 1776. He said he was satisfied with that proposal." Thus for the Doctor.

For my own part I think the terms are most equitable, and am pleased that he is so safely and happily situated. I am informed that he is very diligent, and improves considerably.

I am just returned from my usual Cheshire journey — from whence I have reaped (and I must also include my Sister) considerable benefit. We are in better health, our faculties revived as well as the body, and we hope we have profited in the most essential parts of health and happiness by our recess. I consider it as one of the greatest blessings of my life, and which calls for my deepest gratitude to the Giver. And indeed it strikes everyone who knows it with surprise. I have not yet been a week in town and am just in the same situation in respect to business

459

as when I left it, my time fully taken up. I speak it not boastingly, but thankfully to that Power which disposes of all events, that no other Physicians in this place ever did the like. It has been attempted by several to retire in the summer, but they found such a diminution on their return that they durst not repeat it. Ten years I have followed the favourable inclination of its rectitude, and have reaped the happy fruits of following the line which I trust was pointed out to me by wisdom superior to my own. I retire too far to be followed — too distant for a speedy return of an answer — to a country not abounding with families I am much acquainted with, where the roads are not good, nor anything to induce the curious idler to go in quest for forgetfulness. Yet we want for nothing, and have time to think on those things which ought to be the familiar constant objects of thought to the aged, the young, the noble and plebeian. Now and then I endeavour to do a little work for the public in the line of my profession; to put down a few observations on some particular diseases that have either escaped the notice of others, or seem not to have been properly considered.

Please to tell M. Worley that I have had some letters from her mother, who is extremely anxious to hear from her. I tell her that she is well employed, if it can be so to bring a great number of Rebels into the world! But I dare not propose to Administration to fee her handsomely to kill a good many of them, because I think she would be so much of an American as to refuse the bribe, and thereby place me in a very numerous, though not right honourable, list in your apprehension of Projectors for the Downfall of America. But I see you will take care of yourselves. — There are none who deserve so much and get less compassion than we do. For doing all the good to Society we can, promoting peace, order, industry, and every social virtue, we are hated, and if we are not as bad — that is, as warmly agitated by all the selfish passions as others — we are persecuted and oppressed. I hope this letter will not be deemed treasonable either on this side the water or on yours! I hope it will get safe to thy hands, assure thee of thy Son's welfare,[3] and that I am thy affectionate Friend

J. Fothergill

Ms. autograph letter, William Logan Fox Collection; photostat, HSP.

1. George Logan (1753–1821), after an unsatisfactory period as clerk in the mercantile counting house of John Reynell in Philadelphia, decided to follow a medical career. He sailed for England in May 1775, determined to devote himself to "the

humane art of healing while the other young men of his generation were condemned to learn the savage art of killing." — Frederick B. Tolles, *George Logan of Philadelphia* (New York: Oxford University Press, 1953), 17.

2. Dr. R. C. Sims, physician of Dunmow, Essex, some forty miles from London, had accepted George Logan as apprentice upon recommendation of Dr. Fothergill.

3. Since Dunmow, a market town of 1,500 inhabitants, offered few distractions, George Logan, already independently schooled in Philadelphia by reading textbooks of "physick," was able to devote himself entirely to the practical side of a physician's life. He went with Dr. Sims on sick calls, studied materia medica, and compounded medicines in a small laboratory. In 1776 he entered the medical school of the University of Edinburgh, where from the first he was an outstanding student and a leader in the students' medical society. In 1779, when this society received its charter as the Royal Medical Society of Edinburgh, George Logan was unanimously elected President, the first American to win this honor. He received his medical degree in June 1779, his dissertation being a treatise on poisons.

During his absence in Edinburgh, both his parents died, bequeathing him the family mansion, Stenton. Soon after his return to Pennsylvania, he married Deborah Norris and began to develop Stenton's vast acreage by modern methods of agriculture, continuing and advancing his father's projects. He became a pioneer in scientific farming and was instrumental in establishing an agricultural society which eventually drew favorable attention in Washington from government authorities. He was tireless also in working for the improvement of public education and other progressive causes which he advocated in a series of well-argued pamphlets. Drawn into public service to the exclusion of medical practice, he was honored finally by election to the United States Senate, where he served with distinction from 1801 to 1807, the only Quaker of the old stock to win such public recognition. — Tolles, *George Logan*; Deborah Norris Logan, *Memoirs of Dr. George Logan* (Philadelphia: The Historical Society of Pennsylvania, 1899).

To David Barclay, London, 8 October 1775

Harpur Street, London
8.10.1775

Dear Friend,

I came home last night at ten o'clock extremely fatigued. I could not forbear giving, perhaps, a very strong proof of it. If the enclosed remarks are worthy of the least notice, or any part of them, I wish we could see one another this morning, any time before nine o'clock.

J. Fothergill [1]

[*Enclosure: according to Lettsom a letter "which he wrote in 1775 to a noble Lord"*] [2]

The following sketch will show rather my wishes than my hopes, of

461

seeing the most certain, speedy, and honourable means of effecting the proposed measures.[3]

To send as speedily as possible some person or persons on whom Government may rely, and who are not unknown to some of the leaders of the Congress, and on whose character and probity they may have some dependence, to propose to them:

That an Act shall be passed this sessions, virtually repealing all the blameable acts, by declaring that the Colonies shall be considered as being governed by the same laws, or placed in the same situation as they were in the year 1762.

That in consequence of this declaration, if accepted by Congress, the same persons shall have instructions to the commander in chief to cease all hostilities.

That a general amnesty shall be declared, all prisoners released, the provincial forces be disbanded, and the ports reciprocally opened for both countries.

That these preliminaries being fixed, instructions shall be sent to the several governors, to convene the assemblies, and require them to choose two or more delegates, to meet a proper number of commissioners from England, at New York, and there to settle the due limits of authority on this side, and submission on theirs. The sword will never settle as it ought to be. Submission to force, will endure no longer than superior force commands submission; interest only can make it perpetual: it is the interest of Britain that the union should be perpetual, be the present sacrifice what it may.

The mode of proceeding in the union between England and Scotland may be adopted, so far as circumstances require; that is, the different conditions of the contenders considered. The objects are in most respects very different. From Scotland this country had chiefly in view negative advantages — that the Scots should not be any longer the tools of other powers, to work with to our undoing. From America we have every possible advantage to hope for; not only the benefits of commerce, but their power to protect us. No power in Europe, who knows its interest, and has any possessions in the western world, will choose to offend us, whilst we and America are united; because those possessions are immediately subject to the powers of America, directed by us; what those powers are we now know full well by experience. Every distant possession of every power in Europe, is a pledge for the good behaviour of its owner to Great Britain. — Is any object we are now contending for an equivalent to such an extensive and most certain influence?

It is therefore much to be wished, that some such persons might be pitched upon and sent out rather in a private character as friends of both countries, than with a public authoritative commission; for if those now invested in America with power should *distrust* them, the business is at an end; and this country and that are left exposed to all the distresses, which are only beginning to be felt by both.

Administration may think it an easy matter to avert any storm which may arise from a discovery that they have been misled, misinformed, and grossly abused, by those on whose opinion they had too confidently relied. This, however, may admit of some doubts; and I have too much regard for many of those who compose it, to wish the experiment may ever be made.

Let it be considered, that every provocation we give widens the breach; that the Americans have fully shown us that they are descendants of Englishmen; and if they are warm and impetuous like us, like us also they are placable; and instead of endeavouring to subdue them by force to a condition unworthy of our fellow-subjects, our countrymen, and our relations, let us open the shortest road to a speedy, honourable, and effectual reconciliation.

John Fothergill

Printed in *Works*, ed. Lettsom, III, clxii–clxvi; a somewhat different version printed by Fox, pp. 343 and 400–403.

1. Fox gives his version of the covering letter as from the Barclay Papers, in Dr. Fothergill's hand, dated "7th Inst. (? Oct. 1775)" and endorsed in David Barclay's hand, "From Dr. Fothergill, Copy d-d Ld. Hyde, 8th (I think 12th mo. 1775)."

2. Fox dates the enclosure found in the Barclay Papers "(? Oct. 7th, 1775)"; he says it is written with various emendations in Dr. Fothergill's hand and endorsed in another hand "Letter from Dr. Fothergill to Lord D." Fox's version is somewhat fuller than Lettsom's, which omits five short paragraphs at the beginning and "an alternative paragraph, deleted" at the end. — See Fox, 343, 400–401.

3. Although Lord Dartmouth had told Richard Penn and Arthur Lee that the "Olive Branch" petition would receive no answer, a strong desire persisted in some quarters in both England and America to prevent a final breach between the Mother Country and the Colonies — wishes, if not hope.

To Dr. Lionel Chalmers, Charles Town, South Carolina, 1775

Harpur Street, London
[late 1775]

I could wish Will Bartram would confine his rambles within narrower bounds. My last, which I hope will be properly delivered, will mention my opinion on this subject. I would have him employ all the time he can spare in drawing correctly such new plants as he may discover. These may be preserved until some convenient opportunity offers of sending them — and on this condition I shall continue his salary, and for this he may draw upon me as opportunity may afford.

Thy book [1] is printed — all but the introduction; it is in two octavo volumes. When finished I will send some copies if any [way] offers and pay in the meantime what the bookseller will give me, to the druggist.

The general ignorance in this country of what America is or its consequence to this country prevents any material fluctuation in the national credit. It is not less [*illegible*] than true [*four words illegible*] East India [*half line illegible*] in that country would effect our stocks much more than the news of the loss of all America.[2] Even the people in power are most gravely misled in this respect. I have only time to say that I am

Thy very affectionate Friend
J. Fothergill

Ms. fragment of letter, Charleston Library Society, contributed by Dr. Joseph Ioor Waring of Charleston, South Carolina.

1. Mention of "thy book" indicates the recipient of this letter and approximately its date. Chalmers's book, *An Account of the Weather and Diseases of South Carolina*, seen through the press by Dr. Fothergill, was published by Dilly in London in 1776, regardless of the fact that the American War for Independence was in progress.

2. Investment in enterprises of the British East India Company had already brought extraordinarily high returns, while benefits to be gained in the future by the growth, development, and westward expansion of the North American Colonies were quite beyond conception by the British populace. — P. N. Roberts, *The History of British India under the East India Company and the Crown* (New York: Oxford University Press, 1938).

VIII
1776-1780

I think I see all Europe slowly leaguing
against us . . . In the warmth of my affection
for mankind, I could wish to see engrafted
into this league a resolution precluding the
necessity of general wars — the great object
of universal civilization — by the institution
of a college of Justice where the claims of
sovereigns should be weighed, an award given,
and war only made on him who refused
submission.

To Benjamin Franklin, 25.10.1780

To James Pemberton, Philadelphia, 30 April 1776

Harpur Street, London
30.4.1776

Dear Friend,

This comes to enclose a letter from our Meeting for Sufferings to yours. D. Barclay and D. Mildred were absent as well as some others, or I doubt not they would have signed it.

The interruption of our correspondence may make it necessary for Friends in your Province to establish a regular intercourse with those of our Society in the several provinces in the manner which has heretofore been carried on between us and them. Most probably the circumstance will come under the consideration of our approaching Yearly Meeting, but as it may be long before you receive the result of their deliberations, I wish you would look to this point.

As we have no separate interests from those of the community at large, I hope we shall be permitted, at least, that you will be left at liberty to pursue the great object of our institution without difficulty — helping those of our profession as far as persuasion and entreaty may influence them, from all the disorders that degrade mankind below their natures.

We hope to put this packet under the protection of Lord Howe, who if he is as unfettered as he wishes to be, and the Americans are in their right understanding, we doubt not will return with the olive branch.[1] His knowledge of the ground of these misunderstandings, his regard for the happiness of both countries, his ability to promote them, and the attachment of Americans to his family,[2] gives us hopes — stronger hopes of a reconciliation than anything else that could have been proposed to us. I need not say more than that if the present moment is lost and shadows frighten both sides, if Providence permits that you should be chastised and we undone — who shall say that there is not a cause?

467

While the greatest interests of this extensive Empire are at stake, nothing but diversions are heard of in this metropolis. Can anything be a stronger indication of our folly — or a stronger portent of our calamities?

But let not the review of public difficulties draw our attention from our selves. Public virtue must arise from that of individuals. If we are happy enough to mind above all things the duties of our stations and what we each of us owe to him that made us — we shall so far be in the way of ransoming our own souls, and promoting the good of all — not of our society only but of mankind.

Farewell, my Friend, and let us often remember one another and all the faithful — the society of our departed friends and relatives — and these who yet are wrestling against the most dangerous enemies, those of our own house.

J.F.

Ms. autograph letter, Pemberton Papers, Etting Collection, II, 73, HSP.

1. Vice-Admiral Howe, delayed in departure by Parliamentary debates, reached New York on H.M.S. *Eagle* on 12 July 1776, three days after General Washington's official announcement that "the Continental Congress, impelled by the dictates of duty, policy and necessity" had dissolved "the Connection between this Country and Great Britain." Lord Howe and his brother, Sir William Howe, had Parliamentary appointments as "Commissioners to receive Submission of the Colonies or private persons and to grant Pardons." Members of the Continental Congress distrusted Lord Howe's mission, but in September appointed Benjamin Franklin, John Adams of Massachusetts, and Edward Rutledge of South Carolina "to act as representatives of the free and independent States of America" at a meeting arranged by Lord Howe at his headquarters on Staten Island. Lord Howe welcomed his guests cordially and entertained them at a dinner "with plenty of good wine," after which a serious conference took place, lasting three hours. Lord Howe had no terms of concession to offer; he might confer, advise, or consult with any number of private individuals on disputed questions; he was not empowered to recognize an independent government of united colonies. Return to British allegiance, he averred, would certainly win reconsideration of Parliamentary Acts; the good intentions of the King and Ministry could be counted upon. The Congressional Committee in response assured him that the Declaration of Independence was "the result of long and cool deliberation . . . made by Congress . . . in obedience to the positive instructions of their constituents, every Assembly upon the Continent having instructed their delegates to this purpose." The Declaration having been made, "solemnly ratified and confirmed" by the various Assemblies, action was impossible except as a united independent Nation. To John Adams, the British overtures for peace appeared "to be a bubble, an ambuscade, an insidious manoeuvre." To Lord Howe, no doubt, the outcome of this interview brought new light to the situation as well as genuine disappointment. — *Letters of Members of the Continental Congress*, ed. Burnett, II, 70–93.

2. John Adams relates that "Lord Howe was profuse in his expressions of gratitude

to the state of Massachusetts for erecting a marble monument in Westminster Abbey to his brother [Capt. George Howe] who was killed in America in the last French war . . . That such was his gratitude and affection on that account, that he felt for America as for a brother, and if America should fall, he should feel and lament it like the loss of a brother." — *Ibid.*, 94n.

To Henry Strachey, Secretary to Lord Howe, 1776

Harpur Street, 6th Inst. [1776]

Esteemed Sir,[1]

I beg leave to put the packet that accompanies this under thy protection and wish sincerely that the offers which may be made to the Americans may operate so happily as to enable thee to deliver it to the person it is addressed to.[2]

He has been in England and knows the state of his country pretty thoroughly, and I am sure will be ready to render every kind of office in his power. There is another person likewise of our Profession who is worthy of Notice, viz., James Pemberton for whom Lord Howe is so obliging as to take a letter from David Barclay.

Perhaps the plainness and simple appearance of many of our people in Philadelphia may make no very favourable impression, but in general they are not only inoffensive but they are sensible and judicious, in the line of life to which they have been accustomed.

I shall enclose a little tract which contains in a very short compass, the principal tenets of our persuasion [3] — if I can lay hands on it, Barclay's Apology — these will serve as a key to the principles of a much less known than it deserves to be Society, and their instruction is conducive to the interests and happiness of mankind in general. I may be presumed to be partial, but on the other hand it ought to be granted that I must know them well.

I am much obliged to many persons of respectable character in many parts of America for their partiality to me. It may seem vain to say that in many places of that vast country thee will not fare the worse for saying we are friends. The attachment has grown very sensibly by a mutual intercourse of good offices and I am as well assured that by such means all the colonies may be kept in the bond of perfect allegiance as I am that no force can compel them to it.

I could have wished to have waited upon Lord Howe before his departure, and at some vacant moment please to tell him would risk my head on the possibility of office rather than return without Peace. America, its present power, its future greatness, its consequence to the Kingdom, to all the States in Europe, are literally unknown to those who direct our councils. [*Passage omitted.*]

But why am I writing all this? To convince my friend Lord Howe that I have at heart the union of this country. Accept my best wishes for a prosperous and successful voyage — and believe me to be with great sincerity,

Thy assured friend

J. Fothergill

Ms. autograph letter, Henry Strachey Correspondence, 1776–1783, folios 70–71, Library of Congress, Washington, D.C.; photostat at APS.

1. Henry Strachey (1737–1810), M.P. for Sutton, and later for Bishop's Castle, had been Secretary to Lord Clive in 1764, and subsequently served the government as joint Secretary of the Treasury, under-Secretary of State, and Master of the Household. While Secretary to Lord Howe, Commander of the British naval forces during the American War for Independence, he had an opportunity to become acquainted with colonial conditions and people. — Namier, *The Structure of Politics*, 238, 245.

2. Unidentified.

3. Probably *A Brief Account of the People Called Quakers* — a reprint of the article prepared by Dr. Fothergill and his brother for the first edition of the *Encyclopaedia Britannica* (1769).

To James Hutchinson, London, 9 September 1776

Lea Hall near Middlewich

9.9.1776

Esteemed Friend,

Yesterday I received thy kind letter and have considered it with attention. I see very plainly there is little prospect of any alteration for the better, and therefore readily concur with thy intention to return to America. Of the several modes proposed, I think that by the way of France is most likely, and to take that which comes nearest to Boston or any of the New England Governments.[1] For I imagine when L. H. finds it will be dangerous to attack New York, they will make the best of their way for Philadelphia, which I am afraid has much to endure.[2]

It may not perhaps be difficult to get an account of what ships are at

Bordeaux, and the place of their destination, as speedily as may be, as I think no time should now be lost.

I think, likewise to mention to B. Waterhouse [3] the same route, and I hope he would not be a disagreeable companion. I see it affects his health to be longer absent from his own country, and I think if you were both together, it might be comfortable to you both — whatever happens. — This, however, I shall leave wholly [to yourselves].

In case of going by way of France, it would be of great advantage to take from hence a small medicine chest. Bark, Rhubard, Emet. Tart., Mercurials, Salts and Senna would constitute the greatest part, with Vesicatories [*two words illegible*], and a few other things. They cannot be but very much wanted.

There is no doubt of thy getting into immediate employment — but alas, the Hospital — I wish it may not be in other hands — at least not be filled with the wounded and distressed. — This is one reason that makes me urgent for thy return. Most probably the post of Surgeon to a Regiment may be offered. If it can decently be declined, it would be best, notwithstanding the present advantages. It would be out of character. — In the Hospital thy services would be great, and thy progress though more slow would be more certain. But all this must be left, for alas, we know not whether that great city may not now be in ashes or a heap of ruins!

I think we shall be in London the 29th of this month, being a week sooner than we expected, but some circumstances make it necessary for us to leave this place a few days sooner than we had designed.

[*The fourteen lines which follow cannot be transcribed because the letter is badly blotted, probably from sea water. A portion has been cut away, perhaps by design, since what remains may concern movements of troops, and might therefore have subjected the letter to confiscation if the ship had fallen into enemy hands.*]

the restoration of harmony. If any words occur to thee regarding the proposal I have made, please to let me know — and believe me to be thy assured Friend

J. Fothergill

Ms. autograph letter, Hutchinson Papers, APS, presented by S. Pemberton Hutchinson, 1962.

1. Following Dr. Fothergill's advice, Dr. Hutchinson crossed the Channel to France. At Nantes he met Benjamin Franklin, who entrusted him with important dispatches

to deliver in Philadelphia to the Congress. Sailing on the *Sally* from Nantes on 26 October, he found the passage slow and the food poor and scanty, but he enjoyed the companionship of another physician, Dr. Hugh Williamson. When at last the coast became visible, an American naval vessel, the *Wasp*, made contact with the *Sally*. The officers agreed to transfer the young physicians to the *Wasp*, which would assure their safe arrival in Philadelphia by landing them on the Delaware coast. Welcomed to the hospitality of the naval vessel, the young men feasted on roast pork, garden produce, plenty of claret, and plum pudding. Later they were rowed shoreward in a small boat, launched in a heavy sea. Drenched by waves, they reached shore near Lewes, Delaware, where they were to arrange for transportation to Philadelphia. They were safe; so were Franklin's dispatches, and whatever else Hutchinson carried on his person. The chest of medicines he greatly valued, a small collection of medical books purchased in London, and sixteen notebooks of medical wisdom gleaned in London were left on the *Sally* and were lost, together with his personal belongings, for the *Sally* was captured by the British and taken to New York. — Information in part from Dr. Whitfield J. Bell, Jr., Librarian, American Philosophical Society, Philadelphia.

2. Lord Howe, appointed to command the British fleet sent to the American Colonies, made different plans. He considered New York harbor a more strategic position than the port of Philadelphia on the Delaware River.

3. Benjamin Waterhouse was the grandson of Rebecca Fothergill, a younger sister of John Fothergill, Sr. She married a Yorkshireman, Joseph Proud, and emigrated with him to America, settling in Rhode Island. Their daughter Hannah married Timothy Waterhouse of Newport, Rhode Island, and Benjamin, their son, was born in 1754. Following apprenticeship to a Newport physician, Benjamin Waterhouse at the age of twenty-one had crossed the Atlantic to continue his medical education at Edinburgh. He had ambitious plans for his medical career and was not ready to return to the colonies with James Hutchinson. Remaining in Edinburgh until 1778, he then studied at Leyden for several years, greatly to the eventual benefit of his fellow citizens in the United States.

To [Governor John Penn?], 9 October 1776

London, 9.X.1776

My Honoured Friend: [1]

James Hutchinson of Philadelphia, the bearer of this, has at my request applied himself in a particular manner to the practical and operative part of Surgery in one of our best Hospitals, and under the ablest masters this town affords. From his capacity and incessant application, I have reason to think he returns with qualifications that must be exceedingly useful in these unfortunate times, and as such, I recommend him. I think if he was placed in your Hospital,[2] he would there be much more useful to society by instructing others than by his personal attendance in Camps or Armies. He has preserved an unblemished character so far as I know, and will be able to give some account of

Thy assured, respectful Friend,

John Fothergill

Ms. autograph letter, Hutchinson Papers, APS, presented by S. Pemberton Hutchinson, 1962.

1. This letter, entrusted to Dr. Hutchinson in 1776, omitted the name of the person to whom it was addressed in order to prevent possible incrimination if the letter were intercepted at sea by the enemy. Dr. Fothergill's "Honoured Friend" must have been a person of position and influence, perhaps John Penn (1729–1795), last member of the Proprietary Family to serve as Governor of Pennsylvania (1773–1776). — Shepherd, *Proprietary Government in Pennsylvania*, 571–595.
2. In the autumn of 1776, when Hutchinson returned to Philadelphia, the Pennsylvania Hospital was already troubled because of the uncertainties of war, but Hutchinson was given a staff position in surgery. This was soon exchanged for field work in the Army when Philadelphia in 1777 became headquarters of the British Army of Occupation under command of General William Howe. Hutchinson enrolled as surgeon in the Flying Corps of the Middle Department. His first assignment was to inoculate hundreds of soldiers at Valley Forge to prevent an outbreak of smallpox. After the War for Independence, he was appointed to the chair of chemistry in what is now the Medical School of the University of Pennsylvania. It was a difficult period of transition in College and University organization, but he adjusted to the needs of the time and taught chemistry acceptably through years of upset and change until the University was firmly established. In 1793, when yellow fever in its most virulent form struck Philadelphia, Hutchinson fell victim to the disease. — G. W. Corner, *Two Centuries of Medical Education*, 35–42; *Letters of Benjamin Rush*, ed. Butterfield, I, 289, 571, II, 675.

To Dr. William Hird at Leeds, Yorkshire, for S. Hird, 17 October 1776

Harpur Street, London

17.X.1776

Dear Sally —

My sister, at my request, set out last 2nd day morning for Deal,[1] and she gave me leave to open any letter that might come for her from thee. I hesitated some time, but I did it at last, and informed her of its contents, the day after. I told her, likewise, that I should probably tell thee what I had done, and at the same time acquaint thee with the occasion of her journey, lest it might reach our Friends that indisposition was the cause of it, and give them distress.

473

Though we had a favourable summer in Cheshire, yet her allotment was laborious; she was obliged to see more company than either of us desired, and our return to town was to her anxious and affecting. I perceived a kind of weakness in her voice, and a kind of flutter that was unusual to her. I knew that it was the effect of anxiety and unremitting attention to me, to the family, to everybody, nor could I think of any adequate remedy. It occurred to me one evening that if I could prevail upon her easily to leave home for a week or two, and retire to some seaport where she might bathe if she found it convenient, if not to stay there and enjoy repose, I might possibly contribute more to her advantage than by any other means. — Upon a little consideration, she cheerfully complied being convinced of the necessity. My servant accompanied her thither, left her well and accommodated to her satisfaction. I chose this place, as the most retired I knew — and where she will be as little liable to be persecuted as at any place I knew. I proposed her staying two to three weeks just as she found herself disposed — and we are now likely to be separated longer than we have been for these twenty years or near it. I hope it is the proper plan for her recovery. Her disease was labour, and the cure must be rest. She was sensible of it, and we joined in thankfulness for the intimation.

She is in a family of two persons — the mistress of the house and her maid — is accommodated with everything she wants. There is a small Meeting in the place, and one woman Friend who is [especially] well spoken of; there is also a person of Fortune with servants, to whom she is well known, and who will render her every service in her power, yet without tireing. These little particulars I thought would not be disagreeable to thee to be informed of. I am thankful that I am well and need no such recess at present. — I am of some little use here in one respect or another — and at present, neither busy nor idle.

It was with much reluctance that I consented to be named on such a service as that in which we took a small part; [2] I hope at least to our own help at least — and if we either [were able] to hold up the hands of those who were qualified for the service, or gave proofs that we had the fullest unity with it, we are glad. We find by several accounts that the visit has been well received everywhere, and many testimonies given of its utility. — For my own part, I cannot forbear thinking that times of distress are gradually, imperceptibly advancing. The season may not be in my time, but I wish to be prepared for it — if it should. We must be brought to our senses. I do not know that the present times are worse than the preceding, but if we look about for principle and the people who act from it, where are they? — Perhaps amongst the most despised of our society.

Thy kind present came safe. I will endeavour not to forget my promise in acknowledgement. — But be that as it may — thy attention to us gives us the satisfaction it ought to do. I am sorry to hear that C. Hustler[3] is so much indisposed. I know that no care is wanting — but probably a little quiet retreat from unremitting care of a numerous family might possibly be of some use to her. Why might she not seek it at Scarborough? — though she did not bathe except now and then in a Bath of warm Sea-water. It is as near almost as Buxton — which though a very different Water might be as beneficial — and by this time most of the butterflies and insects are retreated from that place.

I have said not a word to the Dr., to Sally,[4] or our kinsfolk, though I forget none of them. — The Dr. will smile when he hears me talk of making orations at my time of life, but I read one only yesterday to a little society of Physick,[5] on the dignity [befitting] a Physician — and it seemed not to be ill-received. The Licentiates have agreed to bring something every quarter, and this was an introductory, the succeeding will relate to particular subjects of Medicine. If our bodies are less harassed than those of our Brethren in the country, our minds are not always less employed than theirs are. — At present we have a very thin, a very healthy and a very poor town. — The West Indians are returning home in Shoals.

Tell Sally, I think she is in my debt. I believe she promised to say upon paper something like the following — that though I never flattered her, yet she has something like regard for me — and would have no objection to stand fair in my opinion. To obtain this — she must practice all the good rules she has heard inculcated. For her encouragement, I will be content with very little incense, and will promise to repay [regard] when I can fairly. — To my Nephew[6] and his family, say that if they look back frequently to the worthy part of their ancestry with a wish to follow their footsteps, they will be the better for it. Not that we doubt of their care in many respects, but we wish them to be above the middling. — To all the progeny of our worthy Father is the gracious regard of heaven extended, and we ought to be abundantly thankful that so many are preserved from the spots and stains of this life.

Farewell, dear Sally, accept this from the brother of my sister, and believe that they are both your affectionate J. and A. Fothergill.

Ms. autograph letter, Port. 22/98, LSFL.

1. Deal, about eight miles from Dover, once commercially important as one of the Cinque Ports, was at this time a quiet seaside place less frequented than the fashionable resorts.

2. Dr. Fothergill had been appointed by the Yearly Meeting as "one of a committee to make a general visit to the meetings throughout the nation . . . He united with a part of the Committee in visiting the meetings of Friends in Lancashire and Yorkshire, his sister accompanying him in the latter." — Crosfield, *Memoirs*, 532, 534.

3. Christiana Hird Hustler, Dr. Hird's sister.

4. Dr. Hird's adolescent daughter by a previous marriage, who was known by the same name as her stepmother, the "Dear Sally" to whom this letter is written.

5. The society formed in 1767 during the licentiates' unsuccessful agitation for admission to the fellowship in the Royal College of Physicians. Dr. Fothergill was president of this society at the time of his death.

6. Dr. Fothergill's nephew John, Alexander's son, who had married Mary Ann Forbes of London. They now lived in Leeds and were the parents of three children — Mary Ann, John, and a baby, Alexander. — Register of the Fothergill Family, in the papers of the late Miss Mabyn Fothergill of Edinburgh.

To David Barclay, London, 1777?

21st Inst

When I reflect, my dear Friend, on the disregard, call it by no harsher name, with which our opinions have been uniformly treated, though the events have shown them to be not imprudent ones, it affords me but a melancholy proof that everything we can suggest will either be totally neglected or adopted by halves. For these considerations I am against offering any opinion at all, on a strong presumption that what [I] may offer will just share the fate with our former endeavors.

Two years ago, nay, one year, I believe we should neither of us have hesitated to go even to America, and had our powers been *what they ought to have been* — at the former period we should have prevented independency and at the latter [formed] a firm commercial compact and prevented desolations that will, whilst history remains, disgrace the annals of this unhappy country. Treated, however, as we have been, I will please myself with the hope that what may now be suggested by us will be better attended to, and therefore put down the result of our conversation last night as still my opinion.

That the matter is too far advanced for any private person to do any public good is most certain.[1] Perhaps all modes of preventing the approaching calamities will be utterly ineffectual.

I still think that Lord Stormont should leave Paris, as coming home on his private affairs, or to be sent to some other place. That another should be sent in his place — not obnoxious to Versailles, nor unknown to Franklin. That *his* instructions should be only: Say to F———, What measures can at this juncture be adopted, most for the benefit of this country and America? — And these to be adopted by us, *bona fide*.

A single reservation will destroy the whole, and render this attempt as ineffectual as all the expedients have been hitherto.

It requires an amplitude of heart, which I fear is not to be met with, to save us from ruin. But it must be on a ground like this that we can be saved if we are [to be] so. Two months ago a private person thus instructed might have done everything. It must now be the business of a man in a public and responsible character.

I am, thy afflicted Friend,

J.F.

Ms. autograph letter, Barclay Papers, Gurney Collection; printed in Fox, 353–354.

1. This letter, insufficiently dated, was written probably in December 1777, after news of Burgoyne's surrender at Saratoga had reached England. In London there were still advocates of giving the Americans suitable commonwealth standing, and David Barclay had made notes of another plan for conciliation, based on the Hints of 1774 and the Plan of 1775. Franklin, as Commissioner at the Court of Louis XVI in France, did not support this idea. To him, now, it was a war for independence the Americans were fighting; moreover, Franklin and the British ambassador, Lord Stormont, were not able to establish diplomatic accord. Stormont believed Franklin was corresponding under an assumed name with British politicians, while there was evidence that Stormont was himself engaging in secret negotiations with the great continental Powers to partition the American Colonies among them in return for aid in this war, which without allies Britain seemed to be losing. England, according to Stormont's reasoning, would by this plan have been relieved of her intolerable burden of rebellious colonies; the Great Powers would have gained territory in the New World, and the American Colonies, no longer united, would have been reduced to their proper status of dependency. — Fox, 353, 407; Richard B. Morris, *The Peacemakers* (New York: Harper and Row, 1965).

To Benjamin Franklin, 1777–1778?

There is, I doubt [not], one man in this Kingdom who was permitted to be born for its chastisement, if not destruction.[1] By education, by flattery, by disposition, capable of supposing himself superior to every other mortal — unfeeling — unalterable. Persuaded there is no virtuous principle in mankind, and that nobody serves him but for interest — determined to make it their interest to serve him, and with such he is surrounded. Entreaties, petitions are disregarded and their promoters stamped indelibly in the pages of vengeance and disgrace. Vice overlooked, impiety not discouraged, everything overlooked in those who have the will or the ability to flatter and support.

But what has brought us into such a situation? We have long enjoyed the privilege of being as good, as virtuous, and consequently as happy as mortals could be, and we have neglected and forsaken everything that could have made us great and happy.

At the eve of a war with united Nations,[2] the least of whom is at least our match, — we are part of us immersed in pleasures, part in securing their retreat from power with pensions and revenues. Totally disregarding the public good — the few who might be expected to step forward to aid our counsels, disunited, each pursuing his own opinion and opposing that of others, even a trifle superior. From such a state of things what can be hoped for? Nothing. Never was the justice of an Almighty providence more displayed than by thus reducing a powerful, enlightened and yet haughty nation to the threshold of destruction for their impious rejection of every dependence upon it, and plunging into war for causes the most unjust. I forget to whom I am writing, but my heart is full of regard for all that has been connected with Britain, as ever. Save this devoted country from irretrievable ruin if possible — keep back the vengeance of F.[3] as long as can be done. Were the authors of our misfortune to suffer, I should repine the less — but the sword makes no distinction.

Forgive the wretched inhabitants of P.[4] if they sided strongly, from principle some of them and others from inclination, with their present masters; they have been severely chastised for it, and still are. Attribute it to the weakness of their understanding and their honesty — for this was really the case — and not to their hearts. Take no advantage of their mistakes; they are smarting under a rod sufficiently severe; and I find it has made many converts.

We are here of opinion that good fortune still awaits us; that you will quarrel and yet become an easy prey; that the Nation will rise as one man to assert their superiority over every other Kingdom, and though one arm is cut off and the other tied behind her, yet Britain by only showing her teeth will affright every foe. Is not this judicial blindness? From sheer ignorance and imposition the majority here has been against you; but feeling has no fellow, and we now begin to feel in good earnest, but it is only the beginning. Public and private credit are fast, very fast declining, yet one man refuses his consent to any change of measures.

How often have I pleaded with all within my reach to send full powers to treat for a commercial union? I knew my friend's liberality of sentiment, his love to this country and many in it, would make him forget the injuries he had received, and have said that I knew he was incapable of admitting the behaviour of those who had strove to disgrace him, even for a single moment, to prevent him from cooperating for the public lasting benefit of both countries. But where must I end? With the most fervent wishes for the long life and health and immortal happiness of all who are disinterested Friends to the liberties of Morika.[5]

Is it not worth a trial to endeavour to excite the operation of virtuous principle to the benefit of community rather than solely aiming at defending it against the worst parts of human nature? Perhaps a list of fame and another of infamy would operate greatly to the publick good, as China in the best parts of its empire has experienced. Let him who has distinguished himself for virtuous deeds, however humble the objects or his situation, be put on the list of fame for a period proportional to the benefits or exertions. Let him who has behaved amiss be condemned to the list of infamy, and let those be deemed infamous who — not being his immediate relations — countenance him. Cannot at least a part of human malignity be opposed in this manner, in a way more consistent with the reason of man, as well as with the general spirit of the Gospel?

Try one experiment: abolish all oaths and affirmations as the evidence of truth. Let it rest on the simple assertion. Truth ought never to be made so cheap as to have it suspected that under certain formalities it is a crime to forsake her; and that without those formalities she is of no consequence. In short nothing seems to patronize falsehood so much as maintaining a supposition that truth is not at all times of equal reverence. Let falsehood be punished as perjury. The Quakers furnish a proof that oaths are not absolutely necessary, and I know that to some of them the affirmation permitted them in England is considered a reproach and degrading to the dignity of human nature. What, says one of them, have I done to give occasion to suppose that I do not speak truth at all times? Let it be declared that though such kind of formalities are dropped, yet

479

it is expected that a still greater reverence should be paid to truth, and that it should be made a part of universal education; that a deviation would be punished by consigning the transgressor to lasting infamy; and that if parents wished their children to avoid such a sentence, it must be their fixed resolution to keep to truth inviolably. To suggest an idea conducive to support good government on a principle consistent with the dignity of human nature will not be deemed improper, when a plan of government is under consideration of the most extensive and, it is hoped, of the most durable nature.

Would it not be consistent with sound policy to avoid as much as possible enacting any laws for the recovery of debts, and to encourage as much as possible what may be called a ready-money trade? There can be only a certain quantity of commerce in the world: the more equally this commerce is diffused, the more numerous are those who are benefited by it.

A man trusting to the laws for the recovery of his property entrusts a person of reputed credit with a large share of his property. The person so entrusted increases his reputation by this very means, and carries on a share of commerce which would have supported many families. He grows negligent, vicious, extravagant, and squanders, in excess or in injudicious projects, the substance of multitudes — falls into disgrace, and lives on a portion of his spoils, and spreads ruin and distress, even to the unborn. This is the consequence of supposing there are laws by which we can recover our substance, when we have entrusted them to the end of that time where the necessity of self-preservation begins.

In cases of trust such laws should be provided. If A, who has a numerous family of children, trusts B whom he thinks is a man of inflexible integrity with a part of his substance and dies, it is necessary that the children of A should as far as possible be secured from any loss that might arise from their Father's good opinion of B's honor and ability. If in this country all the laws of recovery and the bankruptcy laws were abolished, it would be a happiness to this country. Every man should trade according to his real not reputed ability.

Ms. letter in Dr. Fothergill's hand, Franklin Papers, APS, LVI, pt. 1, no. 12.

1. This letter is unaddressed, undated, and without salutation, conclusion, or signature. It probably reached Franklin in France, and was put away among his papers, which were later sent to Philadelphia; some of its pages may have been mislaid or lost during the packing and unpacking required. The letter, however, gives

evidence of Dr. Fothergill's intense concern for his own country as well as for the American cause. The view of King George III expressed indicates a decided *volte-face* since Dr. Fothergill's letter to J. Pemberton, 2 November 1761 (above), which was filled with admiration for the King upon his accession to the throne.

2. Official word of the Franco-American alliance, signed 6 February 1778, was given to the British Government by the French Ambassador on 13 March. — Van Doren, *Benjamin Franklin*, 594–595.

3. France.

4. Philadelphia. Many of the Pennsylvania Quakers had steadily refused to have anything to do with the war.

5. A rather transparent disguise for America.

To James Pemberton, Winchester, Virginia, 24 April 1778

London, 24.4.1778

Dear Friend,

If this comes to thy hand it may inform thee that I have received, I believe, all thy kind letters together with the Epistle from the Yearly Meeting, an abstract of their Transactions, and a printed copy of your Testimony. These will be laid before our ensuing Yearly Meeting, and whilst the matters contained in them will afford a good degree of satisfaction, will call forth much sympathy and affectionate commiseration.[1]

What intelligence we have received from the several Colonies amounts to this: that like what happened in former times and now happens to you, and may if Providence so permits, be our own lot, affliction though grievous for the present, may work to general good.

Your part is a clear one. Be quiet, mind your own proper business.[2] If your kingdom is not of this world, mind that only which we look for and are taught by the highest Authority to seek. To me it appears that the whole British Empire must be humbled. There is not a nation in the known world that has either been more enlightened in respect to their duties, more at liberty to perform these duties, or less attentive to perform them. Is it not then high time that we should be raised to some attention? Shall we murmur that this is actually coming to pass? Let us then look hither and not at the part we would wish to act, in regard to this party or that. The Kingdom we profess to seek is not of this world — leave the world then to contend for its own.

We are very little sensible yet in this country of the calamities that are gradually and imperceptibly advancing to awaken us from our lethargy. Be more attentive to inculcate a regard to that which has been the cause of this deserved awakening than how to gain the favour of this party or of that. There is a Power above all worldly contrivances. You, many of you, know this and let this be your guide.

We are too little alive in this country to such considerations. But through a degree of divine regard vouchsafed, many are awakened and awakening to better considerations — to prepare to bear the distresses that may be permitted, to be qualified to render help as it may be wanted. I cannot enter into any particulars. My sentiments might give offence to one side or the other — and I am attached to neither, any farther than as the common interests of my country, of my profession, and of mankind in general demand from every reasonable being.

Be quiet and mind your own business; promote every good work, show yourselves subject to that invisible overruling Providence which guides all things for the good of that immortal part which is made to subsist, not only after all the transient outrages are at an end, but through endless Ages.

Farewell, my Friend. My Sister desires to be remembered to all the faithful amongst you, as well as thy Friend,

J. Fothergill

Ms. autograph letter, Pemberton Papers, Etting Collection, IV, 178, HSP.

1. Since September 1777 James Pemberton had been interned at Winchester, Virginia, as one of a group of Quakers found "notoriously disaffected" and "inimical to the patriot cause." Because of religious scruples, many among the older generation of the Society of Friends in Philadelphia had declined to take oath or make affirmation of allegiance to the State. They also refused participation of any kind in the colonists' war effort. Rumors of a Quaker plot to furnish information to the British had alarmed some Congressional leaders, but it was by action of the Council of Safety of Pennsylvania that actual arrest of the suspects was made and their transport to Virginia arranged. Among those taken to Winchester were Israel, James, and John Pemberton; Thomas Gilpin, John Hunt, and Thomas Wharton, Sr. Since many of the exiles were elderly, the winter of 1777–78 brought suffering. Thomas Gilpin and John Hunt died; Israel Pemberton fell severely ill. Through the efforts of Mary Pemberton, Israel's wife, a wagonland of provisions, clothing, and medical supplies was sent to Winchester with General Washington's approval. Mrs. Pemberton, "despite her seventy-five years," had journeyed over rough winter roads to interview Washington and to plead for release of the prisoners. Unfortunately, this was a matter beyond the General's control. He advised application to Congress, then sitting in York during the British occupation of Philadelphia. Congress refused to consider the prisoners under its jurisdiction; it was a question for the Executive Council of the State of Pennsylvania to decide. Release was at last obtained for the exiles, who reached Philadelphia 30 April 1778. — *Letters of Members of the Continental Con-*

gress, ed. Burnett, II, 471, 476–477, 481, 486–487 (Letters 619, 627, 633, 634); Thomas Gilpin, *Exiles in Virginia, with Observations on the Conduct of the Society of Friends during the Revolutionary War* (Philadelphia, 1848), privately published for subscribers by his grandson and namesake Thomas Gilpin III.

2. Dr. Fothergill's favorite Biblical motto: "And that ye study to be quiet, and to do your own business, and to work with your own hands, as we commanded you" (I Thessalonians 4:11).

To an unnamed correspondent, 30 November 1778

Harpur Street, London,
November 30, 1778

This day fortnight I found, on waking out of a short sleep, a forcible inclination to make water, but without the power. I had perceived some heat and unusual difficulty, for a day or two. I immediately got up, took a saline laxative which I had in the house; and found myself so much better next morning, as to go on my usual round of business. In the night I was seized with a total retention. I was bled, had repeated injections instantly but to no effect. I took oily and highly anodyne draughts; and, without the least mitigation of pain, took upwards of 200 drops of Tincture Thebaica [1] in the space of a very few hours, which barely mitigated my distress; till, after repeated and fruitless attempts to draw off the water, with grievous suffering to myself, and no small difficulty to the most experienced operator in Britain, we at length succeeded. I still continue under the necessity of having it drawn off twice a day, not a drop passing without it; but the operation becomes daily rather less painful to myself, and less difficult to my friend Percival Pott,[2] who attends me.

The immediate cause of this difficulty seems to be a great thickening of the neck of the bladder, which was the effect of inflammation. This, being a recent cause, and all fever now removed, will probably ere long give way. — To this another cause is added, which will require attention hereafter, if I am permitted to survive; an enlarged, but not otherwise morbid, prostate gland.[3]

Extract, correspondent unnamed; printed in *Works*, ed. Lettsom, III, 304–305. Dr. Fothergill's medical report of his own illness was probably sent to another physician. The original letter has disappeared.

1. A powerful preparation of opium.

2. Percival Pott (1714–1788), London's most distinguished eighteenth-century surgeon, began medical training when apprenticed at fifteen to Edward Nourse, who supervised his career during seven years in St. Bartholomew's Hospital. Pott's ability and skill won early attention. He also became known for his brilliant lectures; students and doctors from all over London and many intelligent laymen flocked to Barts to hear him. In 1764 he was elected Fellow of the Royal Society of London. His publications include: *A Treatise on Ruptures* (1756); *Some Few Remarks on Fractures and Dislocations* (1769); *Remarks on that kind of Palsy which is found to accompany Curvature of the Spine* (1779), reporting an outstanding discovery. Pott's methods were original and his observation keen. His name was affixed to many conditions because of his thorough and accurate descriptions. "Pott's fracture," "Pott's curvature," and "Pott's aneurysm" are still terms well known to members of the medical profession.

3. Acute urinary obstruction, resulting from hypertrophy of the prostate gland, produced this attack. Two years later, a recurrence of this extremely painful illness caused Dr. Fothergill's death. Three prominent London physicians, Dr. Richard Warren, Dr. (later Sir) William Watson, and Dr. Henry Revell Reynolds, attended the patient, together with his experienced surgeon, Percival Pott. An account of Dr. Fothergill's final illness, with a drawing of the pathological condition found at autopsy, was published by Dr. John Coakley Lettsom in his edition of Dr. Fothergill's *Works* (III, 303–313). Reviewing this case from a modern standpoint, Dr. Willard A. Goodwin, Professor of Urology at the University of California, Los Angeles, comments (personal communication) that it was probably caused by benign enlargement of the median lobe, a not uncommon form of prostatic hypertrophy usually readily cured by modern surgery.

To Catherine Phillips, 5 December 1778

London, 12th Mo., 5th, 1778.

Dear Friend,[1]

Thy very affectionate letter to my sister revived the remembrance of that friendship which has so long subsisted between my brother, thyself, and us, so strongly, that I rather chose to answer it myself. Through unmerited favour, I am in a probable way of recovery, though yet far from well. My disorder was at first a common cold; I struggled with it, under a necessity of great application, till at length it was accidentally increased, and brought on other complaints. I form hopes that by degrees it will give way. My appetite and strength are gradually returning, and though yet unfit for going abroad, I am easy and content.

I cannot express, in a short compass, the feelings of my mind on this trying occasion. I have only to look back to that point when, if I had not been relieved, I must in twenty-four hours have been numbered with the dead, and saw it most clearly, with humbling gratitude for a degree of calm resignation to the Divine will, secretly trusting in his power, goodness, and mercy. And may I never forget the season. Anxiety and fear united, have presented themselves; but I endeavoured to be quiet, and to trust in him who alone is worthy to be confided in for ever. What may now await me I know not. I know too well my own inability to help myself, and to stay me where I ought to remain, without assistance above my own resolutions. I shall wish, however, to detach myself from the world, as occasion may offer, and to which this dispensation may, I hope, contribute. I have not hurried into these numerous engagements, so far as I know of myself, from any other motive than those which urged me on to do the business of the present hour with diligence, whether in the duty of my profession, the common calls of life, or the affairs of the Society.

This plunge will oblige me to make some choice, and its being so generally known will serve me as a just plea for refusing many embarrassing distant engagements. Such are my views and my desires at present, and I humbly trust that goodness and mercy, which has given me my life as a prey, will not leave me. Indeed, the general and cordial regard manifested to me, by Friends and others, lays a strong obligation to gratitude upon me, and would prompt a desire to repay it. But I must not give way. I have hitherto done all I could to serve all within my reach, and it is a satisfaction to feel that I have not served an ungenerous nor ungrateful public.

Thus, my dear Friend, I have endeavored to give thee a just state of our condition. We know thy present desires for our good, and may they be still continued, when access is granted.

J. & A. Fothergill.

Printed in Crosfield, *Memoirs*, 538–540.

1. Catherine Payton, long-time friend and associate of Samuel Fothergill in the Quaker ministry, in 1772 had married William Phillips, a Quaker minister, member of a Cornish family. — *Memoirs of the Life of Catherine Phillips* (London: Printed and sold by James Phillips and Son, 1797), 215.

To Dr. William Hird, Butterworth's Yard, Leeds, 22 December 1778

Harpur Street London 22.12.1778

Dear Kinsman,

It is with much satisfaction that I can inform thee I continue to recover daily. It was near three weeks from the time I was seized before any water was voided spontaneously, and then but a little at a time, and with considerable difficulty. It is now about a week since I had an occasion for manual assistance, and I mend every day in ability to make it; the passibility, the quantity at a time is larger, and I begin to feel the sensations of usual satisfaction. At some time I may perhaps describe this affair more particularly, as a few circumstances attended it that may possibly be useful to others to be made acquainted with. I rose this morning for the first time to breakfast with my family. I see my Friends at home and some patients. I propose to keep to the house this week, and perhaps next I may venture abroad. My sister is daily improving likewise, so that Sally [1] has rather a less gloomy prospect about her than when she first gave us her company. She is well, cheerful and contented at present with her situation. Not but that she has very strong attractions homeward, but with pleasure I believe she at present makes a sacrifice of inclination to duty. We are abundantly pleased with her attention to us, and shall readily give her up when home becomes the most desirable place.

There will, I expect, be a great number of Friends with you next week [2] and many who I know will interest themselves not a little in our welfare. I thought it would be agreeable both to thyself and to them to have it within thy power to inform them that we are both advancing to our usual state of health, and I do not foresee much possibility of a return of this disease, as I hope to take care to guard against it as much as I can.

I think it a great favour that I was preserved during the whole of this afflicting season in patience and resignation, clearly perceiving the danger I was in if relief had not been very seasonably obtained, and at the same time preserving a hope that I might be restored. I hope I may often look back to this critical season with gratitude and reverence, and that it may be a means to shake off some encumbrances. — But this is not wholly in my own power. I trust nevertheless that the instructive season will never be forgot.

I do not long together omit considering the proposition I made, and shall keep it constantly in mind, watching carefully for the proper season of stepping farther. Till then go on cheerfully with business as usual; whenever I can proceed farther with satisfaction, depend upon hearing from me and in the meanwhile consider it as a thing most probably, not immediately, approaching, yet as likely to take place at some future day, when it may be more convenient and agreeable to both sides.[3]

We continue to have mild, temperate weather and neither very wet nor tempestuous. I am so inured to the house that I scarcely know how to face the world again — and at present I have enough cut out for me to acknowledge the kind inquiries of many — my list amounts to near 600!

Remember me to Sally,[4] and tell her I am much obliged to her for her kind concern. I admire her sensibility, it's the companion of an ingenious mind. Some time or other I hope I shall see her and express my acknowledgment in person. My Sister remembers her also affectionately. Tell Christy and her husband[5] I know they have been distressed for us — indeed we have had all our Friends under a heavy contribution — all that we can do is to return a just and grateful sense of it. In retirement I never had more love to Friends than I have now, and I know theirs is reciprocal. I dare not undertake to say what Sally[6] feels, but I know she is full of affection for you all and joins me in this remembrance of it.

Thy
J. & A. Fothergill

Ms. autograph letter, Port. 22/99, LSFL.

1. Dr. Hird's daughter Sally, a girl of seventeen, who was a welcome visitor in the Harpur Street household during Dr. Fothergill's convalescence. — Hird Genealogy, LSFL.

2. Friends assembling for their local Quarterly Meeting.

3. During his illness Dr. Fothergill had apparently considered handing over his practice to Dr. Hird, or at least establishing a partnership.

4. Mrs. Hird, Dr. Fothergill's favorite niece.

5. Dr. Hird's sister Christiana and her husband John Hustler. — Hird Genealogy, LSFL.

6. Reference here is obviously to young Sally, Dr. Hird's daughter.

To Dr. and Mrs. Thomas Knowles, Lombard Street, London, 23 December 1778

Dr. Fothergill presents his kind respects to Dr. & Mrs. Knowles [1] and is much obliged to them for their kind enquiries. He is considerably better, and daily advancing towards his usual state of health.

Harpur Street 23rd Inst.

This note of thanks was one of many gratefully written by Dr. Fothergill in response to letters of felicitation from his friends. Contributed by Miss Ursula Somervell of Cambridge, England.

1. Dr. Thomas Knowles, a Quaker physician of Yorkshire birth, received his medical degree at Leyden in 1772 and was admitted Licentiate of the Royal College of Physicians in 1774 (*Munk's Roll*, II, 342, 343). His wife Mary (1733–1787) was much admired by Dr. Johnson for her animation and conversational powers, as well as for her "subtile pictures" in intricate crewel needlework. — Boswell, *Samuel Johnson*, ed. Ingpen, II, 661, 786–788.

To Alexander Fothergill at Carr End, 4 February 1779

London, 4.2.1779

Dear Brother,

Before this arrives, I hope you will have received from C. Palmer £600 in 6 Bank post bills. — I inclose a bank note of £40 which I hope will come in due time to answer the present exigencies. — I was obliged to borrow the money of C. Palmer, having been obliged to pay away a good deal of money lately, and have scarce any income except from my daily labor — Nobody thinking it ever worth their while to pay me either principal or interest of the money I have lent, and I must now desire thee in good earnest to settle this matter in such a way, as I may receive some benefit from it, for it is impossible for me to last long under the daily labour I undergo to support others — The losses, the expenses, I have had were it only from thy own family, (and I do not mean this by way of reflection) are such, as would have afforded me, with that little I have remaining, some tolerable provision against old age. — I beg therefore that my interest may be considered — and such a produce allowed me as another might reasonably claim.[1] — But I will say little more on this subject farther than that as I do not wish to oppress anyone for my benefit, so I do not think it right, that I should be perpetually laboring at the expense of time, care, anxiety, in the close of life, when I ought to be entitled to some ease for the benefit of those who ought to take some care for themselves. I must desire thee not to make free with riding on horseback — even in a chaise it will retard thy recovery — if not endanger thee more than is expedient. — I have only time to add that we continue tolerably well, and shall be glad to hear of thy continued amendment.

I am almost sorry that William [2] did not close with the proposal I made to him some time since in respect to applying himself to acquire some little knowledge in medicine. — His tenderness makes him wholly unfit for the hardships of Husbandry, at least it seems so by these frequent returns. However, I must leave it with you to act as you think best. — My Sister joins me in warm desires for your welfare in every respect from

thy affectionate Brother

J. Fothergill

Ms. autograph letter, Fothergill Family Papers of the late Miss Mabyn Fothergill, now in the care of her brother, Mr. Edward Fothergill of Edinburgh.

1. Alexander's financial problems were a constant concern to his brother, who had given him considerable financial assistance during his difficulties in 1772 (see manuscript autograph letter from Dr. Fothergill to Alexander Fothergill 29 November 1772, Wallis collection, not included here). In 1762 part of the Carr End property had been mortgaged by Alexander to Thomas Simpson of Richmond, Yorkshire, for £400. On 22 November 1778 Dr. Fothergill had paid £400 to John Newsome, legatee of Thomas Simpson deceased, for the transfer of the mortgage. Now, in February 1779, Dr. Fothergill was sending a further £600 to repay a Richard Seymour to whom the remainder of the property had been mortgaged. The mortgage was then transferred to Dr. Fothergill for £1000. Since both brothers were old and ailing, Alexander recovering from an abscess on the ankle and the doctor from an extremely painful and dangerous illness, it is not surprising that the tone of this letter is uncharacteristically querulous. — Ms. indentures included among the title deeds of Carr End, inspected through the courtesy of Mr. Frank Outhwaite; Ms. letters of Alexander Fothergill to Dr. Fothergill, Port. 38/111; LSFL.

2. Alexander's son, who continued in farming at Carr End.

To Dr. William Hird, Leeds, Yorkshire, September? 1779

Lea Hall near Middlewich, Cheshire

22nd Inst. 1779

My dear Relations,

As we are now preparing to leave this quiet retreat, I could not easily quit it without telling you we often and affectionately remember you, and shall do wherever we are.

Next second day, we propose to go to Buxton, and if Bathing agrees with my Sister to stay there a couple of weeks and then to repair to the busy scene of London. I believe we shall take Hannah Jepson [1] with us, and I hope to her benefit.

We have had but little respite from company ever since we came hither, but it was our Friends' kindness, and we ought to be satisfied with it, and with many we were much so. R. Morris and his wife left us this morning and we were glad of their company. I shall go back to London with a load of writing to do there in the midst of business instead of discharging some unavoidable debts here, which I had fondly expected to have had time here to pay. But I am tolerably well in health, and with other matters I must do the best I can.

My Sister has, I think, improved considerably this last week or ten days and as she is now wholly free from pain, I hope the temperate Baths of Buxton may be serviceable to her. It is a place I do not like, but the time will not be long and if she gets better, everything will be well. We shall have a little [more] chance of quiet now than in the full season, and I think I shall attempt to make use of the waters. I have wrote to Dr. Bullock [2] to desire him to seek us accommodation at the Hall; one bathes there with much the greater convenience.

We are pleased that it so fell out that we had more of your company than I expected when we first set out; and though my Sister was a rather distressing object than otherwise, yet your kindness and ready attention made us feel as if we were at home. We are both sensible of your affectionate concern for us, and we shall hope, if we find ourselves again under your roof, that we neither of us give you any anxiety.

I have been endeavouring to assist Ackworth [3] as well as I could, and have found a young man here who, I hope, may answer as a Schoolmaster.[4] I wish he could be a fortnight under the hands of a Drill Sergeant — to teach him only how to walk — but that is among ourselves. Schoolmasters often strut sufficiently, but they should learn sometimes to do it with a good grace, for the sake of example. But we must take him as he is. I think likewise I have found another person that may be of use to us as a manservant, viz., Samuel Goodwin, perhaps Sally will remember a lad of that name who lived with our dear deceased Brother Samuel at [the time of] his death. He is a sober young man, lives as a servant with his father-in-law in Staffordshire, and wants to be more among Friends. He is nine miles from a Friends Meeting to which he often walks. I hope the business will go on prosperously, however slowly. I have mentioned the persons above mentioned to J. Hustler.[5]

We shall be glad of a line from either of you at Buxton during our stay there, and should be pleased to hear your Quarterly Meeting is to your satisfaction. I could wish to see our Society a little more awake to the difficulties that are approaching, and hastening themselves a little more to seek for a place of shelter when the storm approaches. The idea of pacification is groundless. We are rushing into perdition with a vehemence that renders all counsel of peace fruitless. If affairs should turn out much better than is expected, we shall suffer nothing by being prepared for the worst.

I feel a warmth of affection for you that gives me pleasure. Remember us to Sally — I hear she has thought of a trip to Ireland.[6] In better times I should not have objected to it; I should have wished it. As it is, I wish those who are stationed there by duty, preservation amidst dangers greater than our own.[7] We love you much, and are your affectionate

J. & A. Fothergill

Ms. autograph letter, Port. 21/142, LSFL.

1. Daughter of Dr. Fothergill's brother Joseph.

2. Dr. Bullock is not mentioned in *Munk's Roll*.

3. The new Friends' school which Dr. Fothergill had been instrumental in founding. See Introduction, above.

4. This young man, Joseph Donabend, was given an early appointment at Ackworth and kept his position for thirty-eight years. — Elfrida Vipont, *Ackworth School* (London: Lutterworth, 1959), 31.

5. Dr. Hird's brother-in-law, John Hustler of Bradford, who actively supported construction of the Leeds and Liverpool Canal, served Ackworth School as a trustee for many years.

6. Mrs. Hird had been planning to visit her sister Molly, Mrs. Robert Watson of Waterford, Ireland.

7. Both a French invasion of Ireland and a revolt of the oppressed Irish against the Crown were threatened at this time, while the British army was engaged in America. — Green, *History of the English People*, IV, 266.

To Henry Zouch, Sandal, Yorkshire, 8 October 1779

London, 8th of the 10th mo. 1779

Though I am very apprehensive that the subject of this letter will be of very little consequence, yet I could not easily forego an opportunity of mentioning to thyself [1] some sentiments that have occurred to me in respect to the very important meeting about to be held at York.[2]

I know my voice is feeble and insignificant; but being a native of the county, and having a great regard for it, on this and many other accounts, I think I ought not to be totally silent on so important an occasion, though I know there are so many persons will be present, who, in every respect but one, I acknowledge to be greatly indeed my superiors; — that one is, a disinterested and impartial regard for the good of my native county, and the influence it will hold in the great national business that will come before you.

If the motions made for retrenchments in expence are to be the basis of your deliberations and petitions, I think them altogether unworthy; — all that could be obtained in these retrenchments, either by savings to the public treasury, or abridging the power of the crown, are beneath the notice of such an assembly, even were you sure of obtaining all you have in contemplation. — I am morally certain you will obtain nothing: and every unsuccessful contest disheartens the vanquished, and in proportion adds vigour to the conqueror.

Have we not seen this to be the case, in all the petitions and remonstrances that have been presented? and is it not most certain that the majority will be doubly firm against you, as their interest is so much at stake?

I consider these motions as well intended, and they may be followed by others equally economical and wise; but they will all be rejected, and those who have stood forth in their support be discouraged.

There is one necessary point, which I think you ought in the first place to state most clearly — the general decay of the county — and keep close to your own; manufactures declining, commerce languishing, value of land decaying, all public improvements at a stand, bankruptcies numerous, taxes increasing, multitudes distressed, and, was it not for the late favourable seasons, universal poverty and wretchedness must have taken place. Pray, therefore, that peace may be restored between us and America, as the only means of saving your county from every species of calamity; — the war with that country, and its consequences, having been the general causes of these distresses. — I do not mean that these expressions should be used; you will find much better; but if you do not lay the axe to the root, in vain do you attempt the branches.

Let not a single reflection on the King or the ministry escape you — I mean not to appear in your petition. The acrimony that loaded the American petitions, and disgraced many of our own, have done unspeakable mischief; I beg therefore, and earnestly entreat, that every degree of invective may be shunned. Produce your facts, and state them in the clearest light; but if you mean well to your country, and wish to see an example followed in other counties, shun every thing offensive. As there is no great room for flattery, so neither give way to the reverse temper; — if you do, posterity may load your memories with deserved reproach.

Forgive me for thus offering my sentiments to men much better informed than myself; but it is my firm opinion, from the knowledge I have of the temper of those who must be the judges of your petitions, that so sure as you deviate from a line of language, temperate yet firm, so sure will you shut a door more closely against all that you can urge; — and what must be the consequence? A perseverance in the same measures, to do despite to those who condemned them. Once more, therefore, let me entreat that every thing manifestly offensive in language may be studiously avoided; that no bagatelles may be asked for, but the removal of the great cause of expence — the war with America: the lesser arrangements of economy may then be solicited, and these only to take place at the decease of the present occupants.

Once more excuse me, if I am taking a liberty unbecoming me; — the honour of our county, the good of the country in general, are at stake. If you ask for what is evidently great and right, your example will be followed by all; if you ask for things which you know beforehand will be refused, let your numbers be ever so great, you may possibly meet with many counter-petitions, and an attempt for general reformation be stifled in its infancy.[3]

J. Fothergill

Fothergill, *Works*, ed. Lettsom, III, clxix–clxxiii.

1. Henry Zouch (1725–1795), for many years vicar of Sandal Magna, Yorkshire, and sometime chaplain to the Marchioness of Rockingham, was also a justice of the peace, active in social reforms, and, according to Lettsom, an intimate friend of Dr. Fothergill.
2. Hardships resulting from the war with the American colonies — and since March 1778 with France — had been felt severely throughout the country and had intensified inchoate agitation for economy and the elimination of corruption in governmental spending, for making Parliament more responsive to the electorate, and for thus curtailing the power of the Crown. In Yorkshire, the strongest and wealthiest county

in England, form was being supplied to the movement under the leadership of some two hundred prominent residents. The large meeting of more than six hundred freeholders held at York on 30 December 1779 set an example for other counties, and was a positive step toward the organization of the forces of reform. — George Otto Trevelyan, *George the Third and Charles Fox* (London: Longmans, 1912–1914), II, 206–213.

3. This letter, Lettsom says, "I am informed was read in a committee of the above meeting, and met with the most pointed approbation."

To Joseph Priestley, 24 July 1780

Near Middlewich, 7th Mo., 24th, 1780.

. . . It is my fervent wish that all the professors of Christianity may be more anxious to live Christian lives, than either in advancing the consequence of the sect, or reflecting on our fellow-servants, and our brethren, the sons of the same Father.

I called at Ackworth on my way hither, and find we have made a pretty prosperous beginning. Above 80 girls and 150 boys are assembled, in less than ten months. The head of the house is made for it, and teachers we are making as fast as we can: the children are already moulded into excellent order, and are clean and attentive. The beginning is prosperous, the event must be left. To establish young minds in truth, and erase the prejudices that may have been sown, is a great object with me. Reading, writing, and arithmetic for the boys, and for the girls the addition of necessary female employments, are there taken care of. To give them an early inclination of acting uprightly, doing to all as they would desire others to do to them, even in the most trivial concerns of life, is a matter I very much wish to have *kneaded* into all their instruction. If they can act so as to avoid the reproaches of their own minds in the first place, and then be able to act such a part as to feel from it interior approbation, they never will slide far from the paths of rectitude. The power of Heaven alone can do the rest.

One word more, and I will release thee. Take care of thy health — remit all study — write but little — use moderate exercise; establish good health by these means, then work and welcome.[1]

J.F.

Extract printed in Crosfield, *Memoirs*, 541.

1. The confidential tone of this message suggests the close friendship between Dr.

Fothergill and his patient, Joseph Priestley (1733–1804), the distinguished scientist and liberal theologian. Their acquaintance presumably began at some time when Dr. Fothergill was visiting his brother Samuel in Warrington, where in the 1760's Priestley was a classical tutor at Warrington Academy. Dr. Fothergill for years made an annual financial contribution toward Priestley's studies of the atmosphere, and was instrumental in securing other contributions. — Fox, 215, citing Priestley's *Memoirs*.

To Dr. William Hird, Leeds, 16 September 1780

Lea Hall, near Middlewich, Cheshire
16.9.1780

Dear Doctor,

I received thy acceptable and I may add rather long expected letter. We were anxious to know the situation of our poor Friend who we now understand is no more. We likewise wanted to hear of your welfare. The cloth came safely to hand, but as it is so near our departure I think we shall send it as it is to London and make use of it there.

I am rather expecting we shall see you again on our return home. We propose to leave this place this week, the 23rd, be at Manchester the 24th and by reaching Little Brough get to you on second day night on our way, perhaps with some of thy family, to York Quarterly Meeting. Perhaps we may stay with our relations there some part of the sixth day and get to Pontefract and Ackworth to the committee second day following.[1]

I have been labouring closely with my pen every vacant hour since I came hither, not for myself but on the Yearly Meeting Minutes.[2] I finished all I can do at present, yesterday afternoon. A week's respite to me here would have been pleasing and perhaps useful. But the progress we propose prevents it. As our Friend D.B. has given up so much of his time and wishes I could meet the Friends there, I cannot but yield to his desire, who has sacrificed so much of his time and labour to this very important undertaking.

As soon as we had fully settled, I thought it would be right to give you this information. We would like to be your guests, if you please, and bring with us Dr. Waterhouse. We expect him here by the Coach on third day. He comes that we may have a little more conversation on several points that concern him, on our journey, as he will embark for Holland as soon after our return to London as possible.[3]

495

Our Quarterly Meeting is just finished and our valuable relations from Manchester left us yesterday morning. I have not been able to put down a single note on the business of our profession. Perhaps this will be no loss to anybody.

If I am not prevented or forget it in my hurry on leaving this place, I will endeavour to bring with me a root of the *Convolvulus althaeoides*.[4] I am afraid we shall find you all afloat Parliamentiering.[5] A letter found me out here from H. Buncombe of your county — the only one I have received from any place — not a letter to my content.

The late rains have refreshed us much. The South has had a share, and I hear that my gardener at Upton rejoices much. Indeed we have almost been burnt up here.

We expect C. and A. Whalley this day or tomorrow.[6] Their Sisters left us well about a week ago. Should anything intervene to change our route in any manner, we shall give you timely notice. We shall not be able to reach you before second day evening. I fancy we shall think Elland the shortest road and stop in Brighorn for a breath.

D. Barclay sent me a pretty full account of the affairs at Ackworth, many of which will claim very serious attention.

We salute you all very affectionately,

J. and A. Fothergill

Ms. autograph letter, Port. 21/139, LSFL.

1. This autumn meeting at Ackworth School gave its Country Committee, which supervised daily operation and current needs of the School, an opportunity to meet Dr. Fothergill, his sister, and the London banker David Barclay.

2. Dr. Fothergill did much of the editorial work on *Extracts from the Minutes and Advices of the Yearly Meeting of Friends held in London from its first institution* (1783), an alphabetical arrangement, by topic, of recorded decisions about religious practice. Sponsored by the Yearly Meeting and periodically revised, the compilation came to be known as the Rules of Discipline.

3. Benjamin Waterhouse, having taken his medical degree at Edinburgh, was on his way to Leyden to continue his studies.

4. *Convolvulus altheoides*, the mallow-leaved bindweed, is listed by Lettsom in *Hortus Uptonensis*; see *Works*, III, 90.

5. Parliament had been suddenly dissolved on 1 September and elections were under way.

6. In 1779 Caleb Whalley had married Ann Fothergill (1745–1807), a daughter of Dr. Fothergill's brother Joseph and the last of the six sisters to marry. — *Fothergill Genealogy*, below.

To Benjamin Franklin, Passy, France, 25 October 1780

London, 25.10.1780

When I received my honoured friend's letter by Dr. Waterhouse, little did I expect it would not be in my power to return a more speedy answer. But I will not take up any more of my time in making apologies, as I mean this to be a long letter, but proceed to the business — after entreating my friend to allow me to forget that I am writing to a Minister to one of the first courts of Europe from a state the most promising of any that ever inhabited any part of this globe.

My disorder was not the strangury but the gout. It fell upon the neck of the bladder, swelled the passage, prevented entirely the discharge of any urine, which was drawn off twice a day for a fortnight, or I had perished. The operation was exquisitely painful as passing the instrument through very tender parts occupied by a gouty swelling. At length it gently touched my ankle, left the passage free, and so it has remained ever since.[1]

The strangury is a different disease. It is properly such a kind of heat as attends blisters, creating an inefficient nisus to discharge urine, with a sense of great heat. A solution of gum arabic in water used freely, that is an ounce dissolved in a quart of water, and a spoonful or two of this solution strained and taken in any liquor that is used — or in a little water and milk — often alleviates this disorder, and gives ease by blunting the acrimony of urine. Should a tendency to any difficulty of this kind [recur], pray describe the sensation and symptoms pretty fully, and in return I will say all that occurs to me worth saying on the subject.

I rejoice frankly that I am free from this complaint and yet able in some degree to discharge the duties of a laborious station.

Lady H. is much obliged to my friend for his kind intelligence and will act conformably.[2]

Much horrible mischief would indeed have been prevented had our superiors thought fit to pay any regard to our humble endeavours. But their ears were shut, their hearts hardened, Kings became delirious and the poor Greeks suffered for it.[3]

Still we are all hope, all serenity — nay triumphant — determined to prosecute the same plan. Pride and vengeance are very fallible counsellors — I think I see all Europe slowly leagueing against us, and for

497

two of the strongest reasons in the world and which they cannot but pursue, unless for their sins, they become besotted: to retrench our power, and to increase their own by an open commerce with America.

In the warmth of my affection for mankind, I could wish to see engrafted into this league a resolution precluding the necessity of general wars — the great object of universal civilization — [by] the institution of a College of Justice where the claims of sovereigns should be weighed, an award given, and War only made on him who refused submission.[4] No one man in the world has it so much in his power as my honored friend to infuse this thought into the breasts of Princes, or of those who rule them and their affairs.

Let me touch on a lesser point, in which I also wish to engage a moment of my friend's attention. The most extensive capacity, the greatest human mind, may possibly overlook some humble yet proper object, perhaps as that which I am going to mention. Establish through all the united States, as speedily as possible, one general standard of weights and measures and let this standard be directed, if I may use the expression, by squares. The weights which the apothecaries use are first a grain; 20 make a scruple; 3 scruples, a dram. It is impossible to reduce any of these weights to a unit without a fraction. No more can the foot nor the yard nor measures of capacity [be so reduced]. Let the scruple consist of 16 grains; 4 scruples to make 1 dram; 8 drams, 1 ounce; 16 ounces, 1 pound; and pounds to be reckoned by decimals, if thought more convenient. I rather describe these circumstances to explain my meaning than as the identical rules that ought to take place. Why not institute an American Standard,[5] and at this moment, when your trade is less than it ever will be hereafter while you exist? The diversity and confusion of this Island, not to say in Europe, is a sufficient proof of the need there is for such a reformation; no time more proper for it than the present; no one more capable of forming the basis of such a regulation than my friend; and if proper, I know it will be encouraged.

I sent a long paper on oaths by a gentleman of my acquaintance from Maryland.[6] Pray keep this subject in sight. The Massachusetts Government has adopted such a plan in part; they have allowed those who conscientiously refuse an oath to qualify themselves for offices by an affirmation.[7] This is liberal, and the more to be regarded, as I dare say it sprung from the breasts of those who had the modification of this government committed to them, and not from any solicitation of ours or others who had similar scruples. It is a singular event in the history of the mind that a state heretofore considered as one of the most intolerant should have framed one of the most liberal plans of government ever framed in the world.

My worthy Friend D. Barclay and myself, not being able to influence our Superiors, have become superiors ourselves. We have engaged the Society we belong to to purchase Ackworth schoolhouse in Yorkshire, built as an appendix to the Foundling Hospital. It is converted into a school for a plain English education for the children of such amongst us who are not in affluent circumstances. We have got together near 300 children, boys and girls, in less than a year. We have got people to superintend it diligently. We were there together this autumn and had the satisfaction to see a numerous and orderly family.

I dare not touch upon our situation — but it is tending to the point slowly and certainly which may probably prove extremely advantageous to us — poverty and distress, seldom enemies to virtue. Whilst a single man or a single guinea can be secured, peace is hardly to be hoped for; and while companies and a tribe of devourers are employed, they will always find means to urge a mind not disposed to relent in your favour to proceed with vehemence, however ineffectual. I think your business is to risk nothing. You lose in action for the most part the advantages you reap in patience. The late affair in Carolina [8] is a manifest proof of it, and I fear if you prompt your General to do more than he ought, you may still be sufferers, but I am not a judge of these matters.

Accept my very cordial thanks for thy great kindness to Dr. Waterhouse — a little friend and relation of mine, who I hope will do his country no discredit. After he has had a little experience in the practice of Physic, I think, should the state of Massachusetts ever establish a school of medicine, and such there should be, that if he lives and has his health, he would fill a chair in it very properly.[9] At present he is too young, too inexperienced, but he has collected good material, though I am confident without any such intention for such a purpose.

With cordial regards and undiminished esteem,

I am thy affectionate Friend
J. Fothergill

Ms. autograph letter, APS, Franklin Papers, XX, 138. This is the last letter known to have been written by Dr. Fothergill.

1. Benjamin Franklin had suffered from strangury, a condition characterized by

spasms of the urethra and bladder, caused by a stone, resulting in slow and painful urination. Dr. Fothergill was mistaken in diagnosing his own disease as gout.

2. Selina Countess of Huntingdon, a generous contributor to an orphanage established by the Rev. George Whitefield in the colony of Georgia, had asked if this enterprise was flourishing.

3. *Quidquid delirant reges, plectuntur Achivi* (Horace *Epistolae* I.ii, 14) "For whatever folly kings commit, the people suffer."

4. A very early plea for an organization of nations united to outlaw wars and secure peaceful cooperation for human welfare.

5. Dr. Fothergill was perhaps one of the earliest to suggest that Americans in their new culture might take the lead in securing a uniform standard of weights and measures.

6. The paper on oaths has not been identified.

7. The Massachusetts Constitution of 1780, drafted by a duly elected Constitutional Convention convened 1 September 1779, was presented to the Massachusetts towns on 2 March 1780, for their consideration, and was declared ratified in June. It referred in several places to "oaths or affirmations" and in the penultimate paragraph of Part II, ch. VI, art. I, specifically provided that Quakers declining to take oaths might make affirmation of the substance, omitting the objectionable phrases and substituting, "This I do under the pains and penalty of perjury."

8. The capitulation of Charleston on 12 May 1780 marked the beginning of a series of costly defeats inflicted upon the Colonial forces in the South. The British occupation of Charleston continued until mid-December 1782.

9. Benjamin Waterhouse, in November 1782, soon after his return from nearly seven years of medical study in Europe, was appointed Professor of the Theory and Practice of Physick at Harvard College. He is remembered especially for his untiring campaign to introduce vaccination as a necessary preventative against smallpox, a highly controversial subject in the United States for decades. — John B. Blake, *Benjamin Waterhouse and the Introduction of Vaccination: A Reappraisal* (Philadelphia: University of Pennsylvania Press, 1957); T. E. Moore, Jr., "The Early Years of the Harvard Medical School, Its Founding and Curriculum," *Bulletin of the History of Medicine*, 27 (1953): 53–561.

Dr. Fothergill died on December 26, 1780, having been ill since December 11. The following letter, addressed but without signature, was found among the Miscellaneous Manuscripts of Henry Stevens of Vermont, in the Library of Congress. Although it is not in Benjamin Franklin's hand, it is clearly his tribute to a valued friend.

To Dr. Benjamin Waterhouse, an American at Leyden

Passy, January 18, 1781

Dear Sir,

I received your obliging letter of the 16th past, enclosing one from my dear Friend Dr. Fothergill. I was happy to hear from him that he was quite free of the Disorder that had like to have removed him last summer. But I had soon after a letter from another Friend acquainting me that he was again dangerously ill of the same Malady; and the newspapers have since announced his Death! — I condole with you most sincerely on this occasion. I think a worthier man never lived. For besides his constant readiness to serve his Friends, he was always projecting something for the Good of his Country and of Mankind in general, and putting others who had it in their Power what was out of his own Reach, but whatever was within it he took care to do himself; and his incredible Industry and unwearied Activity enabled him to do much more than can now be ever known, his Modesty being equal to his other Virtues.

I shall take care to forward his letter to Mr. Pemberton. Enclosed is one I have just received under cover from that Gentleman; you will take Care to convey it by some safe opportunity to London.

With hearty Wishes for your Prosperity and Success in your Profession, and that you may be a good Copy of your deceased Relation, I am, Sir.

Yours —

Appendix

Fothergill Genealogy

Manuscript Sources

Selected Bibliography

Index

Appendix
Two Latin Letters

I

To Dr. William Cuming, Dorchester in Dorset

London Anno 1740

[Salutation and opening passage lacking]

Lustratis aliquibus Flandriae, urbibus munitissimis, per magnam Brabantiae partem migravimus; relicto quippe Gandavio ad Bruxellensem, spatiosam splendidamque urbem, nosmetipsos contulimus per oppidulum olim valle et muro vel potius aggere munitum, nomine Ask [Isca], notissimum quidem Brabantiae incolis, quoniam exinde primo Lupulos, horumque colendi modum mutati sunt Angli, in maximum totius Brabanti damnum; utpote olim in hoc mercaturae genere satis celebris. A Bruxelles itur ad Leodiam, hodie Liege Anglorum, Lüttich Germanorum, incolarum vero Luich, urbem ob arcis obsidionem diuturnam satis celebrem, deinde ad oppidulum Spadanum et Aquisgranum, loca quidem toto orbe notissima. Ibi aquas minerales, hic thermales potavi, gustavi, aliqua institutus sum experimenta, sed vulgaria quidem, ob defectum apparatus ad hanc rem idonei. Trajectum ad Mosam, Sylvam Ducis [Bois le Duc], Dordrechtum, iter ad celebre emporium Rotterdamum tenentes, visitavimus; urbem Delphensem, villam splendidissimam Hagensem, urbem Leydam, Haerlemam, pertransivimus ad noblissimam Batavorum civitatem Amstelodamum; urbe deinde perlustrata, per fretum vulgo dictum Dee Zuyder Zee navigamus ad oppidum dictum a Batavis Worcum in Westfrisia, distans viginti praeter propter milliaria a Leeuwardia, nitida satis et bene munita hujus provinciae urbe prima.

Hinc tendimus ad Groningam, et demum per arenosas incultasque regiones, per que urbem Oldenburgum, et villam unam alteramque longe a se invicem

505

dissitam accedimus ad liberam civitatem Bremensem, celebre satis emporium atque dives; hic in cella sub templo maximo cathedrali, corpora aliquot exsiccata, (humana intellige), dura firmaque, natura conservata, peregrinantibus ostenduntur, nullo condimento vel arte qualibet tractata, sed mera qua cellae insit virtute conservatrice; est locus non admodum profundus, et ex uno latere vento perflabilis, sicca est admodum, tota quippe circumcirca regio arenosa est. Sed licet plurimae aliae sunt sub eodem templo hujusmodi cavernae, et etiam sub aliis et vicinis templis, nulla adhuc invenitur quae eadem dote potitur. Corpora circa duodecim habent integra, ex quibus unum duocentos circiter annos habet; alterum, centum et quinquaginta; reliqua, diversarum aetatum et temporum; penitus ex succa videntur et levia, firma tamen adeo ut impositur sub capite manu totum corpus absque minima flexura facile possis erigere. Magnum nitri copiam causam esse asserunt coli, quod in tanta quantitate erui potest, ut singulae librae terrae hujus caverne exhibent uncias duas nitri purissimi.

[*Conclusion lacking*]

Printed in Dr. Fothergill's *Works*, ed. Lettsom, III, xvi–xx, without opening and concluding passages. See translation, above, page 52.

II

Carolo Linnaeo
Johannes Fothergill S.

Londine 4to Ap. 1774

Gratissimus a te litteras nuper accepi. Diu quidem in animo fuerat varias ob causas epistolam tibi mittere. Dubius tamen haerebam ne sine justa ratione otium tibi charum, pretiosum adeo, frustra tererem animum vero addidit, amicissima tua epistolas et que impertiri vellem sic accipe.

Collinsonius noster me plantas amare docuit. Ejus consortio potitus, quis plantas colere non potuit. Quis, qualis, et cetera fuerit dicere non opus est. Hortum instruere suasit. Ipse dedit multa, alia congerrere occasio stimulavit, et sic nata est Gaza haud mediocris plantarum, sub domino Scientia Botanica leviter imbuto, flagrante tamen rei Botanicae amore.

Praxis clinica me fere totum occupit, et dum vires aetate non penitus fractae fuerint, forsan occupabunt. Aegre fatior opem iis ferre recuso, qui mihi fautores, qui sese benignos opitulatores, aetate minore sese ostenderunt.

Forte olim dabitur, ut curis laboribusque confectus, senectutis vitaeque tedium inter amoenos florae Thesauros, tenere possim. Berlinus, brevi postquam Africam adiit, migravit ad plures. Febris ille lethalis, quae in calidis humidisque regionibus, hominem intempestive certo jugulavit. Quum primum morbo correptus fuerat, sua nimis fidens opinione, medicationem experientia diu stabilita prorsus recusavit. Ambiguus et incertus, breve succubuit. Magnum Rei Botanicae et fere irreparabile damnum.

Smeathmanus, spero, inter vivos est. Misit multa et rara insecta. Plantas nullas, nec semina! Ne unicum quidem. Magno nobis infortunio accidit, ut naves nullae aut parcae ab Africa in nostras oras revertunt. Onustae mercibus iniquissisimis hominibus vi surreptis ab eis quae vitam optabilem faciunt, ad Insulas Indiae occidentalis ducuntur; et post moram satis diurnam in Angliam reducuntur. Sic per longam ambagem pereunt omnia. Decrevimus navem conducere, quae sub Smeathmanni gubernatione, si superstes fuerit, quotannis ad Africam eat, redeatque ad nos, ut speramus, immensum rerum naturalium thesaurum apportet. Scripsimus ad Smeathmanum, ad domum quamprimum reverteret, vires refocillet caelo minus ardente et proximo autumno ad Africam redeat. Si quis in celebrissima Linnaea schola juvenis, vegetus, laborum caeli calentis patiens, amoris plantarum Historiae naturalis percitus, socium itineris sese offere velit, ineunte aestate, mihi ut indiceres rogamus. Miror quidem Solandrum animam erga praeceptorem fautorem, adjustorem maximum, tam parum gratiam ostendere. Hoc tamen censendum est. Suae spontis non est. Quod jubet Dominus, id faciendum vel omnino omittendum.

Filium venerandi senis Bartrami misi in Floridas Americae Brittanicae regionum australis, ut planta ibi colligeat. Si quis novas, aut rariores mittat, te participem lubens laetusque faciam. Ex iis oris accepimus Illycium anisatum, quod postrema aetate Millero nostro ad te mittendum dedi.

Quod me etiam autem inter plantarum amatores numerari voluisti, gratias habeo. Quum vero respiciam atque curtam ad modum Scientiae supellecticem, erubesco. Tua vero benignitas debitam apud me semper habebit honorem gratiamque facti recordationem.

Plantam ipsam ad te mittere decrevi, quamprimum, si votis fortuna faveat eo usque ut stolonem vegetum hoc aestate habeam. Vereor ne parum intelliges hanc epistolam. Desuetudo latinae scribendi impromptionem facit. Si quid vero obscurius dictum videatur id quaeso proxime indigites. Utinam viribus otium et rerum cognitione dignarum ea ratione plenum politus essem ut magno Linnaeo, unicum momentum beatius reddere potuissem. Vale vir amicissimus quo nullus forte vixit unquam magis et merito laudatus; etiam habitus inter omnes honore summo.

Vale.

Ms. autograph letter, The Linnean Society, Burlington House, London. See translation, above, p. 409.

Fothergill Genealogy

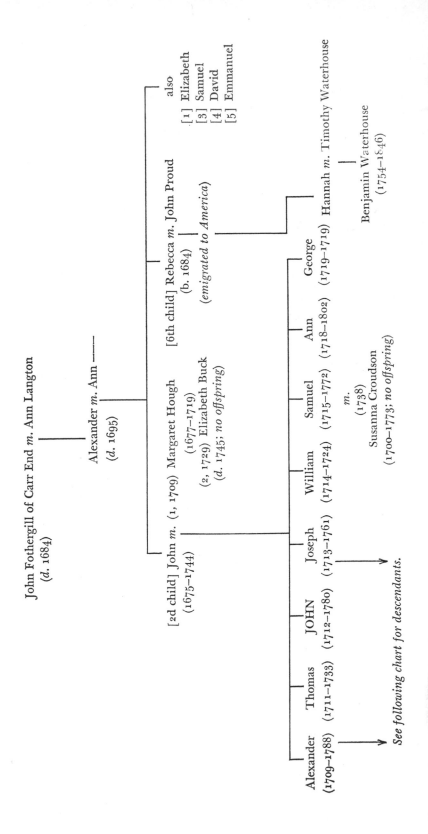

John Fothergill of Carr End *m.* Ann Langton
(*d.* 1684)

Alexander *m.* Ann ——
(*d.* 1695)

[6th child] Rebecca *m.* John Proud
(*b.* 1684)
(*emigrated to America*)

also

Elizabeth [1]
Samuel [3]
David [4]
Emmanuel [5]

[2d child] John *m.* (1, 1709) Margaret Hough
(1675–1744)   (1677–1719)
(2, 1729) Elizabeth Buck
(*d.* 1745; *no offspring*)

Hannah *m.* Timothy Waterhouse

Benjamin Waterhouse
(1754–1846)

Alexander   Thomas   JOHN   Joseph   William   Samuel   Ann   George
(**1709–1788**)   (1711–1733)   (1712–1780)   (1713–1761)   (1714–1724)   (1715–1772)   (1718–1802)   (1719–1719)

m.
(1738)
Susanna Croudson
(1700–1773; *no offspring*)

See following chart for descendants.

Descendants of Dr. Fothergill's Brother Alexander

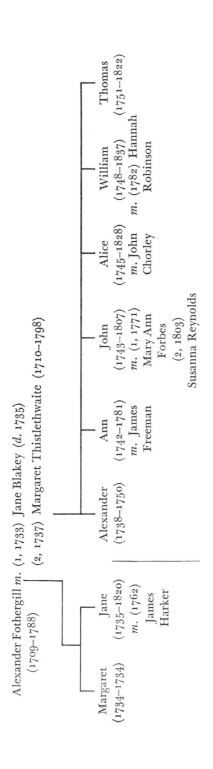

Alexander Fothergill *m.* (1, 1733) Jane Blakey (*d.* 1735)
(1709–1788)   (2, 1737) Margaret Thistlethwaite (1710–1798)

Margaret
(1734–1734)

Jane
(1735–1820)
m. (1762)
James
Harker

Alexander
(1738–1750)

Ann
(1742–1781)
m. James
Freeman

John
(1743–1807)
m. (1, 1771)
Mary Ann
Forbes
(2, 1803)
Susanna Reynolds

Alice
(1745–1828)
m. John
Chorley

William
(1748–1837)
m. (1782) Hannah
Robinson

Thomas
(1751–1822)

Descendants of Dr. Fothergill's Brother Joseph

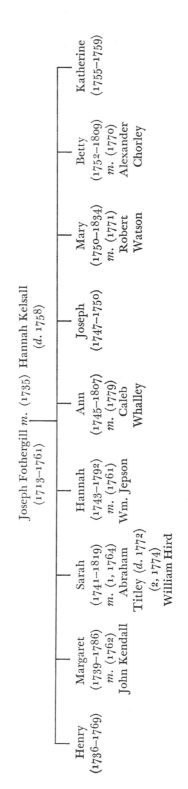

Joseph Fothergill *m.* (1735) Hannah Kelsall
(1713–1761)   (*d.* 1758)

Henry
(1736–1769)

Margaret
(1739–1786)
m. (1762)
John Kendall

Sarah
(1741–1819)
m. (1, 1764)
Abraham
Titley (*d.* 1772)
(2, 1774)
William Hird

Hannah
(1743–1792)
m. (1761)
Wm. Jepson

Ann
(1745–1807)
m. (1779)
Caleb
Whalley

Joseph
(1747–1750)

Mary
(1750–1834)
m. (1771)
Robert
Watson

Betty
(1752–1809)
m. (1770)
Alexander
Chorley

Katherine
(1755–1759)

Manuscript Sources

In England

Library of the Society of Friends, Friends House, London.
Linnean Society, Burlington House, London.
Royal College of Surgeons, London.
Bodleian Library, Oxford.
Dartmouth Papers, Patshull House Collection, William Salt Library, Stafford.
Rockingham Papers, Wentworth-Woodhouse Muniments, Central Library, Sheffield.
David Barclay Papers, in the care of the late Quintin Gurney, Esq., Bawdeswell Hall near Norwich, Norfolk.
Wedgwood Museum, near Barlaston, Staffordshire.
Fothergill Family Papers and Letters, in the care of Mrs. Amy E. Wallis, Darlington, County Durham.
Fothergilliana, held by a collateral descendant, the late Dr. W. Crichton Fothergill, Darlington, County Durham.
Papers in possession of Miss Ursula Somervell, Cambridge.
The Royal Society of London, the British Museum, and the Wellcome Historical Medical Library, London, also possess letters of Dr. Fothergill, which are not included in the present selection.

In Scotland

Fothergill Family Papers held by the late Miss Mabyn Fothergill, now in the care of her brother, Edward Fothergill, Esq., of Edinburgh.
Library of the University of Edinburgh.
National Library of Scotland, Edinburgh.

In the United States

Library of Congress, Washington, D.C.
Richmond Academy of Medicine, Richmond, Virginia.
Charleston Library Society, Charleston, South Carolina.

Philadelphia and Vicinity

American Philosophical Society.
Historical Society of Pennsylvania.
Library Company of Philadelphia (Letter Book of Granville Sharp, now in the custody of the Historical Society of Pennsylvania).
Pennsylvania Hospital Records and Minute Books (now available in microfilm at the American Philosophical Society).
Collection of William Logan Fox, Esq., Philadelphia (letters to William Logan, son of James Logan of Stenton, now available in photostat at the Historical Society of Pennsylvania).
Charles Roberts Autograph Collection, Haverford College.

Selected Bibliography

(Background works, special studies, and titles frequently cited)

Acts of the Privy Council of England (Colonial Series), v. III, A.D. 1720–1745. Edited by W. L. Grant and James Munro. London: H. M. Stationers' Office, 1910.

Adams, John. *The Diary and Autobiography of John Adams.* Edited by Lyman H. Butterfield and others. 4 v. Cambridge, Mass.: Belknap Press of Harvard University Press, 1961.

Adams, Randolph G. *Political Ideas of the American Revolution: Britannic-American Contributions to the Problem of Imperial Organization, 1765–1775,* 3rd ed. New York: Barnes and Noble, 1958.

Andrews, Charles M. *The Colonial Background of the American Revolution.* New Haven: Yale University Press, 1924.

Aubrey's Brief Lives. Edited by Oliver L. Dick. London: Secker and Warburg, 1950.

Barclay, Robert. *An Apology for the True Christian Divinity* . . . Amsterdam, 1676.

Bargar, B. D. *Lord Dartmouth and the American Revolution.* Columbia: University of South Carolina Press, 1965.

Bartram, John. "Diary of a Journey Through the Carolinas, Georgia and Florida, 1765–1766," annotated by Francis Harper. *Transactions of the American Philosophical Society,* 33.1:1–120 (1942).

Bartram, William. "Travels in Georgia and Florida, 1773–1774: A Report to Dr. John Fothergill," annotated by Francis Harper. *Transactions of the American Philosophical Society,* 33.2:121–242 (1943).

———— *The Travels of William Bartram* (London, 1791). Cited from Naturalist's Edition, edited by Francis Harper. New Haven: Yale University Press, 1958.

———— *Botanical and Zoological Drawings, 1756–1788, Reproduced from the Fothergill Album in the British Museum (Natural History).* Edited with an introduction and commentary by Joseph Ewan. Philadelphia: American Philosophical Society, 1968.

513

Beaufoy, Gwendolyn. *Leaves from a Beech Tree.* Oxford, England: privately printed, 1930.

Bell, Whitfield J., Jr. *John Morgan, Continental Doctor.* Philadelphia: University of Pennsylvania Press, 1965.

Besse, Joseph. *A Collection of Sufferings of the People Called Quakers . . .* 2 v. London: Luke Hinde, 1753.

Boswell, James. *The Life of Samuel Johnson, LL.D.* Edited by George Birkbeck Hill, rev. edition by L. F. Powell, 6 v. Oxford: Clarendon Press, 1934–1951.

—— *The Life of Samuel Johnson.* Edited by Roger Ingpen. London, 1907. (Reproduces notes from Malone's edition.)

Bowden, James. *The History of Friends in America,* 2 v. London: C. Gilpin, 1850.

Boyd, Julian P. *Indian Treaties Printed by Benjamin Franklin.* Philadelphia: Historical Society of Pennsylvania, 1938.

Braithwaite, William C. *The Second Period of Quakerism,* 2nd ed., prepared by Henry J. Cadbury. Cambridge, England: The University Press, 1961.

Brett-James, Norman G. *The Life of Peter Collinson.* London: Dunstan and Friends Bookshop, 1926.

Burke, Edmund. *The Correspondence of Edmund Burke.* Volume II: July 1768–June 1774. Edited by Lucy S. Sutherland. Cambridge, England: The University Press; University of Chicago Press, 1960.

Butterfield, Herbert. *George III, Lord North, and the People, 1779–1780.* London: Bell, 1949.

Carlisle, Nicholas. *A Concise Description of the Endowed Grammar Schools in England and Wales.* 2 v. London: Baldwin, Cradock, and Joy, 1818.

A Collection of Memorials Concerning Divers Deceased Ministers and Others of the People Called Quakers in Pennsylvania, New-Jersey, and Parts Adjacent, Philadelphia, 1787.

Corner, Betsy C. *William Shippen, Jr., Pioneer in American Medical Education.* Philadelphia: American Philosophical Society (*Memoirs,* v. 28), 1951.

Corner, George W. *Two Centuries of Medicine: A History of the School of Medicine, University of Pennsylvania.* Philadelphia: Lippincott, 1965.

Crane, Verner W. *Benjamin Franklin's Letters to the Press.* Chapel Hill: University of North Carolina Press, 1950.

Crosfield, George. *Memoirs of the Life and Gospel Labours of Samuel Fothergill.* Liverpool: D. Marples, 1843. The American edition (New York: Collins, 1844) is cited.

Cummings, Hubertus. *Richard Peters.* Philadelphia: University of Pennsylvania Press, 1941.

Darlington, William. *Memorials of John Bartram and Humphry Marshall, with Notices of Their Botanical Contemporaries.* Philadelphia: Lindsay and Blakiston, 1849. Facsimile reprint, with introduction by Joseph Ewan. New York: Hafner, 1967.

Dartmouth Mss. See Historical Manuscripts Commission.

Davis, Joseph. *A Digest of Legislative Enactments Relating to the Society of Friends, commonly called Quakers, in England.* Bristol: Wansbrough and Saunders, 1820.

Dictionary of American Biography. Edited by Allen Johnson and Dumas Malone. 20 v. New York: Charles Scribner's Sons, 1928–1936.

Dictionary of National Biography. Edited by Sir Leslie Stephen and Sir Sidney Lee. Founded in 1882 by George Smith; published since 1917 by Oxford University Press.

Dimsdale, Thomas. *A Tribute of Affection to the Memory of Dr. Fothergill.* London: Privately printed, 1783.

Doncaster, L. Hugh. *Quaker Organization and Business Meetings.* London: Friends Home Service Committee, 1958.

Elliot, John. *A Complete Collection of the Medical and Philosophical Works of John Fothergill, M.D., F.R.S., S.A., with an account of his Life, and Occasional Notes.* London: John Walker, 1781. (Not dependable).

Fothergill, John. *The Works of John Fothergill, M.D.* Edited by J. C. Lettsom. 3 v. London: Printed for Charles Dilly in the Poultry, 1783–1784.

———— *An Account of the Sore Throat Attended with Ulcers,* London, 1748.

———— *An Account of the Life and Travels in the Work of the Ministry, of John Fothergill. To which are added divers epistles to Friends in Great Britain and America, on various occasions.* London: Printed and sold by Luke Hinde, 1753. The 2d ed., London: Mary Hinde, 1773.

———— *Considerations Relative to the North American Colonies.* London: Printed by Henry Kent, at the Printing-Office in Finch-lane, near the Royal Exchange, 1765.

———— *Some Account of the Late Peter Collinson, Fellow of the Royal Society . . . in a Letter to a Friend.* Printed in 1769 without the author's name; handsomely published in 1770, embellished with a full-page engraving.

———— *A Brief Account of the People called Quakers, Their Doctrines and Their Disciplines.* London, 1773.

———— *A Letter from J. Fothergill to a Friend in the Country relative to the Intended School at Ackworth in Yorkshire.* With a plan and Elevation of the Building. London: Printed and Sold by James Phillips, George-Yard, Lombard Street, 1778, 1779.

Fox, R[ichard] Hingston. *Dr. John Fothergill and His Friends: Chapters in Eighteenth Century Life.* London: Macmillan and Co., Ltd., 1919.

Franklin, Benjamin. *Experiments and Observations on Electricity, made at Philadelphia . . . communicated in several letters to Mr. P. Collinson, of London, F.R.S.* 2 v. London: E. Cave, 1751–1753.

———— *Benjamin Franklin's Autobiographical Writings.* Edited by Carl Van Doren. New York: Viking, 1945.

———— *The Writings of Benjamin Franklin.* Edited by A. H. Smyth. 10 v. New York: Macmillan, 1905–1907.

515

―――― *The Papers of Benjamin Franklin.* Edited by Leonard W. Labaree and others. New Haven: Yale University Press, 1959―.

George, M[ary] Dorothy (Gordon). *London Life in the Eighteenth Century,* 3rd ed. London: London School of Economics, 1951.

Gipson, Lawrence H. *The British Empire Before the American Revolution,* 12 v. New York: Knopf, 1958–1965.

Green, John Richard. *A History of the English People.* 4 v. London: Macmillan, 1877–1880.

Guttridge, George H. *The Early Career of Lord Rockingham, 1730 to 1765.* Berkeley: University of California Press, 1952.

Hagberg, Knut. *Carl Linnaeus.* Translated by Alan Blair. London: Jonathan Cape, 1952.

Hale, Helen G. *Westtown Through the Years, 1799–1942.* Westtown, Pennsylvania, 1942.

Hannah Logan's Courtship. Edited by Albert Cook Myers. Philadelphia: Ferris and Leach, 1904.

Hansard, Luke. *Journals of the House of Commons.* London, 1774―.

Harley, Lewis R. *The Life of Charles Thomson.* Philadelphia: Jacobs, 1900.

Hartley, Marie, and Joan Ingilby. *Yorkshire Village.* London: Dent, 1953.

―――― ―――― *The Yorkshire Dales.* London: Dent, 1956.

Hindle, Brooke. *The Pursuit of Science in Revolutionary America, 1735–1789.* Chapel Hill: The University of North Carolina Press, 1956.

Hird, William. *An Affectionate Tribute to the Memory of the Late Dr. J. Fothergill.* London: privately printed, 1781.

Historical Manuscripts Commission. *The Manuscripts of the Earl of Dartmouth,* v. II: *American Papers.* With an introduction by B. F. Stevens. H. M. Stationers' Office, 1895.

Hughes, Edward. *North Country Life in the 18th Century.* London: Oxford University Press, 1952.

James, Sydney V. *A People Among Peoples: Quaker Benevolence in Eighteenth Century America.* Cambridge, Mass.: Harvard University Press, 1963.

Jenkins, James. Manuscript recollections. Library of the Society of Friends, London.

Jones, Mary Gwladys. *The Charity School Movement, a Study of Eighteenth Century Puritanism in Action.* Cambridge, England: The University Press, 1938.

Jones, Rufus. *The Later Periods of Quakerism.* New York: Macmillan, 1911.

Journal of the Commissioners for Trade and Plantations from January 1741/2 to December 1749. Preserved in the Public Record Office. London: H. M. Stationers' Office, 1931.

―――― *1734/5 to December 1741.* London: H. M. Stationers' Office, 1930.

Knollenberg, Bernhard. *Origin of the American Revolution, 1759–1766.* New York: Macmillan, 1960.

Lettsom, John Coakley. *Some Account of the Late John Fothergill.* London:

C. Dilly, 1782. Read before the Medical Society of London 17 July and 23 October 1782. Included in both quarto and octavo editions of the *Works*. Reissued in *Memoirs of John Fothergill, M.D., &c.* By John Coakley Lettsom. The fourth edition. London: Printed for C. Dilly, 1786.

Medical Essays and Observations, 5 v. Edinburgh, 1731–1743.

Medical Observations and Inquiries, 6 v. London: Society of Physicians in London, 1757–1784.

Miller, John. *Illustratio Systematis Sexualis Linnaei. An Illustration of the Sexual System of Linnaeus.* Latin and English, 3 v., folio. London: 1777.

Minutes of the Provincial Council of Pennsylvania, v. VII, VIII. Harrisburg: Published by the State, 1851, 1852.

Montgomery, T. H. *A History of the University of Pennsylvania from its Foundation to A.D. 1770.* Philadelphia: Jacobs, 1900.

Morgan, E. S. *Prologue to Revolution, Sources and Documents of the Stamp Act Crisis.* Chapel Hill: University of North Carolina Press, 1959.

Morgan, Edmund S., and Helen M. Morgan. *The Stamp Act Crisis.* Chapel Hill: University of North Carolina Press, 1959.

Morris, Richard B. *The Peacemakers.* New York: Harper and Row, 1965.

Morton, Thomas G., and Frank Woodbury. *The History of the Pennsylvania Hospital, 1751–1895*, revised edition. Philadelphia: Times Printing House, 1895.

Munk, William. *The Roll of the Royal College of Physicians of London; comprising biographical sketches of all the eminent physicians, whose names are recorded in the annals from the foundation of the College in 1518 to its removal in 1825, from Warwick Lane to Pall Mall east.* 2nd ed. 3 v. London: Published by the College, 1878. Vol. II, 1701–1800.

Namier, Lewis B. *England in the Age of the American Revolution*, 2nd ed. London: Macmillan; New York: St. Martin's Press, 1961.

—— *The Structure of Politics at the Accession of George III.* 2nd ed. London: Macmillan; New York: St. Martin's Press, 1957.

New Cambridge Modern History, VII. Cambridge, England: The University Press, 1907.

Nichols, John. *Biographical and Literary Anecdotes of William Bowyer*, London, 1782.

—— *Literary Anecdotes of the Eighteenth Century.* 9 v. London: Printed for the author by Nichols, Son, and Bentley, 1812–1816.

—— *Illustrations of the Literary History of the Eighteenth Century . . . intended as a sequel to the "Literary Anecdotes."* 8 v. London: Printed for the author by Nichols, Son, and Bentley, 1817–1858. Vols. 7–8 by J. B. Nichols.

Pares, Richard. *King George III and the Politicians.* New York: Oxford University Press, 1953.

Peachey, George C. *A Memoir of John and William Hunter.* Plymouth, England: Brandon, 1924.

Pennsylvania Archives. 8th series: Votes of Assembly. 8 v. (1931–1935), 441.

517

Pennsylvania Colonial Records. See *Minutes of the Provincial Council of Pennsylvania.*

Philosophical Transactions, see Royal Society of London.

Piety Promoted, v. VIII. London, 1775.

Proud, Robert. *History of Pennsylvania.* 2 v. Philadelphia: Printed and sold by Zachariah Poulson, Jr., 1797–1798.

Pownall, Thomas. *The Administration of the British Colonies,* 2nd ed., revised. London: J. Dodsley, 1764.

Raistrick, Arthur. *Quakers in Science and Industry.* London: Bannisdale Press, 1950.

Raven, Charles E. *John Ray, Naturalist, His Life and Works.* Cambridge, England: The University Press, 1950.

Royal Society of London. For scientific papers, consult *A General Index to the Philosophical Transactions from the first to the end of the seventieth volume.* By Paul Henry Maty, M.A., F.R.S., Under Librarian to the British Museum. London: Printed for Lockyer Davis and Peter Elmsly, Printers to the Royal Society, 1787.

Rush, Benjamin. *The Autobiography of Benjamin Rush.* Edited by George W. Corner. Princeton University Press for the American Philosophical Society (*Memoirs,* v. 25), 1948.

———— *The Letters of Benjamin Rush.* Edited by Lyman H. Butterfield. 2 v. Princeton University Press for the American Philosophical Society, 1951.

Shepherd, William R. *History of Proprietary Government in Pennsylvania.* New York: Columbia University, 1896.

Smith, Horace Wemyss. *Life and Correspondence of the Rev. William Smith, D.D.* Philadelphia: Ferguson Brothers, 1880.

Smith, James Edward. *A Selection of the Correspondence of Linnaeus and Other Naturalists, from the Original Manuscripts.* 2 v. London: Longman, Hurst, Rees, Orme, and Brown, 1821.

Smith, William. *A Brief State of the Province of Pennsylvania* . . . London, 1755.

———— *A Brief View of the Conduct of Pennsylvania* . . . London, 1756.

Stephen, Leslie. *History of English Thought in the Eighteenth Century.* 2 v. London: Smith, Elder and Co., 1876. 3rd ed., reprinted. London: John Murray, 1927.

Thayer, Theodore. *Israel Pemberton, King of the Quakers.* Philadelphia: Historical Society of Pennsylvania, 1943.

———— *Pennsylvania Politics and the Growth of Democracy, 1740–1776.* Harrisburg: Pennsylvania Historical and Museum Commission, 1953.

Thompson, Gilbert. *Memoirs of the Life and a View of the Character of the Late Dr. John Fothergill.* London: T. Cadell, 1782.

Thomson, Charles. *An Enquiry into the Causes of the Alienation of the . . . Indians.* London, 1759. (With this was published the first journal of Christian Frederick Post.)

Tolles, Frederick B. *Meeting House and Counting House: The Quaker Mer-*

chants of Colonial Pennsylvania, 1682–1763. Chapel Hill: University of North Carolina Press, 1948.

───── "The Atlantic Community of Early Friends," *Journal of the Friends Historical Society*, Supplement No. 24, pp. 13–34, 1952.

───── *George Logan of Philadelphia*. New York: Oxford University Press, 1953.

───── "America's First Scientist," *Isis*, 47 (1956–57), 20.

───── *James Logan and the Culture of Provincial America*. Boston: Little, Brown, and Co., 1957.

Trevelyan, George Macaulay. *Illustrated English Social History*, v. III: *The Eighteenth Century*, rev. ed. London: Longmans, 1951.

Trevelyan, George Otto. *The American Revolution* [to 1778, concluded by the following]. 3 vols. in 4, London; New York: Longmans, 1899–1907.

───── *George the Third and Charles Fox* [conclusion to *The American Revolution*]. 2 vols. London: Longmans, 1912–1914.

Tuke, James Hack. *A Sketch of the Life of John Fothergill, M.D., F.R.S., Reprinted from the proceedings of the Centenary of Ackworth School*. London: Samuel Harris Sons, 1879.

Van Doren, Carl. *Benjamin Franklin: A Biography*. New York: Viking, 1958.

───── *Benjamin Franklin's Autobiographical Writings*. New York: Viking, 1945.

Vicq d'Azyr, Félix. "Eloge de M. Fothergill," *Histoire de la Société Royale de Médicine*, Paris, 1785.

Vipont, Elfrida. *Ackworth School, from its Foundation in 1779 to the Introduction of Co-education in 1946*. London: Lutterworth Press, 1959.

───── *The Story of Quakerism*. London: Bannisdale Press, 1955.

Wainwright, Nicholas B. *George Croghan, Wilderness Diplomat*. Chapel Hill: University of North Carolina Press, 1959.

Wallace, Anthony F. L. *King of the Delawares: Teedyuscung*. Philadelphia: University of Pennsylvania Press, 1949.

Wallace, Paul A. *Conrad Weiser*. Philadelphia: University of Pennsylvania Press, 1945.

Walpole, Horace. *Correspondence*. Edited by Wilmarth Lewis and others. v. 17. New Haven: Yale University Press, 1954.

───── *Memoirs of the Reign of George III*. Edited by Russell Barker. London: Lawrence and Bullen, 1894.

Watson, J[ohn] Steven. *The Reign of George III, 1761–1815*. The Oxford History of England, XII. Oxford: Clarendon Press, 1960.

Wolff, Mabel P. *The Colonial Agency of Pennsylvania, 1712–1757*. Philadelphia: The author, 1933.

Woolman, John. *The Journal and Essays of John Woolman*. Edited by Amelia M. Gummere. New York: Macmillan, 1922.

519

Index

The following abbreviations are used: *F*, Fothergill; *JF*, Dr. John Fothergill; *n*, note. For brevity and clarity, *Quaker* designates the Religious Society of Friends and its members.

Index

Angus,——, ship captain, 54

Anise: *Anisum (Illicium) stellatum* (star anise), 392, 393*n*, 395; *Illicium floridanum* (purple anise), 401, 403*n*. *See also Illicium*

Anti-militarism, *see under* Quakers

Anti-Quaker feelings, 158, 159, 161*n*

Antiquarian Society, 429

Apology, Barclay's, *see* Barclay, Robert

Apothecaries' Company, Physic Garden, 84, 86*n*

Apothecary: *JF* as, 5, 6; for Pennsylvania Hospital, 284, 288*n*, 321, 322*n*

Arbitrators, in Leeds affair, 348, 349*n*, 350, 352*n*, 362, 363*n*, 366, 380, 384

Areskine, Thomas, *JF*'s landlord, 37, 38, 38*n*, 111, 133

Armistead, William, 4

Askrigg, 130*n*, 229, 229*n*

Assembly, Massachusetts, 288*n*

Assembly, Pennsylvania: sends commissioners to England, 25; opposes governor, 70, 72*n*; appeals to Privy Council, 73, 74, 76*n*; attitude toward Proprietor, 165, 166*n*; bill for militia appropriation, 167, 168, 168*n*, 169, 186*n*, 187*n*; Quakers withdraw from Assembly, 161*n*, 173–175, 179, 184, 195, 198*n*; difficulties with provincial and British government, 210, 215, 254

Association for Regaining and Preserving Peace with the Indians, 196, 198, 199*n*

Augusta, Princess (Dowager Princess) of Wales, 221, 223*n*, 377, 377*n*

Avebury, 94, 95*n*

Avicenna, 93*n*

Badenach, Dr. James, 416, 417*n*, 418*n*

Bainbridge, 229, 229*n*

Balm of Gilead, 43, 44*n*

Balmerino, Arthur Elphinstone, 6th Lord, 118*n*

Balsam, wild, see *Momordica*

Banks, Sir Joseph, 18, 20, 411, 418*n*, 458*n*

Barbados, 118, 119*n*

Barbauld, Anna Letitia, 354*n*

Barclay, David: patient of *JF*, 14; marriage, 123*n*; working for peace with America, 258, 263; handling funds for Pennsylvania Hospital, 329, 387, 388*n*; plans for peace with *JF* and Franklin, 27–29, 434*n*, 443*n*, 444*n*, 445, 496; supports Ackworth School, 31, 496, 499; at *JF*'s deathbed, 33; mentioned, 205*n*, 223*n*, 274, 340, 447, 448, 467, 469, 495, 496
    LETTERS TO, 461, 476

Barclay, Mrs. David (Martha Hudson), 122, 123*n*

Barclay, Elizabeth, *see* Bevan, Mrs. Timothy

Barclay, Robert, *Apology for the True Christian Divinity . . .* , 298, 340*n*, 313*n*, 424, 426*n*, 469

Bark, the, *see* Quinine

Barnard, Thomas, 112*n*

Barnard, Mrs. Thomas, 115, 116, 117*n*

Barnard, Tommy, 116, 117*n*

Barrington, William Wildman, 2d Viscount, 177*n*

Bartlett, Benjamin, apothecary and bookseller, 5, 6, 95*n*, 107, 108*n*

Bartlett, Benjamin II ("Bennie"), 62, 63*n*, 344, 346*n*

Bartlett, Elizabeth (Mrs. John Gurney),
    LETTERS TO, 61, 67, 115

Bartram, John, botanist, 46, 47*n*, 49, 50*n*, 85, 86*n*, 240*n*, 241*n*, 265, 267*n*, 276*n*, 290*n*, 319*n*, 322*n*, 390*n*, 391*n*, 393*n*, 394, 410
    LETTERS TO, 83, 289, 302, 317, 321, 388

Bartram, John, Jr., 415, 416*n*

Bartram, William, artist-naturalist: journeys, 267*n*, 414; drawings commissioned by *JF*, 289, 290*n*, 322, 389, 390, 394, 408, 464; drawings made, 303, 391, 415; *JF*'s directions to, 401, 402, 403*n*; boxes for collecting, 407; studies tortoises, 303, 318, 320; finds Colocasia, 319*n*; finds yellow anise, 319*n*
    LETTERS TO, 391, 401

Baskerville, John, printer, 238, 240*n*

Bath (city), 44*n*, 53*n*, 94

Bathing, *see* Sea bathing

Baths, public, 33

Baume de vie, 291, 366

Bayle, Pierre, 299, 301*n*

Bean, Dr. ——, 106

Beaufoy, Henry, 357

Beaufoy, Mark, 223*n*, 346*n*, 355, 355*n*, 358*n*, 369, 374*n*
    LETTER TO, 373

Beaufoy, Mrs. Mark (Elizabeth Hanbury), 345, 346*n*

Beckford, William, 269, 270*n*

Bee man, *see* Wildman, Thomas

Belgium, *JF* visits, 52, 57

Bell, John, 75, 77*n*

Bentley, Thomas, 335*n*
    LETTER TO, 334

Berkeley, Bishop George, 374*n*

Berlin (Berlinus), Anders, 409, 410*n*, 506

Besse, Joseph, *Collection of the Sufferings of the People Called Quakers*, 96, 97*n*

Index

Index

Index

238. *See also* Edinburgh; Leyden; Medical School

Medical Essays and Observations, 50, 91, 93n

Medical Observations and Inquiries, 172n

Medical School: of the College of Philadelphia, now University of Pennsylvania, 14, 225, 239n, 250, 279, 280, 281n, 310, 399n, 473. *See also* Edinburgh; Leyden

Medical societies, 280; Edinburgh, 49, 50n, 56n, 91, 93n, 361, 461n; Medical Society (of Physicians), London, 33, 170, 172n, 280, 281n, 416n, 457. *See also* College of Physicians

Medical treatment, *see* Drugs and medical treatment

Medicine, JF's practice of, *see under* Fothergill, Dr. John

Medicine, specialization, 238, 239n, 250, 251

Meetings, Quaker: explained, 30. *See also under following heads*

Meetings, Monthly: Edinburgh, 343n; Gracechurch Street, 371; Philadelphia, 128n; Warrington, 340; Westminster, 343n, 372n, 382

Meetings, Particular, Preparatory, 30

Meetings, Quarterly: functions, 30, 121n; Burlington, New Jersey, 148n; Cheshire and Staffordshire, 353, 354n; Cumberland (England), 121n; Leeds, 486, 487n, 491; London, 333n, 343n, 371, 372, 372n, 378, 457, 496; Philadelphia, 148, 158, 165, 167; Scotland, 121n; Warrington, 340; Worcester, 424; Yorkshire, 38, 45, 427, 495

Meetings for Sufferings: 30, 31; London, 69, 77n, 96, 107, 121n, 158, 163, 165, 174, 184, 186n, 192, 202, 226, 331, 424, 445, 446n, 447, 467; Philadelphia, 188, 206n, 214, 222, 222n, 331, 424, 437, 441, 445, 446n, 447, 467

Meetings, Yearly: 30, 31; Chester, 340; London, 23, 30, 31, 38, 74, 77n, 79n, 193, 194, 194n, 198, 201, 243, 310, 341, 343n, 352n, 367, 382, 385, 385n, 467, 495; Philadelphia, 23, 69, 72, 75, 437, 441n

Mennonites, 25

Merchants dealing with America, *see* North America merchants

Merrick, the Misses, 334, 335n

Mesnard, Stephen, ship captain, 152n, 183

Metcalfe, Thomas, 10, 82, 83n, 120, 126, 129, 132, 150, 150n

Middleton Gardens, 408n

Midwife, 412, 413

Miers, Ann, *see* Lettsom, Mrs. John Coakley

Mildred, Daniel, 258, 263, 290, 349n, 467

Militia Act, 23, 192, 193, 194n

Miller, George, 38, 39n

Miller (Müller), Johann Sebastian, 323, 393n, 397, 398n

Miller, Joseph, 43, 44n, 48

Miller, Philip, 274, 276n, 305, 364

Miller, William, gardener, 38, 39n

Miller, William, Jr., 38, 39n

Miller, William, Edinburgh, 345, 357

Millindate, 133

Milne, Colin, 398n

Milner, ———, ship captain, 142

Minera ferri, 48

Mineral waters, 48, 50n, 52, 84, 85, 92, 93n, 94, 250, 291, 292n

Minerals, 55, 82, 84, 85

Minorca, 135, 136n, 142

Minutes (of Meetings): on marriage by priests, 87, 89, 90n; on rebellion of 1745, 107

Misy, 55, 57n

Mohammedan tale, 424, 426n

Mollineaux, J———, 241, 243n

Momordica, 318, 319n

Monro, Dr. Alexander, primus, 7, 41, 42n, 94, 95n

Monro, Dr. Alexander, secundus, 356, 357, 358n, 360, 364

Montague, Lady Mary Wortley, 141n

Montcalm, Louis Joseph, Marquis de, 206n, 216n

Moore, William, Judge, 197, 199n, 200n

Moral reflections, *see* Fothergill, Dr. John: Religious and philosophical reflections

Moravians, 25, 58, 60n

Morgan, Dr. John, 14, 225, 228n, 239n, 251n, 279, 281n

LETTER TO, 250

Morgan, Mrs. John (Mary Hopkinson), 251n

Morris, Gov. Robert Hunter, 161n, 167, 168, 168n, 187n

Morris, R———, 490

Müller, *see* Miller, Johann Sebastian

Mummified bodies, 52, 53n

Museums: Ashmolean, 495, 495n; William Hunter's, 282, 283n

Mushet, Dr. William, 230, 232n

Natural history, proposed work on, 300

Neale, Samuel, Quaker preacher, 52n

Neale, Mrs. Samuel (Mary Peisley), 150, 152n

Neate, Martha, *see* Vanderwall, Mrs. Samuel

Negro slavery, *see* Slavery; Slave trade

Negroes, JF on, 313

Index